THE PRINCIPLES AND PRACTICE OF
Ultrasonography in Obstetrics and Gynecology

THIRD EDITION

edited by

ROGER C. SANDERS, M.A., B.M., B.Ch., M.R.C.P., D.M.R.D., F.R.C.R.

Associate Professor of Radiology, Radiological Science
Assistant Professor of Urology
Department of Radiology
Director of Abdominal Ultrasound
The Johns Hopkins Medical Institutions
Baltimore, Maryland

A. EVERETTE JAMES, JR., Sc.M., J.D., M.D.

Professor and Chairman
Department of Radiology and Radiological Sciences
Professor of Obstetrics and Gynecology
Professor of Medical Administration
Lecturer in Legal Medicine
Vanderbilt University School of Medicine
Nashville, Tennessee

THE PRINCIPLES AND PRACTICE OF
Ultrasonography in Obstetrics and Gynecology

THIRD EDITION

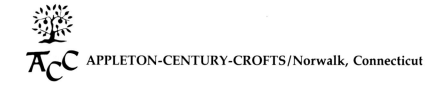
APPLETON-CENTURY-CROFTS/Norwalk, Connecticut

ISBN   0-8385-7956-6

87 88 / 10 9 8 7 6 5 4

Prentice-Hall International, Inc., London
Prentice-Hall of Australia, Pty. Ltd., Sydney
Prentice-Hall Canada, Inc.
Prentice-Hall of India Private Limited, New Delhi
Prentice-Hall of Japan, Inc., Tokyo
Prentice-Hall of Southeast Asia (Pte.) Ltd., Singapore
Whitehall Books Ltd., Wellington, New Zealand
Editora Prentice-Hall do Brasil Ltda., Rio de Janeiro

Library of Congress Cataloging in Publication Data
Main entry under title:

The principles and practice of ultrasonography in
    obstetrics and gynecology.

    Includes bibliographies and index.
    1. Ultrasonics in obstetrics.   2. Generative
organs, Female—Diseases—Diagnosis.   3. Diagnosis,
Ultrasonic.   I. Sanders, Roger C., 1936–
II. James, A. Everette (Alton Everette), 1938–
[DNLM: 1. Genital Diseases, Female—diagnosis.   2. Preg-
nancy Complications—diagnosis.   3. Ultrasonics—
diagnostic use.   WQ 240 U47]
RG527.5.U48U47   1984   618   84–12410
ISBN 0–8385–7956–6

Design: Lynn M. Luchetti

PRINTED IN THE UNITED STATES OF AMERICA

Contributors

Lindsey D. Allen, M.B., Ch.B., M.R.C.P.
Lecturer
Pediatric Cardiology
Guy's Hospital
London, England

Ellis Barnett, F.R.C.R.
Consultant
Department of Diagnostic Radiology
Ultrasonic Unit
Western Infirmary
Glasgow, Scotland

Damon D. Blake, M.D.
Professor of Radiology
Bowman Gray School of Medicine
Winston-Salem, NC

Frank H. Boehm, M.D.
Professor of Obstetrics and Gynecology
Director, Division of Maternal Fetal
  Medicine
Vanderbilt University School of
  Medicine
Nashville, TN

James D. Bowie, M.D.
Associate Professor
Department of Radiology
Chief, Section of Ultrasound
Assistant Professor
Department of Obstetrics and
  Gynecology
Duke University Medical Center
Durham, NC

Albert L. Bundy, M.D., J.D.
Instructor in Radiology
Department of Ultrasound
Brigham and Women's Hospital
Harvard Medical School
Boston, MA

Lonnie S. Burnett, M.D.
Professor and Chairman
Department of Obstetrics and
  Gynecology
Vanderbilt University School of
  Medicine
Nashville, TN

Joan Campbell, R.T., R.D.M.S.
Service Coordinator
Medical Ultrasound Imaging Services,
  Inc.
Baltimore, MD

Stuart Campbell, F.R.C.O.G.
Professor and Head
Department of Obstetrics and
  Gynecology
Kings College Medical School
London, England

Peter S. Cartwright, M.D.
Assistant Professor
Department of Obstetrics and
  Gynecology
Vanderbilt University School of
  Medicine
Nashville, TN

Paul F. Chamberlain, M.B., F.R.C.S. (C)
Fellow, Division of Maternal-Fetal
  Medicine
Department of Obstetrics, Gynecology
  and Reproductive Sciences
University of Manitoba
Winnipeg, Manitoba, Canada

William Clewell, M.D.
Associate Professor and Director of
  Obstetrics
Department of Obstetrics and
  Gynecology
University of Colorado School of
  Medicine
Denver, CO

William J. Cochrane, M.B., Ch.B., F.A.C.O.G.
Associate, Washington Ultrasound
Clinical Professor in Obstetrics and
  Gynecology
George Washington University
Consultant in Ultrasound
Columbia Hospital for Women
Washington, D.C.

Catherine Cole-Beuglet, M.D., F.R.C.P. (C)
Professor of Radiology
Division of Ultrasound and Radiologic
  Imaging
Jefferson Medical College
Thomas Jefferson University
Philadelphia, PA

Virginia L. Corson, M.S.
Instructor
Department of Obstetrics and
  Gynecology
Department of Pediatrics
The Johns Hopkins Medical Institutions
Baltimore, MD

Jack Davies, M.D.
Professor and Chairman
Department of Anatomy
Vanderbilt University School of
  Medicine
Nashville, TN

Greggory R. DeVore, M.D.
Assistant Professor
Department of Obstetrics and
  Gynecology
Division of Maternal Fetal Medicine
University of Southern California
  Medical Center
Los Angeles, CA

David L. DiPietro, Ph.D.
Assistant Professor
Department of Obstetrics and
  Gynecology
Vanderbilt University School of
  Medicine
Nashville, TN

Wylie J. Dodds, M.D.
Professor of Obstetrics and Gynecology
Vanderbilt University School of
  Medicine
Nashville, TN

Stephen S. Entman, M.D.
Assistant Professor of Obstetrics and
  Gynecology
Director, Gynecology Division
Vanderbilt University School of
  Medicine
Nashville, TN

Arthur C. Fleischer, M.D.
Acting Director, Associate Professor
Section of Diagnostic Ultrasound
Department of Radiology and
  Radiological Sciences
Vanderbilt University School of
  Medicine
Nashville, TN

Robert W. Gill, Ph.D. (MSEE)
Research Engineer
Ultrasonics Institute
Sydney, Australia

Lawrence P. Gordon, M.D.
Staff Pathologist
Crouse-Irving Memorial Hospital
Assistant Professor of Pathology
State University of New York
Upstate Medical Center
Syracuse, NY

David Graham, M.D., F.R.C.S. (C)
Department of Obstetrics and
  Diagnostic Ultrasound
The Johns Hopkins Medical Institutions
Baltimore, MD

B.J. Hackelöer, M.D.
Professor of Obstetrics and Gynecology
University Hospital for Women
University of Marburg
Marburg, West Germany

Lynden M. Hill, M.D.
Assistant Professor
Department of Obstetrics and
  Gynecology
Mayo Clinic
Rochester, MN

John C. Hobbins, M.D.
Professor
Obstetrics and Gynecology and
  Diagnostic Radiology
Yale University School of Medicine
New Haven, CT

Charles W. Hohler, M.D.
Director of Perinatology and Perinatal
  Ultrasound
Co-Director, Division of Reproductive
  Medicine
Division of Reproductive Medicine
St. Joseph's Hospital and Medical
  Center
Phoenix, AZ

A. Everette James, Jr., Sc.M., J.D., M.D.
Professor and Chairman
Department of Radiology and
  Radiological Sciences
Professor of Obstetrics and
  Gynecology
Professor of Medical Administration
Lecturer in Legal Medicine
Vanderbilt University School of
  Medicine
Nashville, TN

Burton Johnson, M.D., J.D.
Assistant Professor of Pediatrics and
  Radiology
Georgetown University School of
  Medicine
Washington, D.C.

Michael L. Johnson, M.D.
Associate Professor and Director of
  Ultrasound-CT
Department of Radiology
University of Colorado School of
  Medicine
Denver, CO

Howard W. Jones, III, M.D.
Associate Professor
Department of Obstetrics and
  Gynecology
Vanderbilt University School of
  Medicine
Nashville, TN

Eugene H. Kagan, M.D.
Director of Laboratories
Department of Pathology
Crouse-Irving Memorial Hospital
Syracuse, NY

Haig H. Kazazian, Jr., M.D.
Professor
Department of Pediatrics
The Johns Hopkins Medical Institutions
Baltimore, MD

Theodore M. King, M.D., Ph.D.
Professor and Director
Department of Obstetrics and
  Gynecology
The Johns Hopkins Medical Institutions
Baltimore, MD

Alfred B. Kurtz, M.D.
Professor of Radiology
Associate Professor of Obstetrics and
  Gynecology
Department of Radiology
Jefferson Medical College
Thomas Jefferson University
Philadelphia, PA

Faye C. Laing, M.D.
Associate Professor of Radiology
Chief, Ultrasound Section
University of California San Francisco
San Francisco, CA

Clifford S. Levi, M.D., F.R.C.P. (C)
Assistant Professor
Department of Diagnostic Radiology
University of Manitoba
Winnipeg, Manitoba, Canada

Karen L. Litchfield, R.T., R.D.M.S.
Medical Ultrasound Imaging Services, Inc.
Baltimore, MD

David Little, M.B., M.R.C.O.G.
Consultant
Department of Obstetrics and Gynecology
Birmingham Maternity Hospital
Birmingham, England

Edward A. Lyons, M.D., F.R.C.P. (C), F.A.C.R.
Director of Diagnostic Ultrasound
Department of Radiology
Health Sciences Center in Winnipeg
Winnipeg, Manitoba, Canada

Beatrice L. Madrazo, M.D.
Staff Radiologist
Clinical Assistant Professor of Radiology
Henry Ford Hospital
University of Michigan
Ann Arbor, MI

Maurice J. Mahoney, M.D.
Professor of Human Genetics, Pediatrics, Obstetrics and Gynecology
Department of Human Genetics
Yale University School of Medicine
New Haven, CT

David Manchester, M.D.
Associate Professor of Pediatrics and Pharmacology
Department of Pediatrics and Pharmacology
University of Colorado School of Medicine
Denver, CO

Frank A. Manning, M.D., F.R.C.S. (C)
Head, Division of Maternal-Fetal Medicine
Department of Obstetrics, Gynecology, and Reproductive Sciences
University of Manitoba
Winnipeg, Manitoba, Canada

James Martin, M.D.
Director, Center for Medical Ultrasound
Professor of Medical Sonics
Bowman Gray School of Medicine
Winston-Salem, NC

Paul Meier, M.D.
Assistant Professor
Department of Obstetrics and Gynecology
University of Colorado School of Medicine
Denver, CO

Patricia Morley, M.B., B.S., D.M.R.D., F.R.C.R., M.R.C.P. (G)
Consultant
Department of Radiology (Ultrasound)
Western Infirmary
Glasgow, Scotland

Jennifer R. Niebyl, M.D.
Associate Professor
Director, Division of Maternal Fetal Medicine
Department of Obstetrics and Gynecology
The Johns Hopkins Medical Institutions
Baltimore, MD

Gregory D. O'Brien, M.B., B.S.
Visiting Specialist
Obstetrics and Gynecologic Ultrasound
Royal Womens Hospital
Brisbane, Australia

William D. O'Brien, Ph.D.
Associate Professor
Department of Electrical and Computer Engineering
University of Illinois
Urbana, IL

Maurice Panigel, M.D.
Professor of Reproductive Biology
Universite de Paris VI
Paris, France

J. Malcolm Pearce, F.R.C.S., M.R.C.O.G.
Lecturer
Department of Obstetrics and Ultrasound
Kings College Medical School
London, England

Lawrence D. Platt, M.D.
Associate Professor
Department of Obstetrics and Gynecology
Division of Maternal Fetal Medicine
University of Southern California Medical Center
Los Angeles, CA

Saar A. Porrath, M.D.
Radiologist
Department of Radiology
Santa Monica Hospital Medical Center
Santa Monica, CA

Dolores Pretorius, M.D.
Assistant Professor
Department of Radiology
University of Colorado School of Medicine
Denver, CO

Ronald R. Price, Ph.D.
Associate Professor of Radiology
Associate Professor of Physics and Astronomy
Director, Division of Radiological Sciences
Vanderbilt University School of Medicine
Nashville, TN

John T. Queenan, M.D.
Professor and Chairman
Department of Obstetrics and Gynecology
Georgetown University School of Medicine
Washington, D.C.

E. Albert Reece, M.D.
Department of Obstetrics and Gynecology
Yale University School of Medicine
New Haven, CT

Matthew D. Rifkin, M.D.
Associate Professor of Radiology
Department of Radiology
Jefferson Medical College
Thomas Jefferson University
Philadelphia, PA

Hugh P. Robinson, M.D., M.B., Ch.B., M.R.O.C.G., F. Aust. C.O.G.
First Assistant
Department of Obstetrics and
    Gynecology
University of Melbourne
Melbourne, Victoria, Australia

Roger C. Sanders, M.A., B.M., B.Ch., M.R.C.P., D.M.R.D., F.R.C.R.
Associate Professor of Radiology and
    Radiological Science
Assistant Professor of Urology
Director of Abdominal Ultrasound
Department of Radiology
The Johns Hopkins Medical Institutions
Baltimore, MD

Nancy Smith Miner, R.D.M.S.
Diagnostic Sonographer

Department of Obstetrics and
    Diagnostic Ultrasound
The Johns Hopkins Medical Institutions
Baltimore, MD

Beverly A. Spirt, M.D.
Associate Professor
Department of Radiology
State University of New York
Upstate Medical Center
Syracuse, NY

Gary A. Thieme, M.D.
Assistant Professor
Department of Radiology and
    Radiological Science
Vanderbilt University School of
    Medicine
Nashville, TN

Peter S. Warren, M.B., Ch.B., F.R.A.C.R., Dip. Obst. D.D.U.
Staff Specialist
Department of Diagnostic Ultrasound
Royal Hospital for Women
Sydney, Australia

Thomas J. Withrow, M.S.
Research Biologist
Center for Devises and Radiological
    Health, FDA
Rockville, MD

Marvin C. Ziskin, M.D., M.S. Bm.E.
Professor of Radiology and Medical
    Physics
Department of Diagnostic Imaging
Temple University Medical School
Philadelphia, PA

Contents

Preface

Since publication of the second edition of this text, numerous advances have been made in the discipline of diagnostic ultrasound. Improvements in real-time imaging have greatly facilitated representation of anatomical structure while simultaneously allowing significant physiological information to be obtained.

The relative importance of real-time and static scanning has become better defined in the past few years. It is now apparent that the basic diagnostic modality is "real-time" and that there are various options available with real-time, such as high-frequency small parts instruments, rectal probes, and aspiration transducers. One may elect the additional option to use a static scanner to obtain global views of the entire fetus, uterus, pelvic mass, etc. The role of static scanning appears to be limited to those situations where the demonstration of neighboring anatomical structures will make interpretation of the image possible at a later state or in those instances where the structure or tumor being examined is larger than the field-of-view of the real-time system. In the latter situation, the neighboring anatomical structures cannot be documented on a real-time view but can be delineated by the larger field of view obtained with a static scanner.

In these days of increasing litigation, documentation of sonographic examinations and findings is of great importance. This edition, therefore, continues to contain a number of static scan views, although most images in this text are made with real-time instrumentation. Many real-time views were obtained from linear array systems which provide an excellent method of documenting the many fetal measurements that are presently required and of obtaining accurate depiction of fetal structures that lie close to the skin surface.

Appreciation of the hazard to the developing fetus that occurs with other diagnostic methods used for the evaluation of antenatal problems has given impetus to attempts to define the potential biologic burden with ultrasound. Although one cannot pronounce with finality that ultrasound is completely innocuous, one can offer substantial data to support the position that, at the levels clinically employed, there exists very little significant risk of damaging the fetus. This fortunate circumstance has encouraged clinical use of obstetric sonography.

Several texts have appeared recently in the field of obstetrical and gynecological ultrasound. Most have been overview volumes or atlases. We have attempted to provide the reader with a reference text, as well as one that can be read in its entirety. Several technical advances which have occurred in ultrasound in the last few years are described in the book. Improved transducer construction and the development of better acquisition and processing techniques have markedly increased our ability to achieve more information from ultrasound studies. Using increased computer memory for storage and using programs designed for analyzing sound reflection patterns within structures or organs, tissue signature and characterization is now clinically possible. In this text, improvements that have been shown to be clinically useful are discussed, and techniques with obvious future promise are presented in an introductory fashion. This is new and clinically important information which has resulted in improved health care delivery in obstetrics and gynecology.

We have changed the emphasis of this text to hopefully reflect the changes in the discipline. The diagnosis of the sick fetus in utero continues to represent a diagnostic challenge. A major use of ultrasound is to derive measurements that will allow the determination of fetal maturity and well-being. In the past, this was limited to measuring the biparietal diameter, but now a number of other parameters of fetal well-being are measured routinely, almost constituting a science of their own. Here, real-time ultrasound has become particularly helpful because measurements, such as crown-rump length, are much easier to obtain when one can follow the movements of the fetus. In spite of some initial skepticism, it is apparent that the diagnosis of intrauterine growth retardation can frequently be made by ultrasonic measurements and is of major importance, since this condition, to some extent, can be treated *in utero*. It is likely that thigh measurements will be added in the near future, and some investigators are using intraorbital distance as a further standard to employ in addition to diameter and femur length. To emphasize the many facets of this analysis, there are three chapters devoted to this subject in this text.

Since the last edition, there has been an ever expanding interest in fetal anomalies and in this edition, seven chapters are devoted to this area. Separate chapters describe fetal anatomy, malformations of the central nervous system, limbs, chest, heart, the genitourinary tract, the abdomen, and the face and neck. The number of fetal malformations that have or can be discovered by ultrasound studies increases almost on a daily basis. Additionally, as very high quality real-time systems become available, subtler anomalies will be delineated. Many anomalies can be detected prior to 22 weeks gestation because the fetal anatomical structures become relatively easy to detect from 16 weeks on. Consequently, as a result of diagnostic ultrasound, many elective abortions are being performed for anomalies that are not compatible with life.

In the intervening period between the last edition and this book (three years), there has been a rapid rise and to some extent a subsequent fall of interest in fetal intervention. Most cranial anomalies do not present as isolated phenomena, and although, for instance, one may successfully treat hydrocephalus, the fetus is likely to have some other major anomaly not detectable by ultrasound which can be incompatible with normal life. This technique is described in detail because of the importance of the sonogists' awareness of when fetuses should be referred for interventional therapy to the few centers that specialize in this area.

We have also added as much available material to this third edition regarding the interventional ultrasound procedures as we felt was acceptable for clinical practice at the present time but recognize that this represents an area of future growth. We have attempted to indicate the trend of ever expanding involvement of the ultrasound physician in the dynamic process of therapeutic instrumentation under sonographic guidance. Also, we have tried to place the obligation incurred by the physician's responsibility for this resource in a more societal context. The chapter regarding the legal issues is an attempt to address some of these issues.

We are mindful that the information current at this time of publication can become "dated" in a discipline undergoing such significant changes as is diagnostic sonography. We believe, however, that the new information and the different treatment of present information in this text should render it a clinically useful one at present and a foundation for future understanding of obstetrics and gynecologic ultrasound.

This edition, which we have every reason to believe will be successful, is a reflection of the expertise of the many contributors to whom we are indeed most grateful. They shared knowledge, accepted our editing, and provided appropriate responses to our requests for more information, improved and substituted illustrations, so that the contributions conformed to an overall stylistic format and made a cohesive text. We acknowledge the advice and counsel of the staff of the Departments of Obstetrics and Gynecology under the leadership of Lonnie Burnett and Ted King, at Vanderbilt and Johns Hopkins, respectively.

The experience described in this text could not have been obtained from a single clinic or institution. Those persons who read and offered suggestions regarding chapters in their areas of interest provided expertise that greatly improved the quality of the data contained herein. We are thankful for the assistance from our editoral offices where the manuscripts and galleys were coordinated throughout the publishing process. Finally, we are most appreciative of the confidence and latitude given us by the publisher.

We sincerely hope that the third edition will represent a text that will improve health care delivery through the appropriate application of diagnostic ultrasonography to obstetrical and gynecological problems.

Roger C. Sanders, M.A., B.M., B.Ch., M.R.C.P. D.M.R.D., F.R.C.R

A. Everette James Jr., Sc.M., J.D., M.D.

THE PRINCIPLES AND PRACTICE OF
Ultrasonography in Obstetrics and Gynecology

THIRD EDITION

1 | Basic Physics of Ultrasound

Marvin C. Ziskin

THE NATURE OF SOUND

Sound is the propagation of energy by a mechanical wave through matter. A mechanical wave obeys Newtonian mechanics and requires a mass-containing medium to support its transmission. It, therefore, cannot travel through a vacuum. In contrast, an electromagnetic wave sustains itself by the alternate exchange of energy between electric and magnetic fields and does not require matter for propagation. What the human ear perceives as sound is the pressure change on the eardrum caused by mechanical waves traveling through air.

Any medium that is capable of carrying a mechanical wave (sound) contains mass. The atomic and molecular structure of the medium will determine both the velocity and wave characteristics of the transmitted wave. Let us consider the molecules (or structural units) of this medium represented by rigid spheres. The molecular forces are depicted by coiled springs between adjacent spheres (Fig. 1). A mechanical wave, such as sound, incident upon this medium will cause a displacement of the spheres, so that they move back and forth in relation to one another. This longitudinal motion causes alternate crowding and uncrowding of adjacent spheres. The movement is periodic, with the distance between two bands of compression or rarefactions of the spheres determining the wavelength of the mechanical wave in the supporting medium (Fig. 2). Wavelengths ranging from 0.1 to 1.5 mm are utilized in medical applications. The wavelength is important because it determines the theoretical limit of resolution of the imaging system. Two structures closer than one wavelength apart will not be identified as separate entities in an ultrasound image.

The compressions and rarefactions of the spheres in our hypothetical medium plotted against time describe a sinusoidal curve like the one in the upper portion of Figure 2. Since pressure is proportional to molecular concentration, the local pressure is elevated in regions of compression and reduced in regions of rarefactions. Therefore, sinusoid also describes variations in pressure. The periodic change in pressure on the eardrum is called the frequency of sound. The human ear is capable of hearing frequencies of between 16 and 20,000 cycles per second. The unit of frequency is the hertz, which is equal to one cycle per second, abbreviated Hz. One million hertz equals one megahertz, abbreviated MHz. Ultrasound, by definition, is beyond the range of audible sound and therefore has a frequency greater than 20,000 Hz.

The Speed of Sound

The speed of sound through a medium is dependent upon the density and compressibility of the medium. Materials with heavy molecules will tend to move more slowly than a light-molecular-weight material when there is any given pressure change. Materials that are very compressible, such as gases, will have long excursions of individual molecules and will transmit pressure waves (sound) less rapidly. Therefore, increasing density or decreasing compressibility tends to alter sound transmission. Some materials and their corresponding acoustic speeds are listed in Table 1. There would seem to be a discrepancy in the speeds of liquids if compressibility and density govern speed. Mercury

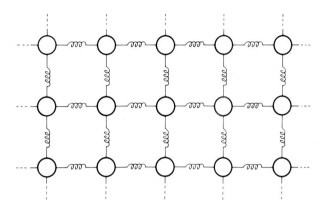

Fig. 1. Organization of matter. From the acoustic viewpoint, matter consists of an array of molecules connected to each of their immediate neighbors by elastic springs.

TABLE 1
Acoustic Speed in Various Tissues

Tissue or Material	Acoustic Speed (Meters/Sec)
Air	331
Fat	1,450
Water	1,495
Soft tissue (mean value)	1,540
Kidney	1,561
Muscle	1,585
Bone	4,080

is 13.6 times denser than water, but its speed is nearly the same. This occurs because mercury's compressibility is nearly 13.6 times less than that of water. Most liquids share this inverse proportionality between compressibility and density and therefore have similar acoustic speeds.

A fixed relationship between acoustic speed, wavelength and frequency exists as follows:

$$C = f\lambda \qquad [1]$$

where C is the speed of sound in conducting material (meters/second), f is the frequency (hertz), and λ is the wavelength (meters). If the acoustic speed within any given material is constant, then as the frequency increases, the wavelength decreases.

Types of Waves
In the previous description, the vibratory motion of molecules is parallel to the direction of propagation. This is referred to as a longitudinal wave and is by far the predominant type of sound wave occurring within the body. A transverse sound wave is a wave in which the vibratory motion is perpendicular to the direction of propagation. Whereas solids, liquids, and gases can support longitudinal waves, only solids can support transverse waves. Surface or Rayleigh waves are waves in which the molecules move in an elliptic pattern. This type of wave occurs at the upper surface of a body of water.

With the exception of compact bone, the longitudinal waves are the only type observed within the body. In bone, both longitudinal and transverse waves can occur.

Intensity of Sound
Intensity is the measure of the "strength" of a sound wave. Consider an imaginary plane positioned perpendicular to a sound wave. Power is then defined as the rate at which energy passes this plane. The unit of power is the watt. Intensity is defined as power per cross-sectional area and is expressed as watts per square centimeter (W/cm²).

Table 2 lists intensities used in various medical applications. Note that intensities employed in diag-

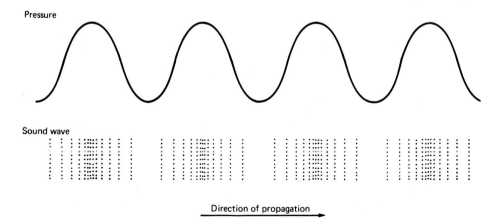

Pressure

Sound wave

Direction of propagation

Fig. 2. Longitudinal sound wave and associated pressure wave.

TABLE 2
Sound Intensities Employed
in Medicine

Medical Usage	Intensity (W/cm²)
Surgical	>10
Therapeutic	1–3
Diagnostic	0.001–0.1

nostic applications are approximately 20 times less than those used in therapeutic applications. Because diagnostic intensities are so small, these are practically always given in units of milliwatts per square centimeter.

Sometimes, instead of absolute measurements, merely a comparison of two intensities is desired. This would normally imply a simple ratio of the two intensities. However, since such a ratio would range from zero to extremely large values, the logarithm of the ratio is used for comparison. Specifically, the intensity of a sound wave relative to some reference sound wave is expressed in decibel units (dB) as given by

$$dB = 10 \log_{10} (I/I_0) \qquad [2]$$

where I_0 is the intensity of the reference sound wave and I is the intensity of the sound wave being compared. Intensity and amplitude ratios are presented in Table 3.

Unless stated otherwise, whenever a sound intensity is expressed in decibel units, it is to be understood that the reference intensity is 10^{-16} W/cm², which is the lowest intensity perceptible to the human ear. Intensities of audible sound waves are most frequently expressed in decibel units. The greater the intensity, the greater the subjective sensation of loudness.

PRODUCTION OF SOUND

In the audible range, sound is usually mechanically produced by means of a loudspeaker, which consists

TABLE 3
Decibel Units and Corresponding Intensity
and Amplitude Ratios

dB	Intensity Ratio	Amplitude Ratio
60	1,000,000	1,000
50	100,000	320
40	10,000	100
30	1,000	32
20	100	10
10	10	3.2
0	1	1
−10	0.1	0.32
−20	0.01	0.1

of a paper cone or diaphragm connected to an electromagnet. An electrical signal, whose voltage varies in accordance with the desired sound pattern, is applied to the electromagnet. This produces a corresponding motion of the diaphragm, which in turn produces a corresponding pressure variation in the air molecules in the vicinity of the diaphragm. This pressure variation propagates through the air and upon reaching the ear is perceived as sound. However, because of their inertia, loudspeakers cannot vibrate rapidly enough to produce ultrasonic frequencies. Consequently, the generation of ultrasound had to await the discovery of piezoelectric crystals.

Most crystals do not possess the property of piezoelectricity. The most important natural crystal possessing this property is quartz. Although quartz has been used in ultrasonic generators for many years, it is now being replaced almost entirely by synthetic ceramic crystals such as barium titanate and lead zirconate, since these synthetic crystals possess better mechanical properties and are easier to fabricate than quartz.

The piezoelectric effect is the generation of an electric voltage when a crystal is compressed (Fig. 3). The voltage generated is proportional to the amount of compression. If the crystal is stretched, a voltage of the opposite polarity is generated. The reverse piezoelectric effect is the compression or expansion of a crystal induced by the application of a voltage (Fig. 4).

Piezoelectric crystals are able to faithfully respond to applied electric signals at high frequencies to produce ultrasonic waves, and they likewise are able to accurately convert ultrasound waves into corresponding electric signals.

In medical application, these crystals are cut into thin wafers (less than 1 mm in thickness) and are mounted on a transducer probe.* The generation of sound waves is illustrated in Figure 5. The top row shows the transducer and the molecules in the surrounding medium at rest. In the next row, an electric voltage has been applied across the piezoelectric crystal. This induces an expansion of the crystal, which causes the molecules closest to the transducer to move toward the right. The resulting greater concentration of molecules is a condensation. The next row shows that, when the electric voltage is removed, the crystal returns to its initial shape and that the condensation continues to move toward the right. The row next to

---

* Technically speaking, a transducer is a device that converts one form of energy into another. In ultrasonics, the piezoelectric crystal is the actual transducer, since it converts sonic energy into electric energy and vice versa. However, in common parlance, the crystal and its housing are referred to as the transducer.

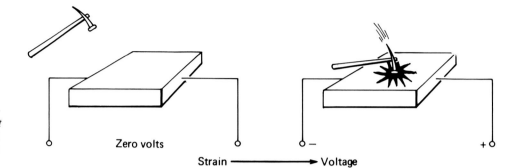

Fig. 3. The direct piezoelectric effect. (*Adapted from Goldberg B et al: Diagnostic Uses of Ultrasound. New York, Grune & Stratton, 1975. By permission.*)

the bottom shows the contraction of the crystal when an electric voltage of opposite polarity is applied. This results in a lesser concentration of molecules in the vicinity of the transducer. When the voltage is removed once more, the crystal returns to its original shape and the condensation and rarefaction continue moving toward the right. A repetitive alteration of the imposed electric voltage therefore generates a continuous sound wave. This is easily accomplished with present-day electronic circuitry.

Types of Transducers

Transducer probes come in a variety of shapes and sizes, each of which is designed for a particular application. Some of the more common types are cylindrical, flat, perivascular, catheter tipped, aspiration, and multitransducer arrays. The cylindrical or pencil-shaped transducer is designed for those examinations requiring scanning or searching for a particular structure. An example is the pencil-shaped Doppler transducer probe that is used to detect the fetal heart.

The flat transducer, in the shape of a disk, is useful for prolonged monitoring since it can be taped to the skin and need not be held throughout the examination period. It is particularly useful in fetal monitoring during labor.

The perivascular type is a cuff that is mounted around an exposed artery or vein at the time of surgery. Very small transducers can be made and mounted on catheter tips, which can then be inserted into blood vessels or the ureters, allowing close inspection of these structures.

The aspiration transducer is essentially a flat transducer with a central aperture through which a hypodermic needle can be inserted. This transducer allows simultaneous viewing of the needle tip location and surrounding anatomic structures and is useful for amniocentesis.

Various multielement transducer arrays are presently available. In these probes, as many as 64 or more individual piezoelectric crystals are mounted on a single unit. Excitation of these crystals in rapid sequence allows real-time viewing of moving internal structures and eliminates the need for manual scanning. "Real-time" implies that one is able to see anatomic movements as they occur.

Sound Beams

Sound beams are classified as divergent, collimated, or focused (Fig. 6). The shape is determined by (a) the sound frequency, (b) the diameter of the transducer, and (c) the presence or absence of an acoustic lens. With a given transducer, the higher the frequency the less the divergence of the beam. In order that the sound beam be sufficiently narrow to be useful in diagnostic applications, the frequency should be greater than 1 MHz. For collimated beams, the beam width is constant and is approximately equal to the transducer diameter.

A narrow, highly directional beam is required for good lateral resolution. Beam pattern is determined by the wavelength and transducer diameter. A characteristic sound beam is depicted in Figure 7. There exists a parallel component, which is the Fresnel or near zone,

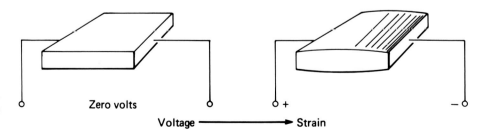

Fig. 4. The reverse piezoelectric effect. (*Adapted from Goldberg B et al: Diagnostic Uses of Ultrasound. New York, Grune & Stratton, 1975. By permission.*)

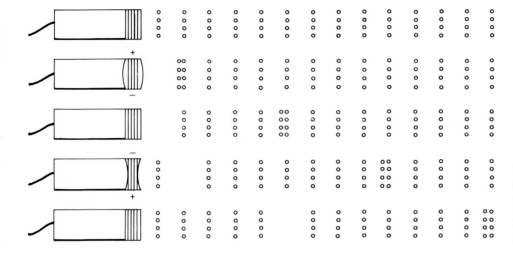

Fig. 5. Generation of ultrasound beam by transducer. Each row represents a successive instant in time. By imposing on oscillating electric signal, the transducer generates a continuous ultrasound beam.

and a diverging component called the Fraunhofer or far zone. The letter T designates the transition point between the Fresnel and Fraunhofer zones. The length of the Fresnel zone may be determined by the diameter of the transducer and the wavelength of the beam by the following relation:

$$T = r^2/\lambda \qquad [3]$$

where T is the length of Fresnel zone (cm), r is the radius of the transducer (cm), and λ is the wavelength (cm). The Fresnel zone is longest for a large transducer and for short wavelength (high frequency) ultrasound. Although both depth resolution and Fresnel zone length are increased with short wavelength (high frequency) ultrasound, the attenuation is so high that deep structures cannot be imaged. Increasing the transducer site also has limitations, as large transducer diameters create wide beams with decreased lateral resolution.

In order to obtain the most resolution in examining deep, internal structures, focused beams are used. They are produced by placing an acoustic lens on the front of the transducer probe. The lens is a thin piece of plastic whose center is thinner than its edges. This lens focuses the sound beam in the same manner as a glass lens focuses light. The focal length of a transducer is the distance from the transducer face to the focal point, which is the narrowest point in the sound beam. A focal length of 9 to 13 cm is used for most obstetric and gynecologic examinations. For examination of more superficial structures, transducers with shorter focal length are preferred. In general, the narrowest part of the beam should occur at the depth where the greatest resolution is desired.

Modes of Operation

There are two modes of transducer operation: continuous and pulsed. In the continuous mode, a sustained electric oscillation is applied to the transducer crystal, and a continuous sound beam is produced. Since this crystal is dedicated to the generation of the sound beam, a second crystal is required to detect returning echoes. The second crystal is normally mounted on the same transducer probe. This mode of operation is used primarily in Doppler units.

The pulsed mode of operation consists of emitting

Diverging

Collimated

Focused

Fig. 6. Beam patterns.

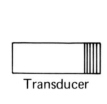

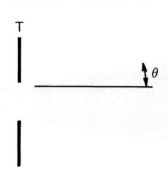

Fig. 7. Characteristic sound beam.

sound in very short pulses and bursts. Between pulses, the transducer is "silent" and able to detect returning echoes. Because the same crystal can act as both a sender and receiver of sound pulses, only one crystal is necessary in this mode of operation.

SOUND TRANSMISSION THROUGH TISSUE

Attenuation
The intensity of a sound beam constantly decreases as it travels through tissue. This decrease in intensity is called attenuation. It is due to three factors: (a) divergence of the sound beam, (b) absorption of sound energy by the tissue, and (c) deflection of sound out of the beam.

Divergence
As a sound beam diverges, its energy is spread over a larger cross-sectional area. Since intensity is proportional to energy per unit area, it decreases in proportion to the divergence of the beam.

Absorption
Absorption is the transfer of energy from the sound beam to the tissue. The energy removed is utilized primarily in overcoming the internal frictional forces of the tissue and is ultimately degraded into heat production. The greater the sound frequency, the more rapidly the tissue molecules must move and the greater the energy expended in overcoming friction. Thus, absorption is proportional to frequency. At 1 MHz, 50 percent of the intensity is absorbed by the time sound travels 2 cm in soft tissue, and less than 1 percent of the original intensity remains after it has traveled 14 cm. At 10 MHz, 50 percent remains at a 0.2-cm depth and less than 1 percent at 1.4 cm. In order to detect deep abdominal structures, the frequency should be less than 3 MHz.

In addition to frequency, the amount of absorption depends on the viscosity of the tissue through which the sound travels. In general, the more rigid the tissue the greater the absorption. Bone absorbs approximately

ten times more than most soft tissues, and these in turn absorb approximately ten times more than body fluids such as blood and amniotic fluid.

Table 4 lists the absorption coefficients and the half-value layers of various tissues for a 1-MHz sound beam. The half-value layer is the distance the sound beam has penetrated into a tissue when its intensity has been reduced to one-half of its initial value.

When sound encounters surfaces or boundaries between structures, a portion of the sound gets deflected out of the beam. Depending upon the dimensions of the surface, the mechanism for the deflection will be that of scattering or reflection. Scattering occurs when the dimensions of the surface are as small or smaller than the wavelength of the sound. The scattered sound leaves the surface in all directions, and is therefore frequently referred to as diffuse reflection. Because the scattered sound is emitted in all directions, the amount going in any one particular direction is very small and requires great amplification in order to be detected in B-scans.

Reflection
Whenever a sound beam reaches a large boundary between two tissues, some of the sound is reflected backward and the remainder is transmitted through the boundary (Fig. 8). This "mirror-like" type of reflection is called specular. The amounts of sound that are reflected and transmitted and the directions in which they travel are determined by certain properties of the

TABLE 4
Absorption Coefficients and Half-Value Layers of Various Tissues

Tissue or Material	Absorption Coefficient (dB/cm)	Half-Value Layer (cm)
Water	0.0022	1,368.00
Blood	0.18	16.72
Fat	0.63	4.78
Liver	0.94	3.20
Kidney	1.00	3.01
Bone	20.00	0.15

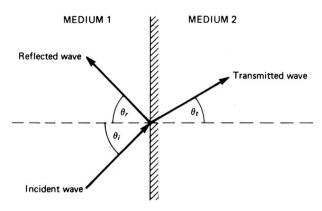

Fig. 8. Reflection and transmission of ultrasound at a boundary. (*Adapted from Goldberg B et al: Diagnostic Uses of Ultrasound. New York, Grune & Stratton, 1975. By permission.*)

TABLE 5
Acoustic Impedances

Tissue or Material	Acoustic Impedance (Rayl × 10⁻⁵)*
Air	0.0004
Fat	1.38
Water	1.48
Blood	1.61
Kidney	1.62
Soft tissue (mean value)	1.63
Liver	1.65
Muscle	1.70
Bone	7.80

* The rayl unit is equivalent to grams per square centimeter second.

two tissues and by the angle at which the incident sound beam strikes the boundary. This incident angle is labeled θ_i in Figure 8. As is true in the case of light, the direction of the transmitted beam is given by Snell's law:

$$\frac{\sin \theta_t}{\sin \theta_i} = \frac{v_2}{v_1} \quad [4]$$

where v_1 is the speed of sound in tissue 1, v_2 is the speed of sound in tissue 2, and θ_t is as defined in Figure 8. The deviation of the direction of the transmitted beam from that of the incident beam is referred to as refraction.

The angle of reflection θ_r equals the angle of incidence. Therefore, in pulse echo techniques, in which one uses the same transducer to both send pulses and receive echoes, the transducer must be positioned so that the sound beam is perpendicular to the boundary, for it is only when the sound beam is perpendicular that specular echoes will be reflected back to the transducer. At any other angle these echoes will be reflected away from the transducer and will not be detected.

The amount of sound reflected is proportional to the difference in the acoustic impedances of the two tissues. Acoustic impedance is the resistance offered by a tissue to the passage of sound and is represented by the symbol Z. It can also be shown to equal the product of the density and the acoustic speed of the tissue

$$Z = \rho v \quad [5]$$

where ρ is the tissue density and v is its acoustic speed.

Table 5 lists the acoustic impedances for various tissues. Note that the acoustic impedance of air is extremely small compared to that of any other item in this list. Therefore, an air–tissue boundary presents such a large difference in acoustic impedances that virtually all of the sound incident on this boundary is reflected. This has several important consequences for diagnostic ultrasound.

The first consequence is that some coupling agent, such as mineral oil or Aquasonic, must be applied to the surface of the skin so that no air exists between the transducer and the skin. The presence of air would cause all the sound to be reflected and prevent any penetration into the patient. The second consequence is that gas within the gastrointestinal tract also blocks any further penetration of a sound beam. Therefore, in order to examine any structure lying beneath a gas-containing intestinal loop, one must move the transducer to a different position to bypass the gas. This also applies to chest examination, where the first air–alveolar boundary effectively blocks any further penetration.

INSTRUMENTATION

Introduction
As mentioned previously, whenever sound enters the body, some of the sound is scattered and reflected backward and the remainder is transmitted through. Both the reflected echoes and the transmitted sound can be detected and analyzed to obtain medical information. This provides for three categories of ultrasonic techniques:

1. *Pulse–echo techniques,* which provide the location of anatomic structures by measuring the transit time for sound to reach the structure and return to the ultrasonic detector.
2. *Doppler techniques,* in which the frequencies of returning echoes are analyzed to determine the velocity of moving structures.
3. *Through-transmission techniques,* in which the sound completely traversing the body is analyzed for transit time, intensity, phase shift, etc.

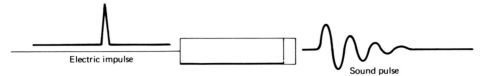

Fig. 9. Shock excitation. A short electric impulse is applied to the transducer crystal to produce the sound pulse. (*Adapted from Goldberg B et al: Diagnostic Uses of Ultrasound. New York, Grune & Stratton, 1975. By permission.*)

Pulse–Echo Techniques

The purpose of a pulse–echo system is to transmit a short ultrasonic pulse and detect all returning echoes. As the transmitted pulse traverses the body, some of its energy is reflected backward at each tissue interface. The amplitude of each echo depends on the orientation of the reflecting surface and the difference in acoustic impedances of the tissues at the interface. Echoes detected by the transducer are displayed on an oscilloscope in either A-mode, B-mode, or B-scan presentations. As the transmitted pulse is approximately 1 microsecond in duration and the pulse repetition rate is typically 1000 per second, the same transducer element is used for both transmitting and receiving.

The generation of each sound pulse is accomplished by applying a short electric impulse, called the excitation wave, to the transducer crystal (Fig. 9). This causes the crystal to "ring" at its natural frequency in a manner analogous to hitting a gong with a hammer. The natural frequency is determined by the thickness of the crystal. In order that the ringing not be too prolonged, damping is employed. This is accomplished by both electronic and mechanical means. In some instruments, a damping control is provided. This should be set so that approximately two complete cycles are contained in each pulse (Fig. 10). If overdamped, too little sound energy is transmitted and echoes are too weak to be detected. If underdamped, the pulse is so long that echoes from neighboring structures tend to overlap and thus resolution is decreased.

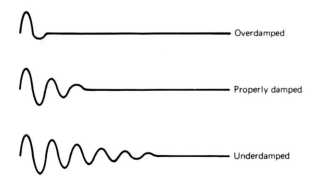

Fig. 10. Effect of damping. (*Adapted from Goldberg B et al: Diagnostic Uses of Ultrasound. New York, Grune & Stratton, 1975. By permission.*)

Returning echoes are converted by the transducer into an electric signal, the amplitude of which is directly proportional to the echo amplitude. The electric signal is processed and amplified in order to produce an adequate display on an oscilloscope (Fig. 11). An oscilloscope is frequently called a cathode ray tube (CRT). Depending on the manner in which the amplified signal is applied to the CRT, any one of several modes or displays can be obtained.

A-Mode. In the A-mode (amplitude modulation), echoes are displayed as vertical deflections along the CRT baseline, with the height of the deflection being proportional to the amplitude of the detected echo (Fig. 12). The distance between the transducer and the reflecting surface is indicated by the position of the deflection on the baseline. Using the value of 1540 m/sec (the mean velocity of sound through soft tissue), the baseline is calibrated so that depth measurements can be made to an accuracy of ±1 mm.

A time-compensated gain is customarily employed to compensate for the decreased amplitude of echoes arising from distant structures.

B-Mode. The B-mode (brightness modulation) differs from the A-mode in that echo information is applied to the Z-axis of the CRT instead of the vertical deflection circuit. Echoes appear as intensified points of illumination along the baseline. The B-mode is not useful by itself but is utilized in the creation of the M-mode and B-scan displays.

M-Mode. The M-mode (motion) display consists of the B-mode in which the baseline is continually raised. A timed photographic exposure records the movements of anatomic structure. This technique has been extremely valuable in studying dynamic changes in the heart. Much of this information, so easily obtained with ultrasound, cannot be attained with any other diagnostic technique. For example, the individual leaflets of cardiac valves are readily identified, and their excursions and velocities measured.

B-Scan. The B-scan provides a two-dimensional, cross-sectional visualization of anatomic structures.

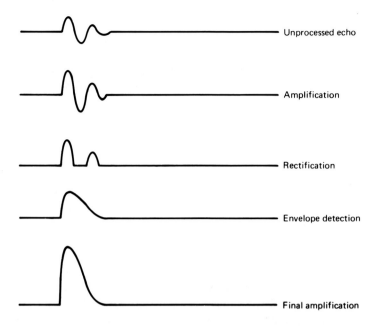

Unprocessed echo

Amplification

Rectification

Envelope detection

Final amplification

Fig. 11 Electronic processing of detected echoes. (*Adapted from Goldberg B et al: Diagnostic Uses of Ultrasound. New York, Grune & Stratton, 1975. By permission.*)

This technique has been very valuable in many medical applications. Of special value is its use in obstetrics, where it is desirable to keep x-ray examinations to a minimum. The B-scan is obtained by moving the transducer over the surface of the body and displaying the echoes in B-mode but with the location and direction of the baseline accurately following that of the transducer (Fig. 13). To accomplish this, accurate, electronic sensing of the transducer position and direction must be maintained throughout the scanning procedure. Scanning is performed mechanically with water bag coupling or manually with contact techniques.

Figure 14 shows a B-scan examination being per-formed utilizing a hanging water bath. The transducer, within the water, is mechanically driven to produce high-quality, reproducible B-scans. Unfortunately, there are many mundane problems associated with this technique. The water has to be kept at a constant temperature and replenished frequently. The weight of the bag causes some discomfort to the patient, and in pregnant patients the pressure on the inferior vena cava may produce syncope. Furthermore, the bag has been known to rupture during an examination. Because of these problems, contact scanning became the preferred technique for clinicians.

In contact scanning, the transducer is mounted

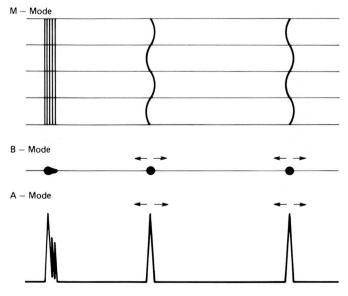

M – Mode

B – Mode

A – Mode

Fig. 12 Comparison of the A-mode, B-mode, and M-mode displays. The small arrows over the A-mode and B-mode displays signify that the indicated echoes move laterally upon direct observation of the CRT face. (*Adapted from Goldberg B et al: Diagnostic Uses of Ultrasound. New York, Grune & Stratton, 1975. By permission.*)

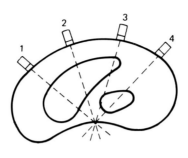
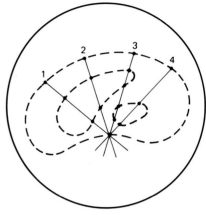

Patient   CRT Face

Fig. 13. Basic principle of the B-scan. The numbers 1 to 4 indicate different transducer placements in an abdominal examination and the corresponding B-scan on the CRT face. (*Adapted from Goldberg B et al: Diagnostic Uses of Ultrasound. New York, Grune & Stratton, 1975. By permission.*)

on a mechanical arm, which permits motion in one plane. Positional sensors are mounted in each articulation of the arm, so that the position and orientation of the transducer can be accurately monitored. An acoustic coupling agent is applied to the skin surface and the transducer is manually moved across the skin (Fig. 15).

Figure 16 shows a standard B-scan of a fetal head in utero. Note that any point in the image is either white or black. There are no intermediate shades of gray. As a consequence, small echoes, such as those arising from the posterior uterine wall or from the vertically oriented side of the fetal head, are not displayed. This results in a discontinuous contour of anatomic boundaries. In many cases, it is quite difficult to decide which displayed echoes should go together to form an anatomic boundary and which neighboring echoes

actually belong to separate structures. This confusion could be greatly reduced, if not totally eliminated, by the display of the smaller echoes. This is providing, of course, that the large echoes are not also increased to the point that they have completely "snowed" the image, making it completely white.

To gain better visualization of small echoes, gray scale capability has been added to B-scan systems. Gray scale refers to the number of distinguishable shades of gray, progressing from the blackest black to the whitest white in an image. The standard B-scan, as seen in Figure 16, has no shades of gray, only white or black. This is due to the imaging limitations of the storage CRT from which this B-scan was photographed. By bypassing the storage CRT and displaying the B-scan on a TV monitor, many shades of gray are obtained (Fig. 17). This is sufficient to provide the

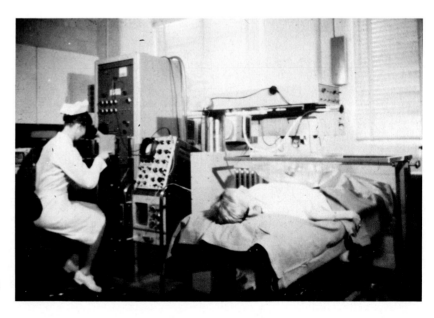

Fig. 14. B-scan ultrasound examination using a hanging water bath coupling technique.

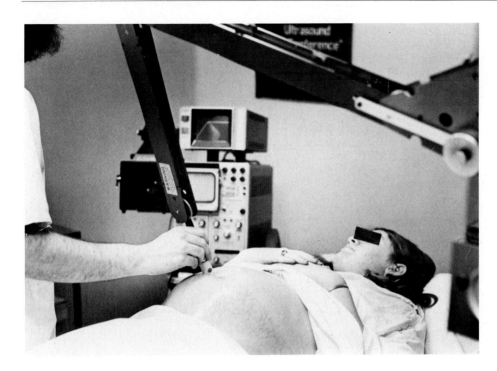

Fig. 15. B-scan ultrasound examination using contact scanning.

eye with an apparent continuously varying gray scale. Gray scale imaging is further enhanced by a nonlinear amplification of echo amplitudes. As seen in Figure 17, this results in the smaller echoes being more highly amplified than the large echoes. The resulting image is a significant improvement, as it displays the small echoes without total whitening by the large echoes.

The value of an apparent, continuously varying gray scale can be seen in the interesting, although somewhat artificial, example illustrated in Figure 18.

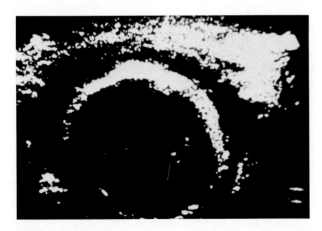

Fig. 16. Transverse B-scan of a pregnant abdomen. The large central ring of echoes represents the fetal head circumference. The large mass of dense echoes represents the anterior uterine wall and overlying skin. The echo-free area surrounding the fetal head is the amniotic fluid.

Close examination shows a 13 × 16 array of blocks. Each block possesses one of five shades of gray. The picture appears to be meaningless. However, if the distinct shades of gray are "smeared" so that the edges of each block appear intermediate in darkness, the picture will appear as though its gray scale were continuously varying. This is easily achieved by viewing the picture at a great distance; by squinting, or, if one wears glasses, by removing them. By so doing, the intended pictorial information is easily recognized.

Figure 19 shows an example of the high quality B-scans that are obtainable using gray scale imaging. This technique clearly provides anatomic information sufficiently detailed for prenatal diagnoses. Further discussion of gray scale generation and perception will follow in Chapter 3.

Real-Time Imaging. A standard B-scan takes approximately 20 seconds to complete. The photographic record of such an examination does not provide any information concerning the motion of structures within the body. To study the dynamic action of moving structures, complete scans must be obtained much more rapidly than one per 20 seconds, and therefore any manual scanning technique is precluded.

By real time, we mean that the examination detects and displays motion as it occurs. Customarily, a frame rate of 15 per second or greater is considered adequate for real-time imaging. Several different automated scanning techniques have been developed to provide real-time imaging. These techniques can be divided

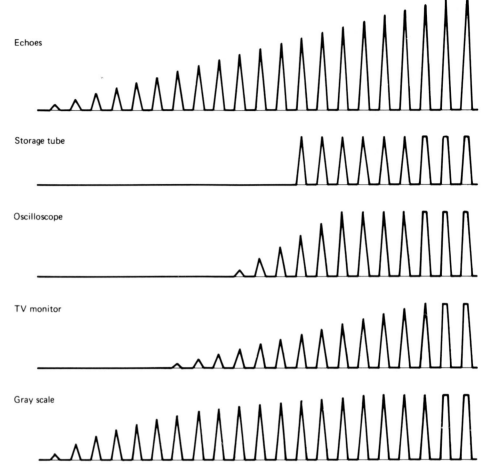

Echoes

Storage tube

Oscilloscope

TV monitor

Gray scale

Fig. 17. Echo display amplitudes. The top row illustrates the range of echo amplitudes detected by the transducer. Echo amplitudes displayed on a storage CRT are either white or black, with no intermediate shades of gray. A conventional oscilloscope and a TV monitor are able to display many shades of gray. Gray scale imaging incorporates nonlinear amplification of echoes, so that small echoes are rendered visible.

into (a) mechanical scanners and (b) multielement transducer arrays.

Mechanical Real-Time Scanners. Mechanical scanners physically move a transducer to scan the area being imaged. The movement of the transducer may be linear, pivoting, or rotational. Each is capable of producing scan rates of 30 frames per second in presently available instruments.

The linear mechanical scanner moves a single transducer back and forth parallel to the skin surface. The excursion of this motion may be several inches. Since the transducer is held fixed such that the sound beam is directed perpendicularly into the body, the resulting scan format is rectangular.

The pivoting mechanical scanner, sometimes called a "wobbler," incorporates a mechanism for rocking the direction of the sound beam to produce a sector (pie-shaped) scan format. In some cases the transducer is rocked; in other cases, the transducer is held stationary and a pivoting acoustic mirror produces the scanning action.

The rotating mechanical scanner is simply a "side looking" transducer mounted on a rotating wheel. If contained within an acoustically transparent housing, this mechanism can scan an entire 360 degree field of view, such as that obtained in a commercially available rectal scanner. Much more commonly, however, the housing is designed to limit the egress of the sound beam to a sector ranging from 60 to 120 degrees. Sometimes two or more transducers may be mounted on the rotating wheel. In this way, it is no longer necessary to wait until the sole transducer rotates all the way back to the acoustic window in order to obtain echo information. Also, the transducer elements may be of differing frequencies or focal distances and thus may increase the amount of diagnostic information obtainable.

Multielement Transducer Arrays. This method of real-time imaging uses many piezoelectric crystals mounted on a single transducer probe and electronically controls the excitation of these crystals such that an entire scan can be completed in a small fraction of a second. Be-

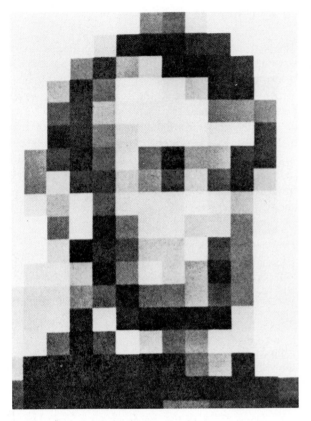

Fig. 18. Portrait of a famous man from history. See text for explanation.

cause there are no moving parts, electronic switching is all that is required to produce frame rates of 60 per second or higher. In fact, the fundamental limitation to the speed of scanning is no longer the instrumentation but the speed of sound. That is, we can employ higher frame rates, but that will not allow sufficient time for sound to travel to deep structures and return prior to the emission of the next ultrasound pulse.

There are two methods of exciting the multielement arrays, multiplexing and phased array. In multiplexed systems, each crystal is excited and following the necessary time for echoes to return to that crystal, the next crystal is excited, and so on until all the crystals have been excited. The total sequence constitutes a single frame. In presently available instruments, four or more crystals are excited at a time for improved beam shaping. The resulting scan pattern or anatomic window is rectangular in shape and has been particularly useful in obstetric applications.

In phased array systems, all of the crystals are excited as a single unit. However, there is a slight delay between each successive crystal, so that the sound pulse leaves the transducer at one end sooner than at the other end. This causes the direction of the emerg-

ing sound beam to deviate from the perpendicular. The amount of deviation is determined by the amount of delay. Rapid changing of the delay pattern can produce rapid beam steering. This electronic beam steering produces a sector type of scan, which has been particularly useful in cardiologic applications.

Image Quality in Real Time. A sonogram is composed of a number of lines of echo information. The larger the number of lines, the greater the spatial resolution and the greater the amount of anatomic detail capable of being displayed. However, the more lines required, the more time it takes to obtain a complete scan. This poses an important limitation for real-time imaging, where the time available for an individual scan frame is short (less than 1/15 of a second).

Each line of echo information requires an adequate time for sound to travel from the transducer to the deepest structures of interest and return. Thirteen microseconds are required for each centimeter of depth. All of the above considerations can be related by:

$$\frac{\text{Frame}}{\text{Rate}} \times \frac{\text{Lines Per}}{\text{Frame}} \times \frac{\text{Image}}{\text{Depth}} = 77{,}000 \qquad [6]$$

This equation is of importance because it states an upper limit on the combination of desirable features in imaging: temporal resolution, spatial resolution, and field of view. For example, an instrument designed to provide a frame rate of 30 frames per second and 200 lines per frame will be limited to an image depth of 12.8 cm. To increase the depth of view it would be necessary to decrease the frame rate or the number

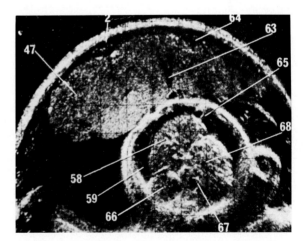

Fig. 19. Transverse B-scan with gray scale of fetus with hydrops. *KEY:* 2, uterine muscle wall; 47, placenta; 58, liver; 59, ascites; 63, lobular divisions of placenta; 64, decidua basalis; 65, falciform ligament; 66, right kidney; 67, fetal aorta; 68, bowel. (*Reproduced with permission from Garrett W. Kossoff G. Lawrence R: Gray scale echography in the diagnosis of hydrops due to fetal lung tumor. J Clin Ultrasound, 3(1): 47, 1975.*)

of lines. Fortunately for obstetric and gynecologic applications, those limitations are not so severe that they prevent excellent visualization of anatomic detail in real time.

Doppler Techniques

Echoes returning from moving structures are altered in frequency. This frequency shift, which under biologic conditions is between 0 and 2000 Hz, is detected and applied to a loudspeaker to produce an audio signal. Its primary use has been to detect and measure blood flow. Backscattered sound from the moving red blood cells provides the effective signal. The standard continuous-wave, nondirectional Doppler technique has been very useful in detecting fetal life (as early as 8 weeks of gestation), detecting nonpalpable arterial pulsations, and evaluating varicose veins.

Directional flow sensing has been provided by use of a single-sideband phasing technique. Pulsed Doppler systems can effectively separate signals from structures at various depths. Velocity profiles within blood vessels have been determined using this technique. Recently, a combined Doppler–B-scan system has been developed that can present images of blood flow patterns.

CONCLUSION

In the past several years, the advancement of ultrasonic instrumentation has been nothing less than spectacular. We are now beyond the point where just any image is acceptable. We have come to expect high-quality images with sufficient gray scale and resolution to provide reliable and accurate diagnostic information. Real-time imaging has provided us with dynamic views of anatomy never obtainable previously. Through-transmission techniques are still in their infancy. Other techniques, presently in the laboratory stage of development, also appear promising. Significant future progress is certain.

BIBLIOGRAPHY

Kremkau FK: Diagnostic Ultrasound: Physical Principles and Exercises. New York, Grune & Stratton, 1980

McDicken WN: Diagnostic Ultrasonics, Principles and Use of Instruments. New York, John Wiley, 1981

Wells PNT: Biomedical Ultrasonics. London, Academic, 1977

Wells PNT, Ziskin MC: New Techniques and Instrumentation in Ultrasonography. New York, Churchill Livingstone, 1980

2 | An Approach to Ultrasonic Risk Assessment and an Examination of Selected Experimental Studies

William D. O'Brien, Jr.
Thomas J. Withrow

INTRODUCTION

It has been more than a decade since the first major efforts to assess the risk of ultrasonic energy were made.[1,2] Since then there have been numerous reviews and assessments.[3-10] Even today, there are projects that have as their aim an assessment of the health risks from diagnostic ultrasound.[11-13] Yet, the basic status regarding risk assessment has remained unchanged during this time, viz. the studies necessary to support a reliable assessment of the risks associated with human exposure to ultrasound have not been undertaken. So, rather than present another broad discussion of ultrasonic risk assessment, it seemed to be much more reasonable to focus upon one ultrasonically induced biologic observation, namely, fetal weight reduction. Prior to a discussion of ultrasonically induced fetal weight reduction, however, let us first consider an approach to risk assessment and then a review of the general trends as they relate to diagnostic level ultrasonic biologic effects. The effect of ultrasound on immunologic function and on sister chromatid exchange frequency will be considered as examples.

APPROACH TO RISK ASSESSMENT

With our current understanding of ultrasonically induced biologic effects, it is difficult to argue against statements such as "diagnostic ultrasound is not harmful to the conceptus." Experimental studies cannot be used to prove diagnostic ultrasound safe. Rather, what such studies will provide, if properly planned and executed, are data that will aid in the overall assessment of risk associated with exposure to ultrasound. Safe implies the complete absence of an effect, that the procedure involves no risk, or the like. It simply is not possible to prove that ultrasound, or for that matter any agent, produces no effect whatsoever at the levels employed diagnostically. Also, the actual use of the word safe is vague since it almost never refers to the absence of an effect. A more useful and workable approach is to examine the "risk" associated with ultrasonic exposure.

Some 35 years after the Curies discovered piezoelectricity in 1880,[14] the first use of ultrasonic energy was developed—underwater acoustic echoes were bounced off submerged objects.[15,16] During the course of this work, the first reported observation was made that ultrasonic energy had a lethal effect upon small aquatic animals.[17] The first extensive investigation of the phenomenon confirmed that ultrasonic energy could kill small fishes and frogs within a minute or two.[18] In perhaps the first review paper of ultrasonically induced biologic effects,[19] the physical, chemical, and biologic effects of ultrasound were evaluated. The effects on cells, isolated cells, bacteria, and tissues were summarized, with a view towards identifying the responsible mechanism. The ultrasonic exposure conditions of this early work were not well characterized but the intensity levels were undoubtedly quite high.

In the early pioneering studies where the ultrasonic exposure conditions were carefully controlled and specified, sciatic nerve paralysis was easily produced in the frog[20,21] and lesions were produced in central nervous system tissue.[22] In addition, high-intensity ultrasound was employed to produce lesions in adult cat and rat brain[23-27]; adult rat and neonatal mouse spinal cord[22,28,29]; adult frog muscle[30,31]; rabbit blood vessel[32]; rabbit kidney and testicle[33]; and rabbit ocular tissue.[34-36] The ultrasonic intensities were very much higher than those utilized in diagnostic ultrasound. For the most part, these studies caused rather severe tissue damage, but they have been extremely important in the elucidation of fundamental interaction processes. In terms of risk assessment, these studies support the view that the employed ultrasonic exposure conditions will more than likely not produce acute, gross irreversible damage.

These high-intensity studies further aid in recognizing the important fact that, at sufficient energy levels, ultrasound is capable of destroying biologic material. Therefore, an approach to the question of assessing the risk from ultrasound is as follows:

1. What biologic systems are most sensitive to ultrasound?
2. What exposure levels impose a significant risk on these systems?

Unfortunately, this approach has its difficulties. How does one determine significant risk? Usually, what is meant by significant risk is that risk that is greater than some upper limit of acceptability. One usually then employs a benefit-versus-risk analysis, which, in principal, is simple but, in practice, is not so easily implemented.

Another important consideration with respect to risk assessment is the extent to which ultrasound is used. Although no statistically based survey had been conducted to document the extent to which ultrasound has been used over the past decade, it is clear that its use is increasing and that a large fraction of the human population will eventually be exposed, especially in utero. As listed in Table 1, in 1971 the Food and Drug Administration's Bureau of Radiological Health surveyed 301 out of 6306 short-term general hospitals in the United States and found that 12 percent of the hospitals used diagnostic ultrasound.[37] The same federal agency reported on the results of its 1974 hospital survey, by which time 35 percent of the surveyed hospitals were using diagnostic ultrasound.[38,39] This represented an almost 200 percent increase between 1971 and 1974, or an annualized increase of 43 percent during this time. The survey further showed that an estimated 16 percent of the obstetric services in the United States used diagnostic ultrasound and that about one-third of all U.S. births for 1974 were delivered in these hospitals.[38,39] Additionally, it was estimated that 470,000 pregnant women were exposed to diagnostic ultrasound in 1974, with about 35 to 40

TABLE 1
Selected Assessment of Diagnostic Ultrasound Usage

Assessment Period	Assessment
1963–1971	Annualized increase in usage via a mail survey about 10 percent[40]
Early 1970s	In the United Kingdom, the number of diagnostic exams doubles every three years (26 percent annualized)[41]
1971	Twelve percent of hospitals use ultrasound[37]
1974	Thirty five percent of hospitals use ultrasound[38,39]

percent of these women being examined more than once.

An international mail survey showed that between 1963 and 1971, there was an average annual increase in use of clinical ultrasound of approximately 10 percent.[40] In the United Kingdom, it had been estimated that in the early 1970s the number of ultrasonic diagnostic examinations was doubling every 3 years,[41] thus representing an annual 26 percent increase.

Although more current use information is not available, sales growth information does indicate that in 1976, the ultrasonic industry annual dollar sales was around $30 million[42] and for the following year about $40 million.[43] In the next four years, estimates of annual sales were $50, $79, $170, and $214 million.[10] Therefore, an increase from $30 to $214 million from 1975 to 1980 represents an average annual increase in sales of approximately 48 percent.

To summarize, if one assumes that at least half of all pregnant women are currently being examined with ultrasound and, additionally, one assumes that its use is increasing at an annual rate of between 10 and 25 percent, then within a few years, virtually every fetus will be examined with diagnostic ultrasound.

GENERAL TREND

Recent reviews[6,9,10,44-49] of the ultrasonic bioeffect literature suggest that as more sensitive biologic endpoints are studied, the ultrasound exposure parameters required to produce measurable effects appears to decrease. Ultrasound diagnostic equipment has been reported to induce biologic effects on immunosuppression, cellular attachment, sister chromatid exchange, platelet aggregation, and phagocytosis.[50-57,59] However, it should be noted that at the lower, sometimes diagnostic, levels of ultrasound, there is no consistent indication of the specific ultrasonically induced biologic alteration. For the two examples to be discussed in detail, immunologic function and sister chromatid exchange, conflicting experimental data exist.

In the first study by Anderson and Barrett,[50] which reported an effect of ultrasound on immunologic function, the splenic area of mice was exposed to ultrasound via a pulsed diagnostic device and it was reported that ultrasound exposure reduced the hemaglutinin and hemolysin response after an injection of sheep erythrocytes. However, another laboratory[50a] could not reproduce these effects and reported that ultrasound had no significant effect on the hemoglutinin and hemolysin response in mice exposed to ultrasound under very similar conditions to that used in the earlier study.[50] Further, in this other experiment at higher spatial average, temporal average, intensities, no effect was produced.[50a]

In a second study, Anderson and Barrett again exposed mice to diagnostic levels of ultrasound, but this time to the liver area.[55] They reported that ultrasound caused a depression of phagocytosis as measured by carbon clearance, and a depression in the ability of peritoneal macrophages from sonicated animals to phagocytose bacteria. In a somewhat similar study,[59] therapeutic levels of ultrasound were applied to the abdominal region of rats, and then the clearance of an injection of radioactive colloid particles was measured. It was reported that the ultrasound caused a slowing in the clearance of the colloid. These studies are very interesting from the standpoint that diagnostic or therapeutic levels of ultrasound may affect immune function. There are, however, many problems in translating these findings to the clinical situations, such as the large difference in area of sonicated versus whole body/organ size in mouse or rat versus man.

Liebeskind and colleagues[51] reported that diagnostic levels of ultrasound increased immunoreactivity to antinucleoside antibodies in cultured cells. This type of effect usually suggests unwinding of the DNA helix, or single-strand breaks, but the authors were not able to identify DNA strand damage. Although this effect is sometimes referred to as an immune effect, it is not an effect on the immune system, but the use of an immune technique as an experimental tool.

Within the last 5 years, a number of experimental studies have been conducted to examine the effect of ultrasonic energy on sister chromatid exchange (SCE) frequency, an indicator of chromosome damage but of which the biologic significance is unclear. The study by Liebeskind et al.[52] has probably received the greatest attention, as it indicated that exposure to a diagnostic ultrasound device caused an increase in SCEs in human lymphocytes and in a human lymphoblast line. In another study, the same authors reported no change in SCEs in a different cell type.[51] There has been only one other positive observation of increased SCEs[57]; here in human lymphocytes at diagnostic levels. However, there have been at least eight other studies,[51,58,60-65] some at diagnostic levels, some at levels much higher than therapeutic levels which have reported no increase in SCEs. The reasons for these differences are not known but could have been due to differences in technique; none of these studies were conducted under identical experimental conditions. Additionally, only the studies of Liebeskind et al.[51,52] included positive controls, a serious omission particularly when reporting negative findings.

One must be cautious in assessing the significance of biologic alterations such as the immune disturbances or increased SCEs as discussed above, or other such observations. They are simply observations, and whether or not ultrasound will be shown to represent a significant risk will depend upon the types of effects observed, the exposure levels at which these effects occur, their dose–effect responses, and the assessment of the mechanism from dose–effect data. These studies are useful, however, in pointing to potentially hazardous or potentially therapeutic interactions of ultrasound and to help understand how ultrasound interacts with biological tissue.

FETAL WEIGHT STUDIES

Over the last few years, and especially within the past year or so, experimental observations have been made that suggest that subtle effects occur in rodent embryos and fetuses when they are exposed to ultrasound in utero. The balance of this chapter selectively examines ultrasonically induced fetal weight reduction in experimental animals. In choosing this topic, an attempt has been made to approach the assessment of risk from ultrasound for this single biologic endpoint. It is not known whether this biologic system is very sensitive (in a chemical and physical sense) to ultrasonic energy but, clearly, it is sensitive in an emotional and political sense. Therefore, it behooves us to understand the experimental data that show that ultrasonic energy does influence fetal weight when the system is exposed to ultrasound in utero.

One of the earliest studies that suggested that in utero ultrasonic irradiation affected prenatal growth and development was reported in experimental animals about 8 years ago.[66] Time-mated mice received continuous wave (1 MHz) ultrasound on the eighth day of gestation under well-controlled and documented exposure conditions.[67] The fetuses were weighed on the eighteenth day of gestation and a statistically significant weight reduction of up to 17.5 percent relative to the control was observed. Two hundred and seventy-two litters (2866 fetuses) were examined in seven separate ultrasound groups, including a sham group. The spatial average, time average intensity ranged from 0.5 to 5.5 W/cm² and the exposure time ranged from 10 to 300 seconds (Table 2).

A detailed account of the initial finding[66] and an extension of the data analysis[68] showed that a dose–effect response was observed. Here the dose–effect response of the exposure condition versus fetal weight was developed by defining the dose parameter I^2t, where I is the exposure intensity (W/cm²) and t is the exposure time (seconds) as listed in Table 2 for each of the seven exposure conditions.

There is a basis for the I^2t dose parameter in the ultrasonic literature and in the literature of other energy forms. Threshold ultrasonic dosages for structural changes in the adult mammalian central nervous system results in a mathematical dependency between the ultrasonic intensity, I, and the exposure duration, t,[24,26,69-71] which is described by the product of I^2 and t equaling a constant value. In other words, if I equals 20 W/cm² ($I^2 = 400$) and t equals 0.5 seconds for the threshold of an ultrasonically induced change, then $I^2t = 200$. This same biologic threshold would occur under the ultrasonic exposure conditions in which I equals 10 W/cm² ($I^2 = 100$) and t equals 2.0 seconds, that is, $I^2t = 200$ again.

A similar type of I^2t dependency has been observed for ultrasonically induced hind limb paralysis of neonatal mice,[26,72] threshold focal lesions in cat liver[73] as well as focal lesions in the rabbit liver, kidney, and testis.[33] In comparison to other forms of energy, a similar dose dependency has been observed for mammary neoplasms at low ionizing radiation doses wherein two x-ray secondary particles (produced by a single neutron) are required to elicit the effect.[74] In photochemical and photobiologic studies, at high energy concentrations, biophotonic excitation (two photons required to produce the effect) has been observed.[75]

What does an I^2t type of dependency for a biologic effect mean? Basically, it means that two energy events are required to produce the biologic effect. However, there is not enough fundamental information available at this time to speculate whether or not the reduced fetal weight observations reported herein can be explained by this dosimetric model. Nevertheless, such a model begins to provide a basis for extrapolating biologic effect observations and such an extrapolation will be done shortly in terms of assessing the potential

for ultrasonically induced fetal weight reduction in humans based upon the mouse data. Thus the following fetal weight observations will be presented in terms of their I^2t dependency.

The observation that in utero ultrasonic exposure can cause weight reduction in the mouse fetuses has been confirmed by two other research groups using two different strains of mice.[76,77] For the data listed in Table 3,[76] relatively high level, pulsed ultrasound conditions were employed. Here the mice were exposed to ultrasound on the eighth day of gestation and the fetuses were individually weighed on the eighteenth day of gestation. A statistically significant 18.8 percent weight reduction was observed for spatial peak, temporal average intensities above 50 W/cm² (spatial peak, temporal peak intensity of 1936 W/cm² and exposure time of 20 seconds) when irradiated on day eight of gestation. At and below a spatial peak, temporal average intensity of 45 W/cm² no statistically significant change in the fetal weight was observed.

The data listed in Table 4[77] show mean fetal weight reductions that range up to 25 percent relative to the sham under continuous wave (2 MHz) exposure conditions at a spatial average, temporal average intensity of 1 W/cm², for exposure times up to 200 seconds

TABLE 2
Summary of CF₁ Mouse* Fetal Weight Study[66,68]

I_{sata} (W/cm²)	t (sec)	I^2t	Percentage Weight Change (Against Sham)
0.5	300	75	− 5.3
2.0	20	80	− 6.1
3.0	10	90	− 6.1
0.7	300	147	− 8.8
3.0	20	180	− 7.9
5.5	10	303	−17.5

* The mice were ultrasonically exposed (continuous wave of 1 MHz) in utero on day eight of gestation and the fetuses were examined on the eighteenth day of gestation.

TABLE 3
Summary of LAF₁/J Mouse* Fetal Weight Study[76]

I_{spta} (W/cm²)	t (sec)	I^2t	Percentage Weight Change (Against Sham)
25.6	20	13,100	− 5.4
35.3	20	24,900	0
45.0	20	40,500	0
50.8	20	51,600	−18.8

* The mice were ultrasonically exposed (pulsed, I_{sptp} = 1936 W/cm², 1 MHz, pulsed repetition frequency = 1 kHz) in utero on the eighth day of gestation and the fetuses were weighed on the eighteenth day of gestation.

TABLE 4
Summary of CFW Swiss Webster Mouse* Fetal Weight Study[77]

I_{sata} (W/cm²)	t (sec)	I^2t	Percentage Weight Change (Against Sham)		
			day 0	day 7	day 12
1	80	80	− 2.7	+ 5.1	− 3.9
1	100	100	+ 1.6	+ 3.9	− 5.6
1	120	120	− 0.4	− 0.4	− 5.3
1	140	140	+ 2.9	− 8.7	−13.3
1	160	160	− 1.8	−11.2	−22.2
1	180	180	−19.1	−11.0	−11.3
1	200	200	−25.1	−11.5	−18.4

* The mice were ultrasonically exposed (continuous wave of 2 MHz) in utero on days 0, 7 or 12 of gestation and the fetuses were weighed on the seventeenth day of gestation.

at gestation ages of 0, 7, and 12. The fetuses were individually weighed on the seventeenth day of gestation. These results compare most directly with the previous finding[66,68] in which similar mean fetal weight reductions were observed.

Figure 1 graphically summarizes in a unified way the three published studies[68,76,77] that reported statistically significant effects of fetal weight reduction from in utero exposure to ultrasound. Here the data from Tables 2, 3, and 4 are represented by the percentage weight change (against control) as a function of the calculated dose parameter I^2t. All three studies graphically show that as the value of I^2t increases the fetal weight (against sham) decreases.

DOSE–EFFECT STUDIES

Dose–effect studies are invaluable for assessing risk.[6] Too often, a communication appears in which a bio-

logic effect is reported under a single ultrasonic exposure condition. When the exposure condition arises from a diagnostic device, we tend to question whether the reported observation is real, or whether the experimental setup produced extraordinary conditions to elicit the effect. In either case, however, there is a tendency to suggest that diagnostic exposure conditions represent a risk to the patient. When the exposure condition is at levels much in excess of diagnostic conditions, we tend to discount their applicability to the clinical situation. The overall problem is that non dose–effect studies are quite difficult to apply to assessing the risk. They do, however, identify biologic endpoint to which dose–effect experimental regimes should then be applied.

Consider the mouse dose–effect fetal weight data shown in Figure 1. If we were to apply this dose–effect curve to a clinical exposure condition for purposes of assessing risk, let us first examine the upper value of the dose parameter I^2t for static pulse echo scanners.[78]

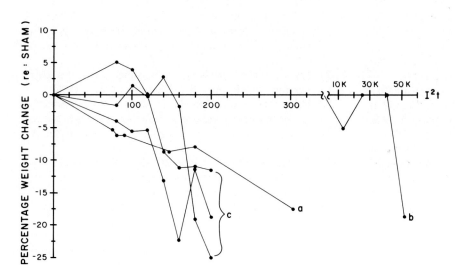

Fig. 1. Summary of fetal weight studies in terms of the dose–effect parameter I^2t. Curves a, b, and c represent data from tables 2, 3, and 4 respectively.

For a single pulse, the spatial peak, pulse average intensity is about 300 W/cm² and the exposure time, here the pulse duration, is about 1 microsecond, yielding an I^2t around 0.09. For the time average case, the spatial peak, temporal average intensity is about 200 mW/cm² and the exposure time, here the length of the exam for maximum effect, is about 30 minutes, yielding an I^2t around 72. Of course, this latter case would require examining the same tissue volume for the entire length of time, which might not be the situation with static pulse echo scanner but is quite possible for a Doppler fetal monitor wherein the spatial peak intensity is about 75 mW/cm². For an exposure time of 1 hour, the I^2t dose parameter calculates to be about 20. The point to be made is that with a dose–effect model, one is in a better position of examining what might be the effect under clinical conditions. The model would have to be validated for such applicability, of course. There is a long way to go with respect to ultrasound.

ACKNOWLEDGMENTS

One of the authors (WDO) acknowledges gratefully the partial support by a grant from the National Institute of General Medical Sciences, National Institutes of Health (GM 30481).

REFERENCES

1. Reid JM, Sikov MR, eds: Interaction of ultrasound and biological tissues workshop proceedings, DHEW Publication (FDA) 73–8008 BRH-DBE. Washington, D.C., U.S. Government Printing Office, 1972
2. O'Brien WD, Shore ML, Fred RK, et al: On the assessment of risk to ultrasound, in deKlerk J (ed), 1972 Ultrasonics Symposium Proceedings. 486–490, IEEE Cat. No. 72 CHO 708–8 SU, New York, 1972
3. Ulrick WD: Ultrasound dosage for nontherapeutic use on human beings—extrapolation from a literature survey. IEEE Trans Biomed Engr BME-21:48, 1974
4. Wells PNT: The possibility of harmful biological effects in ultrasonic diagnosis, in Reneman RS (ed), Cardiovascular Applications of Ultrasound. New York, Elsevier, 1974, pp 1–17
5. Hazzard DG, Litz ML, eds: Symposium on biological effects and characterization of ultrasound sources proceedings, DHEW Publication (FDA) 78–8084. Washington, D.C., U.S. Government Printing Office, 1977
6. O'Brien WD: Safety of ultrasound, in deVlieger M, et al. (eds), Clinical Handbook of Ultrasound. New York, Wiley, 1978, pp 99–108
7. Repacholi MH, Benwell DA, eds: Ultrasound short course transactions. Radiation Protection Bureau, Health Protection Branch, National Health and Welfare, Canada, 1979
8. Repacholi MH: Ultrasound: Characteristics and biological action. National Research Council of Canada, Publication Number NRCC 19244, Ottawa, 1981
9. Dunn F, Frizzell LA: Bioeffects of ultrasound, in Lehmann JF (ed), Therapeutic Heat and Cold. Baltimore, Williams and Wilkins, 1982, pp 386–403
10. Stratmeyer ME, Stewart HF: An overview of ultrasound: Theory, measurement, medical applications, and biological effects. HHS Publication FDA 82–8190. Washington, D.C., U.S. Government Printing Office, 1982
11. Environmental Health Criteria 22. World Health Organization. WHO Geneva Office, Geneva, Switzerland, 1982
12. Biological Effects of Ultrasound: Mechanisms and Clinical Implications. National Council on Radiation Protection and Measurement Document 74. NCRP, Washington, D.C., 1984
13. The Use of Diagnostic Ultrasound Imaging in Pregnancy. National Institute of Child Health and Human Development. NIH Consensus Development Conference process, U.S. Government Printing Office, Washington, D.C., 1984
14. Cady WG: Piezoelectricity. New York, Dover, vol 1, 1946
15. Urick RJ: Principles of Underwater Sound for Engineers. New York, McGraw-Hill, 1967
16. Van Went JM: Ultrasonic and Ultrashort Waves in Medicine. New York, Elsevier, 1954
17. Graber P: Biological actions of ultrasonic waves, in Lawrence JH, Tobias CA (eds), Advances in Biological Physics. New York, Academic, 1953, vol 3, pp 191–246
18. Wood RW, Loomis AL: The physical and biological effects of high-frequency sound-waves of great intensity. Philos Mag 4:417, 1927
19. Harvey EN: Biological aspects of ultrasonic waves: A general survey. Biol Bull 59:306, 1930
20. Fry WJ, Wulff VJ, Tucker D, et al: Physical factors involved in ultrasonically induced changes in living systems: I. Identification of non-temperature effects. J Acoust Soc Am 22:867, 1950
21. Fry WJ, Tucker D, Fry JF, et al: Physical factors involved in ultrasonically induced changes in living systems: II. Amplitude duration relations and the effect of hydrostatic pressure for nerve tissue. J Acoust Soc Am 23:365, 1951
22. Fry WJ: Intense ultrasound in investigation of the central nervous system. Adv Biol Med Phys 6:281, 1958
23. Hueter TF, Ballantine HT Jr., Cotter WC: Production of lesions in the central nervous system with focused ultrasound. A study of dosage factors. J Acoust Soc Am 28:192, 1956
24. Fry FJ, Kossoff G, Eggleton RC, Dunn F: Threshold ultrasonic dosages for structural changes in the mammalian brain. J Acoust Soc Am 48:1413, 1970
25. Pond JB: The role of heat in the production of ultrasonic focal lesions. J Acoust Soc Am 47:1607, 1970
26. Dunn F, Fry FJ: Ultrasonic threshold dosages for the mammalian central nervous system. IEEE Trans Biomed Eng BME-18:253, 1971

27. Robinson TC, Lele PP: An analysis of lesion development in the brain and in plastics by high-intensity focused ultrasound at low-megahertz frequencies. J Acoust Soc Am 51:1333, 1972

28. Dunn F: Physical mechanisms of the action of intense ultrasound on tissue. Am J Phys Med 37:148, 1958

29. Taylor KJW, Pond J: The effects of ultrasound on varying frequencies on rat liver. J Path 100:287, 1969

30. Eggleton RC, Kelly E, Fry FJ, et al: Morphology of ultrasonically irradiated skeletal muscle, in Kelly E (ed), Ultrasonic Energy. Urbana, IL, University of Illinois Press, 1965, p 117

31. Ravitz MJ, Schnitzler RM: Morphological changes induced in the frog semitendinosus muscle fiber by localized ultrasound. Exptl Cell Res 60:78, 1970

32. Fallon JT, Stephens WF: Effect of ultrasound on arteries. Arch Path 94:380, 1972

33. Frizzell LA, Linke CA, Carstensen EL, et al: Thresholds for focal ultrasonic lesions in rabbit kidney, liver and testicle. IEEE Trans Biomed Eng BME-24:393, 1977

34. Colman DJ, Lizzi F, Burt W, et al: Ultrasonically induced cataract. Am J Ophthal 71:1284, 1971

35. Sokollu A: Destructive effect of ultrasound on ocular tissue, in Reid JM, Sikov M (eds), Interaction of Ultrasound and Biological Tissue. DHEW Pub. (FDA) 73-8008. Washington, D.C., U.S. Government Printing Office, 1972, p 129

36. Lizzi FL, Parker AJ, Coleman DJ: Experimental cataract production by high frequency ultrasound. Ann Ophthal 10:934, 1978

37. Landau E: Are there ultrasonic dangers for the unborn? Prac Radiol 1:27, 1973

38. Roney PL, Albrecht RM: Hospital survey of obstetric ultrasound, presented at the Ad Hoc Review Panel on Ultrasound Bioeffect and Measurement meeting, Bureau of Radiological Health, FDA, April 9–10, 1976

39. Roney PL, Albrecht RM: Hospital survey of obstetric ultrasound—United States, 1974, in Hazzard DG, Litz ML (eds), Symposium on Biological Effects and Characterization of Ultrasound Sources Proceedings. HEW Publication (FDA) 78-8048. Washington, D.C., U.S. Government Printing Office, 1977, pp 29–30

40. Ziskin MC: Survey of patient exposure to diagnostic, in Reid JM, Sikov MR (eds), Interaction of Ultrasound and Biological Tissues. DHEW Pub. (FDA) 73-8008. Washington, D.C., U.S. Government Printing Office, 1972

41. Wells PNT: What is the future of ultrasonics? Ultrasonics 11:16, 1973

42. Smith SW: Diagnostic ultrasound: A review of clinical applications and the state of the art of commercial and experimental systems. HEW Publication (FDA) 76-8055. Washington, D.C., U.S. Government Printing Office, 1976

43. Smith SW: Diagnostic equipment and its use. Presented at the 8th Annual National Conference on Radiation Control, Springfield, IL, May 1–7, 1976

44. Stratmeyer ME: Research directions in ultrasound bioeffects—A public health view, in Hazzard DG, Litz ML (eds), Symposium on Biological Effects and Characterizations of Ultrasound Sources Proceedings. HEW Publication (FDA) 78-8048. Washington, D.C., U.S. Government Printing Office, 1977, pp 240–248

45. Frost HM, Stratmeyer ME: In-vivo effect of diagnostic ultrasound. Lancet 1:999, May 7, 1977

46. Nyborg WL: Physical mechanisms for biological effects of ultrasound. HEW Publication (FDA) 78-8062. Washington, D.C., U.S. Government Printing Office, 1978

47. Nyborg WL: Physical mechanisms for biological effects of ultrasound, in Repacholi MH and Benwell DA (eds), Ultrasound Short Course Transactions. Radiation Protection Bureau, Health Protection Branch, National Health and Welfare, Canada, 1979, pp. 84–136

48. Dunn F: Biological effects of ultrasound, in Repacholi MH, Benwell DA (eds), Ultrasound Short Course Transactions. Radiation Protection Bureau, Health Protection Branch, National Health and Welfare, Canada, 1979, pp 51–81

49. Lele PP: Safety and potential hazards in the current applications of ultrasound in obstetrics and gynecology. Ultrasound Med Biol 5:307, 1979

50. Anderson DW, Barrett JT: Ultrasound: A new immunosuppressant. Clin Immunol Immunopath 14:18, 1979

50a. Child SZ, Hare JD, Carstensen E, et al: Test for the effects of diagnostic levels of ultrasound immune response in mice. Clin Immunol Pathol 18:229, 1981

51. Liebeskind D, Bases R, Elequin F, et al: Diagnostic ultrasound: Effects on the DNA and growth patterns of animal cells. Radiology 131:177, 1979

52. Liebeskind D, Bases R, Mendex F, et al: Sister chromatid exchanges in human lymphocytes after exposure to diagnostic ultrasound. Science 205:1273, 1979

53. Siegel E, Goddard J, James AE, et al: Cellular attachment as a sensitive indicator of the effects of diagnostic ultrasound and exposure on cultured human cells. Radiology 133:175, 1979

54. Miller DL, Nyborg WL, Whitcomb CC: Platelet aggregation induced by ultrasound under specialized conditions in vivo. Science 205:505, 1979

55. Anderson DW, Barrett JT: Depression of phagocytosis by ultrasound. Ultrasound Med Biol 7:267, 1981

56. Liebeskind D, Bases R, Koenigsberg M, et al: Morphological changes in the surface characteristics of cultured cells after exposure to diagnostic ultrasound. Radiology 138:419, 1981

57. Haupt M, Martin AO, Simpson JL, et al: Ultrasonic induction of sister chromatid exchanges in human lymphocytes. Hum Genet 59:221, 1981

58. Morris SM, Palmer CG, Fry FJ, et al: Effect of ultrasound on human leukocytes—Sister chromatid exchange analysis. Ultrasound Med Biol 4:253, 1978

59. Saad AH, Williams AR: Effects of therapeutic ultrasound on clearance rate of blood borne colloidal particles in vivo. Br J Cancer 45 (suppl V):202, 1982

60. Wegner RD, Obe G, Meyenburg M: Has diagnostic ultrasound mutagenic effects? Hum Genet 56:95, 1980

61. Zheng HZ, Mitter NS, Chudley AE: In vivo exposure to diagnostic ultrasound and in vitro assay of sister chro-

matid exchanges in cultured amniotic fluid cells. IRSC Medical Science: Biochemistry; Biomedical Technology; Cell and Membrane Biology; Clinical Biochemistry; Developmental Biology and Medicine; Environmental Biology and Medicine; Pathology; Reproduction; Obstetrics and Gynecology 9:491, 1981

62. Au WA, Obergoenner N, Goldenthal KL et al: Sister-chromatid exchanges in mouse embryos after exposure to ultrasound in utero. Mutation Res 103:315, 1982

63. Barrass N, ter Haar G, Casey G: The effect of ultrasound and hyperthermia on sister chromatid exchange and division kinetics of BHK21 C13/A3 cells. Br J Cancer 45 (suppl V):187, 1982

64. Lundberg M, Jerominski L, Livingston G, et al: Failure to demonstrate an effect of in vivo diagnostic ultrasound on sister chromatid exchange frequency in amniotic fluid cells. Am J Med Genet 11:31, 1982

65. Wegner RD, Meyenburg M: The effects of diagnostic ultrasonography on the frequency of sister chromatid exchanges in Chinese hamster cells and human lymphocytes. J Ultrasound Med 1:355, 1982

66. O'Brien WD Jr: Ultrasonically induced fetal weight reduction in mice, in White D, Barnes R (eds), Ultrasound in Medicine. New York, Plenum, 1976, pp 531–532

67. O'Brien WD Jr, Christman CL, Yarrow S: Ultrasonic biological effect exposure system, in deKlerk J (ed), 1974 Ultrasonic Symposium Proceedings. New York, IEEE Catalog No. 74 CHO 896-ISU, 1974, pp 57–64

68. O'Brien WD Jr: Dose-dependent effect of ultrasound on fetal weight in mice. J Ultrasound Med 2:1, 1983

69. Dunn F, Lohnes JE, Fry FJ: Frequency dependence of threshold ultrasonic dosages for irreversible structural changes in mammalian brain. J Acoust Soc Am 58:512, 1975

70. Johnston RL, Dunn F: Influence of subarachnoid structures on transmeningeal ultrasonic propagation. J Acoust Soc Am 60:1225, 1976

71. Johnston RL, Dunn F: Ultrasonic absorbed dose, dose rate, and produced lesion volume. Ultrasonics 14:153, 1976

72. Fry WJ, Dunn F: Ultrasonic irradiation of the central nervous system at high sound levels. J Acoust Soc Am 28:129, 1956

73. Chan SK, Frizzell LA: Ultrasonic thresholds for structural changes in the mammalian liver, in deKlerk J, McAvoy BR (eds), 1977 Ultrasonics Symposium Proceedings. New York, IEEE Catalog No. 77 CH2364-ISU, 1977, pp 153–156

74. Rossi HH, Kellerer AM: Radiation carcinogenesis at low doses. Science 175:200, 1972

75. Wang SY: Introductory concepts for photochemistry of nucleic acids, in Wang SY (ed), Photochemistry and Photobiology of Nucleic Acids. New York, Academic, 1976, vol 1, pp 1–21

76. Fry FJ, Erdmann WA, Johnson LK, et al: Ultrasonic toxicity study. Ultrasound Med Biol 3:351, 1978

77. Stolzenberg SC, Torbit CA, Edmonds PD, et al: Effects of ultrasound on the mouse exposed at different stages of gestation: Acute study. Radiation Environmental Biophysics 17:245, 1980

78. AIUM/NEMA Safety Standard for Diagnostic Ultrasound Equipment. AIUM/NEMA Standards Publication UL1-1981. Available through the American Institute of Ultrasound in Medicine, Bethesda, MD, or the National Electrical Manufacturers Association, Washington, D.C., 1981

3 | Ultrasound Instrumentation and Its Practical Applications

Gary A. Thieme
Ronald R. Price
A. Everette James, Jr.

INTRODUCTION

In recent years, major advances in diagnostic ultrasound technology have resulted in greatly improved image quality and increasingly sophisticated instrumentation. Selection of a satisfactory instrument from the wide variety of equipment available today can be puzzling and time consuming. It is difficult to obtain an unbiased opinion from experts. Although there are no definite guidelines with regard to choice of instrumentation, some general considerations are presented. The discussion will largely be restricted to those aspects of ultrasound imaging technology applicable to abdominal (ABD) and obstetric and gynecologic (OB/GYN) imaging.

In general, it is most helpful to acquire a basic understanding of the physics of ultrasound and a fundamental knowledge of the manner in which the image is formed. These concepts have been presented in Chapter 1. One should also acquire at least a qualitative understanding of the different technologies used in modern instruments. In addition, the patient population must be analyzed because it will largely determine the variety of exams to be performed and the type of equipment necessary. Although many types of exams require the complementary aspects of both static and real-time imaging, some can be adequately performed with real-time imaging alone.

Static-imaging instruments utilize a single transducer attached to a mechanical arm which is manually moved across a body surface. The structures beneath a large, irregularly contoured surface can be imaged to obtain a panoramic view much larger than that pro-

duced by either sector or linear array real-time instruments (Fig. 1). These large cross-sectional images are produced at fixed distance intervals (generally 1 cm) and provide a series of tomographic planes from which the reader can mentally synthesize a three-dimensional concept of the selected region of the body.

Real-time instruments rapidly sweep the ultrasound beam through a sector or rectangular area by either mechanical or electronic means. Frame rates greater than 15 frames per second are required to produce flicker-free images and to observe most moving structures. Because real-time probes are usually not attached to a scanning arm, the sonographer has great flexibility in selecting the image plane orientation. Large volumes of tissue can be rapidly surveyed. Images can be obtained from nearly any patient position and through acoustic windows too small for, or inaccessible to, static scanners. The structural integrity and function of moving structures such as the diaphragm and heart are easily observed. Despite these obvious advantages, the field-of-view provided by all real-time systems is limited, and the appreciation of general anatomic relationships is more difficult when compared to the global view provided by static images.

Both types of instrument systems typically consist of the following:

1. A transducer, which forms a focused ultrasound beam and sweeps it through an image plane by either mechanical or electronic means.
2. A pulser/receiver module, which first energizes the transducer and then amplifies the electrical signal returning from the transducer, applies time-gain

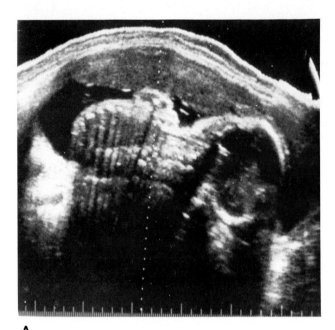

A

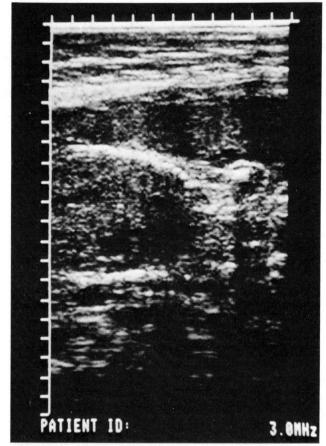

B

compensation (TGC) to compensate for tissue attenuation effects, and transforms the signal into a standard A-mode trace that represents the returning echo amplitudes as a function of tissue depth.

3. A scan converter, which uses position information about the transducer to translate the series of one-dimensional A-mode lines into a two-dimensional B-mode image.

4. Preprocessing and postprocessing controls, which determine the gray scale assignment to the echo amplitudes and affect the user's perception of contrast differences between tissues.

5. A video display unit.

6. A device for permanently recording the images—Polaroid, multiimage format camera, or video tape.

Modern instruments should also have a keyboard for superimposing on the recorded image the patient identification, exam date, and study information.

TRANSDUCER DESIGNS

A transducer is a device that converts one form of energy into another form. For diagnostic ultrasound imaging systems, the transducer is operated in a pulse–echo mode. That is, the transducer converts electrical energy into a short burst of sound energy which is "pulsed" into the body; the reflected sound energy—"echo"—is converted into electrical energy by the same transducer. Strictly speaking, the transducer is the piezoelectric element which performs this function. How-

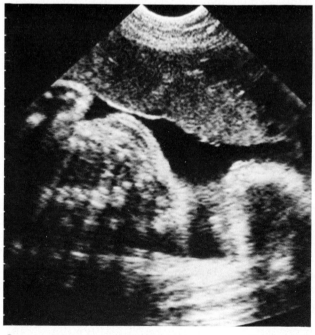

C

Fig. 1. Static, linear array, and sector scans. Fields-of-view are compared for a standard OB examination.

TABLE 1

Frequency (MHz)	Wavelength (mm)
1	1.54
2.25	0.68
3.5	0.44
5	0.31
6	0.26
7.5	0.21
10	0.15

ever, the term is typically used in a broader sense to include the entire scanning head of a real-time system.

Transducers can be characterized by size, frequency, wavelength, axial and lateral resolution, focusing, penetration ability, and sensitivity. These are interrelated variables. Transducer size refers to the diameter of the active element. For routine clinical applications, transducer sizes range from 6 to 19 mm diameter. For special applications such as water-path scanners, transducer sizes up to 10 cm have been employed. In general, the transmitted acoustic power and the received signal strength are directly proportional to the transducer diameter.

Typically, the range of frequencies for diagnostic ultrasound imaging is 2.25 to 10.0 MHz. The commercially specified value is the center (median) frequency. Table 1 lists the corresponding wavelengths at 1540 m/sec (average speed of sound in tissues) for usual transducer frequencies. The spectrum of frequencies emitted is termed the bandwidth and is dependent upon the degree of damping (ringdown). Damping determines the pulse length, which is the actual physical space occupied by the burst of ultrasound (Fig. 2). A heavily damped (short ringdown time) transducer produces a short pulse length and a broad bandwidth. However, the acoustic energy output and sensitivity are much smaller than a moderately damped transducer with a longer pulse length. Most transducers used for diagnostic imaging are damped such that the best compromise between the shortest possible pulse length (a few wavelengths) and the greatest sensitivity is achieved.

Axial resolution is the ability to distinguish two closely spaced structures which lie at different depths along the line of sight of the transducer (Fig. 3A). The shorter the pulse length, the better the axial resolution. The axial resolution is defined as being equal to one half of the spatial pulse length.

Since wavelength is determined by frequency and speed of sound, the following relationship can be stated: increased frequency → decreased wavelength → decreased spatial pulse length → better axial resolution (assuming constant damping factor). Increasing

damping factor → decreased spatial pulse length → better axial resolution (assuming constant frequency). For higher frequency transducers, axial resolution for specular reflectors in tissue equivalent phantom material is typically 0.5 to 2 mm.

Lateral resolution is the ability to distinguish two closely spaced structures which lie along a line that is perpendicular to the line-of-sight of the transducer (Fig. 3B). To resolve two reflectors as separate structures, a sound beam must be narrow enough to pass between them. The major determinant of lateral resolving ability is the beam width; this is governed by the focal zone properties described next. Lateral resolution for specular reflectors in tissue equivalent phantom material is 1 to 2 mm for highly focused, high frequency transducers.

Transducers for static imaging systems have traditionally been single-element, fixed-focus designs (see Chapter 1). Focusing is achieved internally by the transducer element shape or externally by an acoustic lens (Fig. 4A). The depth of the focal region is described as either short (1 to 4 cm), medium (4 to 8 cm), or long (6 to 12 cm) (Fig. 4B). A typical beam diameter in the focused region is 3 mm. As discussed in Chapter 1, the Fresnel zone length is determined by the transducer element diameter and the wavelength of sound. A transducer cannot be satisfactorily focused beyond this depth. A beam profile is used to determine the position, length, and degree of focusing (Fig. 4C). This information provides important guidelines for the proper clinical usage of the transducer and is usually supplied by manufacturers when the transducer is purchased.

Recently, annular array technology has been introduced. This transducer is composed of a series of independent transducer elements, each having the shape of an annular ring. The multiple elements are arranged in concentric rings about a central transducer element (Fig. 5A). Beam formation and focusing is achieved electronically by small time delays in the pulsing of individual transducer elements (Fig. 5B). In addition, when the transducer receives the returning echoes, similar time delays are used to combine the signals from each of the individual elements (Fig. 5C). The result is dynamic focusing during reception and an electronically variable focus for transmission. Focusing is achieved in two dimensions similar to a single focused element; but, unlike mechanical focusing, the focal zone can be altered without physically changing the transducer simply by changing the electronic timing of the individual annular elements. This is joystick controlled or switch selectable. In addition, lateral resolution throughout the field-of-view is substantially improved because a narrower beam diameter over a long path length results from the constructive and destructive interference effects of the sound waves produced by the phased elements. (Fig. 5D). Beam diameters of 1 mm have been quoted.

Transducer sensitivity can be related to its conversion efficiency, which is a measure of how well a transducer converts both the electrical impulse from the instrument pulser into acoustic energy and the received echoes into an electrical signal. To maximize sensitivity, a transducer must be electrically "tuned" to both

the pulser and the receiver. Also, to minimize impedance differences between the human body tissues and the transducer materials, multiple matching layer quarter-wavelength thickness materials are bonded to the surface of the ceramic element. These layers form a gradual impedance transition and help to limit energy losses at the skin–transducer interface (Fig. 6). This, in turn, improves sensitivity by concentrating acoustic energy within the focal zone. A typical value for the sensitivity of transducers in clinical use today is 5 percent.

The depth of the field-of-view is governed by the penetration ability of the transducer. Multiple factors affect the depth of penetration. Of these, the frequency-dependent attenuation of sound in tissues is the most significant factor. For most tissues, this attenuation occurs at a rate of approximately 1 dB/cm/ MHz. For system electronics with a dynamic range of 60 dB, a 3-MHz transducer can be expected to have a penetration depth of 20 cm. Depth of penetration for a 5-MHz transducer would only be 12 cm. A 10-MHz transducer is limited to a depth of penetration of only 6 cm; its use would then be confined to the imaging of superficial structures. Transducer sensitivity and the system electronics sensitivity obviously affect the depth of penetration since they determine the dynamic range (measured in decibels).

In designing transducers, manufacturers have optimized these parameters in order to achieve the highest sensitivity and penetration, optimum focal characteristics, and the best possible resolution—all at the lowest practical acoustic power output levels. In selecting a transducer with optimal properties for the clinical imaging task, the following general points should be considered:

1. Increasing transducer frequency results in enhanced axial resolution, but tissue penetration is reduced.

A

Fig. 2. Transducer bandwidth and pulse length. **A.** This graph of amplitude versus frequency demonstrates the measured bandwidth for a 3.5-MHz transducer. The actual center frequency is 3.0 MHz. The bandwidth is measured at half maximum amplitude and is 1.5 MHz for this transducer. The frequency content ranges from 1.5 to 5.0 MHz. Each small division is 1 MHz. **B.** This transducer has a 6-cycle pulse length of 2.5 μsec. The spatial pulse length is 2 mm at 1540 m/sec speed of sound. This is the physical space occupied by the burst of ultrasound. Structures separated by less than half this distance cannot be resolved.

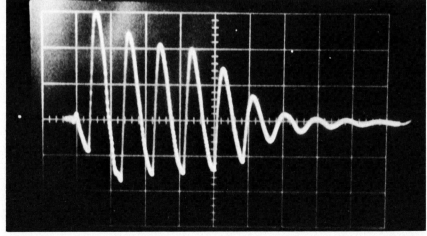

B

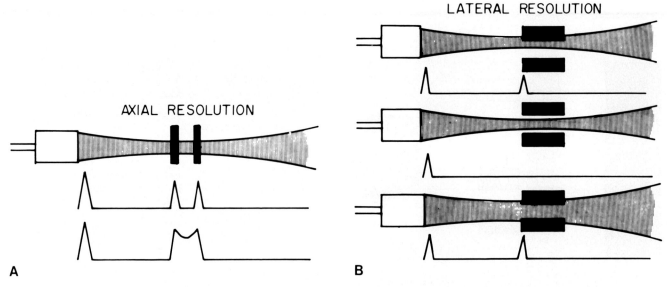

Fig. 3. Demonstration of axial **(A)** and lateral **(B)** resolution of a transducer for objects within focal zone of the ultrasound beam. (*Courtesy of KB-Aerotech*). **A.** The focused beam of the transducer encounters two reflecting structures parallel to the face of the transducer and separated by a short distance. The upper A-mode trace shows two separate spikes for a system with a pulse length short enough to resolve the two structures. The lower A-mode trace shows two spikes merging into one broader spike for a system with a pulse length that is too long to resolve the two structures. **B.** For the narrow-beam configuration, a single spike is produced when the beam encounters the upper reflector and no signal is produced when the narrow beam passes between the two reflectors. For this configuration, each reflector can produce its own signal, and the two reflectors can be resolved as separate structures. For the broad-beam configuration (*bottom*), only a single spike is produced; the two reflectors appear as a single structure to the ultrasound unit.

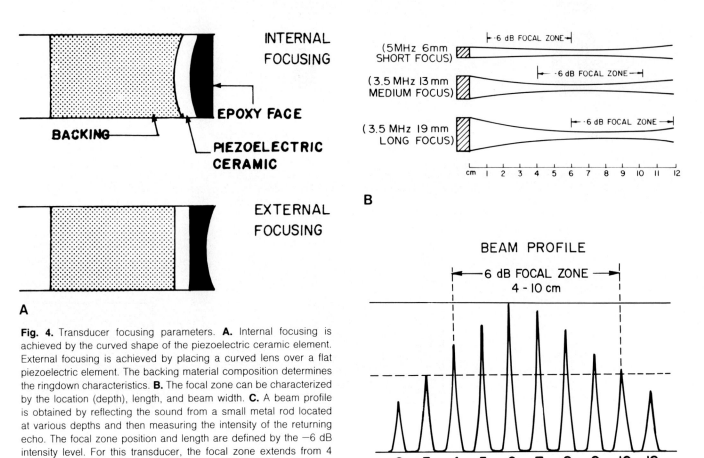

Fig. 4. Transducer focusing parameters. **A.** Internal focusing is achieved by the curved shape of the piezoelectric ceramic element. External focusing is achieved by placing a curved lens over a flat piezoelectric element. The backing material composition determines the ringdown characteristics. **B.** The focal zone can be characterized by the location (depth), length, and beam width. **C.** A beam profile is obtained by reflecting the sound from a small metal rod located at various depths and then measuring the intensity of the returning echo. The focal zone position and length are defined by the −6 dB intensity level. For this transducer, the focal zone extends from 4 to 10 cm.

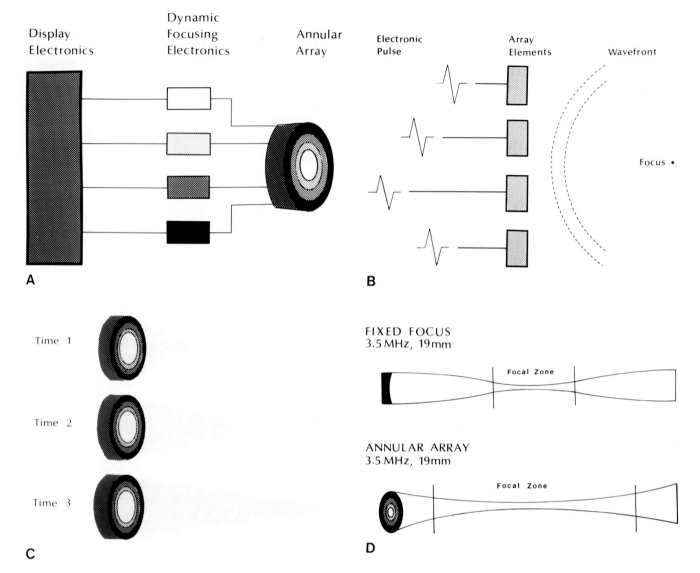

Fig. 5. Annular array transducer. (*Reprinted from Imaging Properties of Dynamically Focused Annular Arrays, Technicare Ultrasound Technology Series. Courtesy of Technicare Ultrasound.*) **A.** The annular array consists of four individual piezoelectric elements. Each element has its own pulsing and receiving circuits. The signals are processed and combined into a standard image. **B.** A focused beam is formed by small delays in the pulsing of individual elements. **C.** Similar delays are used to focus the received echoes dynamically throughout the depth of field-of-view. **D.** The focal zones for a standard fixed-focus transducer and a dynamically focused annular array transducer are compared. A narrower focal zone over a longer length can be obtained with annular array technology as a result of dynamic focusing.

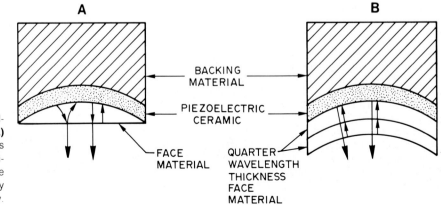

Fig. 6. Construction of a single-element fixed-focus transducer. The standard construction **(A)** does not use quarter-wavelength thicknesses **(B)** of facing material to provide a smoother impedance transition between the ceramic and the skin. Quarter-wave technology improves energy transfer between the transducer and the body.

The highest frequency consistent with adequate tissue penetration should be used.

2. Larger-diameter transducers are better suited to lower frequencies so that good lateral resolution is preserved at depth. They also provide greater acoustic power and sensitivity.

3. Smaller-diameter transducers are better suited to higher frequencies to provide improved lateral resolution over the shorter range. Since the depth of penetration at high frequencies is reduced, a long Fresnel zone is not needed. Power and sensitivity requirements are also reduced.

4. Focused transducers provide improved lateral resolution and sensitivity at the focal zone depth. The choice of the focal zone, therefore, depends upon the depth of structures to be optimally resolved.

The following transducers have proven useful clinically:

1. 2.25-MHz, 19-mm diameter, long-focus transducer for very large adults;

2. 3.5-MHz, 19-mm diameter, long-focus transducer for good penetration on normal size and obese adults;

3. 5.0-MHz, 19-mm diameter, long-focus transducer for standard and smaller adults;

4. 5.0-MHz, 13-mm diameter, medium-focus transducer for more superficial structures; and,

5. 7.5- and 10.0-MHz, 6-mm diameter, short-focus transducers for excellent lateral and axial resolution for thyroid, testicle, and superficial structure visualization.

Similar criteria can be applied to the dynamically focused annular arrays, linear arrays, and steered-beam phased arrays, discussed in the following section.

REAL-TIME TRANSDUCER SYSTEMS

Although the discussion of transducer designs and properties has been primarily in reference to static-scanner imaging systems to this point, the principles are directly applicable to the more sophisticated real-time transducers. A wide variety of designs is available. Basically, the manual function of sweeping the sound beam produced by a transducer at the end of an articulated arm scanner is replaced by an automated mechanical or electronic method of sweeping the sound beam through a sector (pie-shaped) or rectangular area of predetermined, fixed-shape and size.

The multielement, linear-sequenced array transducers produce a rectangular, parallel-line field-of-view. They are most useful for imaging structures requiring a large field-of-view near the skin surface (e.g., an anterior placenta). However, the requirement of a large surface contact area limits the usefulness of linear array transducers when acoustic windows are small or surfaces are curved or irregular (e.g., visualization of the lower uterine segment inferior to the pubic symphysis). The linear array length varies from a few centimeters to as long as 20 cm at 3 MHz. It is a popular design for obstetric scanning.

The linear sequenced array (LSA) transducer is composed of many small piezoelectric elements (M) arranged in parallel (Fig. 7A). A typical 3.5-MHz transducer may have 100 elements spaced at 1.5-mm intervals over 150 mm. The beam produced by such a narrow element will diverge very rapidly after the wavelet travels only a few millimeters. Thus, pulsing of a single individual element would result in poor lateral resolution due to beam divergence and low sensitivity due to the small element size.

To overcome this problem, several adjacent elements (N)—typically 8 to 16—are driven simultaneously. In the subgroup of N elements, pulsing of the inner elements is delayed with respect to the outer elements (Fig. 7B). A focused beam results from the constructive and destructive interference of the N tiny divergent wavelets. The magnitude (time interval) of the delays determines the depth of focus for the transmitted beam and can be changed during scanning. Similarly, the same delay factors are applied to the N elements during the receiving phase; this results in a dynamic focusing effect on the returning signals. In this manner, a single scan line in the real-time image is formed. To generate the next adjacent scan line, another group of N elements is formed by shifting one element position along the transducer array from the previous group (Fig. 7C). The same transmit–receive pattern is then repeated for this set of N elements and subsequently for all other sets along the array, in a cyclic manner.

Electronic focusing in the plane along the direction of the transducer elements improves lateral resolution as well as sensitivity by increasing the amount of energy in the focal zone (constructive interference). Focusing in the direction at right angles to the scan plane determines the slice thickness and is accomplished by use of an external lens (Fig. 7D). The combination of electronic and mechanical focusing is termed "double focusing." A unique advantage of electronically focused transducers is the ability to change the depth of the focal zone simply by changing the magnitudes of the delays applied to the individual elements. Using a joystick or pushbutton control, the focal zone can be scanned through a specified range of depths during the real-time exam. Similar to any single element or annular array transducer, the Fresnel zone limit determines the maximum depth at which the beam can be satisfactorily focused.

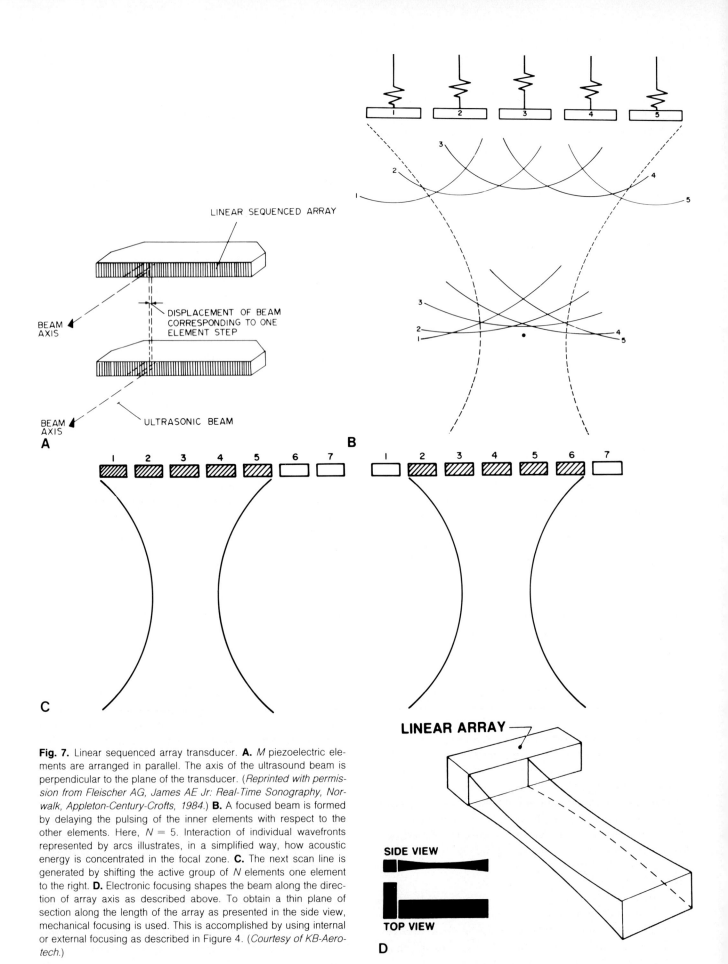

Fig. 7. Linear sequenced array transducer. **A.** *M* piezoelectric elements are arranged in parallel. The axis of the ultrasound beam is perpendicular to the plane of the transducer. (*Reprinted with permission from Fleischer AG, James AE Jr: Real-Time Sonography, Norwalk, Appleton-Century-Crofts, 1984.*) **B.** A focused beam is formed by delaying the pulsing of the inner elements with respect to the other elements. Here, *N* = 5. Interaction of individual wavefronts represented by arcs illustrates, in a simplified way, how acoustic energy is concentrated in the focal zone. **C.** The next scan line is generated by shifting the active group of *N* elements one element to the right. **D.** Electronic focusing shapes the beam along the direction of array axis as described above. To obtain a thin plane of section along the length of the array as presented in the side view, mechanical focusing is used. This is accomplished by using internal or external focusing as described in Figure 4. (*Courtesy of KB-Aerotech.*)

For early linear array designs, off-axis beam artifacts were a significant problem. These appeared as "ghost" structures in clinical images and were the by-product of grating lobes. Both side lobes and grating lobes are secondary ultrasound beams that project off-axis at predictable angles to the main lobe (primary beam) (Fig. 8). Side lobes are usually so small that they do not produce significant artifacts clinically. Grating lobes are unique to multielement array transducers and are caused by the regular, periodic spacing of the small array elements. The energy of grating lobes can be significant relative to the main lobe. When this energy is reflected by off-axis structures and detected by the transducer, the signal produced is artifactual since it is not reflected from any structure along the main beam axis. To overcome this problem, each individual element has been "subdiced," that is, divided into smaller parts, each one a half wavelength wide. This has the effect of "eliminating" the grating lobes by increasing the angle to greater than 90 degrees. Eliminating grating lobes also improves the signal-to-noise ratio by increasing the size of the main lobe energy relative to the background energy. This improves image contrast and, hence, the ability to detect structures that only weakly scatter and reflect sound.

Modern, high-quality linear array transducers utilize subdicing technology and produce artifact-free images under most clinical conditions. Current linear array systems are capable of lateral resolution on the order of 1 to 3 mm. Axial resolution of 1 mm is possible with higher frequency systems. A wide aperture, linear array design that pulses all M elements to form each A-line has been recently introduced. At each A-line, a different delayed pulse sequencing of the M elements is required to form the unique interference pattern, resulting in a highly focused ultrasound beam that is perpendicular to the transducer face. Since a unique delay pattern for the M elements is required to produce each A-line, highly sophisticated computer-controlled electronics are required. Lateral resolution of 0.5 mm has been quoted.

Although linear sequenced array transducer designs tend to be very similar, sector transducer construction varies widely. All designs sweep the ultrasound beam through a pie-shaped wedge or sector with an opening angle ranging from 30 to 100 degrees. The limited view of superficial structures by sector scanners is offset by their high maneuverability and their ability to visualize large areas at greater depths through small acoustic windows. The mechanical designs enclose the transducer in a fluid-filled case with a flexible membrane that provides acoustic coupling with the skin. The properties of the fluid and the membrane must be carefully selected to minimize reverberation arti-

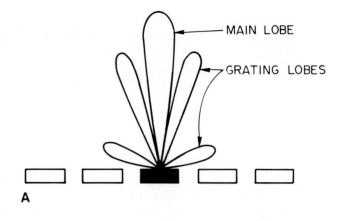

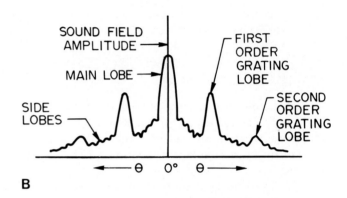

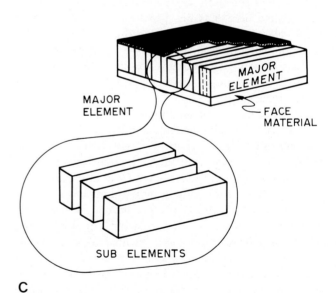

Fig. 8. Grating lobes and subdicing technology. (*Courtesy of KB-Aerotech.*) **A.** The angle of the grating lobe is determined by the center-to-center spacing (pitch) of the array elements. **B.** Grating lobes represent a large off-axis energy component of the ultrasound beam. Side-lobe energy does not contribute to off-axis image artifacts under most clinical imaging circumstances. **C.** To eliminate the grating lobe artifact problem, each major piezoelectric element is divided into subelements. The pitch is then small enough so that the angle θ is greater than 90 degrees. The major element is pulsed as a group of subelements.

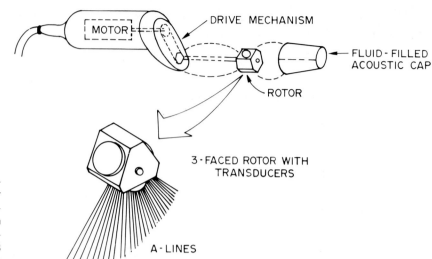

Fig. 9. Rotating wheel mechanical sector transducer. Three transducers mounted on a rotor enclosed in fluid within an acoustic cap are rotated at constant speed by a motor. As each transducer rotates in front of the acoustic window, it is pulsed 128 times to produce 128 evenly spaced scan lines through a 90 degree arc.

facts. Electronically steered, phased array designs require only gel for coupling; the newest designs use multilayer quarter-wavelength impedance matching technology to minimize reverberation artifacts at the skin line.

The mechanical sector is essentially a mechanized extension of the static scanner, with a rapid frame rate and limited field-of-view. Most designs use standard single-element, fixed-focus transducers. Typical element diameters are also similar—13 and 19 mm. We discuss three generic designs for sweeping the ultrasound beam through the sector arc, because of their widespread usage.

One of the most common mechanical designs consists of three single-element, fixed-focus transducers mounted 120 degrees apart on a wheel that is rotated by an external motor (Fig. 9). As the transducers rotate, the pulsing sequence is switched from one transducer to the next, depending upon which transducer has rotated in front of the acoustic window. Because the transducers rotate at a constant speed, angular spacing of lines is uniform throughout the field-of-view. Typically, the scan plane is oriented at a right angle to the axis of the transducer handle. The frame rate of this type of device is determined by the rotational speed of the wheel. For this design, matching the characteristics of three single-element transducers is critical to ensure uniform image quality.

Another popular design oscillates a single-element, fixed-focus transducer through an arc about a fixed point (Fig. 10). The newer electromechanical design eliminates the need for a traditional motor; a changing magnetic field strength powers the transducer

TRANSDUCER (SERVO-SECTOR)

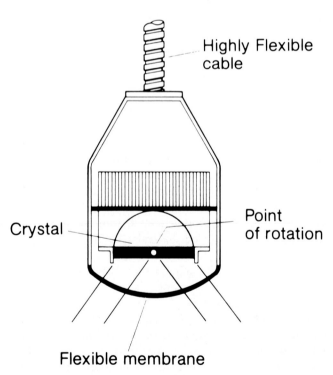

Fig. 10. Oscillating transducer design. A changing magnetic field oscillates the transducer about a fixed point to produce scan lines in a sector format. A flexible membrane is used to enclose the single element crystal in a fluid path. (*Reprinted with permission from Fleischer AC, James AE Jr: Real-Time Sonography. Norwalk, Appleton-Century-Crofts, 1984.*)

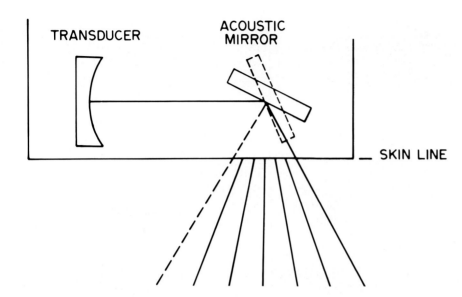

Fig. 11. Oscillating acoustic mirror design. A transducer (either fixed-focus, single-element or variable-focus, annular array) is stationary. A fluid path couples the transducer to oscillating acoustic mirror and the membrane. Scan lines are produced in a sector format radiating from the point of rotation of the mirror. (*Reprinted with permission from Fleischer AC, James AE Jr: Real-Time Sonography. Norwalk, Appleton-Century-Crofts, 1984.*)

motion. This novel design affords a small, lightweight, compact sector transducer. The scan plane is oriented in the same direction as the handle and is commonly referred to as an "in-line" design.

An alternative approach is to keep the transducer stationary and to utilize an oscillating acoustic mirror to move the beam in a sector format (Fig. 11). This design eliminates the need to move an electrically active component (the transducer). Also, the mirror is usually lighter and can be moved more easily and rapidly. The plane mirror only changes the direction of the beam and does not affect the beam focus. Energy loss in the reflection process is negligible. Because the fluid path must be longer (approximately 1 cm) than the rotating wheel and direct oscillating transducer designs, impedance matching and acoustic coupling are especially critical to ensure that reverberation artifacts are minimized in the near-field portion of the image. The size and shape of this design is similar to the rotating wheel types; the scan plane is oriented at a right angle to the axis of the transducer handle. Frame rate is determined by the oscillation frequency.

Until recently, only fixed-focus, single-element transducers were used in the mechanical designs. An annular array transducer has replaced the traditional single-element transducer in the oscillating mirror design. A joystick controller allows the user to change the focal zone electronically instead of having to physically change transducers. Beam steering, however, must be achieved mechanically with this technology (Fig. 11). This design represents a hybrid system and possesses the best characteristics of both the mechanical and electronic designs.

An alternative to the mechanical sector is the electronically steered-beam, phased-array (ESBPA) design. The principles of beam formation are similar to a linear sequenced array (Fig. 12); a simplified diagrammatic version is presented in Figure 13. Its primary use has been in cardiac imaging where low-amplitude echoes from grating lobe and side lobe artifacts can be "rejected" without loss of significant diagnostic information. Unfortunately, these low-amplitude echoes from diffuse scattering events in soft tissues are essential for imaging in the abdomen, pelvis, and gravid uterus. Thus, until recently, the phased-array transducer has not proven satisfactory for general ultrasound imaging.

The development of 64- and 128-element ESBPA systems now appears promising for solving the grating-lobe artifact problem and improving the signal-to-noise ratio. These instruments employ the most advanced designs in array technology. High-quality images have been produced using this technique. Similar to linear sequenced arrays, beam focusing depends upon constructive and destructive interference of the tiny wavelets produced by individual elements (Fig. 13). The electronic complexity is several orders of magnitude greater than that required for conventional LSA systems for two reasons. First, all M elements (64 or 128) must be selectively pulsed to form the wavefront for a single A-line. In contrast, only N elements (typically 8) of M total elements (typically 100) are selectively pulsed to form an A-line for common LSA designs. Second, the LSA system simply moves the same N-element pulse sequence along the M-element array to form parallel focused A-lines. The ESBPA system requires a unique M-element pulse sequence for each

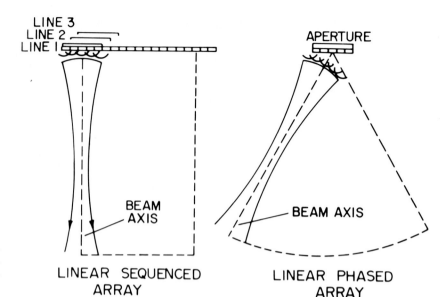

Fig. 12. Comparison of linear and phased array transducers. For the linear sequenced array, the beam position is always perpendicular to the face of the transducer and its position is shifted by using a new set of elements for the next line. For the linear phased array, the angle of the beam with respect to the transducer face changes; all elements are used to form each beam position. Rectangular and sector formats are produced respectively. (*Reprinted with permission from Fleischer AC, James AE Jr: Real-Time Sonography. Norwalk, Appleton-Century-Crofts, 1984.*)

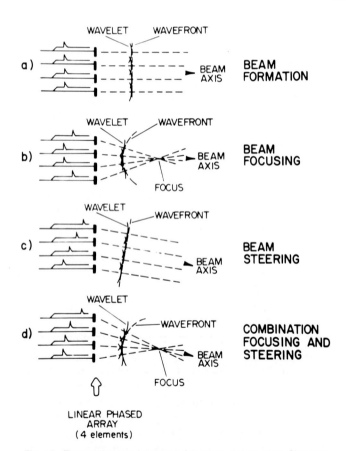

Fig. 13. Electronic beam formation, focusing, and steering. Constructive and destructive interference of the wavelets produced by the tiny transducer elements results in a wavefront with a direction and focal point determined by the delays in the pulse sequence. The pulse sequencing for beam formation in linear sequenced arrays is shown in **a** and **b**. By variations in the pulse sequences shown in **c** and **d**, the beam can be both steered and focused at any angle with respect to the transducer face. (*Reprinted with permission from Fleischer AC, James AE Jr: Real-Time Sonography. Norwalk, CT: Appleton-Century-Crofts, 1984.*)

A-line (typically 128) since each A-line has its own unique angle with respect to the transducer face in the sector format. Whereas, older, simpler LSA and ESBPA systems were "hardwired," the complexity of the newest designs requires sophisticated, high-speed, computer-controlled pulsing of the individual elements—"softwired" circuitry. Electronic focusing on both transmit and receive (similar to annular array designs) provides a longer focal zone with a narrower beam width than conventional single element designs. Similar to LSA designs, focusing in the direction at right angles to the scan plane determines the slice thickness and is accomplished by use of an external lens.

Multiple-layer quarter-wavelength acoustic impedance matching technology improves sound transmission between the transducer and skin surface. Because there are no moving parts, a fluid path is not needed; reverberation artifacts are negligible. Since the beam path is electronically controlled, the direction (vector) of each A-line can be selected at random. This unique advantage over mechanical designs allows the ESBPA system to perform "simultaneous" B-mode imaging and M-mode or Doppler functions.

FRAME RATE, FIELD-OF-VIEW, AND LINE DENSITY

The number of frames displayed per second to define an imaging system as "real-time" is unclear. However, a rate of 10 frames per second would appear to be a minimum, and a rate of at least 15 frames per second is necessary to produce flicker-free images. Frame rate (F), number of A-line per frame (N), and depth of field-of-view (D) are inversely related. The constant limiting parameter is the speed of sound in soft tissues.

The average speed of sound in soft tissue is known to be 1540 m/sec. Thus, 6.5 μsec is required for an ultrasonic pulse to travel 1 cm in soft tissue. Since the same transducer is used to receive as well as to transmit the ultrasonic wave in pulse–echo mode, an additional 6.5 μsec is required for each centimeter of tissue thickness in order to receive the returning echo. Therefore, one must wait 13 μsec for each centimeter of soft tissue thickness being imaged (Fig. 14). The total time (T) required to form a complete image (frame) is then the product of the number of scan lines (N), the depth of field-of-view (D) and the round-trip time ($R = 13$ μsec/cm):

$$T \text{ (sec)} = N \text{ (lines)} \times D \text{ (cm)} \times 13 \times 10^{-6} \text{ sec/cm.}$$

$$[1]$$

The maximum frame rate (F) is simply the inverse of T:

$$F = 1/T \text{ frames/sec.} \qquad [2]$$

These expressions can be reduced to:

$$F \text{ (frames/sec)} \times D \text{ (cm)} \times N \text{ (lines)} = 76{,}923. \qquad [3]$$

It is apparent from this expression that any increase in one parameter requires a decrease in the product of the other two. This restriction is imposed by the speed of sound in tissue.

Another related parameter, pulse repetition frequency (PRF), refers to the rate at which the transducers are activated to form each scan line. PRF (lines/sec) is the product of F (frames/sec) and N (lines/frame). For either the ESBPA or the rotating-wheel mechanical sector, a constant PRF produces constant angular spacing between sector lines (Fig. 14C). Since the oscillating transducer or mirror must reverse direction of motion at the end of each sweep, angular velocity changes throughout the single sweep. A constant PRF would result in closely spaced lines at each end and widely spaced lines in the middle. To overcome this problem, the angular position of the beam is encoded and the pulse repetition frequency is varied so that constant angular spacing is achieved, as in Figure 14C.

After the transducer is activated and the ultrasound pulse directed into the tissue, the transducer is placed into a "listening" mode in order to record the echoes returning from the tissue interfaces. The listening time (L) in microseconds is the product of D (cm) and R (13 μsec/cm). Since the pulse length (P) to produce the burst of ultrasound is usually less than 1 μsec long and since tissue depths of at least 5 cm are imaged, the transducer spends more than 98

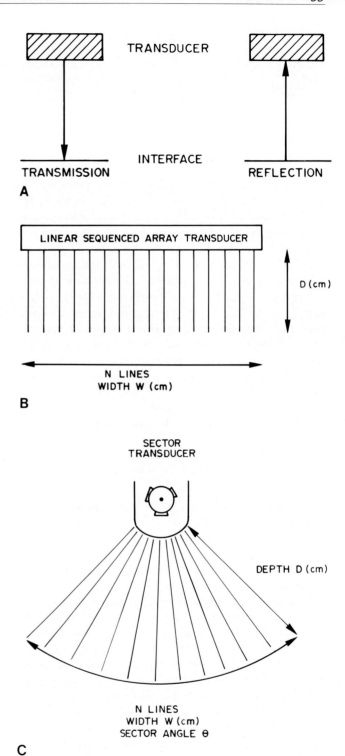

Fig. 14. Physical constraints affecting frame rate and line density. **A.** At 1540 m/sec, the speed of sound in tissue, each direction of travel of the ultrasound pulse requires 6.5 μsec/cm, for a total of 13 μsec/cm. **B.** For a linear sequenced array transducer, a single frame consists of N lines of depth D. The width W in centimeters is constant. Line density LD is N divided by W. **C.** For a sector format, a single frame also consists of N lines of depth D. Angular spacing is constant. However, line density varies as a function of depth D and the sector angle in degrees.

TABLE 2

Depth (cm)	Time (μsec)	15 frames/sec N (lines)	30 frames/sec N (lines)
10	130	512	256
15	195	342	171
20	260	256	128

TABLE 3

Depth (cm)	Time (μsec)	128 Lines F (frames/sec)	256 Lines F (frames/sec)	512 Lines F (frames/sec)
10	130	60	30	15
15	195	40	20	10
20	260	30	15	7.5

percent of its time "listening" (in the receiving mode).

Finally, line density (LD) is determined by the number of lines per frame (N) and the width of the field-of-view (W). For the rectangular field-of-view (Fig. 14B) produced by linear sequenced arrays, line density is constant throughout the depth of field-of-view; the spacing interval between lines is also constant and is determined by both the element size and the subgroup size used to form the beam. Line density is simply N divided by W. For the sector field-of-view (Fig. 14C), line density decreases as depth of field-of-view (D) increases. The width of the field-of-view (W) depends upon both the sector angle (θ) and the depth (D). Minimum acceptable line density must be calculated at depth D; for shallower portions of the image, line density is overdetermined.

Line density (LD) can be expressed as:

$$LD = \frac{N \times 180}{\pi \times D \times \theta \times 2}, \qquad [4]$$

where D is in millimeters and θ is in degrees. In practice, it is desirable to have a line sensitivity of one line per millimeter at depth D. This can be achieved by well-designed real-time scanners under most clinical conditions while maintaining an acceptable field-of-view size and frame rate.

Understanding the interdependence of these parameters enables the sonographer to appreciate the physical limitations imposed upon all real-time systems. Table 2 lists the theoretical limits for lines per image (N) as a function of depth (D); constant frame rates of 15 and 30 per second are assumed. Also listed is the listening time (L). Table 2 describes a "framerate" priority system. It optimizes the ability to "see" structures without noticeable flicker or motion artifacts. At large depths, image information content may be sacrificed because line density is too low. Table 3 lists the theoretical limits for frame rate (F) as a function of depth D; constant values for lines per frame (N) are assumed to be 128, 256, and 512. Table 3 describes a "line number" priority system. It optimizes information content at all tissue depths; this is especially important for visualizing deep structures with long focus transducers. At large tissue depths and high line densities, however, frame rate may be slowed to the point

where motion artifacts become bothersome. In practice, both systems select "middle-of-the-road" values for frame rate and line number in order to optimize image quality at a given depth of field-of-view.

The limits in Tables 2 and 3 are theoretical. Because linear sequenced arrays and electronic steered-beam, phased arrays have no moving parts, these instruments can sweep the ultrasound beam through either a rectangular or sector format at frame rates approaching the theoretical limits. All mechanical designs have "built-in" inefficiencies related to the physical motion of the transducer element or elements. For example, the rotating wheel design with three single-element transducers and a 90 degree sector is acquiring information for only 270 degrees of the 360 degree rotation. Thus, the maximum attainable frame rate can be only 75 percent of the theoretical value. Since the oscillating transducer element or mirror must reverse its direction of motion at the end of each sweep, its angular velocity (speed) changes throughout a single sweep. It will achieve the optimal frame rate only at the center A-line; for all other lines, the frame rate will be less than the theoretical limit. The percent loss in frame rate can be minimized by clever mechanical designs, however.

THE RECEIVER MODULE

The wide variation in transducer designs is contrasted to the uniformity of receiver designs. The low-amplitude signal generated by the piezoelectric effect in the transducer is amplified by the preamplifier that is often located in close proximity to the transducer itself in order to improve the signal-to-noise ratio. This high-frequency signal is conducted through a shielded cable to the main receiver module.

At this point, time gain compensation (TGC) is applied by selectively controlling the degree of signal amplification as a function of time (Fig. 15). This feature is used to compensate for the attenuation of ultrasound energy as a function of tissue depth. Since tissue depth is the product of time-of-flight and speed-of-sound (assumed to be 1540 m/sec), the term depth gain compensation (DGC) is also used to describe this process. The three variables of the TGC are slope rate, delay (slope position), and initial gain (Fig. 16). The slope rate is set so that a uniform echo intensity is produced throughout the depth of field-of-view of a homogeneous tissue. The initial gain is set so that the far end of the slope ramp is positioned at the limit of the depth of field-of-view. Unless there is a fluid path between the transducer and the tissues interrogated, the delay is set to zero. Slope rate is measured in decibels per centimeters, delay in centimeters, and initial gain in decibels.

A constant amplication factor is then applied to the signal to increase its size to a useful level for the system components that follow. Some systems use a large, fixed-amplification factor and then provide stepped attenuator settings to control the overall signal amplitude. The control may be labeled "damping" or "attenuator" and is measured in dB. Other systems provide the user with a variable gain amplifier which provides only the degree of amplification necessary to achieve the desired signal amplitude. Those systems that provide calibrated controls allow the user to do quantitative tissue characterization.

Following these initial steps, this bipolar signal (Fig. 17A) is then converted to a unipolar signal (Fig. 17B) by rectification of the negative components; this is termed "detection." Finally, the "envelope" of the high-frequency signal (Fig. 17C) is produced by a smoothing circuit. The result is an A-mode trace (Fig. 17D), which is proportional to and representative of the echo amplitudes along the line-of-sight of the transducer. Conventional units have performed these functions with analogue circuits. One manufacturer now digitizes the radio-frequency (RF) signal at 22 MHz and performs detection and pixel energy assignment digitally (Fig. 17E). This process improves the signal-to-noise ratio and produces a more accurate image representation of the original RF signal.

To form a two-dimensional gray scale display (B-mode image) from a series of adjacent A-mode traces, an electrical–mechanical unit must sense the orientation and spatial location of the transducer face (Fig. 18). Using this positional information, the A-mode trace can be "projected" along the transducer's line-of-sight. The brightness of the image at each point along that line-of-sight is proportional to the A-mode signal amplitude.

THE SCAN CONVERTER

The device that transforms the one-dimensional A-mode information into a two-dimensional B-mode display is called a "scan converter." In the early analogue systems, scan converter tubes consisting of silicon tar-

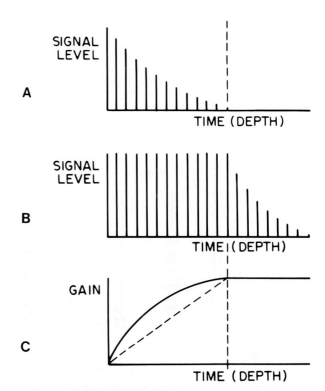

Fig. 15. Time gain compensation function. **A.** The signal level decreases exponentially as a function of time (signal depth) due to the attenuation of sound through absorption and scattering processes. **B.** Amplification of the signal is increased with time (tissue depth) and can be set such that the signal level is uniform throughout the period of compensation. **C.** The gain in signal amplitude (amplification) as a function of time (depth) is displayed as the TGC curve. Signal level is usually measured in decibels, a logarithmic function, rather than amplitude. The gain as a function of depth is then a straight line if exponential attenuation is assumed.

gets were used to store information electronically by "charging" the targets in proportion to the echo amplitude (A-mode voltage). Once the image had been stored, the scan converter tube was "read" and the results were displayed on a video monitor. Each target size could be made imperceptibly small to the eye. A continuous-echo amplitude range could be translated into a relatively infinite gray scale. The result was smooth variations in image intensity and structural boundaries—an "eye-appealing" image.

However, tracking errors and sensitivity to electronic noise limited resolution. These units were very temperature sensitive and required long warm-up periods to assure proper performance. Subtle drifting of image quality was difficult to detect and required frequent periodic alignment procedures.

To solve the stability problems, digital scan converters (DSC) were developed (Fig. 19). In these systems, the analogue voltage levels corresponding to the returning echo amplitudes of each A-mode line are digitized by an analogue-to-digital converter. The gen-

Processing

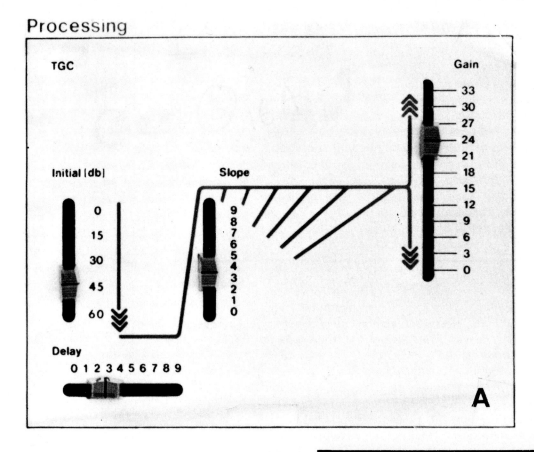

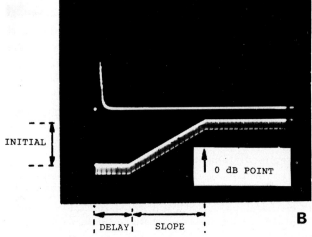

Fig. 16. TGC controls of a static B-mode scanner. **A.** On this model, slide potentiometers are used to control the initial gain (dB), slope (dB/cm), and delay (cm) in a highly descriptive format. The system gain control (dB) is also a part of this control panel. **B.** A graphic display of the TGC curve and the A-mode signal are highly useful features for both understanding and applying TGC to obtain the best possible clinical image.

erated array of values from each A-line are then stored in a digital memory. These discrete digital values are now immune to many of the factors contributing to analogue system drifting problems.

Each individual value stored in the digital memory represents a picture element or "pixel." The memory size determines the number of pixels composing the image. The memory is periodically (typically 60 times per second) interrogated and the image displayed on a video monitor. The brightness of the television signal representing each pixel is controlled by the digital

value stored at each memory location.

The ability of the discrete-form digital image to mimic the "smoothness" of the analogue image is governed both by the number of shades of gray and by the number of pixels used to form the digital image. The number of gray shades is determined by the number of bits in the digitizer. Older versions had 4 bits corresponding to 16 shades of gray. Newer models use 6 bits and provide 64 shades of gray. The human eye can easily distinguish gray level differences when only 16 shades are displayed; gray level differences for 64

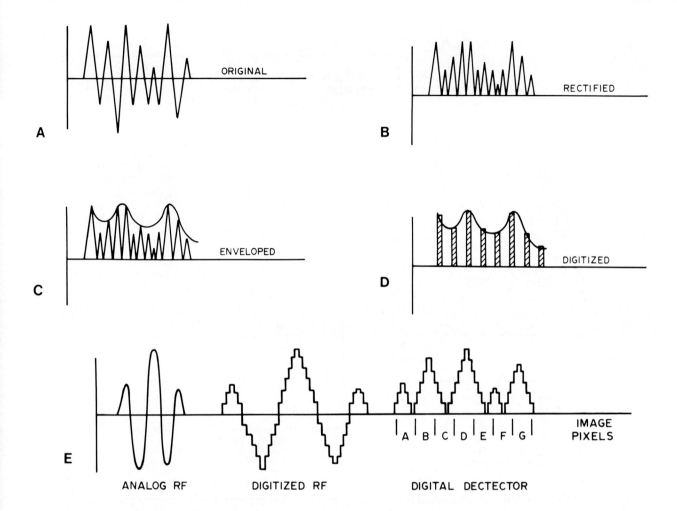

Fig. 17. Processing of the RF signal. **A.** The RF (radiofrequency) signal containing the full spectral content of the echoes received by the transducer is displayed as a function of time (depth). **B.** The signal is rectified to make all components positive; this is termed detection. **C.** A low-pass filter is then applied to produce a smoothed waveform. This is termed enveloping. **D.** The signal is then digitized at 2 MHz to form the A-mode trace, which is sent to the digital scan converter image memory. **E.** An alternative to the predominantly analog process described above is the digital RF processor (DRF). The analogue RF signal is digitized at 22 MHz to 8-bits. Negative components are digitally changed to positive values (digital detection). The digitized and rectified signal is then divided into pixel sizes corresponding to those in the image scan converter. The value of each pixel is proportional to the energy level in the original digitized signal.

shades are almost imperceptible; 128 shades provide the illusion of a continuous variation in gray scale. Digital values for a 4-bit converter range from 0 to 15; for a 6-bit converter, the range is 0 to 63.

The number of pixels used to form the digital image is determined by the size of the memory. Older versions used 128 × 128 digital words (each 4 bits deep). When displayed on a video monitor, this 128 × 128-pixel image has a perceptible "graininess." Newer digital scan converters with 512 × 512 × 6-bit deep memories can indeed mimic the "smoothness"

of analogue scan converters. The bonus, digital stability, translates into minimal maintenance, greater reliability, and very short (minutes) warm-up time.

The scan converter and display monitor quality are certainly important components of an ultrasound system and clearly affect the perceived ultrasound image quality. However, the major determinants of spatial and contrast resolution remain the axial and lateral resolution specifications of the transducer, the signal-to-noise ratio, and the quality of the predisplay electronic signal processing.

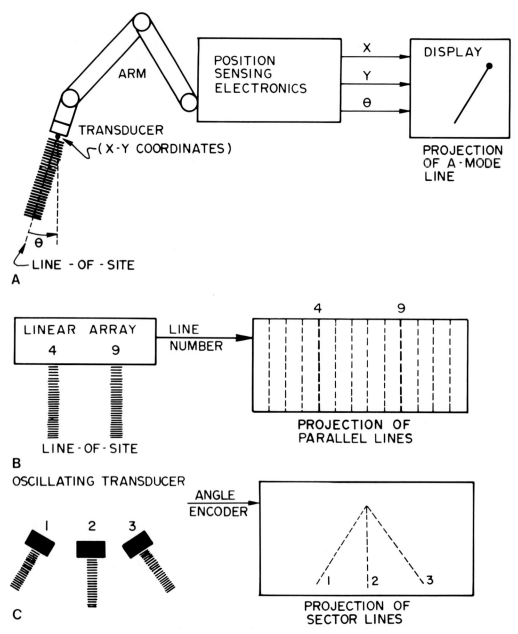

Fig. 18. Relationship of displayed image to transducer line of site. **A.** For a static scanner, the X–Y coordinates and the angle with respect to the vertical are needed in order to accurately display the line-of-site of the transducer. **B.** For a linear array system, only the line number needs to be known to project the line-of-site of the transducer. All lines are parallel. **C.** For an oscillating or rotating transducer, the angle of the line-of-site must be precisely encoded and accurately displayed to obtain a properly proportioned sector image.

PREPROCESSING AND POSTPROCESSING CONTROLS

Preprocessing and postprocessing controls are included on most ultrasound scanners. Preprocessing refers to the assignment of digital levels to the voltage range representing the echo amplitudes (Figs. 19 and 20). This step occurs during the analogue-to-digital conver-

sion and is fixed once the image is obtained ("frozen"). Postprocessing refers to the assignment of the gray levels to the digital values and occurs as the digital scan converter (DSC) information is displayed on the viewing monitor. The postprocessing can be changed after the image has been obtained ("frozen"). Both preprocessing and postprocessing are used to emphasize a selected echo amplitude range and have the effect of changing the contrast differences between tissues.

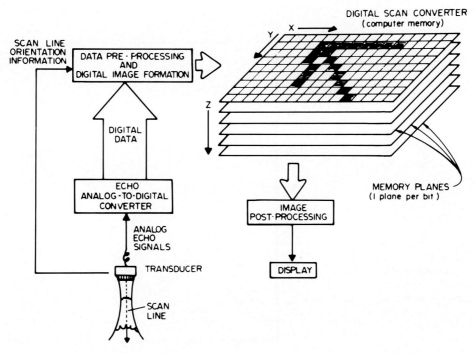

Fig. 19. Digital scan converter. (*Reprinted with permission from Fleischer AC, James AE Jr: Real-Time Sonography. Norwalk, Appleton-Century-Crofts, 1984.*) An analogue-to-digital converter converts the A-mode trace into a digital form. Positional information describing the line-of-site of the transducer is used to project the digitized A-mode signal onto the scan converter memory. The memory consists of a matrix of bits representing the *X–Y* coordinates of each point along the line-of-site of the transducer. The "depth" of the memory is described by the number of bits. The output of the digital scan converter is then processed for display on a video monitor.

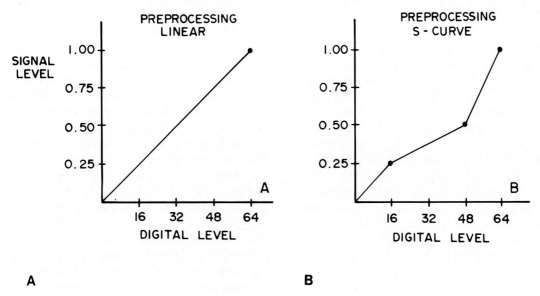

Fig. 20. Preprocessing functions. **A.** Signal levels 0 through 1.00 are evenly distributed over the 64 digital levels. No emphasis is placed on any of the echo amplitudes in linear processing. **B.** For the S-curve, a narrow range of echo amplitudes represented by the 0.25 to 0.50 signal levels are given an expanded digital level range that emphasizes the features of tissues producing these echo levels. Echo levels less than 0.25 or greater than 0.50, representing three-quarters of the signal range, are compressed into one half of the digital levels. Features of tissues producing echoes in these lower and upper ranges are deemphasized.

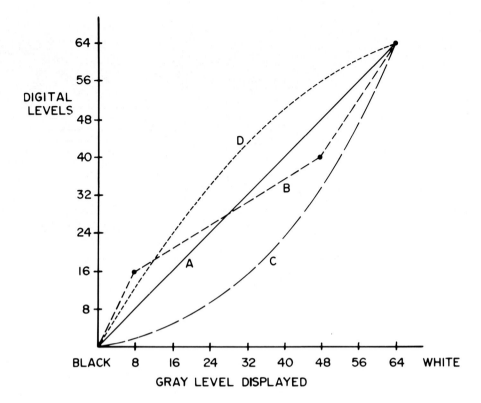

Fig. 21. Postprocessing functions. The assignment of the gray level distribution to the digital levels in the scan converter memory can be changed by the user to enhance certain image features. **A.** For a linear function, the gray level is equal to the digital value. No specific set of values are emphasized. **B.** The S-curve emphasized the lower mid-level echoes by assigning a disproportionately large range of gray levels (8 through 48) to only 32 digital levels (16 through 40). **C.** The low emphasis curve enhances image features represented by low level echoes. **D.** The high emphasis curve enhances image features represented by high level echoes.

Many preprocessing formulas are used. Only the two most common ones, linear and S-curve, are discussed here (Fig. 20). For simplicity, we assume that the signal range for the echo amplitudes displayed in the A-mode trace is from 0 to 1 V and that the DSC has 6 bits (64 levels). A linear assignment means that each digital level represents one sixty-fourth of a volt. Linear preprocessing distributes the digital levels evenly throughout the voltage range (Fig. 20A). In contrast, the S-curve emphasizes the middle-level echo amplitudes by assigning more digital levels to the mid-range voltages than to the low- and high-range voltages (Fig. 20B). The distribution depends upon the shape of the S-curve. For example, one half of the digital levels 16 through 48 might be evenly distributed over the voltage range 0.25 to 0.5 V. Echo amplitudes in this narrow range would have an expanded digital representation. Signal levels at either the low or the high range would be compressed into fewer digital levels. Thus, this S-curve would enhance tissue contrast in the lower middle-echo amplitude range. Since most soft tissues produce echo amplitudes in this range, a curve similar to this is popular for general imaging applications. To change the preprocessing function for a given image, a new image at a similar plane of section must be obtained.

Postprocessing does not alter any of the original digitized values. It only changes the assignment of the gray scale to the digital levels; a new image does not need to be generated (Fig. 19). The four most popular curves are shown in Figure 21. The rate of change from black to white is described by the terms low emphasis, high emphasis, mid (S-curve) emphasis, and linear. Through gray scale assignment changes, the user can visually enhance certain features of the image such as boundaries or tissue texture differences. Several systems now allow the user to program any desired postprocessing curve. Window width and center controls, similar to those used to manipulate CT images, are also provided by some manufacturers.

Both the pre- and postprocessing functions are necessary because the dynamic ranges of the image display system and the human observer are both less than the dynamic range of information contained in the raw echo amplitude signals. The fact that good diagnostic ultrasound images can be obtained using standard settings suggests that for most situations the dynamic range disparity is not as great for ultrasound as for CT and that the clinical usefulness of these functions is limited. Nevertheless, recent improvements in transducer technology and signal processing have extended the system dynamic range and further research on the role of pre- and postprocessing may lead to improved ability to characterize tissue pathology.

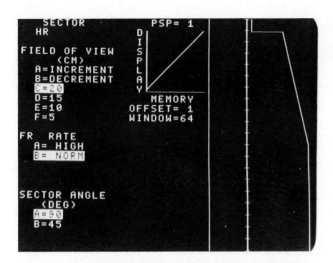
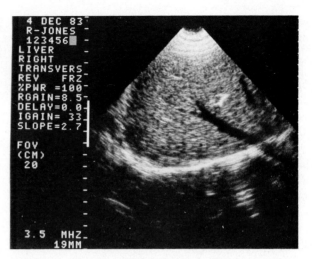

Fig. 22. Display monitor features. This dual display mode provides field-of-view (FOV) size, processing curve, and TGC curve on the monitor. Scan plane orientation, TGC values, and patient information are displayed with the image. Transducer frequency and active element diameter are also specified. Centimeter marker dots are included on the image.

VIDEO DISPLAYS

High-resolution 512 or 1024 line black and white video monitors are currently used to display the B-mode images during scanning (Fig. 22). The A-mode trace should also be displayed on static imaging systems because it is sometimes an aid in setting up the TGC and in distinguishing cystic from solid structures. The A-mode trace changes so rapidly during real-time scanning that it is of little value. A display of TGC informa-tion is essential on all static and real-time imaging systems. Without a visual display of the TGC curve or a listing of the parameter values—initial gain, slope rate, and slope position—it is difficult to set these controls at the proper values for optimal image quality.

The video display should also show the gray bar and scale markers for measuring distances (Fig. 23). Most scale marks are at centimeter intervals; however, marks at finer intervals (5 or 2 mm) certainly are beneficial. Scale marks should be placed in both horizontal

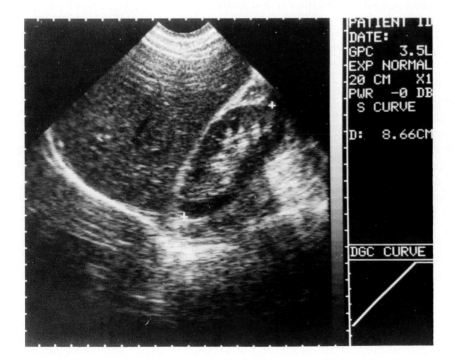

Fig. 23. This display format provides scale markers in both horizontal and vertical dimensions. The TGC curve displayed in the lower right corner is a valuable feature for image set-up even though parameter values are not displayed. Use of measurement calipers is also shown.

and vertical dimensions so that vertical height, horizontal width, and linearity of the video monitor can be periodically checked and adjusted.

All systems should have a character generator to display patient identification, exam date, and study information. Many units also include a battery powered time-of-day and month–day–year display. Digital calipers are also included on most units and allow measurement of linear distances, circumferences, and areas. Many manufacturers are now providing obstetric calculation programs that directly convert the measurements into parameters such as gestational age.

RECORDING DEVICES

Three methods for permanently documenting findings during an ultrasound exam are currently used: Polaroid film, multiimage format film, and video tape.

Polaroid photography has distinct advantages and very definite disadvantages to the user. Operation of the camera itself is simple and images are immediately available for viewing. However, the films are individually separate and must either be mounted or affixed to a flat surface such as cardboard or placed in a plastic holder. Arrangement of these individual views for conferences, consultation with clinical colleagues, teaching, and tutorial sessions can sometimes prove difficult and unwieldy. The gray scale capabilities of Polaroid film are limited compared to multiimage format film. Polaroid imaging is expensive when one considers the cost of an individual picture versus a sheet of transparent film—a consideration that must be weighed against the expenditure for processing equipment and the volume of studies to be performed by that clinic. At current prices, the cost factor can be as great as seven times that for multiimage format film.

Multiimage format film has received rather widespread acceptance in computed tomography, nuclear medicine, ultrasonography, and now, nuclear magnetic resonance. This type of imaging system has become sufficiently utilized so that companies other than those primarily involved in ultrasound instrument manufacturing sell multiimage format recording cameras. This type of image presentation is the most uniform if regarded as a part of the overall imaging department and has distinct advantages for consultation, conference presentation, image correlation, and storage. Radiologists and other physicians who have had previous experience with radiographs are familiar with this type of presentation and viewbox demonstration. Film manufacturers have developed a number of special types of films for ultrasound recording. In choosing an appropriate film, one should be particularly attentive to the stability of response and reproducibility of density. This is especially of concern in recording low-level "texture" echoes. The latitude, or ability to depict a wide range of gray scale levels, of transparency film is greater than that obtained with Polaroid film.

Although the initial cost of a multiimage format camera (about $9000) is many times the cost of a good Polaroid system, this cost difference is quickly recovered in reduced film cost, even for small volume clinics, if processing equipment is also used for other standard radiologic studies. It is advisable to purchase a compact camera design because it may be mounted directly on the ultrasound machine to maintain portability. For most systems, the 9-on-1 format produces an adequate image size for viewing and measurement purposes. If a larger recorded image size is desired, the 6-on-1 format should be chosen.

Videotape recorders allow the real-time study to be recorded as it was performed; movement of structures, such as the fetal heart, can be documented. This modality has greatly increased the acceptance of real-time imaging by referring physicians and has been made practical by the availability of compact, high-quality, inexpensive videotape recorders that can be mounted directly on the ultrasound instrument cart. Most video recorders have one or two audio channels that can be used by the operator during scanning to record the orientation of the transducer and to describe the findings that are presented by the images. This format is particularly useful for study reviews and teaching purposes. A microphone, amplifier, and speaker are needed to record and playback the spoken portion of the videotape.

Videotape units utilizing one-half inch, VHS standard videotape are relatively inexpensive, can be purchased for less than $1500, and are capable of storing up to 2 hours of real-time video on a single tape (at a cost of approximately $15 each). These units generally include a slow–fast motion playback mode, still-frame replay mode, and automatic search capabilities.

For both Polaroid and multiimage format cameras, a program to ensure maintenance of optimum image quality is mandatory. Videotape systems require few adjustments once they are properly installed.

OPERATION OF AN ULTRASOUND SCANNER

Both a full understanding and the correct use of the controls of an ultrasound scanner are imperative in order to achieve optimal instrument performance and good diagnostic images. Misuse of the controls will result not only in poor quality images but can also

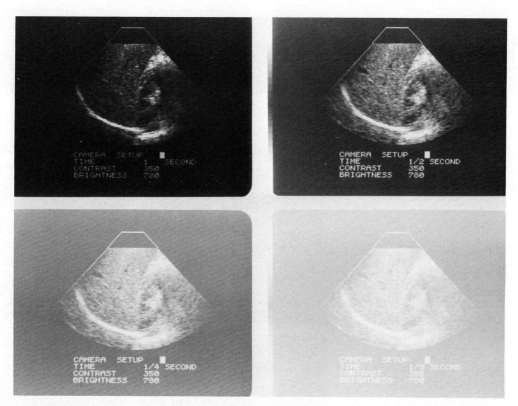

Fig. 24. Multiimage format camera adjustment. **A.** Contrast has been set to the recommended value by the manufacturer. Image brightness has been adjusted on the video monitor for optimum appearance of the reverse image. The exposure control has been varied to obtain a first-order adjustment of background density. The best choice is ½ second (*cont.*).

lead to missed or incorrect diagnoses. Each scanner has a slightly different control panel layout and, in some instances, the same control may be labeled differently from machine to machine. It is important, therefore, that users thoroughly understand the operating manual for the scanner to ensure that they are familiar with the function of each machine control. In addition, technical assistance is usually available from the manufacturer's applications specialist.

At first sight, the controls on any B-scanner appear formidable. However, if they are divided into functional groups, they are much easier to understand and use.

1. The image display controls (brightness, contrast, and processing), which determine the gray scale display of the final image.
2. The scale, zoom, and center controls, which set the size of the image and its relative position on the display screen.
3. The gain and TGC controls, which vary the amplitude of the echo signals.

Before attempting to scan a patient, a number of preliminary adjustments need to be made on the ma-

chine. First, the brightness and contrast of the viewing monitor should be adjusted to display an optimal clinical image and smoothly varying shades of the gray bar from black to white. The monitor is best viewed under subdued lighting conditions. Once set, these controls should require little further adjustment from day to day.

Second, the controls affecting the hard copy device should be set for the type of film being used. The brightness and contrast controls on the camera video monitor should be adjusted to obtain a smoothly varying gray bar pattern and satisfactory image background density. The exposure time control on the camera can then be adjusted so that the image on the film approximates that on the display monitor. Film contrast response may not exactly match the monitor display. Further adjustments of the hard copy system should be made using both the gray bar test pattern and a typical clinical scan. Fine tuning by iterative adjustments of brightness and contrast settings may be needed before a satisfactory hard copy image is obtained (Fig. 24). By following the step-by-step instructions in the camera manual, the complete process of matching the hard copy display controls to the film

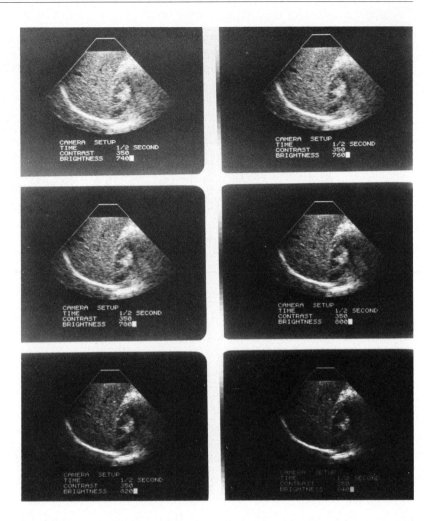

Fig. 24. cont. B. Small variations in the brightness control are then used to select the final image brightness. A brightness setting of 780 seems best. If contrast adjustments are necessary, a similar panel of pictures can be taken with stepped changes in contrast.

type can be accomplished in less than 1 hour and after the exposure of several films. Following the initial setup, the images should be checked periodically for drift, and appropriate adjustments should be made.

At the start of each patient examination, one of the first adjustments to be made is the scale control. This control determines the size of the field-of-view; it should be adjusted so that the image just fills the display screen. Setting the field-of-view too large effectively minifies the image; this results in a loss of image resolution (Fig. 25A). Setting the field-of-view too small will result in loss of peripheral portions of the scan (Fig. 25B). An image with the correct scale setting is shown in Figure 25C, for comparison.

Confusion sometimes arises as to the correct use of the scale and zoom controls. The zoom control is occasionally used at the completion of a scan to magnify selected portions of the image or to recenter an off-center image in static systems only. It is important to understand that the "read" zoom control in no way improves image resolution since it merely interpolates between existing data. This control should, therefore, not be used to magnify an image obtained by setting the field-of-view too small since suboptimal image resolution will result. The correct procedure for setting the field-of-view is to use the scale control, as described above, and rescan the region of interest. Some units have a "write" zoom control that enables selected portions of an image to be magnified during the scanning process; this technique does not result in loss of information content because real information is used to form the image. For real-time scanners, the write zoom feature requires a slower frame rate since the line density must be proportionately increased to achieve the same resolution.

The system gain, power, and TGC controls are the next to be adjusted. The TGC has three components: slope rate, delay, and initial gain (Fig. 16). These are used to produce a balanced image in which the echo amplitudes are uniform throughout the field-of-view. The delay control determines the depth (in centimeters) at which the slope begins. Its primary use is to shift the slope to a deeper position beyond a nonattenuating medium, such as urine in the bladder. Normally, it is set to zero.

The slope setting is used to compensate for the frequency-dependent attenuation of ultrasound; an approximate value for most tissues is 1 dB/cm/MHz. For diagnostic ultrasound frequencies from 1 to 10 MHz, the attenuation coefficient dependence upon frequency is approximately linear. If the tissue is homogeneous throughout, there is a unique slope setting that will produce a uniform echo amplitude distribution throughout the depth-of-field. The initial setting (in decibels) determines the tissue depth over which the slope is effective; beyond this depth the TGC curve is flat and echo amplitude rapidly declines (Fig. 15).

The system gain and power control should be set initially at about two-thirds of the maximum value. For most instruments, the voltage applied to the transducer is constant, and, thus, so is the power output. The system gain determines the overall amplification of the echo amplitudes, is constant with respect to tissue depth, and is independent of the TGC operation. A few instruments determine echo amplitude range by adjusting the voltage applied to the transducer, rather than varying the system gain.

These guidelines can be used as a starting point for adjusting the TGC and system gain and power controls. Even though this textbook is primarily concerned with OB/GYN ultrasound applications, the most appropriate organ to use for instrument setup is the liver since it provides a long segment of homogeneous tissue with attenuation of about 1 dB/cm/MHz. It is good scanning practice to initially use the liver for TGC setup (Fig. 26). The TGC settings in Figure 26B produce uniform echogenicity throughout the depth of field-of-view and result in an optimal quality image.

Because attenuation of sound by tissues in the pelvis and gravid uterus is similar to the liver, this TGC setup can be applied to these scanning situations with good results. Overall brightness of the image can be altered by varying the system gain and power controls (Fig. 27). For scanning through the urine-filled bladder, the delay control can be used to compensate for the nonattenuating property of urine in the bladder. An alternative approach is to leave the delay control set to zero and simply decrease the system gain and power levels.

Although most static scanners have TGC and system gain controls, these fundamental features have been omitted or greatly abbreviated on real-time systems produced by some manufacturers, especially for the smaller "office-sized" units. This is most unfortunate as it leaves the novice and marginally trained users

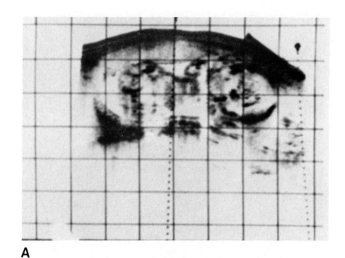

A

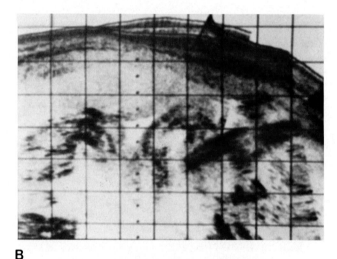

B

C

Fig. 25. Field-of-view comparison. **A.** The field-of-view setting is too large. **B.** The field-of-view setting is too small. **C.** The region of interest should just fill the display screen for optimum viewing.

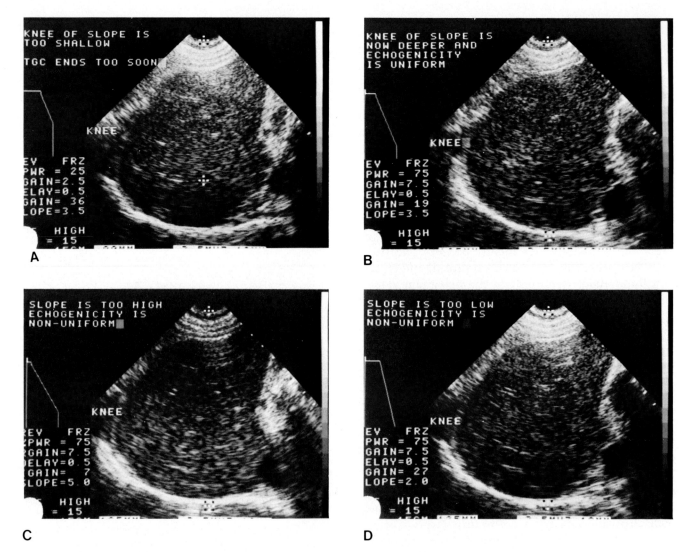

Fig. 26. TGC set-up using the liver as a homogeneous medium. **A.** For a 3.5-MHz transducer, the slope is initially set to 3.5 dB/cm. Power (%PWR) and system gain (RGAIN) are set to one-quarter maximum. Delay is set to zero since there is no fluid path. Initial gain has been adjusted so that satisfactory image brightness is achieved. The slope length is insufficient and echoes from deep portions of the liver are lost. **B.** Increasing PWR and RGAIN to 75 percent of maximum while decreasing IGAIN lengthens the slope and improves visualization of deeper portions of the liver. These settings produce an optimal image. **C.** Increasing the slope to 5.0 dB/cm overcompensates for attenuation of sound by the liver and results in increasing echo brightness with depth. **D.** Decreasing the slope to 2.0 dB/cm undercompensates and results in decreasing echo brightness with depth.

with little more than a "twiddle-the-knobs" approach for obtaining satisfactory images. Some of these instruments present challenging setup problems even for experienced ultrasonographers.

The operator's skill in making these adjustments to obtain optimal image quality clearly influences the physician's ability to recognize normal anatomy and pathology. In turn, these factors clearly influence the level of diagnostic certainty.

Two additional features, preprocessing and post-processing, impact significantly upon the viewer's interpretation of the image. These functions have been extensively described in the instrumentation section. With respect to their clinical application, the preprocessing S-curve that emphasizes the mid-range echoes characteristic of soft tissues should be chosen initially. The linear or mid-emphasis postprocessing curve should be tried first. In general, the operator needs to find the combination that best optimizes boundary definitions and tissue texture features.

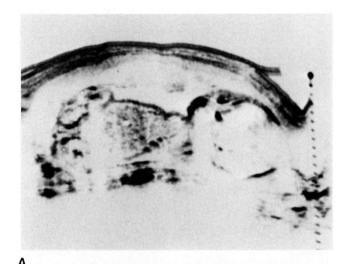

A

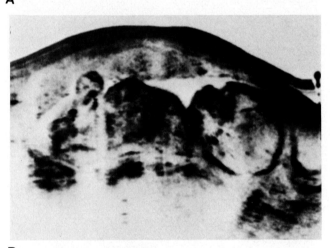

B

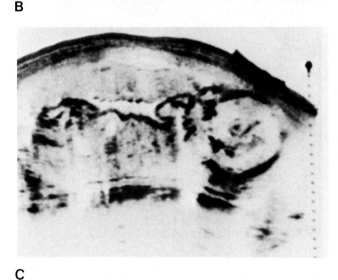

C

Fig. 27. The effect of the system gain control is illustrated in these longitudinal images of a 32-week pregnancy. **A.** The gain setting is too low, resulting in loss of detail, especially the placenta. **B.** The gain setting is too high. **C.** Properly set gain demonstrates the fine detail of the placenta and fetus.

SCANNING TECHNIQUE

The art of good ultrasound scanning takes many months of daily practice and is best acquired by spending the initial training period working under the direct guidance of an experienced ultrasonographer. A task force of the American Institute of Ultrasound in Medicine (AIUM) has recommended that training for real-time scanning be a minimum of 1 month of initial learning mode plus an additional 2 months of experience. Although good scanning technique can only be acquired by constant practice, the following are some general guidelines that, if followed, will save the novice practitioner considerable time and frustration.

One of the first requirements of performing any scan is that the ultrasound beam be able to easily penetrate body tissue to the region of interest. Scanning is, therefore, greatly facilitated by the use of "acoustic windows" in the body, which permit ultrasound to easily pass through them so that scans of underlying structures may be obtained. In obstetric and gynecologic work, the single most useful window is the full urinary bladder, which permits easy passage of ultrasound so that scanning of the uterus and adnexa is feasible (Fig. 28A). Loss of image detail is readily apparent when the same scan is performed without using the acoustic window, that is, when the patient has a partially filled bladder (Fig. 28B). The right lobe of the liver is another example of an acoustic window that can often be used to facilitate visualization of the underlying right kidney (Fig. 28C).

In principle, acoustic windows may be found in many regions of the body, but the presence of either air or bone will effectively eliminate the acoustic window. A large acoustic impedance mismatch is encountered at an interface between soft tissue and either air or bone; virtually all of the ultrasound beam is reflected and very little penetrates to regions beyond the interface (see Chapter 1). This fact has a number of practical implications. Any air that is trapped between the transducer and the skin surface of the patient acts as a barrier to ultrasound and prevents the sound energy from penetrating even to the most superficial tissues. For this reason, a coupling medium, such as a commercially available ultrasonic scanning gel, must be liberally applied to the patient's skin in the region of interest before attempting to scan. The coupling gel serves to eliminate the tiny air bubbles that would otherwise be trapped between the transducer and the patient's skin. This facilitates easy passage of the ultrasound beam into the patient.

Unfortunately, air in the bowel of the patient has the same effect, that is, almost total blockage of the

50

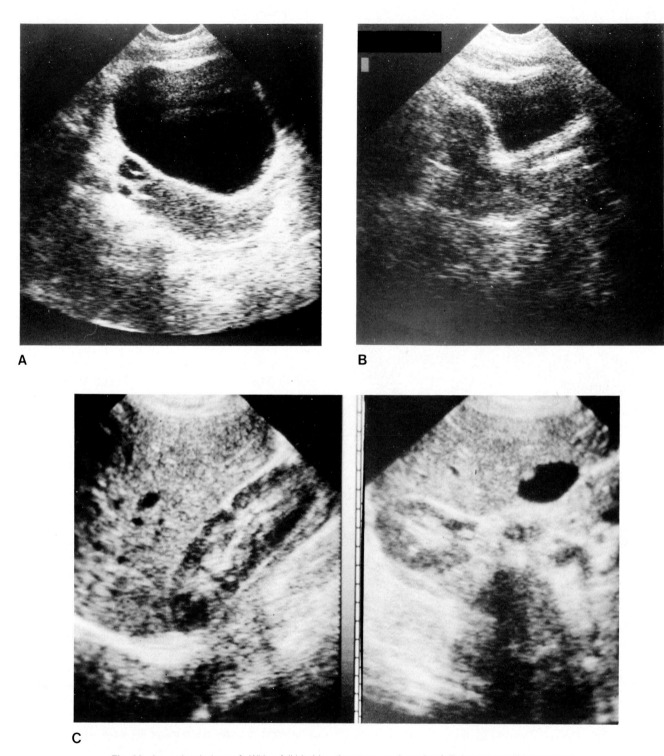

A

B

C

Fig. 28. Acoustic windows. **A.** With a full bladder, the uterus and ovarian follicles are readily visualized. **B.** With only a partially filled bladder, the uterus is difficult to identify and the follicles can not be seen. **C.** The right kidney is best seen through the right lobe of the liver. The liver also provides a window to the gallbladder.

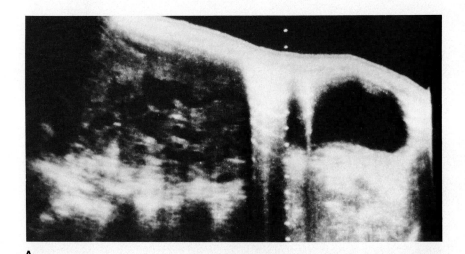

A

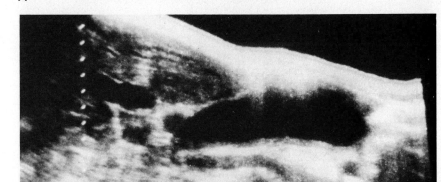

B

Fig. 29. Bowel gas artifacts. **A.** Mulitple intense reverberation echoes are produced by gas in the bowel. The bowel is interposed between the dilated gallbladder and the liver which has dilated bile ducts. **B.** A section ½ cm medial avoids the bowel gas.

sound beam, and is often the cause of many technically poor abdominal and pelvic scans. Bowel gas often results in artifacts called reverberations, which are produced by multiple internal reflections of the ultrasonic beam between the air pocket and the transducer (Fig. 29A). It should be noted that any image detail lying directly underneath the site of the air pocket is artifactual, and no amount of gain or TGC increase will be sufficient to "blast" the ultrasound through the air pocket. It is sometimes possible to scan around the air pocket (Fig. 29B), but in many instances it is necessary to rescan the patient a day or two later in the hope that bowel gas has disappeared. If this is the case, it may be advisable to reduce bowel gas production by requesting the patient to refrain from eating, drinking carbonated liquids, and smoking for at least 24 hours prior to the exam. The administration of any of the commercially available simethicon-containing drugs, such as Mylecon, which is available without a

prescription in tablet form, is also helpful in eliminating bowel gas. Filling the lumen of the gas-containing structure (usually the stomach, duodenum, or rectum) with water or a dilute solution of methylcellulose has also been effectively employed (Fig. 30).

A second barrier to the passage of ultrasound is bone. For this reason, one should never attempt to scan through a rib during abdominal studies. Instead, the transducer should be angled either underneath the rib cage or through the intercostal spaces. In this sense, the intercostal space can be considered an acoustic window while scanning the liver, kidney, and other abdominal organs. If a rib is inadvertently scanned over, a shadow or reverberation-type artifact will be produced (Fig. 31).

Once a suitable acoustic window has been found, the actual method in which the transducer is scanned over the region of interest during static scanning is very important. There are two basic types of scanning

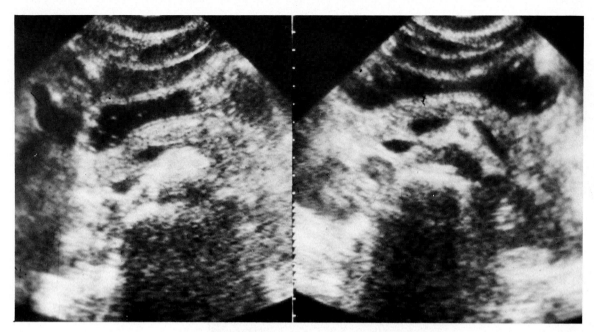

Fig. 30. Water (w) in the stomach is used to displace gas and provide an acoustic window to the pancreas.

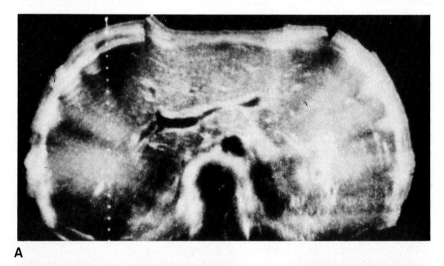

A

Fig. 31. Rib artifacts. **A.** Although scanning over the ribs provides an outline of the body contour, the sound is reflected by the ribs and underlying internal detail is obscured. A linear scan through the left lobe of the liver from an anterior approach shows the architectural detail of the liver. **B.** Using a real-time sector scanner, it is possible to orient the plane of section through an intercostal space to obtain an unobstructed view of the right lobe of the liver and right kidney.

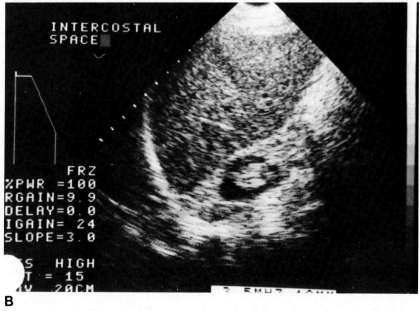

B

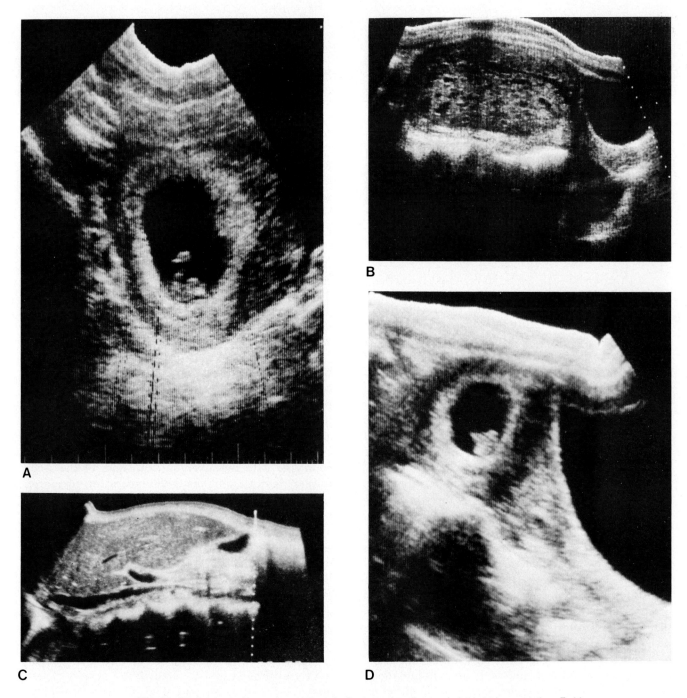

Fig. 32. Basic types of scanning motion. **A.** Sector scan of an early intrauterine gestation. **B.** Linear scan of hydatidiform mole. **C.** Linear scan of an enlarged right lobe of the liver. **D.** A combination of linear and sector scanning has been used to image the early gestation and lower uterine segment (through the bladder).

motion: the sector scan (Fig. 32A) and the linear scan (Figs. 32B,C). Most clinical scans are produced by combining these two basic types of motion (Fig. 32D). The sector scan involves pivoting the transducer about its face in a sector motion and is used in scanning regions of the body that have restricted access to the sound beam. For example, sagittal images of the upper portion of the right lobe of the liver may be obtained by angling the transducer up, underneath the rib cage. The linear scan involves moving the transducer in a straight line, without pivoting, and is used in situations where the acoustic window is unrestricted, such as scanning the pregnant uterus, large pelvic masses, and the inferior portions of the liver.

54 THE PRINCIPLES AND PRACTICE OF ULTRASONOGRAPHY IN OBSTETRICS AND GYNECOLOGY

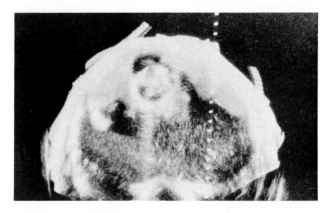

Fig. 33. Compound scanning. This large abdominal mass could only be satisfactorily imaged by scanning it from multiple angles.

The successful interpretation of gray scale images relies heavily on evaluating the gray scale texture of the scans. To produce an image with a reliable gray scale texture, the transducer should be smoothly and uniformly scanned over the region of interest and no region should be scanned more than once. This method is termed "single pass" scanning, as Figure 32 illustrates. Scanning over a region more than once distorts the gray scale texture and results in a loss of spatial resolution since registration is imperfect and minor movements of the patient are unavoidable. There are, however, situations in which compound scanning is useful to demonstrate the general features of a large mass. Multiple sweeps from several angles are needed to form such a large image (Fig. 33).

The role of early real-time imaging was to supplement the panoramic images provided by static scanning. The flexibility of scan plane orientation and the ability to observe moving structures led to the rapid acceptance of real-time imaging. Views of structures that were difficult or impossible to obtain with static imaging systems are often rather easily produced with real-time transducers (Fig. 34). Many ultrasound imaging centers now use real-time as the initial exam mode and static scanning as a supplementary technique when global views are needed.

Real-time imaging has greatly increased access to tissues underlying small acoustic windows. Bowel gas can often be "pushed aside" to view underlying structures, such as the abdominal aorta. Fast-frame rates allow artifact-free imaging of moving structures, such as the diaphragm, pulsating vessels, and fetal heart. Large portions of the liver can be visualized through the intercostal spaces and the inferior margin of the liver.

Real-time imaging is especially useful for distinguishing true masses from pseudomasses, such as peri-

stalsing bowel, seen on static images. It can be used to rapidly survey a large volume of tissue. Freeze-frame images should be recorded on film to document not only pathology, but also normal structures. These images should be properly labeled with the name of the structure and orientation of the image, since the limited field-of-view of real-time images provides few clues to the global relationships displayed by static imaging.

The sector format is especially valuable for visualizing the lower uterine segment and cervix and for obtaining a BPD on a fetal head that is low in the pelvis. Sector imaging is clearly the modality of choice for evaluating the female pelvis through the urine-filled bladder. The sector provides a larger field-of-view through a smaller acoustic window and is less prone to encountering critical angle problems at the bladder wall than the parallel scan line format of the linear array. The wide view and scanning flexibility allow the sonographer to rapidly survey the pelvis and obtain optimal views of the uterus, cervix, adnexa, and pelvic sidewalls.

The linear array format provides better visualization of superficial structures when large, relatively flat acoustic windows are available. It has been especially popular for second and third trimester obstetric scanning because of its large field-of-view for picturing anterior structures such as an anterior placenta. Since the scan lines are parallel, critical angle problems encountered with the diverging scan lines of the sector format are not a problem when measuring circumferences of oval structures such as the fetal abdomen and head (Fig. 35). Fields-of-view as wide as 20 cm are available, but the large size of the transducer clearly limits maneuverability. Thus, access to desired views of the fetus is restricted when compared to the small, lightweight sector scanners. Comparison of the more popular 10-cm wide linear array with a typical 90 degree sector format shows that the linear array is only advantageous for the first 5-cm depth. Thereafter, the sector format provides a wider field-of-view (Fig. 36).

Both linear array and sector real-time imaging have greatly increased our knowledge of normal fetal anatomy and structural pathology. Observation of fetal movement patterns provide information about fetal well-being. Real-time imaging provides a rapid means of surveying the gravid uterus for abnormalities with a flexibility unattainable by static scanning. Most exams prior to 16 weeks of menstrual age can be satisfactorily performed with real-time imaging alone since the field-of-view is usually large enough to include most of the uterus in a single frame. Thereafter, static scans are a useful adjunct for assessing and documenting fetal position, placenta location, amniotic fluid volume, and any uterine wall abnormalities such as fibroids. It is important for the sonographer to develop

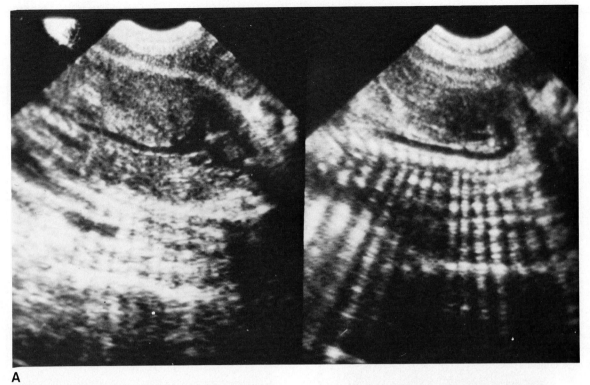

A

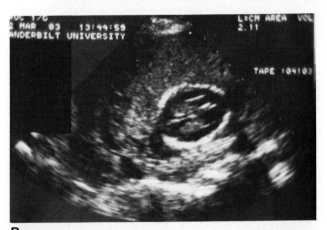

B

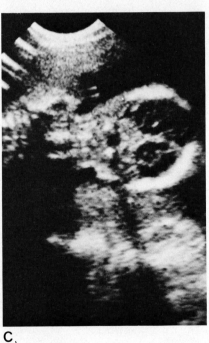

C.

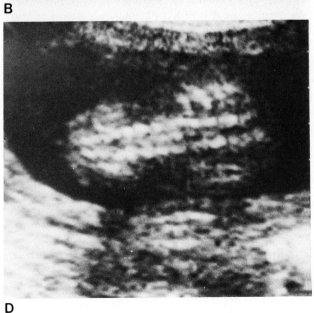

D

Fig. 34. High-detail sector real-time images. **A.** On the left, the fetal inferior vena cava is seen to enter the right atrium. On the right, the fetal thoracic aorta and aortic arch are clearly seen. **B.** The choroid plexus within each lateral ventricle is seen at 16 weeks of menstrual age. Both the lateral and medial walls of the nearer lateral ventricle are beautifully demonstrated. The falx and the lateral wall of the more distant lateral ventricle are well visualized. **C.** This coronal view of the fetal skull demonstrates the cerebellar hemispheres and the occipital horns of the lateral ventricles surrounded by normal occipital lobe brain. **D.** This coronal view of the fetal spine at 16 weeks clearly shows the posterior elements of the fetal spine (lower thoracic, lumbar, and sacral). Ribs, iliac wings, and portions of vertebral bodies are also seen.

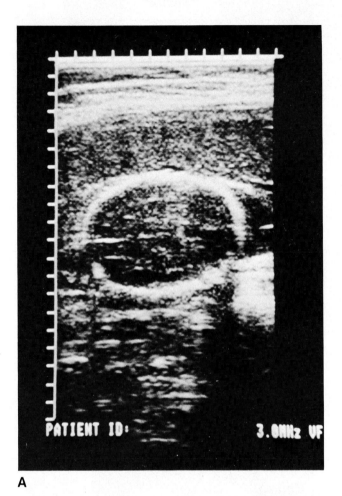

A

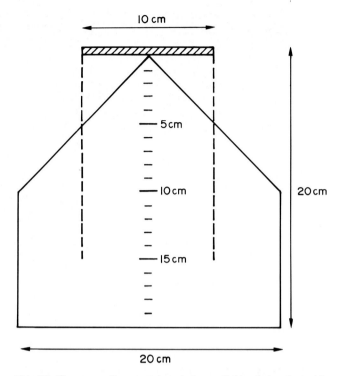

Fig. 36. Diagrammatic comparison between fields-of-view for a 10-cm wide linear array and a 90-degree sector transducer. For the first 5 cm, the linear array provides a wider field-of-view. Thereafter, the sector field-of-view is larger. Only when the width of the linear array is 15 or 20 cm does it provide a substantial advantage over the sector format.

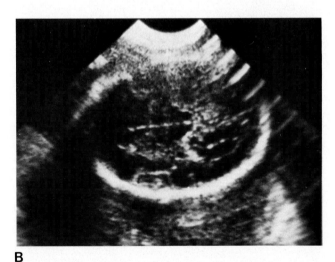

B

Fig. 35. Comparison of sector and linear array images of the fetal head. **A.** Parallel lines of the linear array provide sharp definition of the frontal and occipital aspects of the skull. **B.** For fetuses near term, measurement of the length of the skull may not be possible with a sector scanner because of the critical angle problem. Here, the front of the skull cannot be imaged.

an organized approach to scanning so that all features of the gravid uterus and adnexa are examined.

Finally, M-mode capability is a clearly desirable feature for evaluating fetal cardiac anomalies (Fig. 37). It is especially valuable for evaluating arrhythmias and then monitoring the effects of pharmaceuticals administered to the mother to correct the arrhythmia. The two-dimensional echocardiographic portion of the fetal heart exam for structural defects can be performed with any high quality real-time instrument; however, the sector scanners with a narrow angle (45 degree) format clearly provide the greatest flexibility for obtaining the special viewing angles required.

In conclusion, both linear array and sector scanners have been successfully used for obstetric and gynecologic exams. However, intelligent application requires that the sonographer understand the advantages and disadvantages of each for the specific clinical situation. Often, the best exam can be performed by using a combination of both sector and linear array images. In addition, static scanning is still very important because it provides a global view.

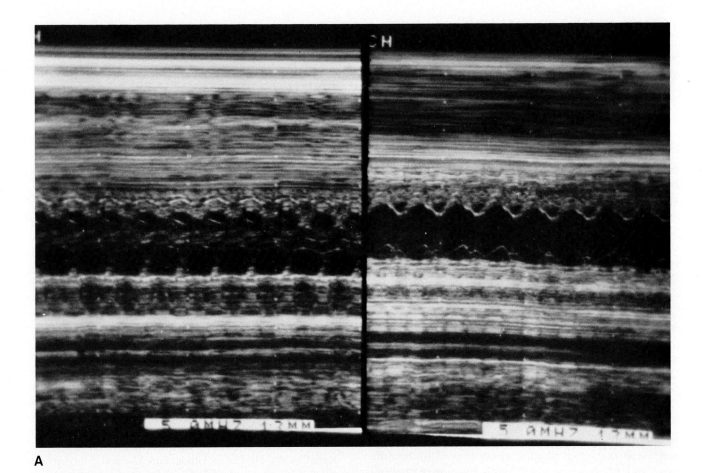

A

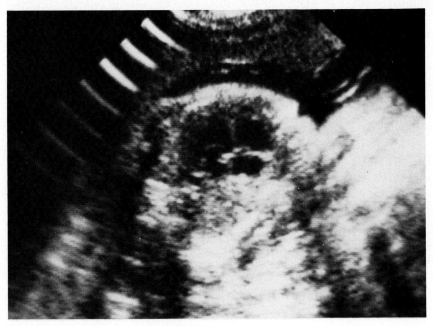

B

Fig. 37. Fetal heart imaging. **A.** The M-mode trace shows a normal rate and rhythm. The left tracing is made through the aortic root. The right tracing is made through the left ventricle. **B.** Transverse four-chamber view of the fetal heart shows four chambers and mitral and tricuspid valves.

TRENDS IN OB/GYN IMAGING

Since the writing of the previous edition of this book, advances in imaging technology have produced a wide variety of high-quality real-time imaging instruments. These have revolutionized the practice of obstetrics and gynecology.

High-detail (single sweep by definition) views of the fetus, difficult or impossible to obtain by static technique, are routinely obtained. Abnormalities of the fetus and its environment are more clearly depicted, enabling better diagnosis. Not only can the structural aspects of the fetus be studied, but also the functional aspects of the fetus can be evaluated. The study of various fetal movements and activity patterns provide information about fetal well-being within its environment. Both the structural and functional information are used to guide the clinical decision-making process.

Real-time imaging has become a valuable method for problem solving on the labor and delivery ward and for monitoring such procedures as versions and delivery of multiple fetuses. It is also valuable for periodically monitoring fetal activity during labor when a compromised fetus is suspected.

Traditionally, routine obstetric and gynecologic ultrasound exams have been performed in hospital-based or outpatient radiology suites with sophisticated static and real-time imaging systems, and by technicians and physicians with extensive training in imaging techniques and their limitations. The emphasis has been on thorough examinations and complete documentation of both normal anatomy and pathology. For obstetric exams, there has been a trend toward routine evaluation of the fetus for anomalies and a multiple-parameter approach to estimation of gestational age. This has required that both technicians and physicians have both a sophisticated knowledge of normal variations and pathologic conditions and the technical abilities to obtain the necessary views.

It is the opinion of these authors that ultrasound imaging is a sophisticated technique requiring extensive training of physicians and technicians performing the exams. We need to ensure that users understand the principles of operation of the instruments and that scanning techniques are adopted that are of maximum benefit to the patients. It is hoped that this chapter will contribute to these goals.

ACKNOWLEDGMENT

The authors gratefully acknowledge the assistance of Mary Henry in the preparation and editing of this chapter and John Bobbitt for his excellent photographic reproductions.

BIBLIOGRAPHY

Instrumentation

Banjavic RA: Design and maintenance of a quality assurance program for diagnostic ultrasound equipment. Semin Ultrasound 4(1):10, 1983

Carson PL: Diagnostic ultrasound emissions and their measurements, in Fullerton GD, Zagzebski JA (eds), Medical Physics of CT and Ultrasound. New York: AAPM Monograph No. 6, 1980, pp 550–577

Dietz D, Johnson M: Imaging Properties of Dynamically Focused Annular Arrays. Technicare Ultrasound Corporation. 90 Inverness Circle East, Englewood, CO 80112

Dick DE, Carson PL: Principles of auto scan ultrasound instrumentation, in Fullerton GD, Zagzebski JA, (eds), Medical Physics of CT and Ultrasound. New York: AAPM Monograph No. 6, 1980, pp 322–341

Eggleton RC, Feigenbaum M, Johnston KW, et al: The visualization of cardiac dynamics with real-time B-mode ultrasonic scanner, in White D (ed), Ultrasound in Medicine, New York: Plenum, 1975, Vol 1, p. 385

Griffin JM, Henry WL: A sector scanner for real-time two dimensional echocardiography. Circulation 49:1147, 1974

Keil O: Ultrasound and its various modes in use, Part II. Real-time scanners. Med Instru 16(2):107–110, 1982

Kremkau FW: Diagnostic Ultrasound: Physical Principles and Exercises. New York: Grune and Stratton, 1980

McDicken WN: Diagnostic Ultrasonics: Principles and Use of Instruments. New York: Wiley, 1981

McKeighen RE: Basic transducer physics and design. Semin Ultrasound 4(1):50, 1983

Powis RL: Ultrasound Physics . . . for the fun of it. Unirad Corporation (Technicare Ultrasound Corporation), Denver, CO.

Thickman D, et al: Effect of Display Format on Detectability. J Ultrasound Med 2:117, 1983

Wilkinson RW; Principles of real-time two dimensional B-scan ultrasonic imaging. J Med Engin Technol 5:21, 1981

Winsberg F: Physical and design considerations in real-time ultrasonography. Semin Ultrasound 4(1):44, 1983

Zagzebski JA, et al: Focused transducer beams in tissue-mimicking material. J Clin Ultrasound 10:159, 1982

Zwiebel WJ: Review of basic terms used in diagnostic ultrasound. Semin Ultrasound 4(1):60, 1983

Linear Arrays: Theory of operations and performance. Aero-Tech Reports, Vol. 1, No. 2, KB-Aerotech, Lewistown, PA 17044

Lateral Resolution: Aero-Tech Reports, Vol. 1, No. 3, KB-Aerotech, Lewistown, PA 17044

One-quarter Wavelength Theory and Application: Aero-Tech Reports, Vol. 1, No. 2, KB-Aerotech, Lewistown, PA 17044

Multiple Matching Layer Theory and Application: Aero-

Tech Reports, Vol. 1, No. 2, KB-Aerotech, Lewistown, PA 17044

Sensitivity I: Aero-Tech Reports, Vol. 1, No. 3, KB-Aerotech, Lewistown, PA 17044

Axial Resolution: Aero-Tech Reports, Vol. 1, No. 1, KB-Aerotech, Lewistown, PA 17044

Clinical Applications

Bartrum RJ, Crow HC: Real-Time Ultrasound: A Manual for Physicians and Technical Personnel, 2nd ed. Philadelphia: Saunders, 1983

Birnholz J: The art of dynamic imaging. Editorial. Am J Roentgenol 137:1284, 1981

Goldstein A: Range ambiguities in real-time ultrasound. J Clin Ultrasound 9:83, 1983

Goldstein A, Madrazo B: Slice-thickness artifacts in gray scale ultrasound. J Clin Ultrasound 9:365, 1981

Laing FC: Commonly encountered artifacts in clinical ultrasound. Semin Ultrasound 4(1):27, 1983

Sample WF, Erikson K: Basic principles of diagnostic ultrasound, in Sarti DA, Sample WF (eds), Diagnostic Ultrasound Text and Cases. Boston: G. K. Hall, 1980, pp 3–61

Skolnick M: Real-time ultrasound imaging in the abdomen. New York: Springer, 1982

Sommer F, Filly R, Minton M: Acoustic shadowing due to refractive and reflective effects. Am J Roentgenol 132:973, 1979

Wicks JD, Howe BA: Fundamentals of Sonographic Technique. Chicago: Year Book, 1983

Winsberg F, Cooperberg P (eds): Real-time ultrasonography. Clinics of Diagnostic Ultrasound. New York: Churchill-Livingstone, 1982

Ziskin M, Thickman D, Goldenberg N, et al. The comet tail artifact. J Ultrasound Med 1:1, 1982

4 | Sonographic Depiction of Pregnancy During Embryonic Development

Arthur C. Fleischer
A. Everette James, Jr.
Jack Davies
Wylie J. Dodds
Maurice Panigel
Hugh P. Robinson

Continued improvement in the resolution of sonographic imaging devices has allowed detailed depiction of the anatomic changes that occur in the embryonic period of pregnancy. This period is regarded as extending from fertilization of the ovum to development of the fetus.[1] It is thus generally considered to extend to the end of the seventh week after conception (7 weeks' gestational age) or 9 weeks' menstrual age, by which time all major structures of the fetus have begun to develop.[1]

During the embryonic period of pregnancy, the developing human undergoes a great number of morphologic changes. Only those changes that can presently be depicted by sonography are emphasized in this chapter. This discussion is organized according to the approximate time of occurrence of a particular developmental sequence.

Menstrual age, as used by most obstetricians, refers to the weeks of gestation, starting with the first day of the last menstrual cycle. When embryologists refer to the gestational age of pregnancy, they are beginning with the time of fertilization. For this reason there is usually a 2-week difference between the menstrual age and gestational age of a fetus. However, variation in the time of ovulation from the usual 14-day interval from the first day of menses can cause a discrepancy between the menstrual and gestational age. Although there is often a 2-week interval between the first day of the menstrual cycle and ovulation, this phenomenon can occur any time between the eighth and twentieth day.[2] Thus, an embryo that may be 6 weeks by menstrual age can actually vary from 5 to 7 weeks by gestational age. The time of ovulation seems to have a more consistent temporal relation to the next menstrual period than to the previous menses. Although most detailed embryologic descriptions utilize gestational age, this discussion describes embryologic development according to menstrual age because this convention is generally used in clinical circumstances.

EARLY EMBRYONIC DEVELOPMENT

Fertilization to Fourth Gestational Week

Although a multitude of changes occur during the first few weeks of gestation, few can be delineated by currently available sonographic scanners. During this time the ovum is fertilized; usually this occurs in the ampullary portion of the fallopian tube. While the ovum travels through the fallopian tube toward the intra-uterine lumen, the fertilized zygote undergoes several mitotic divisions to form a cluster of cells called the morula (Fig. 1). The morula usually reaches the uterine cavity 3 days after fertilization and remains unattached within the uterine lumen for 3 to 4 more days. During this time, the number of cells increases and a central fluid cavity develops to form a blastocyst (Fig. 2). The blastocyst consists of an inner cell mass that gives rise to the embryo, a blastocyst cavity, and an outer layer of trophoblastic cells that surrounds the inner cell mass and the blastocyst cavity. About 7 days after fertilization (3 weeks' menstrual age), the blastocyst implants on the uterine endometrium. However, up to 3 days variation in time between fertilization and implantation can occur.[1]

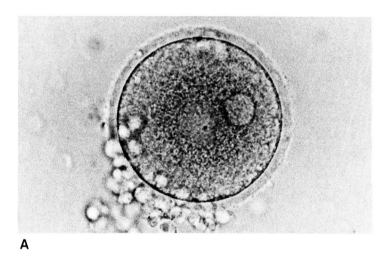
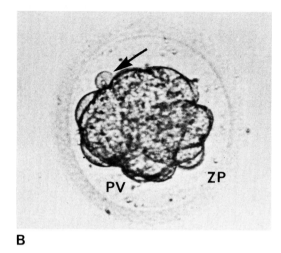

A   B

Fig. 1. A. Human oocyte in process of fertilization (×420). **B.** A preimplantation baboon embryo (similar to the human) as the morula is transforming into a blastocyst. Arrow, column segmentation cavity; PV, perivitelline space; ZP, zona pellucida.

At the point of attachment to the endometrium, the trophoblastic cells that surround the conceptus invade the endometrial epithelium and stroma. The embryonic entoderm begins to form from the ventral surface of the inner cell mass. These cells constitute one of the first germ cell layers of the embryo. By the end of the first week of embryonic development, the blastocyst is superficially implanted in the endometrial lining of the uterus (Fig. 3).

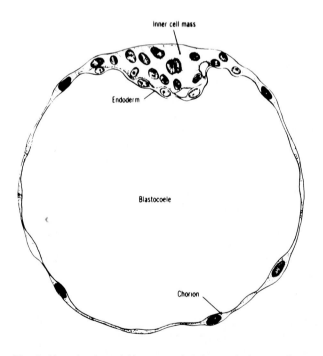

Fig. 2. Line drawing of blastocyst showing early inner cell mass and trophoblast. (*Reprinted with permission from Davies J: Human Developmental Anatomy, New York, Ronald, 1963.*)

During the second week of gestation (4 weeks' menstrual age), there is rapid proliferation and differentiation of the trophoblast into an inner single cell layer of cytotrophoblasts and an outer multicellular layer of syncytotrophoblasts. Fingerlike processes of the syncytotrophoblasts grow into and invade the endometrial decidua. Vascular lacunae develop around the conceptus and soon fuse to form the lacunar networks (Fig. 4). The trophoblasts erode maternal sinusoids within the endometrium. Blood and secretions from eroded endometrial glands seep into the lacunar networks to form a primitive uteroplacental circulation. Primary villi grow from the chorionic plate. At this time, the implanted conceptus becomes embedded entirely within the endometrium (Fig. 5).

The endometrium surrounding the implanted conceptus undergoes decidual changes. Recent articles describe the sonographic appearance of the decidua in intrauterine pregnancies during the early embryonic period prior to sonographic depiction of an embryo.[3,4] Sonographic demonstration of decidual development can be helpful in distinguishing intrauterine from extrauterine pregnancies, prior to the sonographic delineation of an embryo.

Decidual development occurs in the presence of a blastocyst in a sensitized endometrium. Production of chorionic gonadotropin by trophoblasts serves to prolong the life of the corpus luteum. The corpus luteum secretes progesterone that further supports the implanted conceptus.

After the blastocyst embeds within the endometrium, the decidua closes over the conceptus and is termed the decidua capsularis. The part of the decidua between the conceptus and the uterine muscle wall is termed the decidua basalis. Subsequently, this por-

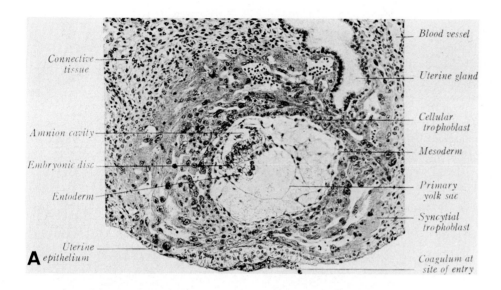

Connective tissue

Amnion cavity

Embryonic disc

Entoderm

Uterine epithelium

A

Blood vessel

Uterine gland

Cellular trophoblast

Mesoderm

Primary yolk sac

Syncytial trophoblast

Coagulum at site of entry

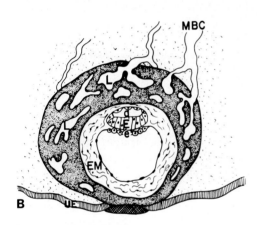

MBC

L

a
E
e

EM

B   UE

Fig. 3. A. Section of 11-day human embryo showing cellular and syncytial trophoblast. (*Reprinted with permission from Arey B: Developmental Anatomy, Philadelphia, Sanders, 1962.*) **B.** The first stages of embryonic development, 12-day implanted embryo; a, amnion and amniotic cavity; E, embryonic ectoderm; e, embryonic entoderm; EM, extraembryonic mesenchyme; L, maternal blood lacuna in the trophoblast; Ue, uterine epithelium; MBC, maternal blood circulation. (*Redrawn by Panigel: in Grasse' (ed), Traité de Zoologie, Masson, 1976. Reprinted with permission from Hertig and Rock[17] and from Starck.*)

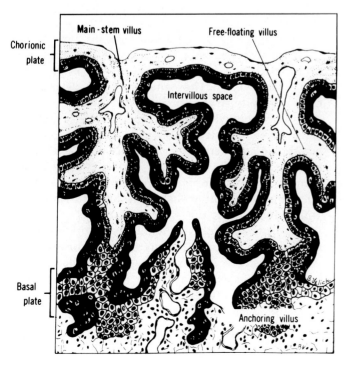

Chorionic plate

Main-stem villus   Free-floating villus

Intervillous space

Basal plate

Anchoring villus

Fig. 4. Cross section of early human placenta that demonstrates portions of the villous tree and stem villi anchored to the decidua basalis. (*Reprinted with permission from Davies J: Human Developmental Anatomy, New York, Ronald, 1963.*)

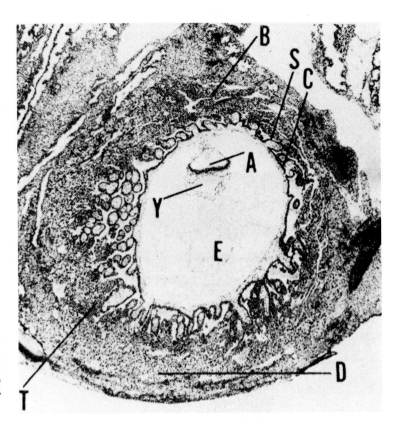

Fig. 5. Cross section though an early (16 day) gestational sac. B, decidual basalis; D, decidual capsularis; T, cytotrophoblast; C, chorion, S, secondary villus; A, amnion, Y, yolk sac; E, exocoelomic cavity. (*Reprinted with permission from Gruenwald P: The Placenta, 1st ed, Baltimore, University Park, 1975.*)

tion of the decidua combines with the chorion frondosum to form the mature placenta. The part of the decidua that lines the remainder of the uterus is termed the decidua parietalis or decidua vera.

As the developing embryo and surrounding cavities develop, the gestational sac protrudes into the uterine lumen and penetrates deeper into the endometrium. Because the developing conceptus is surrounded by two layers of decidua, the sonographic demonstration of concentric decidua can be used as a means to differentiate the decidual reaction that occurs with an intrauterine pregnancy from that occurring with the single layered decidual reaction associated with an ectopic pregnancy (Figs. 6A,B,C,D). As discussed in Chapter 30, the term "decidual cast" is derived from the appearance of the passed decidua of an ectopic pregnancy when it is shed in a more or less complete state.

The chorion represents the trophoblasts and fetal mesenchyme that provides nutrition for the developing embryo. Initially, from the third week of gestation (fifth menstrual week), the chorion is covered with villous stems that are continuous peripherally with the trophoblastic shell and in close apposition to the decidua capsularis and basalis. As the gestational sac continues to expand, the decidua capsularis is progressively stretched and thinned. Thus, its circulation

is gradually reduced. This process continues until the chorion, located beneath the decidua capsularis, becomes smooth and is termed the "chorion laeve." In contrast, the villous stems of the disc-shaped region of the chorion in contact with the decidua basalis increase greatly in size and ramify to form the chorion frondosum. The decidua basalis and chorion frondosum constitute the beginnings of the true placenta.

Sonographically, the decidua basalis and chorion frondosum appear as an area of localized thickening of the choriodecidua along the periphery of the gestational sac (Fig. 8); The embryonic pole develops in close proximity to the chorion frondosum.

Concurrent with the development of the choriodecidual layers, the developing embryo forms an extraembryonic mesoderm, with the endoderm eventually forming the primitive yolk sac. At this point of development, the extraembryonic coelom forms the major volume of the gestational sac. The amniotic cavity begins to form as the inner cell mass begins to develop into a bilaminar embryo. At this stage, the bilaminar embryo is less than 1 mm in size and consists of a ventral layer of cuboidal cells and a double layer of high-columnar cells or epiblasts (Fig. 7). The ventral cells face the blastocystic cavity or primitive yolk sac and develop into the endodermal germ layer that subsequently forms the gastrointestinal tract. The epiblasts

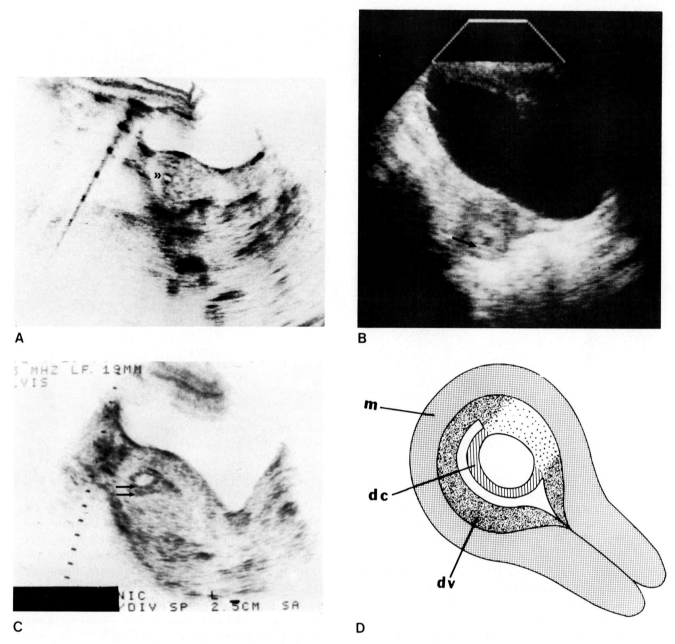

Fig. 6. Sonographic depiction of pregnancies of 3 to 5 weeks' menstrual age. **A.** Longitudinal static sonogram showing a rounded 5-mm cystic structure (*arrowheads*) in upper uterus that corresponds to the exocoelomic cavity of a pregnancy of 4 weeks' menstrual age. **B.** Longitudinal real-time sonogram of 5 weeks' intrauterine pregnancy demonstrating concentric decidual layers (*arrow*). **C.** Longitudinal static sonogram showing decidua capsularis (*crossed arrow*) and decidua vera (*arrow*) of pregnancy of 5 weeks' menstrual age. **D.** Diagram of decidual layers depicted in **C.** m = myometrium, dc = decidua capsularis; dv = decidua vera.

that are in contact with the floor of the amniotic cavity give rise to the embryonic germ layers of mesoderm and ectoderm.

During the middle of the third week of gestation (5½ weeks' menstrual age) the embryonic disc differentiates into a trilaminar embryo composed of three primary germ layers—ectoderm, intraembryonic meso-

derm, and endoderm. At this stage, the length of the developing embryo is only 2 to 3 mm, a size that is at the limits of resolution of most ultrasound devices (see Chapter 3). During the third week of gestation, the neural tube begins to form, as well as blood islands on the yolk sac and heart tubes.

By the end of the early phase of embryonic devel-

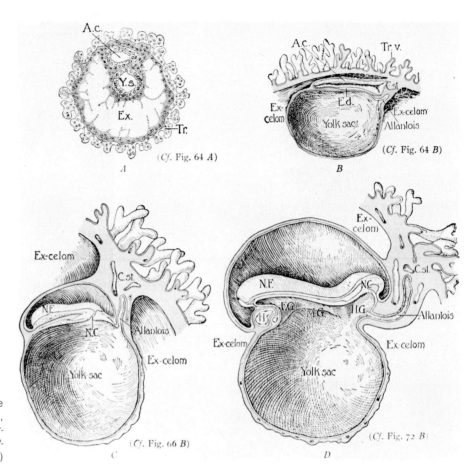

Fig. 7. Diagrams showing progressive growth (**A** through **D**) of the amniotic sac, yolk sac, and embryo. (*Reprinted with permission from Arey B: Developmental Anatomy. Philadelphia, Saunders, 1962. p 89.*)

opment (4 to 5 weeks' menstrual age) the choriodecidua that surrounds the gestational sac chorionic tissue appears on sonography as a concentric ring of echogenic tissue (Figs. 9A–C). This structure is referred to as a "gestational sac." The inner ring corresponds to the decidua capsularis, whereas the outer ring corresponds to the transformed endometrium or the decidua vera. The embryo itself is usually too small to be consistently visualized by sonography. At 4 weeks' menstrual age, the gestational sac measures only 2 mm in diameter, but grows to approximately 1 cm at 5 weeks.

LATE EMBRYONIC DEVELOPMENT

Fourth Through Seventh Week of Gestation
During the latter portion of embryonic development, sonographic scanning can depict the gestational sac, developing embryo, some of its surrounding membranes, and the choriodecidua. During this period, the organogenesis of most body viscera occurs. Growth and maturation of the organs proceeds during the fetal period of development.

During the fourth week of embryonic develop-

ment (6 weeks' menstrual age), the embryo is approximately 3 to 4 mm in length (Fig. 8A). The neural tube is closed in its midportion but open at the rostral and caudal ends. The branchial archs form and the somites develop as rounded surface elevations. Forty-two of 44 somites form: these paired structures eventually give rise to the axial skeleton and associated musculature. The heart produces a large ventral prominence in the C-shaped embryo. The arm and leg buds also appear during the fourth gestational week.

During the fifth week of development (7 weeks' menstrual age), the developing embryo grows from 6 to 11 mm in crown–rump length (Fig. 8B). During the fifth week, head growth is extensive, resulting mainly from rapid development of the brain. The limb buds show considerable differentiation and the elbow and wrist regions form. The yolk sac is relatively large and the amniotic cavity continues to expand its size. The yolk sac can be depicted sonographically and has an important function in early hematopoiesis.

During the sixth week of embryonic development (8 weeks' menstrual age), the head is large, relative to the trunk, and is bent over the heart prominence. This position of the head results in an overall bending

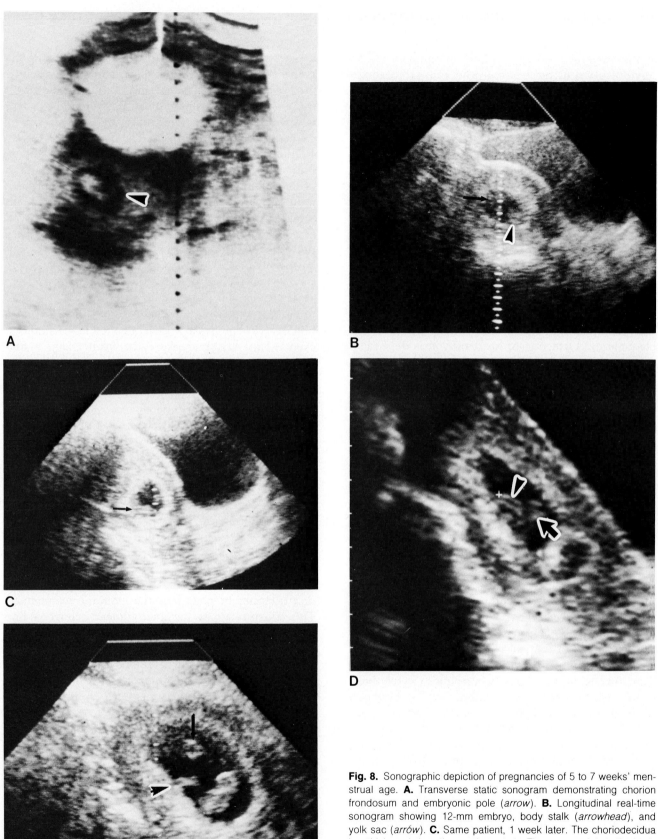

Fig. 8. Sonographic depiction of pregnancies of 5 to 7 weeks' menstrual age. **A.** Transverse static sonogram demonstrating chorion frondosum and embryonic pole (*arrow*). **B.** Longitudinal real-time sonogram showing 12-mm embryo, body stalk (*arrowhead*), and yolk sac (*arrow*). **C.** Same patient, 1 week later. The choriodecidua has thickened since the previous study. The arrow points to the body stalk. **D.** Longitudinal magnified real-time sonogram showing body stalk (*arrowhead*) and 14-mm embryo (*large arrow*). These findings correspond to a 6- to 7-weeks' menstrual age embryo. **E.** Transverse real-time sonogram of 18-mm embryo. The yolk sac (small arrow) and umbilical stalk (*arrowhead*) are also shown.

of the embryo or cervical flexure in the area of the cervical region of the embryo. The yolk sac becomes progressively smaller and its extraembryonic portion narrows into a yolk stalk. The intestines enter the extraembryonic coelom, beginning the normal process of umbilical herniation. During the sixth week of gestation, the embryo grows from 14 to 21 mm in crown–rump length (Fig. 8C).

By the end of the seventh week of gestational age (9 weeks' menstrual age), the embryo has attained human features discernible on sonography (Fig. 8D). The head is rounded and erect, but remains large. The neck region is established and the eyelids are formed. The fingers and toes are well differentiated.

Sonographically, fetal heart activity is detected consistently at 5 weeks' gestational age (7 weeks' menstrual age). Inability to detect fetal heart motion at this gestational age suggests the possibility of a nonviable embryo.[5] Detection of heart motion is dependent upon scanning with a real-time scanner that has a high frame rate (over 20 frames per second) and a transducer that is focused optimally. Occasionally, it is difficult to discriminate fetal heart motion from "flickering" or noise that is encountered with real-time scanning (see Chapters 3 and 15). In most cases, one should follow a "conservative" approach when fetal heart motion is not seen. Repeat examination in 1 to 2 weeks may prevent inadvertent termination of a normal pregnancy.

Besides depiction of the embryo and choriodecidua, sonography can also delineate changes as the connecting body stalk develops into the umbilical cord. In particular, sonography will demonstrate the presence of the yolk sac that appears as a rounded structure, floating within the extra embryonic coelom. The yolk sac is best observed between 5 and 7 weeks' menstrual age (Fig. 9A,B). The connecting stalk initially connects the caudal end of the embryo to the chorion but later fuses with the allantois to form the umbilical cord. The proximal part of the stalk surrounds the relatively short allantoenteric diverticulum, but is traversed throughout its length by the umbilical vessels. The dorsal surface of the body stalk is covered with the amnion and its ventral surface is bounded by the extraembryonic coelom. Concurrent with the folding of the embryo and enlargement of the amnion, the attachment site of the connecting body stalk migrates to the ventral surface of the embryo. The embryonic mesoderm approaches that of the yolk sac and its stalk. With continued enlargement of the amnion, the extraembryonic coelom becomes progressively obliterated and its only remaining part surrounds the elongated yolk stalk and sac. During this phase, the yolk stalk and its contained entodermal duct and accompanying

vessels gradually elongate to keep pace with the increase in length of the umbilical cord. The vitelline duct and vessels degenerate and usually disappear by midpregnancy. The entodermal allantoic duct, which is confined to the proximal end of the growing umbilical cord, elongates and thins. The remnants of the allantoic duct may persist as a series of epithelial strands until term. At the umbilicus, the proximal strand is often continuous with the urachus. The embryonic right umbilical vein disappears by the sixth or seventh week of gestation. A weakness of the abdominal wall at the base of the umbilical cord can occur in the location of the embryonic right umbilical vein and may be the site of gastroschisis.

Several reports describe the sonographic appearance of the yolk sac.[6,7] The yolk sac appears as a rounded sonolucent structure floating within the gestational sac. The yolk sac, which lies outside the amniotic cavity (Figs. 8D,E), measures between 2 and 5 mm in diameter, and is connected to the umbilicus via a narrow stalk. The yolk sac appears during the fifth menstrual week of pregnancy and attains its greatest size of about 5 mm by the seventh menstrual week. It floats freely within the gestational sac until approximately the eleventh menstrual week, when the expansion of the amniotic sac compresses the yolk sac against the chorion and the uterine wall.

During sonographic examination, it is important not to include the yolk sac in measurement of the crown–rump length. The yolk sac should also not be mistaken for the fetal cranium or a fetal anatomic anomaly, such as an omphalocete (Figs. 10A,B; 11A,B; 12A,B).

Another structure that can be recognized in the first trimester pregnancy is the amniotic membrane.[8] This structure appears as a curvilinear, echogenic line within the fluid surrounding the developing embryo (Fig. 12C). As the amnion enlarges, it gradually surrounds the embryo and later fills the entire uterine cavity. The amniotic membrane is best imaged when it is perpendicular to the incident ultrasonic beam. The amniotic membrane remains unfused to the chorion until approximately 16 menstrual weeks. Thus, during the seventh through the twelfth week of pregnancy, a considerable separation may exist between the chorion and amnion.

DISCUSSION

The division between the embryonic and fetal periods of prenatal development is somewhat arbitrary. The fetal period of development is generally considered to extend from the eighth gestational week to birth. Dur-

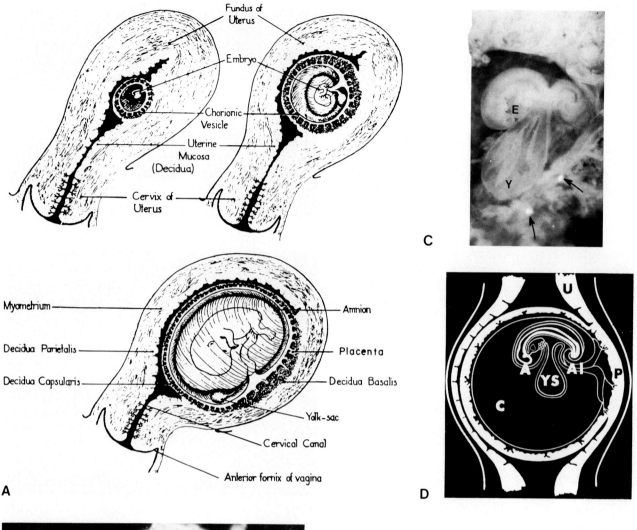

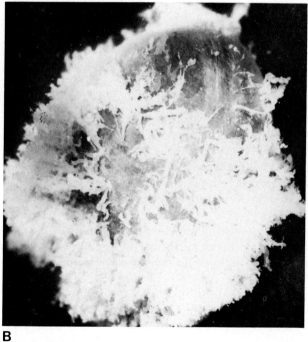

Fig. 9. **A.** Diagrams in cross section of uterus at 6, 8, and 10 weeks' menstrual age showing embryonic membranes and their development. **B.** The external surface of a human chorionic sac showing both the chorion frondosum and chorion laeve areas. **C.** 10-mm embryo, E; yolk sac, Y; and the chorionic villi (*arrows*). **D.** Diagram of **C** showing 10-mm human embryo with its membranes and surrounding villous trophoblast. C, amniotic cavity; P, placenta; U, uterus; YS, yolk sac. (*Redrawn by Panigel: in Grasse'* (*ed*), *Traite de Zoologie, Masson, 1976. Reprinted with permission from Stark.*)

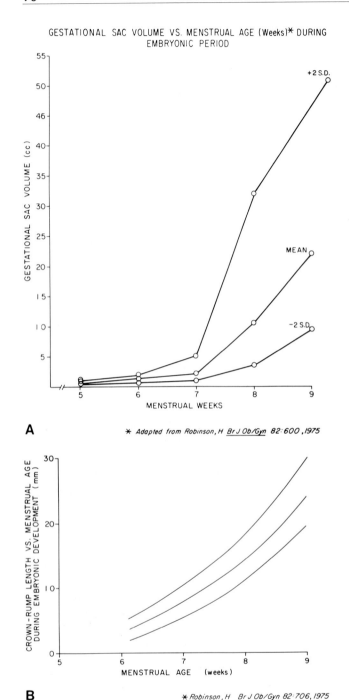

A

B

Fig. 10. Gestational duration estimates by sonographic measurements. **A.** Graph depicting gestational sac volume during embryonic period. **B.** Graph showing crown–rump length during embryonic period.

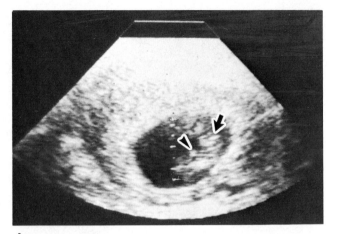

A

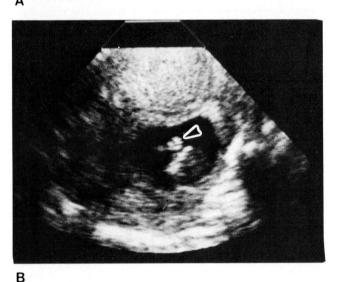

B

Fig. 11. Sonographic depiction of 8- to 9-week fetus. **A.** Transverse real-time sonogram showing 22-mm fetus (*arrow*) corresponding to a 9-week (menstrual age) fetus. The head (*arrow*), body, and arm (*arrowhead*) can be discerned. **B.** Transverse real-time sonogram of 9-week fetus showing fetal hand (*arrowhead*), with fingers near face.

ing the embryonic period, an undifferentiated mass of cells develops into the homunculus—the beginning of a recognizable human being (Figs. 11A,B). Development during the fetal period consists mainly of growth and maturation of organs and tissues that began to develop during the embryonic stage. Only a few new structures appear during the fetal period. As the structures within the embryo enlarge during the fetal period,

many of them can be depicted by sonography. The imaging of fetal structures by sonography is considered in subsequent chapters.

During the embryonic phase, estimates of gestational age can be made by measurement of gestational sac volume. Because the degree of bladder distension can affect the size of the gestational sac in its sagittal dimension, we recommend the use of volumetric rather than linear measurements of the gestational sac. In order to calculate gestational sac volume, inner boundaries of the greatest long, transverse, and anterior posterior dimensions are multiplied together and the product halved. This method is based on the geometric approximation of a prolate ellipsoid and is similar to gestational sac volumetric determinations performed by serial sonograms taken in 0.5 or 1.0 cm intervals

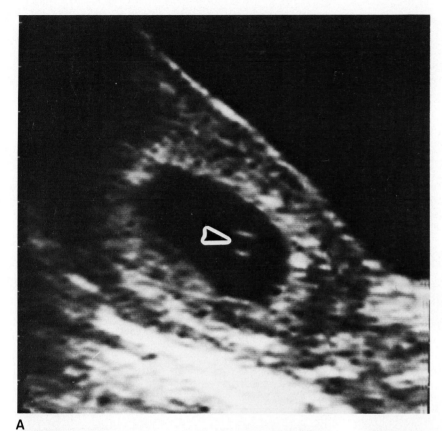

A

Fig. 12. Extraembryonic structures. **A.** Yolk sac depicted at 6 weeks' menstrual age. **B.** Transverse real-time sonogram of diamniotic twin pregnancy at 9 weeks showing two yolk sacs (*arrowheads*). **C.** Transverse real-time sonogram demonstrating linear interface (*arrow*) in upper position of gestational sac corresponding to the amniotic membrane. As the amniotic cavity enlarges and the extraembryonic coelom regresses, the amniotic membrane can be delineated.

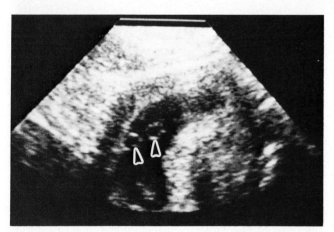

B

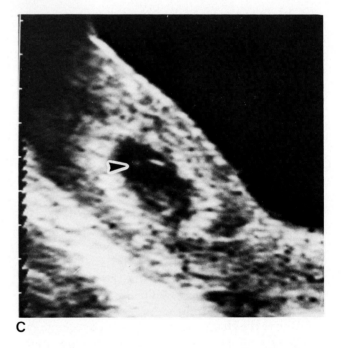

C

used by Robinson.[10] The accuracy of this method is approximately ± 1 week.[10]

Calculation of gestational sac volume can also be helpful in evaluating incomplete abortions or suspected ectopic pregnancy. If the approximate gestational age is known, the appropriate gestational sac size can be estimated or predicted from established nomograms. When seen in association with an ectopic pregnancy, the sonolucent intraluminal structure between the decidua does not attain the volume expected for a normal intrauterine pregnancy. Similarly, if there is a greater than 4-week discrepancy in gestational sac size in a patient with first trimester bleeding, an incomplete

abortion is likely to have occurred. One should correlate anatomic features, such as the presence of a double decidual layer with gestational sac volume measurements, before establishing a specific diagnosis.

Occasionally one has difficulty in satisfactorily demonstrating a gestational sac that is located within a markedly anteflexed uterus. Since the gestational sac

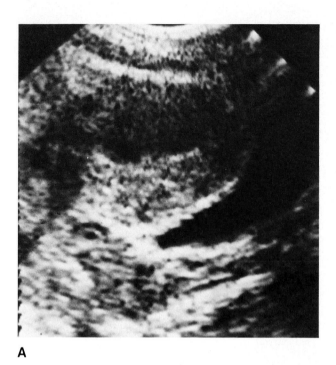

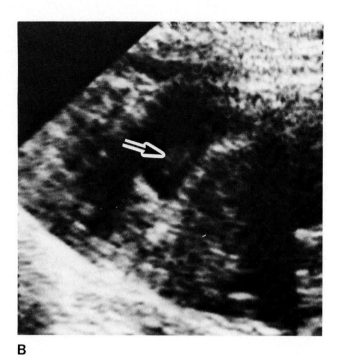

A

B

Fig. 13. Technical factors. **A.** Reverberations project into the gestational sac of an anteflexed uterus. Reverberations that occur in the near field can hamper adequate depiction of the contrast of the gestational sac. **B.** Same patient scanned with transducer water bag placed on abdomen. The anteriorly located gestational sac and embryo are more clearly delineated.

can be located immediately beneath the skin, technical problems that result from reverberation artifacts projected in the near field may hamper the sonographic demonstration of superficial sacs. In these circumstances, it may be helpful to use an intravenous (IV) bag filled with saline as a water path delay. The bag is placed on the maternal abdomen and the transducer on top of the bag (see Chapter 3). This arrangement minimizes the problem of near-field reverberations that may detract from images of an anteriorly located gestational sac (Figs. 13A, B).

Although estimation of the gestational age can be made by calculating gestational sac volume, the use of anatomic parameters described in this chapter and summarized in Table 1 for the assessment gestational age is recommended. In those patients in which the amniotic membrane is depicted, one should realize that the measurement of the gestational sac includes both the amniotic cavity and the extraembryonic coelom.

During the later stages of embryonic development, sonographic measurement of the crown–rump length is an accurate method to estimate gestational age (see Table 2 and Figure 15). Crown-rump measurements have a standard deviation of less than 1 week (±4 days).[11] The greatest length of the embryo in its long axis should be obtained. One should be careful not to include the yolk sac in this measurement.

Estimates suggest that as many as 70 percent of

fertilized zygotes fail to develop into viable offspring.[9] Disorders that occur during the embryonic period of pregnancy often become clinically manifest by causing abnormal uterine bleeding. Sonographic delineation of the expected findings for a particular gestational age confirms normal embryonic development. Conversely, discovery of abnormal findings on sonography can influence clinical management.[12]

One should be aware that vaginal bleeding can be experienced in uncomplicated pregnancies during the first weeks of pregnancy related to the process of implantation. A minor episode of vaginal spotting may occur during implantation, 3 to 4 weeks after the first day of the last menstrual period. This bleeding can be misconstrued by the patient as bleeding associ-

TABLE 1
Sonographic Embryologic "Milestones"

Menstrual Age in Weeks (±1 wk)	Sonographic Feature
3–4 weeks	Double decidual rings
4–5 weeks	Chorion frondosum and embryonic pole develops
5–6 weeks	Embryo, umbilical stalk, and yolk sac are identifiable
5–7 weeks	Heart motion first discernable by real-time scanning

TABLE 2
Crown–Rump Length versus Menstrual Age

Crown–Rump Length (mm)		Menstrual Age	
Mean	2 SD	Weeks	Days
6.6	2.9	6	2
7.3	3.0	6	3
8.0	3.1	6	4
8.7	3.3	6	5
9.4	3.4	6	6
10.2	3.5	7	0
10.9	3.7	7	1
11.8	3.8	7	2
12.6	4.0	7	3
13.5	4.1	7	4
14.4	4.2	7	5
15.3	4.4	7	6
16.3	4.5	8	0
17.3	4.6	8	1
18.3	4.8	8	2
19.4	4.9	8	3
20.4	5.1	8	4
21.6	5.2	8	5
22.7	5.3	8	6
23.9	5.5	9	0

Adapted from Robinson H: MD. Thesis, University of Glasgow, 1978.

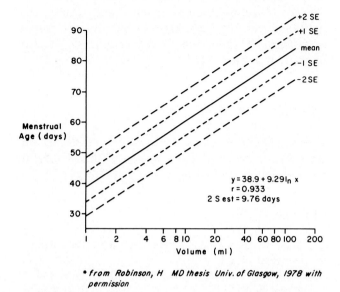

GESTATIONAL SAC VOLUME VS. MENSTRUAL AGE*

$$y = 38.9 + 9.29 \ln x$$
$$r = 0.933$$
$$2\,S\,est = 9.76\ days$$

* from Robinson, H   MD thesis Univ. of Glasgow, 1978 with permission

Fig. 15. Sonographic estimation of gestational duration during embryonic period. Chart showing crown–rump length vs. menstrual age. (*Adapted from Robinson H, Fleming J: A critical evaluation of sonar crown-rump length measurements. Br J Ob/Gyn, 82:702, 1975.*)

ated with a normal period. In uncomplicated pregnancies, sonographic identification of an anechoic space adjacent to the gestational sac most likely represents the unobliterated lumen of the uterus. However, if significant bleeding occurs, this sonographic finding may represent a so-called blighted twin (Figs. 14A,B).[13,14]

Future developments in sonography will undoubtedly enable even better depiction of the embryo and its related structures not yet presently possible. However, one must consider that the chance for possible production of a congenital defect by exposure of the embryo to sonography during this critical time of organ formation remains, even though the chances for

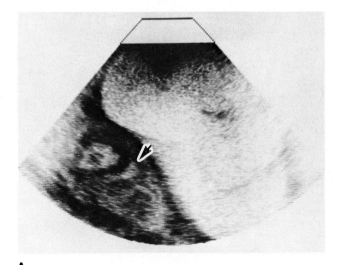

A

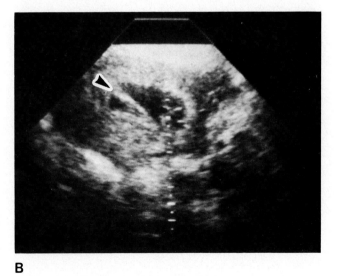

B

Fig. 14. Sonographic variants. **A.** Hypoechoic space (*arrowhead*) between decidua capsularis and vera in a patient with first trimester bleeding. This hypoechoic space probably represented blood between the two decidual layers, but could correspond to a portion of the uterine lumen that was unobliterated by the enlarging gestational sac. **B.** Hypoechoic area (*arrow*) around the gestational sac that most likely resulted from an implantation bleed.

significant harm are probably miniscule or nonexis-tent.[15,16] Therefore, the use of sonography during the embryonic period of development should continue to be restricted to only those situations in which it is clinically indicated.

ACKNOWLEDGMENTS

We are grateful to Doctors Howerton and Weinstein, who participated in the preparation of this chapter in the first and second editions of this textbook.

REFERENCES

1. Moore K: The Developing Human, 1st ed. Philadelphia, Saunders, 1973
2. Hellman J, Prichard J (eds): The ovarian cycle and its hormones, in William's Obstetrics. New York, Appleton-Century-Crofts, 1971, p 66
3. Bradley W, Fiske C, Filly R: The double sac sign of early intrauterine pregnancy: Use in exclusion of ectopic pregnancy. Radiology 143:223, 1982
4. Nyberg D, Laing F, Filly R, et al: Ultrasonographic differentiation of the gestational sac of early intrauterine pregnancy from the pseudogestational sac of ectopic pregnancy. Radiology 146:755, 1983
5. Anderson S: Management of threatened abortion with real-time sonography. Obstet Gynecol 55(2):259, 1980
6. Mantoni M, Pedersen J: Ultrasound visualization of the human yolk sac. J Clin Ultrasound 7:459, 1979
7. Sauerbrei E, Cooperberg P, Poland B: Ultrasound demonstration of the normal fetal yolk sac. J Clin Ultrasound 8:217, 1980
8. Jeanty P, Renoy P, Kerkem J, et al: Ultrasonic demonstration of the amnion. J Ultrasound Med 1:243, 1982
9. Biggers J: In vitro fertilization and embryo transfer in human beings. N Engl J Med 304(6):336, 1981
10. Robinson H. Gestational sac volume as determined by sonar in the first trimester of pregnancy. Br J Obstet Gynecol 82:100, 1975
11. Robinson H, Fleming J: A critical evaluation of sonar crown–rump length measurements. Br J Obstet Gynecol 82:702, 1975
12. Robinson H: The diagnosis of early pregnancy failure by sonar. Br J Obstet Gynecol 82:849, 1975
13. Finberg H, Brinholz J: Ultrasound observations in multiple gestations in first trimester bleeding: The blighted twin. Radiology 132:137, 1979
14. Lyons E, Levi C: Ultrasound in the first trimester. RCNA 20(2):259, 1982
15. Bolson B: Question of risk still hovers over routine prenatal use of ultrasound. JAMA 247(16):2195, 1982
16. Barnett S: The influence of ultrasound in embryonic development. Ultrasound Med Biol 9(1):19, 1983
17. Hertig AT, Rock J: On the division of the early human ovum with special reference to the trophoblast of the pre-villous stage; a description of seven normal and five pathologic human ova. Am J Obstet Gynecol 47:149, 1944

5 | Doppler Monitoring Techniques in Pregnancy

Jennifer R. Niebyl

THE DOPPLER PRINCIPLE

To explain the apparent differences in the color of stars, a professor of physics at the University of Vienna in 1842, Christian Doppler, formulated the principle that now bears his name. He postulated that the apparent frequency of light or sound waves depends on the relative motion of the wave source and the observer. In other words, sound waves reflected back from a moving object return to the transmitting source at a slightly altered frequency. Furthermore, the magnitude of the frequency change is proportional to the target's velocity. Movement of the reflecting object toward the sound source results in an apparent increase in the frequency of the reflected sound, and movement away from the source results in a decrease.[1,2]

CLINICAL APPLICATIONS

General Considerations

The Doppler principle provides us with a technique for detecting and studying *movement* of the parts of patients that cannot be seen or palpated. The flow of blood cells through vessels, the opening and closing of heart valves, and peristaltic waves of bowel all constitute movements that would cause a change in the frequency of a sound wave sent in their direction and reflected back to the transmitting source. To detect those movements, one needs an apparatus capable first of transmitting a sound of constant frequency and then instrumentation that is able to determine changes in the frequency of the reflected sounds. If the apparatus

were sufficiently sophisticated to detect the magnitude of the frequency alteration, one could determine the velocity of the movements. Also, if increases in frequency could be distinguished from decreases, one could measure the movement toward or away from a transmitter. Equipment with at least some of these capabilities is routinely available at present.

The machinery devised to apply the Doppler principle to obstetrics consists of an abdominal wall transducer containing both ultrasonic transmitting and receiving crystals. The detected frequency changes are recorded in a central unit which can translate the signals into any of several output formats: audible sounds, waves on an oscilloscope screen, or a tracing on a continuously moving paper chart (Table 1).[3]

Obstetric Applications of the Doppler Instrument

Within the abdomen of a pregnant woman, movements from many sources produce detectable Doppler shifts (Table 2).[3-7] When translated into audible sounds, the fetal heart signal has a biphasic, galloping rhythm with a rate of 120 to 160 beats per minute. The first component represents atrial contraction and the second reflects atrioventricular (AV) valve closure and semilunar valve opening. Pulsatile blood flow in the umbilical and other fetal vessels produces monophasic sounds that are higher pitched than the fetal heart signal. The umbilical sound is characterized also by frequent changes in location. The placental sound is complex, combining a wind-like sound at the maternal pulse rate (70 to 90) and the umbilical signal at the fetal rate (120 to 160). The characteristic placental sound

TABLE 1
Components of a Doppler Ultrasound Unit

Transducer	Central Unit	Output
A. Transmitting crystal(s) (Constant frequency)	Frequency changes detected	A. Visual 1. Oscilloscope 2. Strip chart
B. Receiving crystal(s)		B. Audible sounds

is generated only in the area of umbilical cord insertion and cannot be detected over the remainder of the placenta.[6]

The sounds produced by blood flow in maternal vessels (aorta, uterine arteries, etc.) may be distinguished by their rate and their synchrony with the radial pulse. Movement of the fetal body or of an extremity produces an abrupt, short, large-amplitude signal. Other detectable movements include fetal hiccups and breathing and maternal bowel peristalsis.[7]

At any time, combinations of sounds may be detected, and a false placental sound may be produced by the combination of maternal arterial and maternal venous signals. The sound of the maternal venous system can be altered significantly by increasing intraabdominal pressure with a Valsalva maneuver, which can assist in distinguishing the true placental sound from the false.[6]

Clinical situations in which the Doppler instrument has been found to be useful include early detection of pregnancy,[1-3,5,6,8-10] diagnosis of fetal death in utero (FDIU),[2,4] detection of a remote fetal heart (in the mother with obesity or hydramnios), intermittent observation of the rate and rhythm of the fetal pulse (during the antenatal examinations), placental localization,[6,11] diagnosis of multiple pregnancy,[6] the differential diagnosis of vaginal bleeding during pregnancy,[2,6] and fetal monitoring in the third trimester and during labor (Table 3).

Early Diagnosis of Pregnancy. The Doppler ultrasound transducer provides a rapid, simple method of

TABLE 2
The Maternal Abdomen: Movements Detectable by Doppler Ultrasonic Devices

Origin	Rate	Characteristics
Fetal		
1. Heart	120–160	Rate, biphasic, pitch
2. Umbilical cord	120–160	Rate, monophasic, frequent changes in location
3. Fetal vessels	120–160	Rate, monophasic
4. Movement	isolated	Abrupt, large amplitude
5. Hiccups	5–20	Abrupt, large amplitude
6. Breathing	30–90	Rate, rushing noises with smooth rise and fall
Placenta		
Souffle		
Fetal	120–160	Complex sound
Maternal	79–90	
Maternal		
1. Aortic flow	70–90	Rate, synchronous with radial pulse
2. Uterine artery flow	70–90	Rate, synchronous with radial pulse
3. Pelvic veins	70–90	Rate, altered by valsalva
4. Breathing	15–25	Slow rate
5. Bowel peristalsis	isolated	

Reprinted with permission from Boyce ES, Daneo GS, Gough JD, et al: Doppler ultrasound method for detecting human fetal breathing in utero. Br Med J 2:17, 1976.

TABLE 3
Obstetric Applications of Doppler Ultrasound

Early diagnosis of pregnancy (detection of fetal life)
Diagnosis of fetal death in utero (FDIU)
Detection of remote fetal heart
Intermittent observation of rate and rhythm of fetal pulse
Placental localization
Diagnosis of multiple pregnancy
Differential diagnosis of vaginal bleeding during pregnancy
Fetal monitoring
  Labor
  NST, OCT (CST)

establishing the presence of an early pregnancy during the initial examination. Furthermore, since the Doppler instrument detects either fetal movements or fetal heart activity, it provides evidence not only of a pregnancy but also of a living fetus. This latter point indicates one advantage of this method over chemical pregnancy tests: human chorionic gonadotropin (hCG) can be detected in the maternal urine after demise of the fetus as long as some viable trophoblastic tissue remains.[10,12] Detection of a fetal heart rate does not guarantee a normal pregnancy, however. A normal fetal heart signal has been reported from a still viable ectopic pregnancy.[12]

In one study, the fetal heart rate was detected in all patients 12 or more weeks after the last menstrual period (LMP), except in three patients in whom intrauterine fetal death had occurred.[8] With more than one examination by different observers, 100 percent accuracy can be approached as early as 10 weeks of pregnancy.[12] Occasional reports appear that claim detection of fetal heart activity as early as 7.5 weeks after the LMP.[10] The few false negative findings in large series of patients are due to too early a gestational age, obesity, or hydramnios. In most instances where a viable pregnancy is suspected on physical examination but not substantiated by Doppler investigation of the abdomen, the ultimate diagnosis is fetal demise in utero (FDIU), uterine myomata, hydatidiform mole, or ovarian tumor. Of importance is the fact that most investigators report *no* false positive results.[6,10,12]

An incidental discovery attributable to use of the Doppler instrument was that the average frequency of the fetal pulse was found to be 170 to 179 per minute in the 8th to 11th week of pregnancy and to slow to an average of 149 by the 16th week.[12]

Diagnosis of Fetal Death In Utero. Confirming FDIU is a difficult obstetric problem (see Chapter 32) in which the Doppler instrument has been helpful. Severe limitations were encountered with older methods of

determining fetal death (Table 4). Detection of FDIU by physical examination is possible only in the second half of pregnancy and requires both failure to palpate fetal movements and failure to auscultate fetal heart sounds on two examinations separated by a 1-week interval. Radiographic evidence of FDIU (also available only in the second half of pregnancy) is unobtainable until 7 to 10 days after fetal demise, and errors in interpretation are frequent.[6] Detection of the fetal ECG establishes that the fetus is living, but negative results with that test are unreliable.[6] Urine hCG excretion, as mentioned, can continue after fetal death occurs. Examination with the Doppler instrument has been more dependable and can be used as early as 10 weeks after the LMP.

When a Doppler examination was performed on 40 patients in whom no fetal heart beat could be detected with a stethoscope, 23 had a fetal heart signal detectable by Doppler shift, confirming the presence of a living fetus. In the remaining 17 patients, no fetal heart activity could be detected and FDIU was subsequently confirmed at delivery.[3] In another study, 152 patients were examined because of suspected FDIU. Fetal life was detected in 116. In 35 patients, no evidence of fetal life could be detected and fetal death was later confirmed. In one patient, no fetal heart motion was detected initially, but a subsequent examination disclosed the presence of fetal heart activity. Thus, with two examinations, 100 percent accuracy was achieved.[4]

Where real-time ultrasonic scanning is available, failure to find a fetal heart signal with the Doppler instrument can be substantiated by failure to detect fetal heart movement on direct visualization of the fetal chest.

TABLE 4
Detection of FDIU

Methods reliable only in second half of gestation:
  Clinical detection
    Auscultation of fetal heart
      Two negative exams at 1-week interval
    Palpation of fetal movement
  X-ray
    Evidence unobtainable until 5 to 10 days after fetal death
    Frequent errors in interpretation
  Fetal ECG
    Unreliable if negative
hCG tests
  Excretion continues after fetal death
Doppler ultrasound
  100 percent accuracy with two exams
Real-time ultrasound
  Method of choice when available

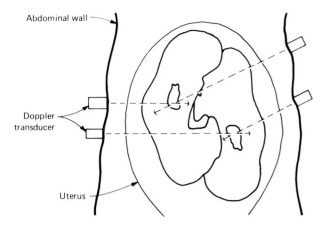

Fig. 1. Detection of multiple pregnancy with Doppler ultrasound.[6] Representation of the use of triangulation to diagnose multiple pregnancy with the Doppler ultrasonic instrument. Each fetal heart signal is located from two separate locations on the maternal abdomen and the point where those two beams would cross is marked on the anterior abdominal wall. All fetal hearts must then be detected within a 5-second interval.

Remote Fetal Heart and Multiple Pregnancy. Doppler ultrasound can be most helpful in situations in which detection of the fetal heart with a stethoscope is difficult, as is the case with polyhydramnios or obesity.[6]

Multiple pregnancies can be diagnosed by a method of triangulation which utilizes the directional nature of the Doppler ultrasound beam (Fig. 1). Each

fetal heart is located from two separate positions on the maternal abdomen. The point at which the two beams would intersect is then projected to the anterior abdominal wall and marked. After the other fetal hearts have been located and marked in a similar manner, the transducer is placed over each marked point and all fetal hearts are displayed one after the other within a total of 5 seconds.[6]

However, this method has essentially been replaced by use of real-time ultrasound because of the difficulty of accurately directing the Doppler beam. The diagnosis and characterization of twin pregnancies by other ultrasound techniques will be discussed in Chapter 24.

Placental Localization. Localization of the placenta is important prior to amniocentesis and in determining the etiology of third trimester bleeding. Because of the relatively directional nature of the Doppler ultrasound beam, the placental sound can be detected over only a small area of the anterior abdominal wall when the placenta is anterior in location and over a much larger area when the placenta is posterior (Fig. 2). Also, when the placenta is posterior in location, angulation of the transducer permits the observer to determine that the fetal heart signal is anterior to the placental sound.[6]

There are numerous limitations to placental localization by the Doppler technique. The overall accuracy

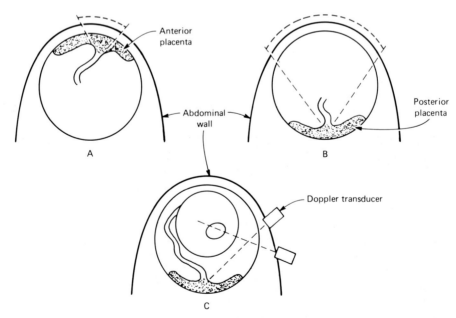

Fig. 2. Placental localization by Doppler ultrasound.[6] **A.** With anterior position of placenta, the placental signal is heard over a relatively small area of the anterior abdominal wall. **B.** With posterior placenta, signal is heard over large area. **C.** With posterior placenta, fetal heart signal is located anterior to placental signal.

has been only about 60 percent,[3] and the technique cannot be used before 24 weeks.[3] For these reasons, other ultrasonic techniques are generally used when the placenta must be accurately located (see Chapters 25 and 26).

Fetal Monitoring

Labor. Uterine contractions result in decreased perfusion of the intervillous spaces and thereby intermittently interfere with maternal–fetal exchange.[13,14] Although fetuses in a stable intrauterine environment tolerate these transient insults well, a fetus in a compromised situation could become hypoxic and even acidotic under the added stress of labor. However, with traditional monitoring of labor by auscultation of the fetal heart rate (FHR) with a stethoscope, the fetal heart generally cannot be heard during contractions. Brief reactions of the FHR to uterine contractions cannot be detected and only profound and prolonged bradycardia or tachycardia is noticed. Often, the fetal condition during labor is unknown and can only be inferred from evaluation of the newborn immediately after birth.[15]

Fetal monitoring can be done with the attachment of an electrode to the fetal scalp, which permits monitoring of the fetal ECG both during and between contractions. However, such internal monitoring requires that the fetal membranes be ruptured. This can be accomplished only when the cervix is sufficiently effaced and dilated to admit the electrode. The procedure requires skilled personnel and cannot be used with such complications as placenta previa and premature labor or for monitoring the second twin.

To overcome the limitations of internal monitoring and still have a continous fetal heart record, various forms of external monitoring (phonocardiography, surface fetal electrocardiography, and Doppler ultrasound) have been developed (Table 5). Of these, the Doppler transducer has proven to be the most reliable overall.[16,17] The ultrasonic transducer is attached to the maternal abdomen by a belt or tape over the area of the fetal heart and the instantaneous FHR is continuously recorded on a strip chart. Uterine contractions can be recorded simultaneously by an external tocodynamometer or, after the membranes have ruptured, by a catheter placed between the cervix and the fetal head. Simultaneous tracings with Doppler external monitoring and electrocardiographic internal monitoring document that the Doppler apparatus allows accurate interpretation of FHR patterns (Fig. 3).[16]

The components of the FHR patterns which have been investigated include decelerations, tachycardia, bradycardia, baseline variability, and accelerations.

TABLE 5
Advantages of External Doppler Monitor

Can be used when cervix not dilated
Fetal membranes need not be ruptured
Can be operated by nursing staff
More reliable than fetal ECG or phonocardiography
Can be used when internal monitoring is contraindicated
   Premature labor
   Prolapsed cord
   Placental abruption
   Placental previa
   Monitoring second twin

Decelerations have been categorized as early, late, and variable.

Decelerations. The early deceleration (Fig. 4) is of uniform shape, reflecting the shape of the associated uterine contraction, and has its onset early in the contraction. It is thought to be due to fetal head compression and to be an innocuous FHR pattern. Its main clinical significance is that it must be distinguished from the more ominous late deceleration.[15]

The late deceleration (Fig. 5) is also of uniform shape, reflecting the shape of the uterine contraction. However, its onset is late in the contraction, occurring at or after the peak of intrauterine pressure. It is thought to represent uteroplacental insufficiency due to decreased maternal–fetal exchange. This may be seen in high-risk pregnancies and may be caused by uterine hyperactivity or maternal hypotension. The deceleration may be alleviated by decreasing uterine activity (i.e., if oxytocin is being used its infusion should be decreased or stopped), correcting maternal hypotension, changing the maternal position, or administering oxygen to the mother.[15] Although this pattern is an ominous one and is associated with progressive depression of the fetal pH, it usually occurs with the baseline FHR in the normal range.[18]

A variable deceleration (Fig. 6) changes both in its shape and in the timing of its onset. Its shape does not reflect the smooth rise and fall of intrauterine pressure and its onset shows no consistent relationship to the contraction. It is probably due to umbilical cord occlusion and is usually markedly alleviated by maternal position change.[15] Pulsed Doppler with simultaneous imaging may allow proof of this etiology. Fetal pH falls slightly in response to transitory variable decelerations but recovers within 1 to 2 minutes if there is no added insult.[18]

Tachycardia and Bradycardia. A baseline FHR above 160 is considered tachycardia and has been associated with

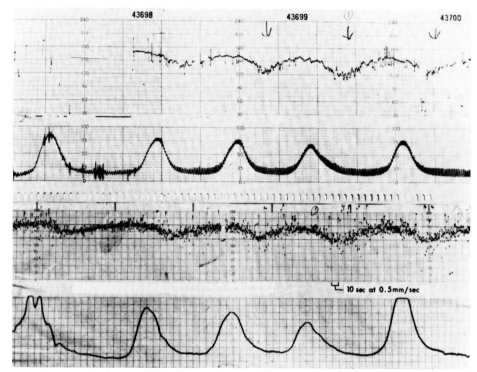

Fig. 3. Tracings demonstrating late decelerations, comparing fetal electrocardiogram (*top*) and Doppler (*bottom*). (*Reprinted with permission from Shenker L, Kane R: Doppler ultra sonic fetal heart monitoring during labor. Obstet Gynecol 39:613, 1972.*)

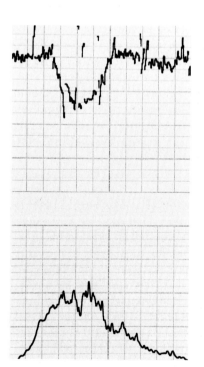

Fig. 4. Early deceleration.

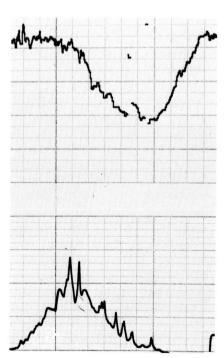

Fig. 5. Late deceleration.

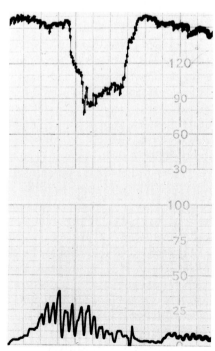

Fig. 6. Variable deceleration.

TABLE 6
Causes of Fetal Tachycardia

Maternal	Fetal/Placental
Drugs	Fetal distress[37]
Epinephrine	Cardiac arrhythmias
Atropine[34]	Paroxysmal atrial tachycardia[38]
Scopolomine	Atrial flutter[39]
Isoxsuprine	Ventricular arrhythmias[40]
Pyrexia[35]	Hyperthyroidism[36]
Anxiety[34]	Chorangioma of the placenta[41]
Hyperthyroidism[36]	
Cigarette smoking[34]	

many maternal and fetal conditions (Table 6). However, when the monitoring records of large numbers of patients have been reviewed, baseline tachycardia has been found to be neither a reliable nor a constant sign of severe antepartum fetal hypoxia or impending fetal demise.[19]

Persistent bradycardia below 120 is not a sign of fetal hypoxia or impending FDIU unless it is associated with marked FHR decelerations.[19] It has been associated with congenital heart lesions and complete AV block.[20]

Variability. Baseline irregularity of the FHR (Fig. 7) reflects normal interaction of the fetal sympathetic and parasympathetic nervous systems, and the presence of reasonable variability (6 to 10 beats per minute difference in the "peak-to-valley," long-term [3 to 6 cycles per minute] oscillations) is equated with a functionally responsive fetal autonomic nervous system.[21] Decreased variability has been observed with fetal asphyxia but also occurs with immaturity and administration to the mother of such drugs as diazepam.[22] In the normal fetus, there may be periods of decreased variability lasting up to 20 minutes, and it is believed that these episodes represent fetal sleep—wake or

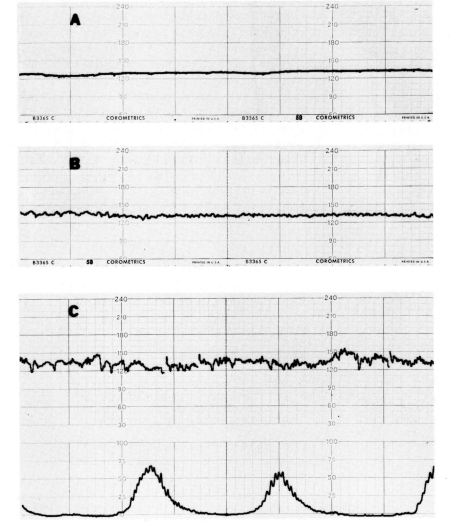

Fig. 7. Baseline variability. Doppler ultrasonic external monitoring tracing from three labor patients. **A.** No variability **B.** Minimal irregularity (2 to 5 bpm) **C.** Average (6+ bpm). Although the absence of variability in such tracings is considered reliable, the appearance of normal variability may be due to artifact.

rest—activity cycles rather than fetal compromise.[19,23] In the healthy fetus, variability will increase with fetal movements, uterine contractions, and fetal manipulations such as the obtaining of a scalp blood sample for pH determination (Table 7).[21]

A very ominous type of altered variability of the baseline FHR is the sinusoidal pattern observed in severely affected fetuses of pregnancies complicated by Rh isoimmunization. This undulating FHR pattern is thought to represent virtual absence of CNS control over the FHR; and, in one series, it was associated with a 50 percent perinatal mortality rate.[19]

Because of background noise in the recording of the FHR by the Doppler instrument, the interpretation of the baseline variability in the ultrasonic tracing has been difficult.[17,24] If the baseline FHR appears smooth, the true FHR probably does have decreased variability. When normal or increased irregularity is seen, the variability may be real or artifactual.[14] However, a recent improvement in the Doppler system permits electronic selection of the frequency changes produced by movements either toward or away from the transducer. This directional Doppler technique produces a more identifiable signal with a higher signal-to-noise ratio, and the accuracy of the recorded baseline variability is very similar to that obtained by fetal scalp ECG.[24]

Antepartum Monitoring. As the significance of the various changes in the FHR became known and as fetal monitoring during labor became more widespread, the perinatal outcome in many large medical centers improved, especially for high-risk pregnancies.[25] However, the obstetrician was still faced with the fact that fetal compromise and even death occur in some complicated cases before the onset of labor. The next step was to learn to use the Doppler ultrasonic equipment to monitor the fetal status in the weeks preceding labor.

TABLE 7
Variability of Baseline FHR

Decreased
  Fetal immaturity
  Fetal inactivity or "sleep"
  Maternal drug administration
  Fetal asphyxia
Increased
  Fetal movements
  Uterine contractions
  Fetal manipulation

Reprinted with permission from Paul RH, Suidan AK, Yeh S, et al: Clinical fetal monitoring: VII. Am J Obstet Gynecol 123:206, 1975.

TABLE 8
Protocol for OCT

Semi-Fowler's position (to avoid supine hypotension)
Maternal BP and pulse every 10 minutes
IV infusion
External monitor
Baseline recording of FHR: 20–40 minutes
Oxytocin infusion (if spontaneous uterine activity is insufficient)
  Start: 1 mU/min
  Increments: 1 mU every 10–20 minutes
  Endpoint: 3 contractions in 10 minutes, each lasting 40–60 seconds

Reprinted with permission from Freeman RK: The use of oxytocin challenge test for antepartum clinical evaluation of uteroplacental respiratory function. Am J Obstet Gynecol 121:481, 1975.

Oxytocin Challenge Test or Contraction Stress Test. As late decelerations of the FHR occurring in response to uterine contractions during labor were known to be associated with signs of uteroplacental insufficiency such as fetal acidosis, low Apgar scores, FDIU, and asphyxia neonatorum,[26] it was postulated that such decelerations would also occur (in a sufficiently compromised fetus) in response to spontaneous or induced contractions occurring prior to labor. It was this logic which led to the development of the oxytocin challenge test (OCT) (Table 8).[17,26-30] In performing the OCT, only external monitoring is used. Hence, this test can be performed at any time in the third trimester (as early as 26 weeks gestation in some centers[23]), as long as there are no contraindications to the administration of oxytocin.

Negative results (Table 9) with the OCT have proven to be extremely reliable as a predictor of fetal condition, with fetal death rarely occurring within a week of a negative OCT.[17] Even when other factors

TABLE 9
Results of OCT

Negative
  Adequate contraction pattern, no late decelerations
Positive
  Persistent late decelerations
Equivocal
  Occasional late decelerations
Hyperstimulation
  Late decelerations occurring with:
    a. Contractions closer than every 2 minutes
    b. Contractions lasting longer than 90 seconds
    c. Apparent rise in baseline tone
Unsatisfactory
  Tracing inadequate for interpretation
Repeat test in 24 hours when results are other than "positive" or "negative."

Reprinted with permission from Freeman RK: The use of oxytocin challenge test for antepartum clinical evaluation of ultraplacental respiratory function. Am J Obstet Gynecol 121:481, 1975.

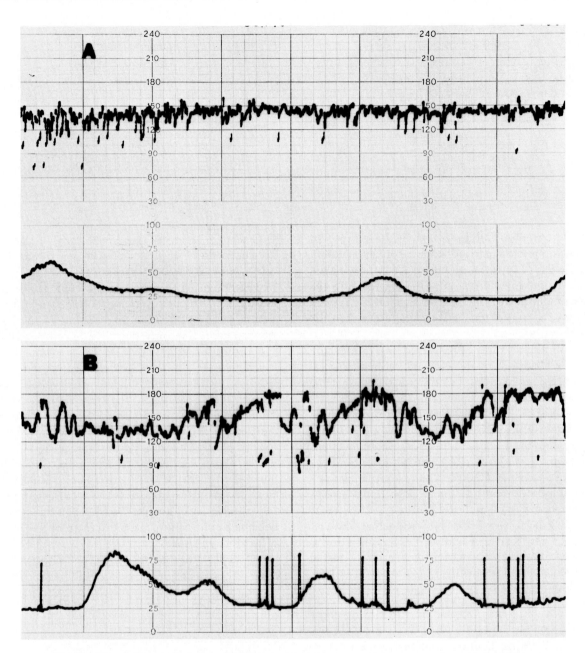

Fig. 8. Acceleration of FHR in association with fetal movement. **A.** Tracing during period of fetal inactivity. **B.** Marked accelerations with fetal movements (same patient). Vertical lines in uterine activity tracing indicate individual fetal movements.

(low or falling estriols, meconium in amniotic fluid, lack of uterine growth) point to fetal risk, a negative weekly OCT has frequently allowed the delay of intervention until fetal maturity is achieved. Despite the reliability of a negative OCT in indicating that the fetus will survive in utero for one more week, a negative test does not predict the subsequent performance of a fetus during labor: a significant number of patients with only negative tests will develop late decelerations in labor.[17]

Positive results with the OCT have been less reliable. In many reported series, most of the fetuses demonstrating late decelerations during an OCT will show evidence of significant compromise (low Apgar scores, FDIU). However, there also is approximately a 25 percent incidence of false positive tests, with a number of fetuses showing no late decelerations in labor following clearly positive tests.[17,23]

To distinguish the false positive from the true positive OCT, the clinician must look for other evidence

TABLE 10
Protocol for NST

Semi-Fowler's position
Maternal BP and pulse every 10 minutes
External monitor
20-minute recording
If nonreactive:
    Stimulate fetus during abdominal or vaginal exam
    Additional 20-minute recording

Reprinted with permission from Nochimson DJ, Turbeville JS, Terry JE, et al: The nonstress test. Obstet Gynecol 51:419, 1978.

TABLE 12
Contraindications for Use of Oxytocin

Previous classical cesarean section
Placenta previa
Multiple gestation
Incompetent cervix
Premature rupture of membranes

Reprinted with permission from Freeman RK: The use of oxytocin challenge test for antepartum clinical evaluation of ultraplacental respiratory function. Am J Obstet Gynecol 121:481, 1975.

of fetal compromise. Good results have been reported by those who intervene in a premature pregnancy only if both the OCT is positive and the daily urinary estriol excretion is low or falling.[17] Another approach to the problem of identifying the false positive OCT has been to examine features of the FHR tracing other than the late decelerations.

One of the features investigated was the occurrence of accelerations of the FHR in response to fetal movements (Fig. 8).[19,23,28,31-33] In one series of 1570 OCTs on 565 high-risk antepartum patients, 8 tests were classified as falsely positive in that no stigmata of placental insufficiency was noted during the delivery of the fetuses. Six of these fetuses had demonstrated accelerations of more than 10 beats per minute in response to movement. On the other hand, 90 percent of the fetuses with minimal or no accelerations showed some evidence of placental insufficiency and the most depressed fetuses were from the group that showed complete lack of FHR acceleration.[33] In another study, no patients showing acceleration of the FHR greater than 20 beats per minute with fetal movement during the baseline observation period before oxytocin infusion subsequently had a positive OCT.[32]

Nonstress Test. The significant correlation between the presence of FHR accelerations and the negative OCT led to the development of the nonstress test (NST) (Table 10). In this test, if in a 20-minute period FHR

TABLE 11
Results of NST

Reactive (in 20 minutes):
    a. At least 4 accelerations of
    b. At least 15 bpm and
    c. Lasting 15 or more seconds
Nonreactive
    Any of the above conditions not met
Unsatisfactory
    Tracing inadequate for interpretation

Reprinted with permission from Nochimson DJ, Turbeville JS, Terry JE: The nonstress test. Obstet Gynecol 51:419, 1978.

is "reactive" to fetal movements with four or more accelerations of at least 15 bpm above the baseline and lasting at least 15 seconds (Table 11), an OCT need not be performed.[23] If the NST is nonreactive and remains so during an additional 20-minute observation period (the additional period is necessary to prevent recording only during a "sleep" cycle, which can last up to 20 minutes), an OCT is obtained.[23]

The value of the NST is twofold. First, it is a simpler test than the OCT (see protocols above) and requires less time. Thus, the NST represents an economic saving to the hospital. Second, when certain conditions obtain (Table 12), the administration of oxytocin is inadvisable and the NST provides a noninvasive means of evaluating the fetus. An additional possibility is that if the patient is experiencing sufficient spontaneous uterine activity (as often happens, for example, after an amniocentesis[17]), the NST might become a contraction stress test despite the avoidance of oxytocin usage.

The presence of progressive loss of baseline variability also correlates well with poor fetal outcome,[19,21,32] but with Doppler ultrasonic monitoring, the routine interpretation of baseline irregularity will have to await the availability of the more sophisticated equipment discussed previously.

The occurrence of spontaneous fetal heart rate decelerations during antepartum nonstress testing is associated with intrauterine growth retardation in over 60 percent of cases.[34] Nonreactive nonstress tests and nonreactive positive contraction stress tests are associated with significantly increased morbidity and mortality.[43] The presence of persistent late decelerations (positive contraction stress tests) is an earlier warning sign of fetal deterioration than the loss of reactivity.[35]

SAFETY

Women who experience difficult and protracted labors may find themselves and their fetuses continuously exposed to Doppler ultrasound for many hours. Doppler is to traditional ultrasound roughly what fluoroscopy is to x-ray, i.e., it is a relatively continuous, low-intensity energy beam. Doppler ultrasound, like the rest of diagnostic ultrasound, employs intensities several orders of magnitude lower than therapeutic ultrasound. Doppler is continuous in nature, however, and therefore, the dose rises over time.

Takemura et al.[36] have observed in vitro hemolysis of maternal erythrocytes exposed to continuous direct irradiation by diagnostic levels (2.25 MHz) of ultrasound for 6 hours or more. Hemolysis was observed to increase in proportion to time.

In our study,[37] maternal erythrocyte fragility was studied in 16 women exposed to Doppler ultrasound monitoring during labor and eight controls. Blood samples were taken before and after Doppler monitoring and no significant change in erythrocyte fragility was seen, although there was a trend toward increased fragility in patients exposed continuously for over 7 hours. In general, however, Doppler ultrasound is considered to be safe, and there is no reason to question its overall safety in diagnostic use.[38]

SUMMARY

Equipment that allows the application of the Doppler principle in obstetric practice has proven to be valuable clinically. A Doppler ultrasonic device with audible output permits early diagnosis of pregnancy and simple verification of fetal life on subsequent examinations. In high-risk pregnancies, fetal status in the third trimester can be followed by serial NST/OCTs. In labor, perinatal outcome can be improved by Doppler monitoring of the FHR, which warns the physician of developing fetal compromise and thereby enables intervention before severe fetal asphyxia or death occurs. As electronic capabilities advance, the signal-to-noise ratio will improve and the Doppler ultrasonic monitoring will reveal even more information regarding fetal condition.

REFERENCES

1. Bernstine RL, Callagan DA: Ultrasonic Doppler inspection of the fetal heart. Am J Obstet Gynecol 95:1001, 1966
2. Barton JJ: Evaluation of the Doppler shift principle as a diagnostic aid in obstetrics. Am J Obstet Gynecol 102:563, 1968
3. Bishop EH: Obstetric uses of the ultrasonic motion sensor. Am J Obstet Gynecol 96:863, 1966
4. Brown RE: Detection of intrauterine death. Am J Obstet Gynecol 102:965, 1968
5. Pystynen P, Ylostalo P, Ojala A: Detection of foetal heart action by ultrasound transformed into audible signals. Ann Chir Gynaec Fenniae 57:607, 1968
6. Brown RE: Doppler ultrasound in obstetrics. JAMA 218:1395, 1971
7. Boyce ES, Daneo GS, Gough JD, et al: Doppler ultrasound method for detecting human fetal breathing in utero. Br Med J 2:17, 1976
8. Johnson WL, Stegall HF, Lim JN, et al: Detection of fetal life in early pregnancy with an ultrasonic Doppler flowmeter. Obstet Gynecol 26:305, 1965
9. Muller K, Osler M: Early detection of foetal life by "Dopplerophonia." Acta Obstet Gynecol Scand 48:130, 1969
10. Resch B, Herczeg J, Altmayer P, et al: The efficiency of Doppler-technique in the first trimester of pregnancy. Ann Chir Gynaec Fenniae 60:85, 1971
11. Pystynen P, Ojala A, Ylostalo P, et al: Placental localization by different methods. Acta Obstet Gynecol Scand 48:158, 1969
12. Jouppila P: Ultrasound in the diagnosis of early pregnancy and its complications. Acta Obstet Gynecol Scand 50:1, 1971
13. Ramsey EM: Uteroplacental circulation during labor. Clin Obstet Gynecol 11:78, 1965
14. Greiss FC, Anderson SG: Uterine blood flow during labor. Clin Obstet Gynecol 11:96, 1965
15. Hon EH: An introduction to fetal heart rate monitoring. New Haven, CT, Yale Cooperative, 1971
16. Shenker L, Kane R: Doppler ultrasonic fetal heart monitoring during labor. Obstet Gynecol 39:609, 1972
17. Freeman RK: The use of the oxytocin challenge test for antepartum clinical evaluation of uteroplacental respiratory function. Am J Obstet Gynecol 121:481, 1975
18. Hon EH, Khazin AF: Biochemical studies of the fetus: Part 1—The fetal pH—Measuring system. Obstet Gynecol 33:219, 1969
19. Rochard F, Schifrin BS, Goupil F, et al: Nonstressed fetal heart rate monitoring in the antepartum period. Am J Obstet Gynecol 126:699, 1976
20. Sokol RJ, Hutchinson P, Krouskop RW, et al: Congenital complete heart block diagnosed during intrauterine monitoring. Am J Obstet Gynecol 120:1115, 1974
21. Paul RH, Suidan AK, Yeh S, et al: Clinical fetal monitoring: VII. The evaluation and significance of intrapartum baseline FHR variability. Am J Obstet Gynecol 123:206, 1975
22. Beard RW, Filshie GM, Knight CA, et al: The significance of changes in the continuous fetal heart rate in the first stage of labour. J Obstet Gynaecol Br Commonw 78:865, 1971
23. Nochimson DJ, Turbeville JS, Terry JE, et al: The nonstress test. Obstet Gynecol 51:419, 1978
24. Lauersen NH, Hochberg HM, George MED, et al: Technical aspects of ranged directional Doppler: A new Doppler method of fetal heart rate monitoring. J Reprod Med 20:77, 1978
25. Paul RH, Hon EH: Clinical fetal monitoring: V. Effect on perinatal outcome. Am J Obstet Gynecol 118:529, 1974
26. Ray M, Freeman R, Pine S, et al: Clinical experience

with the oxytocin challenge test. Am J Obstet Gynecol 114:1, 1972

27. Spurrett B: Stressed cardiotocography in late pregnancy. J Obstet Gynecol Br Commonw 78:894, 1971

28. Schifrin BS, Lapidus M, Doctor GS, et al: Contraction stress test for antepartum fetal evaluation. Obstet Gynecol 45:433, 1975

29. Ewing DE, Farina JR, Otterson WN: Clinical application of the oxytocin challenge test. Obstet Gynecol 43:563, 1974

30. Chik L, Sokol RJ, Rosen MG: "Prediction" of the one-minute Apgar score from fetal heart rate data. Obstet Gynecol 48:452, 1976

31. Lee CY, DiLoreto PC, O'Lane JM: A study of fetal heart rate acceleration patterns. Obstet Gynecol 45:142, 1975

32. Trierweiler MW, Freeman RK, James J: Baseline fetal heart rate characteristics as an indicator of fetal status during the antepartum period. Am J Obstet Gynecol 125:618, 1976

33. Farahani G, Fenton AN: Fetal heart rate acceleration in relation to the oxytocin challenge test. Obstet Gynecol 49:163, 1977

34. Freeman RK, Anderson G, Dorchester W: A prospective multi-institutional study of antepartum fetal heart rate monitoring. I. Risk of perinatal mortality and morbidity according to antepartum fetal heart rate test results. Am J Obstet Gynecol 143:771, 1982

35. Pazos R, Vuolo K, Aladjem S, et al: Association of spontaneous fetal heart rate decelerations during antepartum nonstress testing and intrauterine growth retardation. Am J Obstet Gynecol 144:574, 1982

36. Takemura H, Suehara N: The present status of the safety of ultrasound diagnosis in the area of obstetrics: Studies on the hemolytic effect of clinical diagnostic ultrasound and the growth rate of cultured cells using a calibrated ultrasound generating system. Ultrasonic Med (Japan) 4(1):32, 1977

37. Bause GS, Niebyl JR, Sanders RC: Doppler ultrasound and maternal erythrocyte fragility. Obstet Gynecol 62:7, 1983

38. Lele PP: Safety and potential hazards in the current applications of ultrasound in obstetrics and gynecology. Ultrasound Med Biol 5:307, 1979

6 | Doppler Measurement of Umbilical Blood Flow

Robert W. Gill
Peter S. Warren

The well-being and normal development of the fetus in utero depend on the supply of oxygen and nutrients from the mother. In normal pregnancies, this intra-uterine support is considered to have considerable reserve capacity. However, fetal growth retardation and fetal hypoxia are often attributed to failing intrauterine support, as indicated by the use of terms such as "placental insufficiency."

Although a number of risk factors (such as maternal hypertension) associated with this failure of fetal support have been identified, the causes are not well understood. It has been stated, however, that for the majority of such cases ". . . the type of pathology . . . implies that the cause is extrinsic rather than intrinsic to the fetus, something that affects his supply lifeline somewhere from the uterine vascular supply, through the placenta, to the umbilical blood flow . . ."[1] A study of the blood flow in the umbilical cord was therefore undertaken to determine whether changes in the rate of this flow occur in pregnancies with complications, and if so whether measurement of the flow may have diagnostic value.

Newly developed ultrasonic Doppler techniques have made possible this measurement in utero without trauma to the mother or fetus.[2] Previously, information on the fetal circulation was obtained largely in animals[3] or in the human fetus at abortion[4,5] or immediately following delivery.[6,7] This chapter reviews the results to date obtained using the Doppler technique to measure umbilical blood flow in normal and high-risk pregnancies.

INSTRUMENTATION

The method of flow measurement involves a combination of B-mode ultrasonic imaging and pulsed Doppler ultrasound.[2] The imaging system used in this study was a UI Octoson,* a multitransducer water-coupled B-scanner. The patient lies prone on a plastic membrane forming the top of the water bath (Fig. 1)[8] and the eight large-diameter, focused transducers inside the bath are scanned mechanically to produce simple or compound images with high resolution.

The operator first adjusts the plane of scan to obtain a longitudinal image of the umbilical vein within the fetal trunk (Fig. 2). Care is taken to ensure that the point of measurement is in the umbilical vein proper, and not in left portal vein or the ductus venosus.[9] Caliper markers are then placed on the inner edges of the vessel walls to determine both the lumen diameter and the spatial orientation of the vessel (Fig. 3). The sonographer then selects one of the eight transducers for Doppler measurement, ensuring that it has a clear ultrasonic path and a suitable angle of approach to the vessel. The selected transducer is then automatically directed towards the vessel, and the range-gate of the pulsed Doppler adjusted so that it spans the vessel at the point of measurement (Fig. 3). The pulsed Doppler unit is then activated, and the average Doppler shift at each instant is electronically measured.[10]

It has been shown that the average Doppler shift

---

* Ausonics P/L, 16 Mars Road, Lane Cove, N.S.W., Australia.

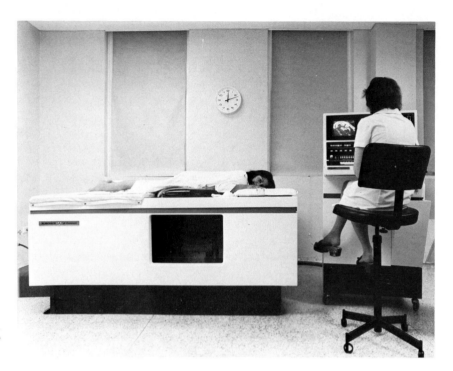

Fig. 1. The UI Octoson. The patient lies prone, with the transducers scanning from below through the water tank.

is directly related to the average blood velocity in the vessel if the "sample volume" of the Doppler is large enough to uniformly insonify the entire lumen of the vessel.[2] For the UI Octoson with the Doppler system operating at 1.5 MHz, this is true for vessels up to 10 mm in diameter, as indicated in Table 1. (For larger vessels, flow estimation is still possible but with reduced accuracy.)

The total rate of blood flow in the vessel is then simply obtained by multiplying this average velocity by the cross-sectional area of the vessel:

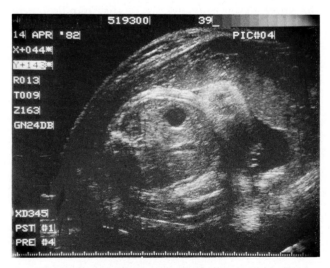

Fig. 2. Approximately transverse section of a fetal trunk at term, showing a longitudinal section of the umbilical vein and left portal vein.

Flow = (Average Velocity) × (Lumen Area)

$$= \left\{ \frac{2.46\ FD^2}{\cos \theta} \right\} \text{ml/min (for 1.5 MHz Doppler)}$$

where F is the average Doppler shift (Hz), D is the internal diameter of the vessel (cm), and θ is the angle of approach of the Doppler ultrasound beam to the vessel. Both D and θ are automatically calculated from the caliper positions, permitting the machine to continuously compute and display flow values using the above equation (Fig. 4).

The 5-second flow trace on the display can be "frozen" at any time for averaging and for other detailed measurements. Several readings are normally obtained in each patient, resetting the calipers and (whenever possible) using different angles of approach in order to average out random errors. The total examination time may vary from 10 to 30 minutes, with minimal inconvenience to the patient. Table 1 summarizes the specifications of the Doppler system. The figures for accuracy are based on initial theoretical calculations subsequently confirmed by in vitro tests of absolute accuracy and in vivo tests of repeatability.[2]

NORMAL PREGNANCIES

Initially, umbilical venous flow was measured in 47 normal patients with single pregnancies (ranging from 22 weeks gestation to term).[11] These pregnancies were uncomplicated at the time of the study, and the patients were subsequently delivered of babies with birth

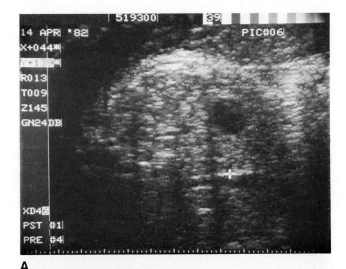

A

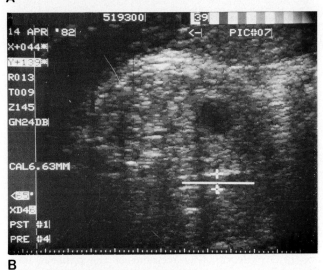

B

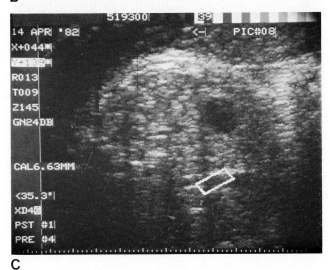

C

Fig. 3. Sequence of images showing placement of the caliper markers to measure the vessel diameter. The second marker in **B** is positioned so that the line segment is parallel to the vessel walls; this indicates the orientation of the vessel to the machine. In **C** the "sample volume" of the pulsed Doppler is indicated by the superimposed rectangle.

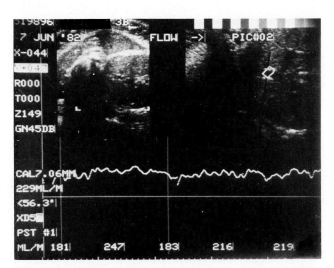

Fig. 4. Typical output display. The flow data in the lower half of the picture have been "frozen" for measurement. The average value of flow over the 2-second segment defined by the vertical marks is indicated on the left (229 ml/min), together with the vessel diameter (7.06 mm) and the angle between the vessel and the ultrasound beam (56.3°). This flow value is at approximately the 10th percentile for gestational age (37 weeks). Fetal growth, as indicated by serial BPD measurements, had virtually stopped.

weights appropriate for gestational age, and with no perinatal morbidity. These data have since been supplemented by values obtained in a further 71 pregnancies (selected using the same criteria), giving a total of 118 subjects as a basis for defining the normal range.

The results are shown in Figure 5. The rate of umbilical venous flow increases steadily with increasing gestational age, parallelling fetal growth, until a maximum is reached at 37 to 38 weeks, after which there is a reduction. A similar reduction near term has been reported in uterine flow in the rabbit,[12] and in human maternal serum estriol and HPL levels.[13]

To account for variations in fetal size, the rate of flow *per kilogram of fetal weight* can be calculated. The results for the initial group of 47 normal pregnancies described above are shown in Figure 6. Fetal weights were estimated by extrapolating back from the birth weights along the appropriate centile lines, using locally derived fetal growth charts.[14] The umbilical flow rate per kilogram is seen to be essentially constant

TABLE 1
Doppler Specifications

Ultrasonic frequency	1.5 MHz (or 3.0 MHz)
Angle of approach to vessel (for best accuracy)	30°–65°
Vessel diameter (for best accuracy)	4–10 mm (at 1.5 MHz) 4– 7 mm (at 3.0 MHz)
Standard error of measurement	10%–15%
Typical examination time	15–30 min

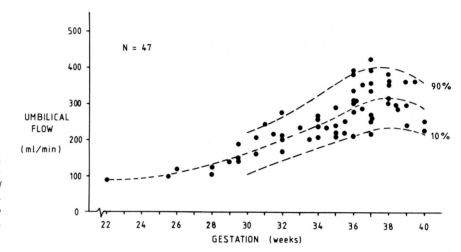

Fig. 5. Umbilical venous blood flow as a function of gestational age in normal pregnancies. (*Reprinted with permission from Gill RW, et al: Fetal umbilical venous flow measured in utero by pulsed Doppler and B-mode ultrasound. I. Normal pregnancies. Am J Obstet Gynecol 139:720, 1981.*)

until 35 weeks, averaging 120 ml/min/kg. Beyond 35 weeks a gradual decrease is seen, falling to an average value of 90 ml/min/kg at 40 weeks. Dawes has reported a similar decrease in umbilical flow per unit weight in the fetal lamb near term.[3]

Table 2 provides a summary of the umbilical flow values per unit weight in the human fetus as reported by various authors. The values agree closely, with the exception of the thermodilution measurements made in the cord immediately after delivery, where lower values were recorded.[6] This discrepancy is not surprising in light of the dramatic changes that occur in the fetal circulation at birth.

HIGH-RISK PREGNANCIES

Following the determination of umbilical flow rates in normal pregnancies, a group of high-risk pregnan-

cies was studied to investigate the potential of this measurement for diagnostic use. The group consisted of 124 patients hospitalized either because of complications of pregnancy (hypertension, preeclampsia, maternal diabetes, suspected fetal growth retardation, Rh-isoimmunization, maternal bleeding, or the like) or because of poor obstetric histories. Gestational ages ranged from 22 weeks to term, with 94 of the patients being studied within 2 weeks of delivery. The flow studies were made in conjunction with conventional B-mode examinations [including measurement of the biparietal diameter (BPD)], generally at weekly intervals from admission to parturition. The number of flow studies in each patient averaged 2.4, ranging from a minimum of one (in 55 patients) to a maximum of six (in 3 patients). Management of the patients was not influenced by the umbilical flow data, with the results being analyzed following delivery.

Several approaches to the analysis of the flow

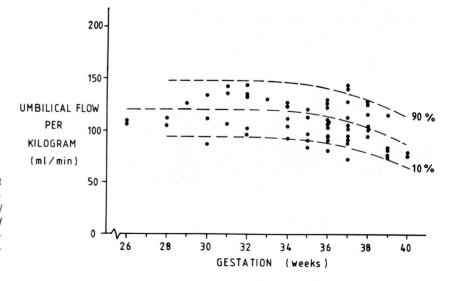

Fig. 6. Umbilical flow per kilogram of fetal weight as a function of gestational age in normal pregnancies. (*Reprinted with permission from Gill RW, et al: Fetal umbilical venous flow measured in utero by pulsed Doppler and B-mode ultrasound. I. Normal pregnancies. Am J Obstet Gynecol 139:720, 1981.*)

TABLE 2
Umbilical Flow Per Unit Fetal Weight— Normal Pregnancies

Authors	Method	Number of Subjects	Gestational Age	Average Flow/kg	Ref.
Assali et al. (1960)	Electromagnetic (at abortion)	12	10–28 wk	110 ml/min	4
Stembera et al. (1965)	Thermodilution (after delivery)	17	term	75 ml/min	6
Rudolph et al. (1971)	Microspheres (at abortion)	11	10–20 wk	110 ml/min	5
Gill et al. (1980)	Doppler (in utero)	27 / 20	26–35 wk / 36–40 wk	120 ml/min / 106 ml/min	11
Eik-Nes et al. (1980)	Doppler (in utero)	20	32–40 wk	110 ml/min	15
Jouppila and Kirkinen (1982)	Doppler (in utero)	101	30–36 wk	100 ml/min	16
Kurjak and Rajhvajn (1982)	Doppler (in utero)	63	30–41 wk	107 ml/min	17

values were examined. First, values were classified as "low," "normal," or "high," depending on whether they fell, respectively, below the 10th percentile, between the 10th and 90th percentiles, or above the 90th percentile of the previously established range for normal pregnancies (Fig. 5). Secondly, the flow per unit fetal weight was estimated, as described above. With this group of patients where fetal growth was frequently abnormal, the weight estimates were based on serial BPD measurements in addition to the birth weight and fetal growth charts. Thirdly, normalized flow (and flow per kilogram) values were calculated by dividing the measured values by the median values for normal pregnancies of the same gestational age.

Figure 7 shows the distribution of the normalized flow values for this group of high-risk pregnancies in comparison with normal pregnancies. A significantly wider spread of values was found in the high-risk group. More than half the patients had some flow values outside the normal range, with approximately equal numbers having "low" and "high" values.

HIGH FLOW VALUES

The figures given in Table 3 show that several complications of pregnancy were associated with consistently high values. In 10 of the 11 patients with antepartum hemorrhage, high flow values were recorded within 1 week of maternal bleeding, with the flow returning to normal within 2 weeks of the cessation of bleeding. In the two patients with Rh-isoimmunization, extremely high flow values were recorded, increasing further following intrauterine transfusion. In one of these

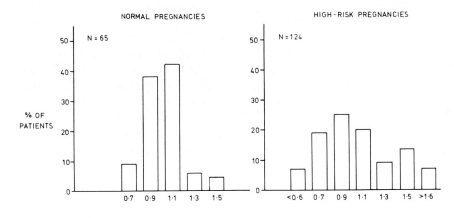

Fig. 7. Average (normalized) flow values in normal and high-risk pregnancies. The high-risk group showed a significantly wider spread of flow values.

patients the umbilical flow rate following transfusion was more than double the median value for normal pregnancies, this being the highest flow rate measured in the entire series of patients. The fetus died in utero the following day, the only intrauterine death in the series.

These findings in Rh disease have been largely confirmed by Kirkinen et al, who studied 18 pregnancies complicated by Rh-incompatibility.[18] They went further, demonstrating a negative correlation between umbilical flow rates and cord blood hemoglobin levels, which suggests that compensation for the impaired oxygen-carrying capacity of the fetal blood is occurring. The increased umbilical flow may therefore be useful as a guide to the severity of the disease.

Another finding that was associated with significantly high values of flow (and flow per kilogram) was abnormal ultrasonic appearance of the placenta. In a total of 37 patients the placenta was heavily calcified or infarcted; high flow values were observed in almost half of these (46 percent). Again this suggests that compensation may be occurring, in this case for impaired placental function. Clavero-Nunez has reported a similar result, using radioisotope techniques to measure relative flow rates in the umbilical and uterine circulations.[19] With more experience it may prove possible to use the high flow values observed in these patients to recognize when such compensation is occurring, possibly even to assess whether the compensation is adequate.

Table 3 also shows high flow values in pregnancies complicated by maternal diabetes. However, the average flow per kilogram was normal in these patients, suggesting that the high flow values simply reflected the larger than average size of these babies.

LOW FLOW VALUES

Approximately 40 percent of the patients with flow values below the normal range were suspected of in-

trauterine growth retardation or "placental insufficiency." In the following sections, low flow values are correlated with fetal growth retardation, fetal hypoxia, and neonatal morbidity and mortality.

UMBILICAL BLOOD FLOW AND INTRAUTERINE GROWTH RETARDATION

Intrauterine growth retardation (IUGR) and its association with greatly increased fetal morbidity and mortality are discussed in Chapter 11. Although ultrasonic size measurement of the fetus and uterus provides an effective method for detecting growth retardation in the majority of cases, a need still exists for a test that can detect IUGR (preferably near its onset) with high sensitivity and accuracy.

In this section the relationship between reduced umbilical flow and IUGR will be discussed for the group of high-risk patients described above. For these purposes, IUGR was defined as having occurred if the birth weight was below the 10th percentile (using locally derived figures on normal birth weights[14]). In twin pregnancies a correction was made for the lower birth weights normally found in twins.[20] Pregnancies complicated by maternal diabetes were not included because of difficulties in establishing normal birth weights for this group. Patients in whom the last flow measurement was made more than 2 weeks before delivery were also excluded.

A total of 81 high-risk pregnancies remained, 11 of which proved to be cases of IUGR. Ultrasonic BPD measurements correctly predicted growth retardation in only 7 of these 11 and wrongly predicted it in a further 15. In comparison, 9 of the 11 cases of IUGR recorded at least one low value of umbilical flow, with 7 having low values on at least two successive occasions. Looking at the exclusion of IUGR on the other hand, 55 of the 57 patients in whom no low flow values were recorded delivered babies with normal birth weights.

Similar results have been reported by other authors. Kurjak and Rajhvajn found low flow values in each of seven IUGR fetuses,[17] whereas Jouppila and Kirkinen found 34 percent of the umbilical flow readings in 74 IUGR fetuses were low.[16] In the sheep, experimental embolization of the uteroplacental circulation has shown that umbilical flow decreased with time in those that subsequently became growth retarded, while it increased with time in the control animals which had not been embolized.[21] The reduced flow in the growth-retarded animals was shown to be related to increased vascular resistance in the umbilical circulation.

TABLE 3
Increased Umbilical Flow

	N	Average Flow*	Average Flow/kg*
Antepartum hemorrhage	11	+17%†	+30%†
Rh-Isoimmunization‡	2	+65%†	+27%†
Pathologic placenta	37	+16%†	+23%†
Maternal diabetes	16	+20%†	− 5%

* Compared with median value for normal pregnancies.
† Significant at $p < 0.01$ level.
‡ One fetus died in utero.

These results suggest that reduced umbilical flow is strongly associated with growth retardation, to the extent that there is potential diagnostic value in the measurement of umbilical flow, both for the diagnosis of IUGR and for its exclusion. Table 4 compares umbilical flow (considered as a hypothetical test for IUGR) with the other routine tests used in our institution at the time of the study: BPD measurement and maternal urinary estriols and HPL. In this group of high-risk patients, low umbilical flow would have predicted IUGR with higher sensitivity than either hormones or BPD measurements. Three of the four cases of IUGR that were missed on the basis of serial BPDs had low flow values (indeed they had low values on at least two successive occasions) and so would have been correctly diagnosed on the basis of flow. Similarly, of the 15 patients wrongly thought on the basis of BPD measurements to be growth retarded, 10 would have been correctly diagnosed as normal on the basis of flow; the other 5 each had a single low flow value, with none having two successive low flows. Thus, flow would have correctly classified 13 of the total of 19 cases that were misdiagnosed on the basis of BPD. If the diagnostic criterion for IUGR had been the recording of two successive low flow values, the flow test would have performed even better.

Table 4 indicates a high false positive rate for umbilical flow (and indeed for BPD measurement), as reflected by the low positive predictive value. This warrants further comment. First, if as suggested above the diagnostic criterion was changed to require the recording of low flow values on two successive occasions, the positive predictive value for flow would have been 58 percent. Secondly, if the growth pattern of the remaining ten "false positives" is examined more closely, it is found that three were cases of marginal growth retardation (with birth weights below the 20th percentile), while another five were cases of late flattening of fetal growth (where prompt delivery presumably

prevented the birth weights falling below the 20th percentile). Thus, only two of the "false positives" in fact had normal growth.

The two false negatives (i.e., cases of IUGR where low flow values were not recorded) also require further discussion. One of these patients had umbilical flow values and maternal estriol levels that were within the normal range but falling consistently on serial measurement. Presumably flow may well have fallen below normal if the pregnancy had been allowed to continue. The second was a case of flattened growth, with growth ceasing abruptly at 31 weeks' gestation. Flow values could not be obtained at either 31 or 32 weeks due to inability to image the umbilical vein.

This failure to visualize the vein occurred in a total of four patients in the series, all of whom were preeclamptic. Three of the four subsequently delivered babies with birth weights below the 10th percentile, suggesting that the inability to image the vein could be caused by severe narrowing of the vessel, probably in association with considerably reduced umbilical flow. Jouppila and Kirkinen have reported a similar inability to measure flow in approximately 7 percent of their cases of growth retardation.[16]

Where fetal growth flattened, it is of considerable interest to examine the relative timing of any reduction in umbilical flow. In those cases where flow did fall below the normal range, the first low value was detected either at the same time as BPD measurements first indicated flattened growth, or up to 3 weeks *before* the reduced growth was discovered. On average, the low flow values were detected 1 week before BPD measurements first revealed the flattening of fetal growth.

UMBILICAL FLOW PER KILOGRAM AND RISK

Having demonstrated that low umbilical flow values were found in most cases of IUGR, a significant question remains: was the flow simply reduced in proportion to the reduced size of the fetus, or was the reduction more severe than this? Calculation of the umbilical flow per unit fetal weight provides the answer to this question. Of the 11 cases of IUGR discussed above, 7 had some low values of flow per kilogram. Two had consistently low values to the extent that the *average* flow per kilogram was below the normal range. Both of these babies were severely growth retarded, and both died within a week of birth. These were the only neonatal deaths in the entire series of 124 patients, suggesting that low values of flow per kilogram may be useful as predictors of high risk.

TABLE 4
Diagnosis of IUGR

	Umbilical Flow*	Maternal Es, HPL*	Ultrasonic BPD
N =	81	34	81
Sensitivity	82%	64%	64%
Specificity	79%	91%	79%
Pos. Pred. Value	38%†	78%	32%
Neg. Pred. Value	96%	84%	93%

* Test considered positive if any reading below normal.
† Where two successive low flow values are recorded, positive predictive value rises to 58%.

Table 5 provides a summary of all patients in whom flow was measured within 2 weeks of parturition, classified into four groups on the basis of whether any low values of flow or flow per kilogram were measured. Consider first the nine patients with low values of flow but not of flow per kilogram (i.e., the last column in Table 5). By definition, these were all small babies, with four of the nine having birth weights below the 10th percentile. However, the incidence of antenatal hypoxia [indicated by abnormal fetal cardiotocograph (CTG) records] was low, and there were no cases of significant neonatal morbidity and no neonatal deaths. In short, this was a group of small but healthy babies. Significantly, all showed the "low profile" pattern of growth retardation, which Campbell and Dewhurst have reported to be associated with a low risk of asphyxia at birth.[22]

In contrast, the group in which low values of both flow and flow per kilogram were recorded had a very high incidence of antenatal fetal hypoxia. Two babies died, and a significant number developed serious neonatal complications (such as respiratory distress syndrome). Seven of the 33 babies in this group suffered IUGR, six of them displaying the late flattening pattern of growth retardation. Again it is interesting to note that Campbell and Dewhurst reported high incidences of perinatal asphyxia and neonatal hypoglycemia in association with the late flattening growth pattern.[22] Jouppila and Kirkinen have also reported consistently low values of flow per kilogram in babies that suffered fetal distress.[16]

The group of patients with no low values of flow or flow per kilogram contained only one case of IUGR (that discussed earlier where flow and hormones were falling but remained within normal limits). The incidence of antenatal hypoxia and neonatal complications was also low in this group. Finally, the babies with normal flow values but with low values of flow per

kilogram were (by definition) larger than average. They did not differ significantly from those with normal flow and flow per kilogram in the incidence of perinatal complications.

Thus, all but one of the IUGR babies fell into the "low flow" category (i.e., the last two columns of Table 5), again indicating that low flow would have been a good predictor of IUGR. However, of potentially more significance for the management of patients is the fact that the flow per kilogram enabled separation of the IUGR babies (indeed of all the "low flow" babies) into two groups, one with a high incidence of perinatal problems, the other with relatively low incidence. This suggests that flow as a diagnostic test may be useful not so much for the prediction of IUGR as for the identification of those fetuses with a high risk of perinatal complication.

Thus, in Table 6, low flow in conjunction with low flow per kilogram is analyzed as a hypothetical predictor of antenatal hypoxia and neonatal morbidity and mortality. Comparison is made with IUGR considered as a predictor of risk. (Indeed, the great interest shown in IUGR is due precisely to its association with increased risk.) The second column of Table 6 refers to "suspected IUGR" since not all cases of IUGR were correctly diagnosed antenatally, while the third column refers to the ideal situation which would have applied if IUGR was itself predicted with 100 percent accuracy.

TABLE 5
Flow and Flow per Kilogram

Flow Flow/kg	Normal* Normal	Normal Low†	Low Low	Low Normal
N‡ =	43	9	33	9
Antenatal hypoxia	8%	14%	48%¶	13%
Neonatal morbidity	9%	11%	15%	0%
Neonatal mortality	0%	0%	6%¶	0%
IUGR	2%	0%	21%¶	44%¶

* "Normal" means no low values recorded.
† "Low" means the recording of any low flow values, or inability to image the umbilical vein.
‡ All babies delivered within 2 weeks of last flow reading.
¶ Significant at $p < 0.05$ level.

TABLE 6
Flow and IUGR as Predictors of Risk

	Flow*	Suspected IUGR	Actual IUGR
A. Prediction of antenatal fetal hypoxia (N = 78)			
Sensitivity	69%	39%	37%
Specificity	81%	80%	86%
Positive predictive value†	48% (62%)	37%	47%
Negative predictive value	91%	81%	80%
B. Prediction of neonatal morbidity (N = 94)			
Sensitivity	50%	40%	33%
Specificity	67%	79%	87%
Positive predictive value†	15% (29%)	18%	22%
Negative predictive value	92%	92%	92%
C. Prediction of neonatal mortality (N = 94)			
Sensitivity	100%	100%	100%
Specificity	66%	78%	87%
Positive predictive value†	6% (14%)	9%	11%
Negative predictive value	100%	100%	100%

* Diagnostic criterion for high risk—at least one low value of both flow and flow/kg, or inability to image umbilical vein.
† When two successive low flow values recorded, figure in brackets applies.

The most striking observation is that umbilical flow would have been a more sensitive predictor of antenatal hypoxia and neonatal morbidity than IUGR. Thus, for example, 69 percent of the cases of antenatal hypoxia had met the flow criteria for "high-risk," but only 37 percent were growth retarded.

For a single flow reading the "false positive" rate for flow would have been similar to that for IUGR. However, where serial flow measurements were made and low values were recorded on at least two successive occasions, flow would have had a lower false positive rate than IUGR in all three categories. Looking at the exclusion of risk, where the flow criteria for "high-risk" were not met the likelihood of serious compromise of the baby was less than 10 percent, giving a false negative rate equal to or better than that of IUGR.

Finally, the subject of timing arises again. On average, low flow values were measured 1 week before BPD measurements first indicated the onset of growth retardation; low flow values similarly preceded the first indication of fetal hypoxia (on the CTG records), again by an average of 1 week. Thus it appears that umbilical flow offers a comparatively accurate and timely warning of risk to the fetus, superior in many respects to that given by fetal growth retardation.

UMBILICAL ARTERY FLOW WAVEFORM ANALYSIS

An alternative method for the study of the umbilical circulation, using somewhat different instrumentation, has been described by several authors.[23-25] Doppler signals are obtained from the umbilical arteries within the cord, using either continuous wave or pulsed Doppler. These signals are processed by a frequency analyzer to produce a "spectrogram" which shows the arterial flow waveform (Fig. 8). Since neither the diameter nor the orientation of the vessels is known, the spectragram cannot be quantified in terms of blood velocity or flow. However, the shape of the waveform, which is independent of the angle between the ultrasound beam and the cord, does provide information regarding the resistance offered to blood flowing in the umbilical circulation. As mentioned above, animal experiments have suggested that the reduced umbilical flow seen in IUGR is associated with increased resistance to flow. These changes should therefore be reflected in changes in the arterial flow waveform.

Normal umbilical artery flow waveforms, and their variation with gestational age, have been described.[24,25] An increased diastolic flow component is observed as

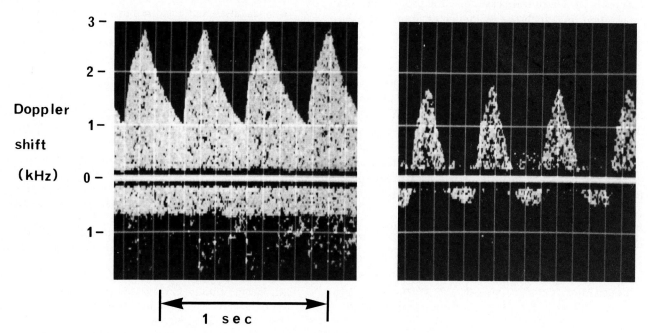

Fig. 8. Sonogram displays of Doppler signals obtained from the umbilical cord using continuous wave Doppler. The tracing on the left, from a normal pregnancy at 34 weeks' gestation, shows signals from both the umbilical artery (above the zero line) and the umbilical vein (below the zero line). The umbilical artery tracing on the right was obtained from a pregnancy with severe IUGR and an abnormal CTG (at 34 weeks). Notice the reversal of flow during diastole. (*Courtesy Dr. B.J. Trudinger, Fetal Welfare Laboratory, Westmead Centre, N.S.W., Australia.*)

pregnancy progresses, reflecting a reduced resistance to flow. In pregnancies with complications, on the other hand, abnormal waveforms indicative of high flow resistance have been observed in connection with fetal compromise and death.[23,25] Further data are required to establish the relationship between the information obtained from umbilical artery flow waveforms and that given by quantitative umbilical flow measurement.

SUMMARY

Failing intrauterine support of the fetus can lead to fetal growth retardation, and it is associated with a high risk of neonatal morbidity and mortality. In this chapter results have been presented from a study of the umbilical blood circulation, which forms a vital part of the intrauterine support of the fetus. These show that abnormal flow values occurred frequently in pregnancies with complications. High flow values were found in connection with maternal bleeding, Rh-isoimmunization and pathologic placentas, with the increased flow in these patients appearing to represent a compensation mechanism.

Low flow values, on the other hand, were found in association with a high incidence of IUGR. In some cases, the flow was reduced only in proportion to the reduced size of the fetus (i.e., the flow per kilogram was normal). These were cases of "low profile" growth retardation, in which the incidence of antenatal hypoxia, neonatal morbidity, and mortality were low. In others, however, umbilical flow was more severely reduced so that the flow per kilogram was also low. In this group there was a high incidence of "late flattening" IUGR, and of fetal hypoxia and neonatal morbidity, and two babies with extremely low flow values died shortly after birth. These findings are consistent with failure of the intrauterine support of the fetus.

The results of this study thus suggest that umbilical flow is not only capable of use as a predictor of IUGR, but that it may also be able to identify which of the IUGR fetuses are at risk. Further, it may be a better and more timely predictor of risk than is IUGR itself.

Additional work is required to evaluate umbilical flow as a diagnostic test for high-risk pregnancies. It is hoped that contributions can also be made to improved understanding of the pathophysiology of the processes involved.

REFERENCES

1. Usher RH: Clinical and therapeutic aspects of fetal malnutrition. Ped Clin N Am 17:169, 1970
2. Gill RW: Pulsed Doppler with B-mode imaging for quantitative blood flow measurement. Ultrasound Med Biol 5:223, 1979
3. Dawes GS: Foetal and Neonatal Physiology. Chicago, Year Book, 1968
4. Assali NS, Rauramo L, Peltonen T: Measurement of uterine blood flow and uterine metabolism. VIII. Uterine and fetal blood flow and oxygen consumption in early human pregnancy. Am J Obstet Gynecol 79:86, 1960
5. Rudolph AM, Heymann MA, Teramo KAW, et al: Studies on the circulation of the previable human fetus. Ped Res 5:452, 1971
6. Stembera ZK, Hodr J, Janda J: Umbilical blood flow in healthy newborn infants during the first minutes after birth. Am J Obstet Gynecol 91:568, 1965
7. McCallum WD: Thermodilution measurement of human umbilical blood flow at delivery. Am J Obstet Gynecol 127:491, 1977
8. Kossoff G, Carpenter DA, Radovanovich G, et al: Octoson: A new rapid multi-transducer general purpose water-coupling echoscope, in Kazner E, de Vlieger M, Muller HR, McCready VR (eds), Proceedings of the Second European Congress on Ultrasound in Medicine. Amsterdam, Exerpta Medica 1975, pp 90–95
9. Chinn DE, Filly RA, Callen PW: Ultrasonic evaluation of fetal umbilical and hepatic vascular anatomy. Radiology 144:153, 1982
10. Gill RW: Performance of the mean frequency Doppler demodulator. Ultrasound Med Biol 5:237, 1979
11. Gill RW, Trudinger BJ, Garrett WJ, et al: Fetal umbilical venous flow measured in utero by pulsed Doppler and B-mode ultrasound. I. Normal pregnancies. Am J Obstet Gynecol 139:720, 1981
12. Barcroft J: In Keele CA, Neil E (eds), Sampson Wright's Applied Physiology, 10th ed. London, Oxford University Press, 1961, p 533
13. Taylor ES: Obstetrics and Fetal Medicine. Baltimore, Williams and Wilkins, 1977, p 32
14. Betheras FR, White JG, Betheras GW: Intrauterine growth in an Australian population. Aust N Z J Obstet Gynaecol 9:153, 1969
15. Eik-Nes SH, Brubakk AO, Ulstein MK: Measurement of human fetal blood flow. Br Med J 280:283, 1980
16. Jouppila P, Kirkinen P: The role of fetal blood flow measurements in obstetrics, in Kurjak A (ed), Measurements of Fetal Blood Flow, C.I.C., Rome, 1983
17. Kurjak A, Rajhvajn B: Ultrasonic measurements of umbilical blood flow in normal and complicated pregnancies. J Perinat Med 10:3, 1982
18. Kirkinen P, Jouppila P, Eik-Nes S: Fetal blood flow in Rh-incompatibility, in Kurjak A, Kratochwil A (eds), Recent Advances in Ultrasound Diagnosis 3. Amsterdam, Excerpta Medica, 1981, pp 243–245
19. Clavero-Nunez JA: Uteroplacental blood flow in pregnancy at term, in Aladjem S, Brown AK, Sureau C (eds), Clinical Perinatology. St. Louis, Mosby, 1981
20. Ounstead M, Ounstead C: On Fetal Growth Rate. Suffolk, Spastics International Medical Publications, 1973, p 17

21. Clapp JF, Szeto HH, Larrow R, et al: Umbilical blood flow response to embolization of the uterine circulation. Am J Obstet Gynecol 138:60, 1980
22. Campbell S, Dewhurst CJ: Diagnosis of the small-for-dates fetus by serial ultrasonic cephalometry. Lancet 2:1002, 1971
23. McCallum WD, Williams CS, Napel S, et al: Fetal blood velocity waveforms. Am J Obstet Gynecol 132:425, 1978
24. Stuart B, Drumm J, FitzGerald DE, et al: Fetal blood velocity waveforms in normal pregnancy. Br J Obstet Gynaecol 87:780, 1980
25. Giles WB, Trudinger BJ, Cook CM: Fetal umbilical artery velocity waveforms. Proceedings of the 27th Convention of AIUM. J Ultrasound Med 7 (Suppl): 98, 1982

7 | Normal Anatomy of the Female Pelvis: Ultrasound with Computed Tomography Correlation

Alfred B. Kurtz
Matthew D. Rifkin

INTRODUCTION

In the female pelvis, ultrasound is 82 to 91 percent accurate in detecting abnormalities.[1-4] Accuracy is dependent upon proper technique, including distension of the urinary bladder, which serves as an acoustic window to visualize adjacent structures and displaces the small bowel and mesentery out of the pelvis. When the rectosigmoid colon is concomitantly filled with fluid, more complete evaluation of the intervening and posterior structures can be made.[5,6]

This chapter concentrates on an analysis of the structures of the pelvis. The bones, muscles, blood vessels, ureter, urinary bladder, vagina and uterus, adnexa, rectosigmoid colon, and the potential peritoneal spaces are systematically evaluated. Transverse computed tomograms are shown to emphasize cross-sectional anatomy. Ultrasound techniques that enhance diagnostic accuracy are stressed.

PELVIC SKELETON

The pelvis is a bony ring consisting of two bilateral symmetrical hipbones and a sacrum.[7] Each hipbone is composed of three parts, the ilium, ischium, and pubis, which unite at a large cup-shaped articular cavity termed the acetabulum. The ilium is the most superior bone. It is broad and expanded cranially, articulating with the sacrum posteriorly (Fig. 1). The pubis, the most anterior bone, extends medially from the acetabulum to articulate in the midline at the pubic sym-

physis with the hipbone from the opposite side (Fig. 1). The ischium is the most inferior bone and is strongest of the three. Cross-sectional images at various pelvic levels reveal specific bony shapes. Because of the symmetry, comparison between the bony contours of one side to the other can be made (Figs. 2–5).[8]

Anatomically, the pelvis can be further divided into the greater and lesser pelvis by an oblique line termed the pelvic brim. This invisible line passes through the prominence of the sacrum posteriorly, the arcuate and pectineal lines laterally, and the superior margin of the pubic symphysis anteriorly.[7] The greater or false pelvis that is situated above this line is bound posteriorly and laterally by the iliac bones. It is incomplete anteriorly, but communicates cranially with the remainder of the abdomen and caudally with the lesser pelvis. The lesser or true pelvis is situated below the pelvic brim and has more complete bony walls. It resembles a bowl tilted backward approximately 50 to 60 degrees from the vertical.[7] This bowl is bound anteriorly by the pubic symphysis and superior pubic rami, laterally by the acetabulum and posteriorly by the pelvic surfaces of the sacrum and coccyx. The lesser pelvis communicates superiorly with the greater pelvis and is enclosed inferiorly by a group of muscles termed the pelvic diaphragm.

Computed tomography (CT) is a good technique for imaging the outlines and internal architecture of the pelvic bones, including the soft tissue surrounding the bones (Figs. 2A,3A,4A,5A).[8] Gas in either the large or small bowel does not affect adequate imaging of the pelvic structures; for this reason, bladder distension

100

Key to Abbreviations for Illustrations

A	= Anus		LK	= Left Kidney
AC	= Acetabulum		O	= Ovary
ACDS	= Anterior Cul-De-Sac		OA	= Ovarian Artery
Ao	= Aorta		OIM	= Obturator Internus Muscle
APS	= Anterior Peritoneal Space		OV	= Ovarian Vein
B	= Urinary Bladder		P	= Peritoneum
BG	= Bowel Gas		PCDS	= Posterior Cul-De-Sac
BL	= Broad Ligament		PD	= Pelvic Diaphragm
CIA	= Common Iliac Artery		PIM	= Piriformis Muscle
CIV	= Common Iliac Vein		PM	= Psoas Muscle
CM	= Coccygeus Muscle		PU	= Pubis Bone
Co	= Coccyx		QLM	= Quadratus Lumborum Muscle
Cx	= Cervix		R	= Rectum
EIA	= External Iliac Artery		RAM	= Rectus Abdominus Muscle
EIBV	= External Iliac Blood Vessels		RK	= Right Kidney
EIV	= External Iliac Vein		RL	= Round Ligament
F	= Fallopian Tube		S	= Sigmoid Colon
GMM	= Gluteus Maximus Muscle		SA	= Sacrum
I	= Iliac Bone		SMA	= Superior Mesenteric Artery
IIA	= Internal Iliac Artery		SP	= Symphysis Pubis
IIV	= Internal Iliac Vein		U	= Urethra
IL	= Inguinal Ligament		Ur	= Ureter
ILM	= Iliacus Muscle		Ut	= Uterus
IMA	= Inferior Mesentery Artery		UtBV	= Uterine Blood Vessels
IPL	= Infundibulopelvic Ligament		V	= Vagina
IPM	= Iliopsoas Muscle		VBV	= Vesicular Blood Vessels
IVC	= Inferior Vena Cava		(H)	= Toward Patient's Head
LAM	= Levator Ani Muscle		(R)	= Toward Patient's Right Side

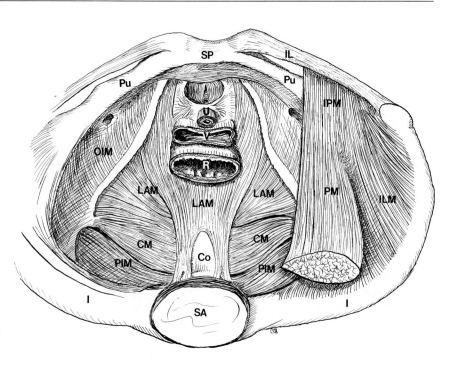

Fig. 1. Diagram of the pelvic musculature and bones seen from above.

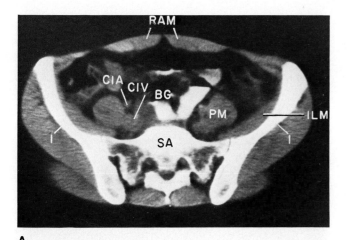

A

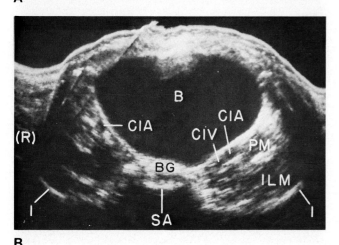

B

Fig. 2. Paired transverse pelvic images in different patients at the level of the upper sacrum (SA). **A.** Computed tomogram with nondistended urinary bladder. **B.** Ultrasound. Only one of the common iliac veins (CIV) is imaged due to overdistension of the urinary bladder (B). Also note displacement of bowel gas (BG) posteriorly by the distended bladder.

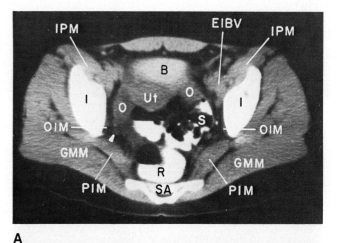

A

B

Fig. 3. Paired transverse pelvic images in different patients at the level of the lower sacrum (SA). **A.** Computed tomogram. Arrowhead shows rounded soft tissue densities posterior to the ovary (O), which are most likely a combination of internal iliac artery and vein, ureter and normal lymph nodes. **B.** Ultrasound. The external iliac veins are not seen due to compression by a rounded but overdistended urinary bladder (B). The left piriformis muscle (PIM) is not visualized due to gas in the rectum (R) and sigmoid colon (S).

is not necessary. There are, however, some limitations to CT:

1. The failure to separate soft tissues having similar attenuation coefficients, particularly in those patients where there is a paucity of interposed fat.
2. The limitation imposed by the analysis of transverse images when the long axis of many structures is either longitudinal or oblique.
3. The inability to separate true masses from fluid-filled bowel without introducing water-soluble contrast or air by mouth or rectum, or by the use of pelvic compression.[9]
4. The inability to distinguish blood vessels or ureters without the use of intravenous contrast.
5. The beam-hardening artifact, which degrades the

image between two dense bony structures such as the acetabulae.[10]

By contrast, ultrasound can image the pelvic structures in any plane and is able to distinguish subtle differences in all soft tissues that have different densities and velocities of transmitted sound. This is referred to as acoustical impedance. Although ultrasound is not able to penetrate bone, the anterior skeletal surfaces can be clearly distinguished so that the posterior boundary of the overlying soft tissues may be carefully analyzed (Figs. 2B,3B,4B,5B). If scans are performed

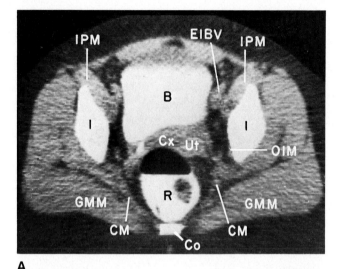

A

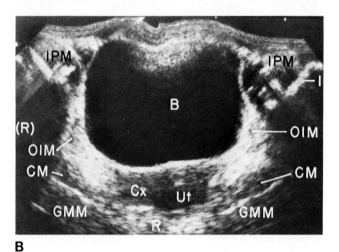

B

Fig. 4. Paired transverse pelvic images in different patients at the level of the coccyx (Co). **A.** Computed tomogram. **B.** Ultrasound. The urinary bladder (B) is indented by the prominent iliopsoas muscles (IPM).

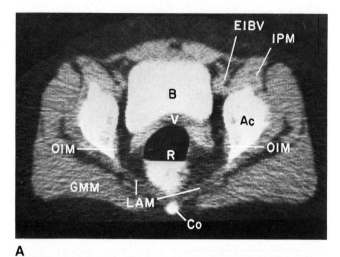

A

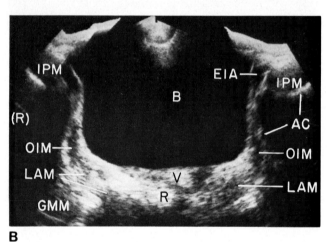

B

Fig. 5. Paired transverse pelvic images in different patients at the caudal aspect of the coccyx (Co) demonstrating a square-shaped bladder (B) due to the acetabelum (Ac). **A.** Computed tomogram. **B.** Ultrasound. The obturator internus muscle (OIM) is inseparable from the levator ani muscle (LAM) laterally. The posterior part of the levator ani muscle and the sacrum are obscured by a gas filled rectum (R).

from the anterior, lateral, and posterior surfaces of the pelvis, the outer boundaries of the bones and the overlying soft tissues can be imaged.[11] Gas-filled bowel presents difficulty in imaging because gas reflects sound back to the transducer, causing inadequate penetration. Although a good deal of the small bowel is displaced out of the lesser pelvis by distension of the urinary bladder, small bowel still persists in the greater pelvis and in the posterior cul-de-sac of the lesser pelvis. Additionally, gas may be present in the large bowel. If the small intestine is superficial, gentle pressure while scanning will frequently displace the bowel, allowing visualization of underlying structures. If gas in the rectosigmoid colon limits visualization, this can often be eliminated by the introduction of fluid per rectum.[5]

PELVIC MUSCULATURE

The pelvic muscles like the previously mentioned pelvic bones, are paired structures and are usually quite symmetrical, allowing contralateral comparison. Although these muscles are routinely seen by CT,[8] they are less likely to be completely imaged with ultrasound (Figs. 2–5). In the greater pelvis, the iliopsoas muscle is a combination of the psoas major and the iliacus muscle.[12] The psoas major muscle is a long, thick muscle originating in the paralumbar vertebral region and coursing caudally, anteriorly and laterally (Fig. 6). Upon entering the greater pelvis, it lies anterior and medial to the iliacus muscle, which arises from the superior two-thirds of the anterior surface of the iliac

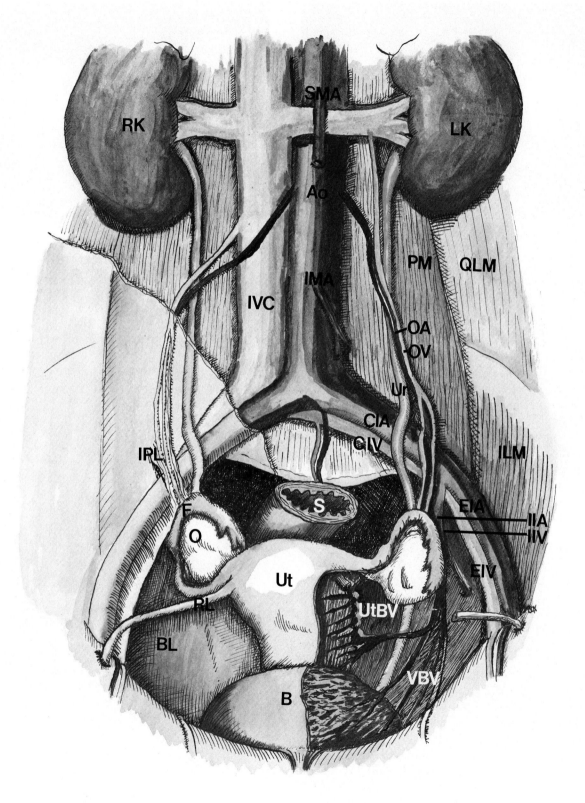

Fig. 6. Anterior diagram of the lower abdomen and pelvis showing the retroperitoneal structures, the ovaries (O) and urinary bladder (B). The left ovary has been moved anteriorly and part of the left side of the uterus (Ut), bladder and broad ligament has been removed to show the position of the adjacent blood vessels and ureter.

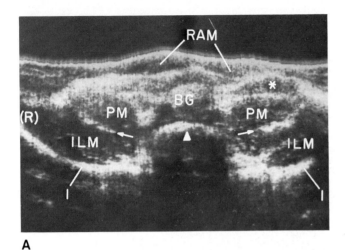

A

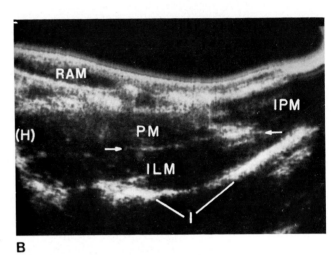

B

Fig. 7. Ultrasound images of the greater pelvis. **A** is the transverse, **B** the longitudinal oblique along the long axis of the iliopsoas muscle from midline toward hip. Arrows denote hyperechoic line separating the psoas (PM) from the iliacus (ILM) muscles. An asterisk indicates collapsed descending colon. An arrowhead indicates anterior surface of fifth lumbar vertebral body.

bone (Figs. 1,6). These two muscles join to form the iliopsoas muscle, which continues caudally, anteriorly, and laterally to its tendinous insertion on the lesser trochanter of the femur (Fig. 1).

On ultrasound examination, particularly in thin, muscular people, the psoas major muscle, the iliacus muscle, and the combined iliopsoas muscle may be seen, and are relatively hypoechoic with distinct margins (Figs. 2B,3B,4B,5B).[13] The separation of the psoas major and iliacus muscles is frequently possible in the upper part of the greater pelvis due to an interposed thin, hyperechoic line that is a combination of the fascia surrounding the muscles, interposed fat, and the large femoral and smaller nerves (Fig. 7).[8,14] The cranial portion of these muscles is often incompletely visualized due to overlying gas-filled bowel. The more anteriorly located caudad part is more commonly imaged, however, due to fewer interposed bowel loops, and may be imaged in oblique scans through the distended urinary bladder. To obtain long axis views of the iliopsoas muscle, an oblique longitudinal image is needed. This is obtained by scanning from the midline toward the hip (Fig. 7B). The muscles can also be segmentally imaged in transverse and true longitudinal projection.

There are four major muscle groups of the lesser pelvis: the levator ani and coccygeus (termed the pelvic diaphragm), the obturator internus, and the piriformis (Figs. 1, 8).[15] The obturator internus and the levator ani muscles are closer to the distended urinary bladder and are more routinely imaged. The piriformis and coccygeus muscles are situated more deeply, posteriorly and cranially, and are less commonly identified by ultrasound.

The obturator internus muscle covers a large portion of the inner surface of the anterior and lateral walls of the lesser pelvis (Fig. 1).[15] It is surrounded by the obturator fascia, which serves as tendinous insertion for the levator ani muscle.[15] On ultrasound ex-

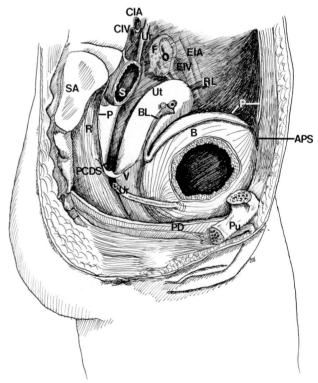

Fig. 8. Sagittal pelvic diagram lateral to midline. The intact midline organs and structures of the opposite lateral pelvic sidewall are shown.

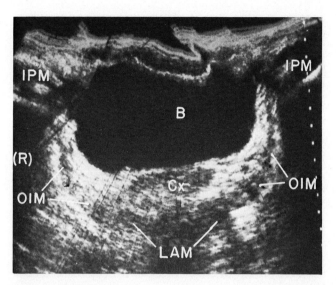

Fig. 9. Cranially angled transverse pelvic scan imaged from pubic symphysis toward head. Note the more prominent obturator internus (OIM) and less prominent levator ani (LAM) muscles.

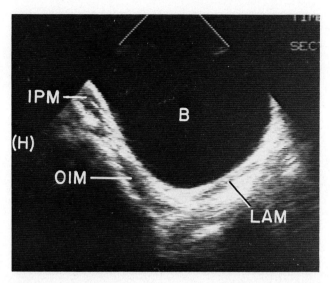

Fig. 10. Longitudinal pelvic ultrasound scan angled from midline toward pelvic sidewall showing the normal sidewall muscles.

amination, this muscle is imaged through the distended urinary bladder as an elongated and relatively hypoechoic ovoid muscle surrounded by the bright reflector of the obturator fascia.[11,13,16] The muscle is most easily recognized in true anteroposterior transverse view (Figs. 4B,5B) and may be accentuated by transverse scans angling cranially from just above the pubic symphysis toward the head (Fig. 9).[17] In addition, it has been suggested that all structures of the lesser pelvis may be imaged more effectively in the transverse plane by scanning through a distended bladder from the opposite side, thus permitting more perpendicular scanning of sidewall structures.[16] The obturator internus muscle may also be seen in longitudinal scans angled from the midline or opposite side toward the pelvic sidewall (Fig. 10).

The levator ani muscle stretches across the pelvic floor like a hammock, separating the pelvis from the perineum (Figs. 1, 8),[15] and is the most caudal structure of the abdominopelvic cavity. In lower animals, the levator ani muscle can be subdivided into its two components, the pubococcygeus and iliococcygeus muscles, but this separation is not as distinct in man.[15] On ultrasound examination, the levator ani muscle is imaged as a relatively hypoechoic curvilinear band situated posterior, medial, and caudal to the obturator internus muscle (Fig. 5B). These two muscles are frequently inseparable laterally because of their major attachment to the fascia surrounding the obturator internus muscle (Figs. 5B,11). The levator ani muscle is less completely seen than the obturator internus. Even with a distended urinary bladder, interposed loops of gas-filled small bowel and rectosigmoid colon may obscure the muscle.

Although the levator ani muscle is routinely imaged in the true anteroposterior transverse plane, it may be accentuated by transverse scans angled caudally from the superior aspect of the urinary bladder toward the feet (Fig. 11).[17] This caudally angled view, while maximizing the size of the levator ani muscle, minimizes the size of the adjacent but more superiorly located obturator internus muscle. On occasion, the levator ani muscle may be imaged on longitudinal scans, angled toward the pelvic sidewall (Fig. 10).

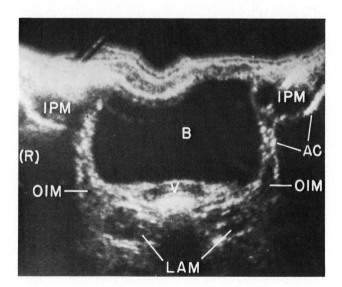

Fig. 11. Caudally angled transverse pelvic ultrasound scan imaged from top of urinary bladder toward feet. The levator ani muscle (LAM) is more prominent while the obturator internus muscle (OIM) is less. Note the difficulty in separating their lateral margins.

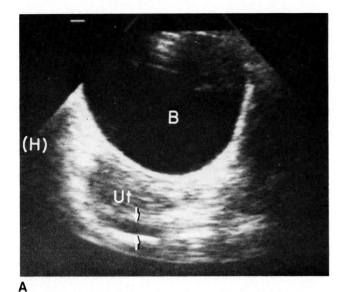

A

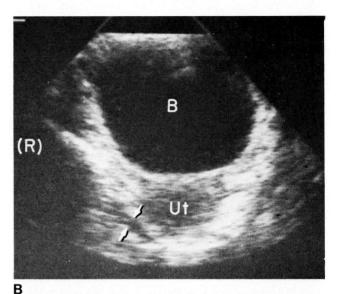

B

The coccygeus and piriformis muscles are less commonly identified by ultrasound because of overlying gas-filled small bowel and sigmoid colon. When the urinary bladder is overdistended, however, these loops may be displaced, allowing visualization on transverse scans, either true anteroposterior or angled cephalad. Both muscles appear acoustically similar to the other muscles, i.e., relatively hypoechoic bands surrounded by the distinct hyperechoic fascial margins. The coccygeus muscle, slightly cranial to the levator ani muscle, appears as a thin, ribbon-shaped muscle (Fig. 4B). The piriformis muscle, seen even deeper and more superiorly, is triangular in shape with the apex of the triangle pointed toward the sacrum (Fig. 3B). Although it has been stated in the past that the piriformis muscle can be mistaken for the more anterior but adjacent ovary,[13,18] we have not found this to be the case. Rather, on occasion, this hypoechoic muscle can be mistaken for fluid slightly eccentrically placed within the cul-de-sac (Figs. 12A,12B). To confirm that the hypoechoic area is the piriformis muscle, we have found that transverse scans angled superiorly from the pubic symphysis toward the head may more clearly define the piriformis muscle (Fig. 12C). Lastly, when transverse scans image the coccygeus, piriformis, and levator ani muscles, the gluteus maximus muscles may also be imaged more posteriorly through the greater sciatic foramen (Figs. 3–5).

PELVIC BLOOD VESSELS

The blood vessels of the pelvis, as the pelvic musculature, can be divided into those predominantly of the greater or lesser pelvis. The common iliac arteries, after

C

Fig. 12. Normal piriformis muscle (PIM) mimicking eccentrically placed fluid in the cul-de-sac. **A.** Longitudinal ultrasound image 2 cm to right of midline showing a hypoechoic area (*arrows*) posterior to uterus (Ut). **B.** Transverse ultrasound image 3 cm above pubic symphysis showing same area (*arrows*) to right of midline. **C.** Cranially angled transverse ultrasound image defining the hypoechoic region as the medial portion of the piriformis muscle.

arising from the bifurcation of the abdominal aorta at the lower lumbar spine, diverge laterally and caudally to enter the greater pelvis, coursing along the anterior medial aspect of the iliopsoas muscle (Fig. 6).[19] In the cranial portion of the greater pelvis, the common iliac arteries bifurcate into the external and internal iliac arteries. The external iliac artery continues its course along the anterior medial aspect of the iliopsoas muscle, and passes behind the inguinal ligament to become the femoral artery in the thigh (Fig. 6). The internal iliac artery, after its origin, immediately passes over the pelvic brim and descends sharply into the lesser pelvis, posterior and slightly lateral to the ovary and ureter (Fig. 6). It continues in a predominantly posterior direction and divides into visceral and parietal branches.[19] The common, external, and internal iliac veins and their branches follow the same course as their companion arteries except that the veins are more posteriorly and usually more medially positioned (Figs. 6, 8).[19]

The ovarian artery and vein enter the greater pelvis anterior to the common iliac artery and vein through the infundibulopelvic ligament and then descend into the lesser pelvis to reach the ovaries via the mesovarium (Fig. 6).[19,20] The ovarian artery and vein are at first superior and lateral to the ovary, then course posteriorly to enter the ovary on its medial aspect at the ovarian hilum. Although the diameter of these vessels is between 3 and 10 mm,[20] the vessels are too small to be routinely imaged except perhaps at the time of ovulation when these vessels may enlarge.

Ultrasound examination of the iliac arteries and veins shows them to be tubular structures, centrally anechoic surrounded by hyperechoic walls. Usually, the arteries can be distinguished from the veins by their more anterior position and with real time by their radial pulsations with each heartbeat. The common iliac artery and vein are either incompletely imaged or nonvisualized superiorly in the greater pelvis primarily due to their deep position with overlying gas-filled bowel. In thin patients with a paucity of bowel gas or in patients with overdistension of the bladder, they may be imaged (Fig. 2B). More inferiorly, the external iliac artery and vein can be more routinely imaged because of their anterior position, particularly through a distended urinary bladder (Figs. 3B,4B,5B,13).[11,13] The precise point at which the common iliac ends and the external begins cannot be defined unless the origin of the internal iliac artery or vein can be identified. On occasion, bladder distension may compress the common and external iliac veins so that only the common and external iliac arteries are imaged (Figs. 2B,3B). When this occurs, partial bladder emptying will allow the veins to reexpand. In addition, if the veins are still difficult to identify, leg raising may allow increased distension. For long-axis imaging of the common and external iliac artery and vein, the same projection as that used for imaging the iliopsoas muscle should be performed, i.e., from the midline toward the hip (Fig. 13B). Transverse and true longitudinal views give only a segmental analysis of the vessels. Further evaluation of these blood vessels can be made by determining their flow patterns with pulsed range-gated doppler.

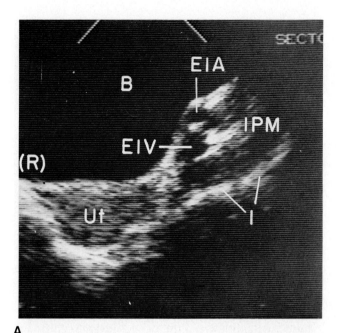

A

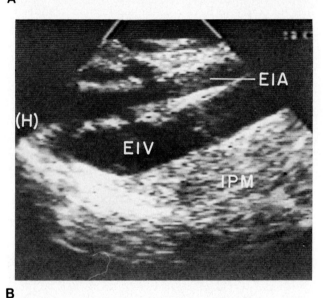

B

Fig. 13. Pelvic ultrasound scans of the left external iliac artery (EIA) and vein (EIV). **A** is the transverse and **B** the longitudinal oblique along the long axis of the blood vessels from midline to hip. The vessels are at the medial margin of the iliopsoas muscle (IPM), with the artery anterior and lateral to the vein.

Ultrasound cannot usually visualize the internal iliac artery and vein at their origins in the superior aspect of the greater pelvis (Fig. 14). They can be routinely imaged posterior and slightly lateral to the ovary and ureter (Figs. 15,16A).[11,16] Not infrequently, these blood vessels can be traced posteriorly and caudally to their bifurcation into vaginal and uterine branches. Their long axis can be imaged in the lesser pelvis primarily on longitudinal scan, angled from the midline

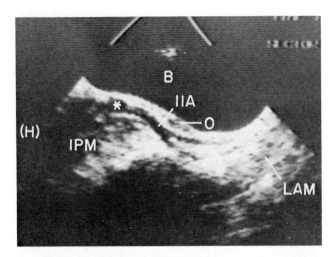

Fig. 14. Longitudinal pelvic ultrasound scan angled from midline toward pelvic sidewall showing the origin (*) of the internal iliac artery (IIA) at the medial margin of the iliopsoas muscle (IPM).

or opposite side toward the pelvic sidewall. Although it is necessary to have a distended urinary bladder to optimally image these vessels, overdistension may sometimes compress the internal iliac vein so that only the artery is seen (Fig. 15A). Partial emptying of the bladder will allow the vein to reexpand (Fig. 15B).

Computed tomography can also image the blood vessels (Figs. 2A,3A,4A,5A).[8] Usually, however, CT is not able to distinguish between the artery and the vein except (1) if intravenous or intraarterial contrast has been given, (2) if a catheter has been placed within a blood vessel, or (3) if calcification in the iliac arteries is present.

The detection of lymph nodes, which lie alongside the artery and vein, is better appreciated with CT than with ultrasound.[8,14] Although adenopathy greater than 2 to 3 cm can be routinely imaged with ultrasound, normal pelvic lymph nodes have not been seen.[16] Computed tomography can identify normal lymph nodes and has been shown to detect subtle adenopathy as small as 1 to 2 cm in size.[21,22]

URETER

The ureters, originating from the kidneys, initially lie anterior to the psoas muscles, and upon entering the greater pelvis, run anterior to the common iliac artery and vein (Fig. 6).[23] They then pass over the pelvic brim, descend into the lesser pelvis, continuing both posterior to the ovaries and also medial and anterior to the internal iliac vessels (Figs. 6, 8). The ureters then continue caudally to insert into the trigone on both sides of the cervix at the region of the upper portion of the vaginal canal (Fig. 8).[23]

The ureters cannot be imaged within the greater pelvis due to their small size and overlying gas-filled bowel. They can be routinely seen in the lesser pelvis through a distended urinary bladder.[11,13] The ureters can be followed from the region posterior to the ovary, parallel to the posterior margin of the urinary bladder (Figs. 16A,16B), and occasionally to their insertions into the bladder trigones (Figs. 16D,16E). The ureter is best imaged in its long axis, with scans performed from the midline or opposite side toward the pelvic sidewall (Figs. 16A,16B,16D), but may also be seen in transverse view (Fig. 16C). The ureter has hyperechoic walls, usually brighter than the walls of the adjacent internal iliac artery and vein, with an anechoic

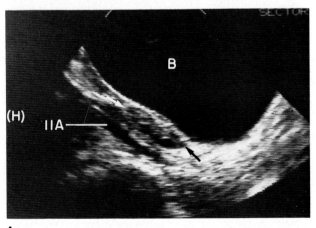

A

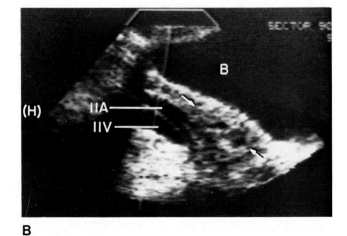

B

Fig. 15. The effect of urinary bladder (B) distension on the internal iliac vein (IIV). Longitudinal pelvis scans angled from midline toward pelvic sidewall. In **A,** with an overdistended urinary bladder, only the internal iliac artery (IIA) was imaged. In **B,** after partial voiding, the internal iliac vein reexpanded posterior to the artery. Arrows denote edge of normal ovary.

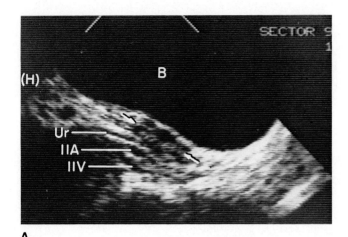

A

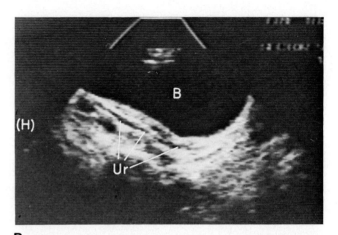

B

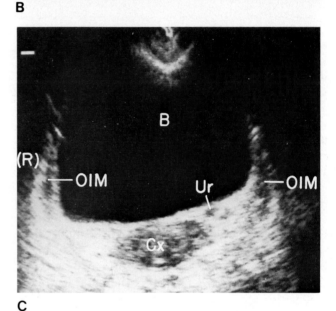

C

Fig. 16. Pelvic ultrasound scan of the ureter (Ur). **A.** Longitudinal scan angled from midline toward pelvic sidewall showing the ureter anterior to the more laterally positioned internal iliac artery (IIA) and vein (IIV). Note the ureteric walls are more hyperechoic than those of the artery and vein. **B.** Longitudinal scan angled from midline toward pelvic sidewall showing ureter parallel to posterior margin of bladder. **C.** Transverse scan showing the left ureter adjacent to the cervix (Cx). On occasion, uterine blood vessels may be imaged in this region so that a long axis view is also needed to confirm that the structure is the ureter (*cont*).

center (Fig. 16A). Real-time examination allows imaging of normal peristalsis within the ureter as a sparkling pattern of intermittent echoes without change in the inner diameter of the ureter.[17] When imaged posterior to the normally placed ovary, the ureter is usually anterior and medial to the internal iliac vessels (Fig. 16A). To date, there has not been a measurement determining the ureter's upper limits of normal.

As the ureter inserts into the urinary bladder, occasionally a small papilla, visualized as a slight rise in the bladder wall, can be seen (Figs. 16E,16F). Within the urinary bladder, as within the ureter, intermittent showers of echoes can be imaged as the urine passes from the ureter into the bladder (Figs. 16E,16F).[24,25] This is termed the "ureteric jet phenomenon." It is best appreciated with real time in a caudally angled transverse view as a bright intermittent hyperechoic stream originating from the ureteric orifice and extending in a straight line for approximately 3 cm toward the opposite lateral wall of the bladder before dissipating. When both ureters discharge urine into the bladder simultaneously, the bilateral jets criss-cross. Each jet averages approximately 3.5 seconds in duration and has a frequency of between 2 and 4 per minute.[25] It is felt that the jet effect results from differences in specific gravity as the urine passes from ureters into the bladder.[25]

In the pelvis, the ureters pass close to the ovaries and to the cervix (Figs. 6,8,16C,16D). Any abnormality of these structures may potentially obstruct the ureter on that side, leading to ureterectasis and hydronephrosis. Therefore, if an abnormality is seen in the ovary or cervix, the ipsilateral ureter should be sought. If the ureter cannot be visualized, if it is felt to be slightly enlarged or if persistalsis is not seen, the ipsilateral kidney should be examined for possible hydronephrosis. Additionally, due to the position of the ureters as they pass over the pelvic brim, any enlargement

of the uterus may potentially obstruct the ureters, leading to bilateral hydronephrosis.

URINARY BLADDER

Within the lesser pelvis, the urinary bladder is the most anterior of the midline unpaired organs, anchored caudally by the urethra and the trigone (Figs. 6,8,17).[23] In its nondistended state, the bladder is collapsed

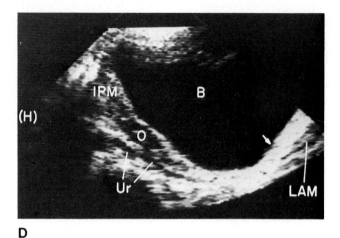

D

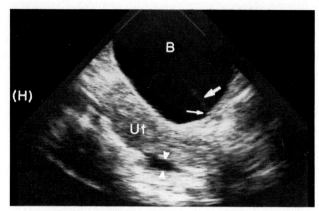

E

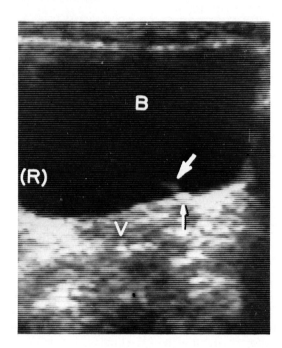

F

against the urethra and trigone. When the bladder fills with urine, its anterior and superior surfaces distend, displacing a significant amount of small bowel and mesentery out of the lesser pelvis. Since the rectum and vagina are midline unpaired structures posterior to the bladder and also anchored in the pelvic diaphragm, they are not displaced by the distended urinary bladder. Bladder distension, however, bows the vagina posteriorly and affects the position of the more cephalic structures of the lesser pelvis—the uterus, sigmoid colon, and adnexa (Fig. 17).

On ultrasound examination, the distended urinary bladder is an anechoic structure with smooth, thin walls. There are predictable contours to the urinary bladder in both transverse and longitudinal views. In transverse sections, the superior portion of the urinary bladder is rounded (Figs. 2B,3B). When prominent iliopsoas muscles are present, the lateral walls are straightened and indented in both longitudinal and transverse projections (Figs. 4B,18).[17] This same phenomenon has been described on CT (Fig. 4A).[26] More inferiorly, the lateral walls of the urinary bladder are squared due to the parallel walls of the acetabulum (Figs. 5,11).[17] In its long axis, the urinary bladder is usually triangular in shape, both in the midline and laterally, with the lower or caudad surface parallel to the vagina, the anterior surface parallel to the anterior abdominal wall, and the third side extending obliquely from the superior aspect of the vagina toward the umbilicus (Fig. 19). These normal shapes cannot be overemphasized. Although all normal structures cause slight indentation on the urinary bladder, it is highly unusual for indentation to occur from any other structure, including normal bowel, except when fecal impaction is present.[17] For this reason, except in cases where previous bladder or pelvic surgery has been performed, any shape that differs from those described above, especially if asymmetry is created, should be

Fig. 16. cont. D. Longitudinal scan angled from midline toward pelvic sidewall showing the ureter posterior to the ovary (O). Arrow denotes ureteral insertion into bladder (the superior portion of the trigone) initially identified by detecting a ureteric jet originating from that point. **E.** Longitudinal scan angled from midline toward pelvic sidewall showing a papilla (*small arrow*) at the insertion of the ureter into the bladder. Large arrow denotes ureteric jet extending from papilla into bladder. Arrowheads denote fluid in posterior cul-de-sac. **F.** Transverse scan angled toward feet showing a small papilla (*small arrow*) at the insertion of the left ureter into the bladder. This is the superior portion of the trigone. Large arrow denotes a ureteric jet extending from papilla into bladder.

considered abnormal and a mass at the place of distortion should be carefully sought.

The technique of using at least moderate urinary bladder distension is also very important. In addition to the displacement of small bowel out of the pelvis,

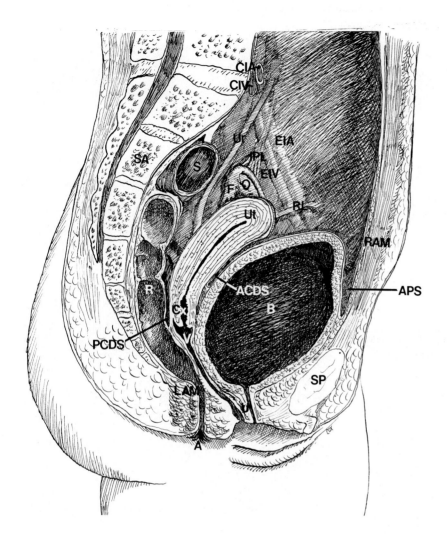

Fig. 17. Sagittal midline pelvic diagram showing the cut sections of midline organs and intact structures of opposite pelvic sidewall.

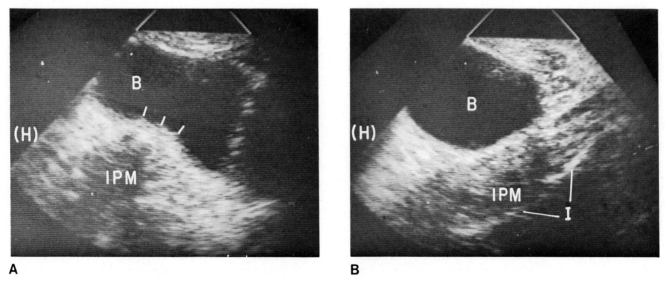

A   B

Fig. 18. Normal iliopsoas muscle (IPM) indenting urinary bladder. **A.** Longitudinal pelvic ultrasound scan 4 cm to left of midline showing an indentation (*denoted by lines*). **B.** Longitudinal oblique ultrasound scan angled along the long axis of the muscle, showing that the indentation was caused by the adjacent iliopsoas muscle.

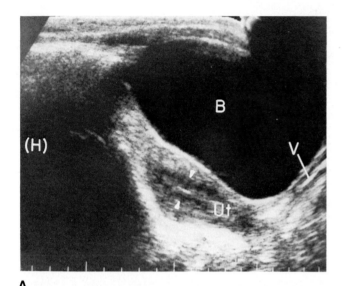

A

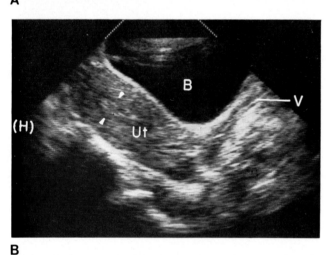

B

Fig. 19. Nulliparous uteri. Longitudinal midline pelvic ultrasound scans of uterus (Ut) and vagina (V) in two postpubertal-premenopausal women. The echogenicity of vagina is greater than that of the uterus. The urinary bladders (B) are triangular in shape. **A.** Uterus in preovulatory (proliferative) phase showing a thin hyperechoic endometrial canal surrounded by hypoechoic endometrium (*arrowheads*). **B.** Uterus in postovulatory (secretory) phase showing a slightly thicker and less hyperechoic endometrial interface surrounded by a thicker hypoechoic granular endometrium (*arrowheads*).

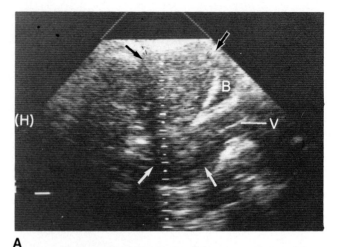

A

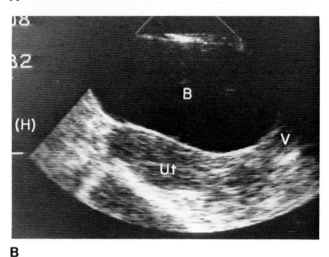

B

Fig. 20. The effect of urinary bladder (B) distension on vaginal shape and on uterine shape and position. **A.** Longitudinal midline pelvic ultrasound scan with an almost empty bladder showing an anteverted uterus (*arrows*). Note thickness of vagina (V). **B.** Longitudinal midline pelvic ultrasound scan with a very distended bladder in the same patient showing a thinner elongated vagina bowed posteriorly and a compressed uterus (Ut) displaced horizontally.

which to compare the echopatterns of the normal pelvic organs and pelvic masses.[11]

VAGINA AND UTERUS

The vagina is a midline structure with an overall length of 7 to 10 cm, situated between the caudal portions of the urinary bladder anteriorly and the rectum posteriorly (Figs. 8,17).[27] The uterus and its most caudad portion, the cervix, is a thick-walled hollow muscular organ contiguous with and superior to the vagina (Figs. 6,8,17).[27] The most common uterine position is midline and anteverted, forming an angle of between 45 and

the distended bladder serves as an acoustic window to optimally image the adjacent structures. Although moderate to marked distension of the urinary bladder may cause anatomic distortion of the vagina and uterus, the ovaries, and sigmoid colon, interpretation is rarely hindered (Fig. 20). When the bladder is not distended, however, the normal structures may not be completely imaged or on occasion may be misinterpreted as masses (Figs. 21,22). The distended urinary bladder also serves as a fluid-filled reference with

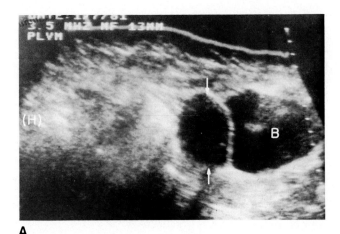
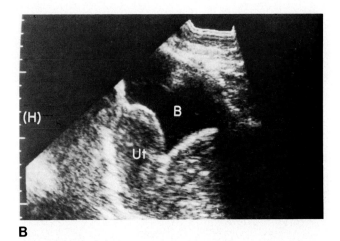

Fig. 21. The value of urinary bladder (B) distension on uterine visualization. **A.** Longitudinal midline pelvic ultrasound scan through incompletely filled bladder showing apparent hypoechoic mass (*arrows*) superior to bladder. **B.** Longitudinal scan in same patient through well-distended bladder showing the "mass" to be a normal anteflexed uterus (Ut).

90 degrees with the vagina (Fig. 17).[18] The uterus may instead extend normally to the right or left of midline and be anteflexed or retroflexed (see Chapter 38).

On ultrasound examination, the vagina is imaged posterior to the lower part of the urinary bladder. It normally appears as a collapsed tube with a central high amplitude linear reflector from the apposed surfaces of the vaginal mucosa (Fig. 19).[18] This bright reflector is surrounded by the thin anterior and posterior hypoechoic vaginal walls, which should not have an overall thickness of greater than 1 cm.[13] It has been stated that the posterior fornix in transverse scan may

be misinterpreted as a hyperechoic bullseye or pelvic mass.[13] In our experience, this situation rarely causes diagnostic confusion. If fluid accumulates in the vagina, an anechoic area may be imaged within the vagina, instead of the usual hyperechoic apposed mucosa. When this occurs, the anterior and posterior vaginal fornices surrounding the lower aspect of the cervix are visualized.[17] In the adult, this is usually due to recently menstruated blood, whereas in children the anechoic area is usually urine secondary to either physiologic or pathologic incontinence.[13,14]

The uterine size and shape varies with age, parity,

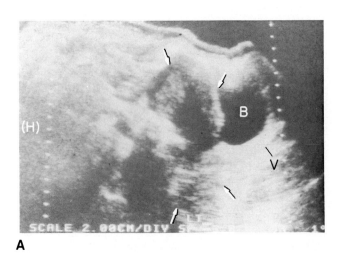
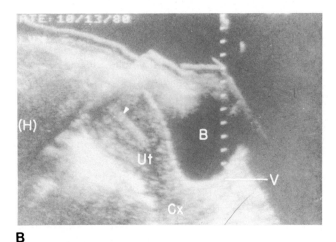

Fig. 22. The value of urinary bladder (B) distension on uterine visualization in a multiparous woman. **A.** Longitudinal midline pelvic ultrasound scan through incompletely filled bladder showing an apparent mass (*arrows*) of mixed echogenicity. **B.** Longitudinal scan in same patient through well distended bladder showing the "mass" to be a prominent anteverted uterus (Ut). The prominent uterus, measuring 13 cm in long axis, was otherwise normal. Arrowhead = endometrial canal.

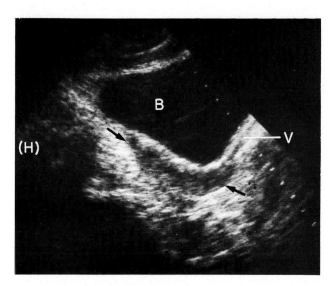

Fig. 23. Infantile uterus. Longitudinal midline pelvic ultrasound scan showing a small tubular uterus (*arrows*) with thin fundus.

and time of the menstrual cycle.[18] At birth, the uterus is small but has an adult shape secondary to maternal hormonal stimulation.[14] After this stimulation disappears, the cervix occupies two-thirds to five-sixths of the total uterine length with the diameter of the uterine corpus less than the diameter of the cervix (Fig. 23). During this prepubertal period, the average uterine length is 2.5 cm and anteroposterior diameter is 1 cm.[16] When menarchy begins, the uterine corpus grows predominantly in width and thickness, assuming a pear-shaped appearance, measuring no greater than 8 cm in its long axis (from the base of the cervix to the top of the fundus), 5.5 cm in width and 3 cm in anterior posterior dimension in the nulliparous woman (Fig. 19).[16,28] In the multiparous woman, the length of the uterus in its nonpregnant state may enlarge at least 1.5 to 2.0 cm (Fig. 22B). Postmenopausally, the uterus undergoes atrophy and decreases to a size no greater than 6.5 cm in long axis and 2 cm in anterior posterior dimension.[29] It also assumes less of a pear shape but does not revert to the infantile form.

During the post pubertal–premenopausal period, three areas within the uterus can be identified by their echogenicity: (1) an area of low- to medium-level echogenicity throughout the myometrium, (2) a hyperechoic central interface, corresponding to the apposed endometrial linings, brighter than the myometrium, and (3) a thin, interposed, rim, corresponding to the endometrium (Fig. 19).[11] The endometrial canal can be imaged in almost all patients, except in retroverted and retroflexed uteri, and is typically less bright than the midline vaginal echo (Figs. 19,22B).[30] The prominence of the endometrium and the size of the uterus

are related to the stage of the menstrual cycle in three ways. First, the thickness and brightness of the endometrial lining is not constant. During the proliferative phase (preovulatory), the endometrial lining is thin and bright, while during the secretory phase (postovulatory), the lining is usually slightly thicker, less well-defined, and slightly less hyperechoic (Fig. 19). Second, the hypoechoic zone surrounding the endometrial lining, corresponding to the endometrium, has been shown to become more prominent just prior to menstruation.[31] Third, the uterine size progressively enlarges slightly during each cycle from the time of menstruation until it reaches a maximum by the twenty-seventh day of the cycle.[28]

The degree of bladder distension may greatly affect the vagina and uterus. With a full bladder, while the overall vaginal position is unchanged, it may be elongated, thinned, and bowed posteriorly (Fig. 20). The uterine position and, on occasion, the shape, are also affected by bladder distension. Most commonly, when the bladder is empty, the uterus is sharply anteflexed (Fig. 20A). When the urinary bladder is distended, the uterus is frequently displaced from an anteverted toward a horizontal position. Occasionally the full bladder causes additional uterine compression and elongation (Fig. 20B). If the sacrum is also horizontal, the uterus may be further compressed between it and the bladder. We have also noted that the echogenicity of the endometrial canal may be affected by urinary bladder distension. It must be reemphasized that although urinary bladder distension may create anatomic distortion of the uterus, a full bladder will allow more complete visualization of the uterus (Fig. 20). When the urinary bladder is not adequately distended, the uterus may not be fully imaged and on occasion the fundus may be mistaken for a mass (Figs. 21,22).

The vagina and uterus are usually imaged best in a true longitudinal plane. However, if the uterus extends to the right or left of the midline, transverse scans are sometimes necessary to define the true axis of the uterus (Fig. 4B).[16] When the uterus is not midline, scans should be performed in an oblique longitudinal direction to include the vagina with the full extent of the uterus. To allow for correct orientation of the adnexa in these patients, longitudinal scans laterally to the right and left of midline should be performed without changing the scanning angle.

The normal uterine shape, echogenicity and endometrial echoes are routinely imaged in the anteverted and horizontally placed uterus. All of these findings may be greatly distorted in the more posteriorly positioned retroverted and/or retroflexed uterus, which assumes a globular shape, a decreased echogenicity, and a loss of the identifiable endometrial echo due to

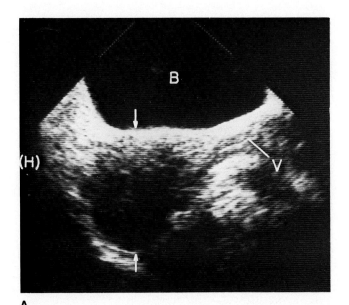

A

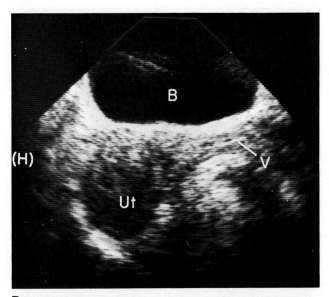

B

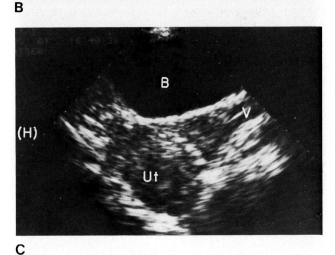

C

Fig. 24. Retroverted and retroflexed uteri. **A.** Longitudinal midline pelvic ultrasound scan showing a globular hypoechoic area (*arrowheads*) occupying the body and fundus of the uterus at normal signal amplification. **B.** Longitudinal scan in same patient as scan **A** but with increased signal amplification. The normal echogenicity of the retroverted uterus (Ut) is now apparent. **C.** Longitudinal midline pelvic ultrasound scan in a second patient at high signal amplification showing a retroflexed uterus (Ut) with normal echogenicity.

change in uterine angulation even after bladder emptying (Fig. 24).[17,30] Although the globular shape cannot be explained, the decreased echogenicity is probably due to absorption of the ultrasound beam as it traverses more uterine muscle. Increasing the overall signal amplification will allow more penetration of the uterus and will show the normal uniform uterine echogenicity, eliminating the possible misdiagnosis of a fibroid (Figs. 24A,24B).[17]

Computed tomography cannot consistently define the vagina and uterus (Figs. 3A,4A,5A). Frequently the vagina can only be demonstrated when an air-containing tampon is inserted.[8] The uterus can only be inferred by its position directly superior and contiguous with the vagina. If the urinary bladder is not distended, the uterus may be misdiagnosed as a mass with a very large anteroposterior dimension. Since the cranial–caudal extent is narrow, however, a rounded mass could not be present, and thus the correct diagnosis can at least be inferred.

ADNEXA

The adnexa consist of the fallopian tubes, broad ligaments, mesosalpinges and ovaries (Figs. 6,8).[27] The fallopian tubes extend serpiginously from the fundal aspect of the uterus, a distance of 7 to 14 cm, finally terminating at the ovaries (Fig. 6). The ovaries are the only truly intraperitoneal adnexal structures, and in the nulliparous woman lie in a shallow depression named the ovarian fossa (Fig. 8).[27] This fossa is on the lateral wall of the pelvis, bound by the external iliac vessels, the obliterated umbilical artery and the

ureter. The ovary is suspended in the pelvic peritoneum by the mesovarium, the mesosalpinx, and by the broad, ovarian, and the infundibulopelvic ligaments, so that the usual ovarian position is lateral to the superior aspect of the uterine body. During the first pregnancy, however, it is displaced from the ovarian fossa and probably never returns.[27] In addition, ovarian position is affected by the position of the uterus, by urinary bladder distension, and occasionally by rectal fullness

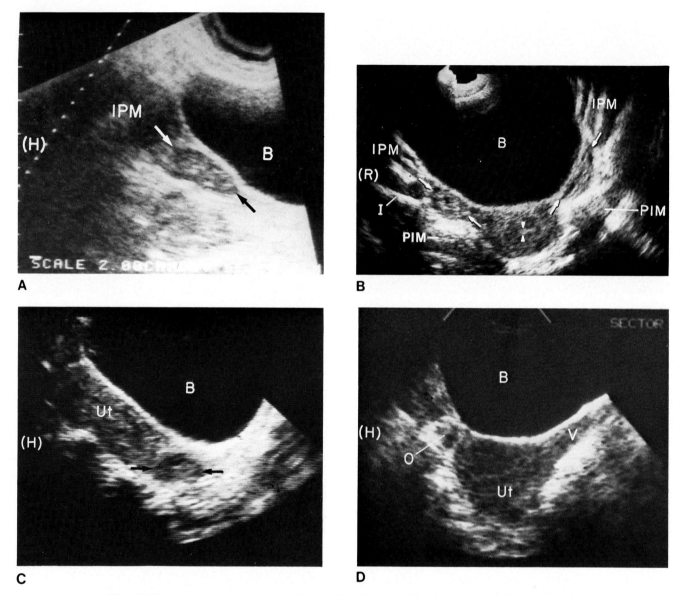

Fig. 25. Variations in normal ovarian position. **A.** Longitudinal pelvic ultrasound scan 3 cm to left of midline showing the normal ovary (*arrows*) in long axis. **B.** Transverse pelvic ultrasound scan in the same patient at the superior aspect of the uterine body showing both ovaries (*arrows*) and the intervening uterus with a well-defined endometrial canal (*arrowheads*). The scan was performed from the right toward the left pelvic sidewall. Note the ovaries are one-third to one-quarter the size of the adjacent uterus. Part of both piriformis muscles are imaged. **C.** Longitudinal pelvic ultrasound scan 2 cm to right of midline in another patient showing the uterus (Ut) deviated to the right and the ovary (*arrows*) posterior in the cul-de-sac. **D.** Angled longitudinal pelvic ultrasound scanned from the midline slightly toward the left in a third patient showing a retroverted uterus with the left ovary (O) superior to the fundus near the midline.

so that the ovaries may lie instead posterolateral, directly posterior, or even superior to the uterus.[11,13] Of all of these, the position of the uterus seems to be of particular importance in determining ovarian position. This is due to the ovarian ligament, which connects the ovary to the uterine fundus and is shorter and more dense than the infundibulopelvic ligament.

The ovary, therefore, tends to follow the uterus. When the uterus is normally anteflexed and midline, the ovaries are usually directly lateral or posterolateral to it (Figs. 25A,25B). When the uterus is deviated to one side, the ipsilateral ovary is frequently superior to the uterine fundus, but may on occasion be imaged within the cul-de-sac posteriorly (Fig. 25C).[16] When the uterus

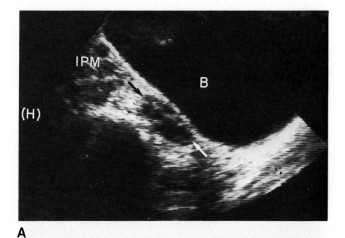

A

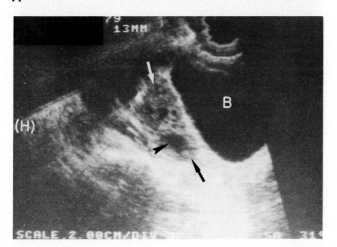

B

Fig. 26. Serial longitudinal pelvic ultrasound scans of the right ovary in their most common position lateral to the uterus. **A.** Ovary (*between arrows*) with multiple immature follicles 5 days postmenses. **B.** Same ovary (*between arrows*) just prior to ovulation. There is one dominant cyst (*arrowhead*) measuring 20 mm.

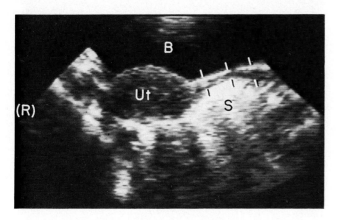

Fig. 27. Transverse pelvic ultrasound scan at level of uterine fundus (Ut). The left adnexal structures (*lines*) including the fallopian tube, ligaments, mesosalpinx, and mesovarium can be identified between the urinary bladder (B) and the sigmoid colon (S).

is retroverted and midline, both ovaries are commonly lateral, superior, and close to the uterine fundus near the midline (Fig. 25D).

On ultrasound examination, the ovaries are routinely imaged as ovoid structures, with their longest axis cranial–caudal along the same axis as the internal iliac artery and vein (Fig. 25A).[16] Because of great variability in normal ovarian shapes, all three dimensions should be obtained to determine if the ovary is enlarged, with the best analysis of ovarian size made by calculating a volume based on a simplified formula for a prolate ellipse, (length × width × height)/2.[16] In the prepubertal period, below the age of 2, the ovaries are rarely imaged and should be less than 1 cm³ in volume.[16,32] Between the ages of 2 and 12, still in the prepubertal period, the ovarian volume enlarges but should still be less than 1 cm³. In the post pubertal-premenopausal period, the ovary enlarges to measure 3 × 2 × 1 cm on the average, with the longest axis occasionally measuring 5 cm.[11] The largest volume is expected, however, not to exceed 6 cm³.[16] Another approach to ovarian size is to image the ovary and the adjacent uterus in transverse projection; usually the normal ovary is between one-third and one-quarter the uterine size (Fig. 25B).[33]

Although it is generally felt that in the postmenopausal patient the atrophic ovary can rarely be identified,[16] a recent study comparing ultrasound of the pelvis to laparotomy detected 84 percent of normal ovaries in this age group.[34] This study found the normal ovary to have a mean volume of 4 to 5 cm³, not significantly different from that of premenopausal ovaries, with some as large as 10 cm³. The mean difference between the volumes of the right and left ovaries was only 1 to 2 cm³. It was suggested that if an ovary were twice the average volume or twice the size of the contralateral ovary, neoplasm should be suspected.

The ovary demonstrates an echogenicity that is higher in amplitude but with a fewer number of reflectors than that of the uterus (Figs. 25A,25B). However, in the postpubertal–premenopausal period, multiple cysts or follicles normally develop during each menstrual cycle, distorting the ovarian size, shape and echogenicity (Fig. 26). Although a detailed analysis of follicular development or abnormal cystic changes of the ovaries will not be dealt with in this chapter, the follicles generally develop in the early part of the menstrual cycle, with one dominant follicle reaching an average size of 18 to 25 mm by the time of ovulation (Fig. 26B).[35-37] Within seconds of ovulation, a rapid reduction in follicular size with irregular outlines and increased internal echogenicity can be seen, occasionally with simultaneous free fluid imaged in the cul-de-sac.[18]

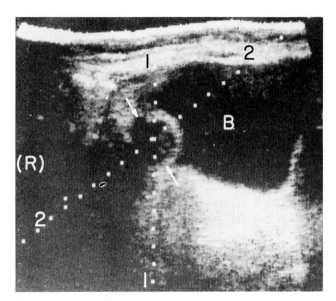

A

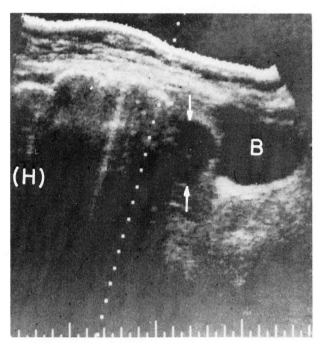

B

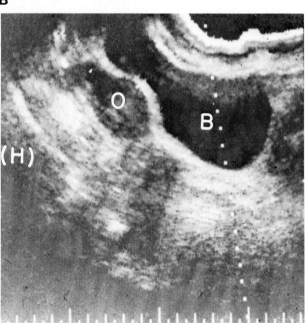

C

The remainder of the adnexa is only infrequently identified on ultrasound examination. When imaged, it is best seen in transverse view as a thin, moderately hyperechoic area no greater than 5 mm in maximum thickness arising from the uterine fundus (Fig. 27). It is on occasion difficult to separate the normal adnexa from the adjacent wall of the urinary bladder. Abnormality of the fallopian tubes, however, can be suggested if an abnormality can be traced to the fundus of the uterus, particularly if the area is thicker than 5 mm, is tubular with an anechoic center, or is rounded.

The urinary bladder should always be distended when imaging the ovaries. Although this technique may change the ovarian position, utilization of the filled bladder is often the only adequate way to visualize the ovaries with ultrasound, and is particularly helpful when the ovary is superior to the urinary bladder.[16] When the ovary is far lateral to the uterus or at the superior aspect of the urinary bladder, transverse and longitudinal images directly over the ovary may not be adequate to fully define the ovary (Fig. 28). Scans angled from the opposite side in both longitudinal and transverse projections will frequently image more of the ovary using the urinary bladder as an acoustic window.[11,17]

Computed tomography is usually not of great value in imaging the adnexae or normal ovaries (Fig. 3A). Other soft tissue densities such as blood vessels, lymph nodes, and even fluid-filled bowel can be imaged adjacent to the uterus, making separation of the adnexae from these structures difficult.

Fig. 28. Technique for ovarian scanning. **A.** Transverse pelvic ultrasound scan superior to uterus showing rounded structure (*arrows*) at the right superior margin of the bladder (B). Dotted lines, numbers 1 and 2, denote position of longitudinal planes in **B** and **C. B.** Longitudinal scan along dotted Line 1 showing the same rounded structure (*arrows*) at superior margin of bladder (B). No further definition of this structure can be made. **C.** Longitudinal scan obliqued from the left side toward the right pelvic sidewall along dotted line 2. The ovary (O) can now be clearly defined. Note that this scanning plane allowed more bladder to be imaged anterior to the ovary, allowing better visualization.

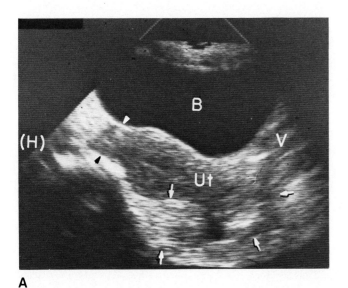

A

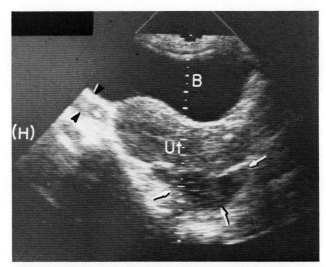

B

RECTOSIGMOID COLON

In the lesser pelvis, the rectum is fixed retroperitoneally in the midline directly posterior to the vagina (Figs. 8,17). It is continuous with the sigmoid colon cranially at the level of the third sacral vertebral body, extending caudally to end in the anal canal (Figs. 6,17).[38] The sigmoid colon originates at the descending colon at the left superior aspect of the lesser pelvis and forms one or two loops in the lesser pelvis before becoming continuous with the rectum inferiorly. It is completely surrounded by peritoneum and is attached to the pelvic wall by an extensive mesentery termed the sigmoid mesocolon.[38] This mesocolon allows the sigmoid colon to be quite redundant in certain patients and may extend far to the right or left of midline or may remain centrally located. It also permits considerable range of movement in its central portion.[38]

Ultrasound descriptions of the colon have shown various patterns, depending upon the amount of gas, fluid, and feces present. Since peristalsis is not common in the colon, only infrequently can movement within the bowel allow differentiation of true pelvic mass from a fluid and feces pseudotumor of the rectosigmoid colon.[6] For this reason, when there is any doubt that a suspected mass might be a pseudotumor, particularly in the regions posterior or posterolateral to the uterus and ovaries, water should be introduced into the rectum to define the position and extent of the rectosigmoid colon (Figs. 29A,29B).[5,6] This water enema examination clearly images the distended rectum in longitudinal and transverse planes immediately posterior to the vagina and bladder (Fig. 29B). The sigmoid colon can also be imaged, but is usually more difficult

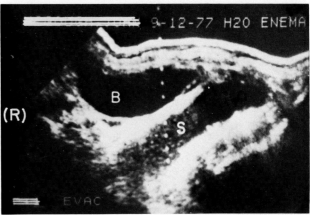

C

Fig. 29. Normal rectosigmoid colon. **A.** Longitudinal pelvic midline scan showing two ill-defined areas that may be pseudotumors of the rectosigmoid colon. One area is posterior to the uterus (Ut) denoted by arrows and the other is superior to the uterus denoted by arrowheads. **B.** Longitudinal midline scan in same patient after introduction of water into the rectum showing the two areas to have changed in shape and echogenicity. The posterior area is rectum and the superior area is sigmoid colon. **C.** Transverse scan in another patient at dome of urinary bladder (B) showing water-filled sigmoid colon (S) after water enema. The echogenic material within the colon represents feces.

to appreciate. In general, longitudinal scans to the left of midline or transverse oblique scans from the right hip toward the left shoulder at the dome of the urinary bladder will often image the sigmoid colon (Figs. 29B,29C). It is preferable to do this examination under continuous real-time supervision through a partially distended urinary bladder. Lukewarm water is introduced in small increments to minimize patient discomfort and to allow for quick and accurate identification of the rectosigmoid colon.

RETROPERITONEAL REFLECTIONS

The peritoneal surface covers the superior aspect of the urinary bladder, uterus and rectum (Fig. 8). With distension of the urinary bladder, three potential peritoneal spaces are formed: the anterior peritoneal space between the anterior peritoneum and the urinary bladder, the anterior cul-de-sac between the bladder and the anterior aspect of the uterus, and the posterior cul-de-sac between the uterus and rectum (Figs. 8,17). The latter compartment is the largest of these spaces and the most posteriorly located, extending caudally to at least the upper one-quarter of the vagina, frequently containing normal small bowel and mesentery. Because of its posterior position, it is the most common pelvic site for peritoneal collections to accumulate. The other two compartments are much smaller and are only infrequently involved with pathogenic processes.

ACKNOWLEDGMENT

The authors wish to thank Mr. Larry Waldroup for his technical expertise and Ms. JoAnn Anderson and Mrs. Rosemarie K. Boccella for their editorial assistance.

REFERENCES

1. Cochrane WJ, Thomas MA: Ultrasound diagnosis of gynecologic pelvic masses. Radiology 110:649, 1974
2. Fleischer AC, James AE Jr, Millis JB, et al: Differential diagnosis of pelvic masses by gray scale sonography. Am J Roentgenol 131:469, 1978
3. Lawson TL, Albarelli JN: Diagnosis of gynecologic pelvic masses by gray scale ultrasonography: Analysis of specificity and accuracy. Am J Roentgenol 128:1003, 1977
4. Walsh JW, Taylor KJW, Wasson JFM, et al: Gray-scale ultrasound in 204 proved gynecologic masses: Accuracy and specific diagnostic criteria. Radiology 130:391, 1979
5. Rubin C, Kurtz AB, Goldberg BB: Water enema: A new ultrasound technique in defining pelvic anatomy. J Clin Ultrasound 6(1):28, 1978
6. Kurtz AB, Rubin CS, Kramer FL, et al: Ultrasound evaluation of the posterior pelvic compartment. Radiology 132:677, 1979
7. Gray H: Osteology, in Goss CM (ed), Gray's Anatomy, 28th ed. Philadelphia, Lea & Febiger, 1966, pp 236–245
8. Balfe DM, Peterson RR, Lee JKT: Normal abdominal anatomy, in Lee JKT, Sagel SS, Stanley RJ (eds), Computed Body Tomography. New York, Raven, 1983, pp 131–165
9. Rubin CS, Kurtz AB, Bancks NH, et al: Abdominal compression: A new technique for improved computed tomographic images. Radiology 132:751, 1979
10. Revak CS: Mineral content of cortical bone measured by computed tomography. J Computer Asst Tomogr 4(3):342, 1980
11. Green B: Pelvic ultrasonography, in Sarti DA, Sample WF (eds), Diagnostic Ultrasound. Boston, MA, G.K. Hall, 1980, pp 502–589
12. Gray H: Muscles and fasciae, in Gross CM (ed), Gray's Anatomy, 28th ed. Philadelphia, Lea & Febiger, 1966, pp 490–507
13. Sample WF: Gray scale ultrasonography of the normal female pelvis, in Sanders RC, James AE (eds), The Principles and Practice of Ultrasonography in Obstetrics and Gynecology, 2nd ed. New York, Appleton-Century-Crofts, 1980, pp 75–89
14. Sample WF, Sarti DA: Normal anatomy of the female pelvis: Computed tomography and ultrasonography, in Rosenfield AT (ed), Genitourinary Ultrasonography. New York, Churchill Livingstone, 1979, pp 191–205
15. Gray H: Muscles and fasciae, in Goss CM (ed), Gray's Anatomy, 28th ed. Philadelphia, Lea & Febiger, 1966, pp 434–438
16. Sample WF, Lippe BM, Gyepes MT: Gray-scale ultrasonography of the normal female pelvis. Radiology 125:477, 1977
17. Kurtz AB, Rifkin MD: Normal anatomy of the female pelvis, in Callen PW (ed), Ultrasonography of Obstetrics and Gynecology. Philadelphia, Saunders, 1983, pp 193–207
18. Deutsch AL, Gosink BB: Normal female pelvic anatomy. Semin Roentgenol 17(4):241, 1982
19. Gray H: The arteries, in Goss CM (ed), Gray's Anatomy, 28th ed. Philadelphia, Lea & Febiger, 1966, pp 628–656
20. Hackeloer BJ, Nitschke-Dabelstein S: Ovarian imaging by ultrasound: An attempt to define a reference plane. J Clin Ultrasound 8:497, 1980
21. Walsh JW, Amendola MA, Konerding KF, et al: Computed tomographic detection of pelvic and inguinal lymph-node metastases from primary and recurrent pelvic malignant disease. Radiology 137:157, 1980
22. Glazer GM, Goldberg HI, Moss AA, et al: Computed tomographic detection of retroperitoneal adenopathy. Radiology 143:147, 1982
23. Gray H: The urogenital system, in Goss CM (ed), Gray's Anatomy, 28th ed. Philadelphia, Lea & Febiger, 1966, pp 1287–1296
24. Dubbins PA, Kurtz AB, Darby J, et al: Ureteric jet effect: The echographic appearance of urine entering the bladder. Radiology 140:513, 1981
25. Kremer H, Dobrinski W, Mikyska M, et al: Ultrasonic in vivo and in vitro studies on jet phenomenon. Radiology 142:175, 1982
26. Wechsler RJ, Brennan RE: Teardrop bladder: Additional considerations. Radiology 144:281, 1982

27. Gray H: The urogenital system, in Goss CM (ed), Gray's Anatomy, 28th ed. Philadelphia, Lea & Febiger, 1966, pp 1316–1334

28. Piiroinen O, Kaihola HL: Uterine size measured by ultrasound during the menstrual cycle. Acta Obstet Scand 54:247, 1975

29. Miller EI, Thomas RH, Lines P: The atrophic postmenopausal uterus. J Clin Ultrasound 5(4):261, 1977

30. Callen PW, DeMartini WJ, Filly RA: The central uterine cavity echo: A useful anatomic sign in the ultrasonographic evaluation of the female pelvis. Radiology 131:187, 1977

31. Kelley D, Hall D, Hann L, et al: Sonographic morphology of the normal menstrual cycle. Presented at the 24th Annual Meeting of the American Institute of Ultrasound in Medicine, San Diego, CA, 1978

32. Haller JO, Schneider M, Kassner G, et al: Ultrasonography in pediatric gynecology and obstetrics. Am J Roentgenol 128:423, 1977

33. Zemlyn S: Comparison of pelvic ultrasonography and pneumography for ovarian size. J Clin Ultrasound 2(4):331, 1974

34. Campbell S, Goessens L, Goswamy R, et al: Real-time ultrasonography for determination of ovarian morphology and volume. Lancet 1(8269):425, 1982, pp 425–426

35. Hall DA, Hann LE, Ferrucci JT Jr, et al: Sonographic morphology of the menstrual cycle. Radiology 133:185, 1979

36. Hill LM, Breckle R, Coulam CB: Assessment of human follicular development by ultrasound. Mayo Clin Proc 57:176, 1982

37. Fleischer AC, Daniell JF, Rodier J, et al: Sonographic monitoring of ovarian follicular development. J Clin Ultrasound 9:275, 1981

38. Gray H: The digestive system, in Goss CM (ed), Gray's Anatomy, 28th ed. Philadelphia, Lea & Febiger, 1966, pp 1234–1245

8 Fetal Anatomy

Roger Sanders
Nancy Smith Miner
James Martin

Ultrasound has provided physicians with a method to study all phases of a pregnancy after the first 2 to 3 weeks following conception. We will present a review of the ultrasonic features of the fetal organs as they develop.

GESTATION PERIOD

Fetal structure is morphologically visible during the embryonic period from the second to the eighth week of fetal development.[1] This corresponds with the fourth through the tenth week from the last menstrual period. This is the most sensitive developmental phase, when the blastocyst is converted into a C-shaped cylindrical embryo (as discussed in Chapter 4). Fetal appearances change rapidly during the early formation of the brain, liver, somites, ears, limbs, nose, and eyes. Most congenital anomalies are evident by pathologic examination during this period but are not identifiable sonographically.

The first sonographic evidence of a fetus is a small group of echoes within the gestational sac. As soon as one delineates the fetus at about 5 to 5½ weeks after the last menstrual period, cardiac motion can be visualized. At approximately the same time and for the subsequent 2 to 4 weeks the yolk sac can be seen as a small cystic structure adjacent to the fetus.[2-4] Over the next few weeks fetal anatomy gradually becomes more distinct as a definite head, trunk and fetal limbs emerge (Figs. 1, 2). By about the 10th week after the last menstrual period, it is possible to make out a definite intracranial sonolucent area with a midline falx.

Pertinent fetal ultrasound observations in the first trimester of pregnancy include: (1) observation of cardiac activity which establishes fetal viability; (2) counting the number of fetuses; (3) monitoring of the fetal head, limb, and trunk growth; (4) distinction of the yolk sac and cord from the fetus.

FETAL PERIOD

The fetal period begins with the ninth week of gestation and terminates with the delivery of the fetus. By the tenth gestational week, most of the organs are ultrasonically recognizable and have assumed their final anatomical position. During this period ultrasound studies can be used to determine whether an organ system is normal or abnormal. Visualizing anatomy in sufficient detail to diagnose fetal anomalies is difficult until 14 weeks after the last menstrual period, apart from gross anomalies such as anencephalus or omphalocele.

TECHNIQUE OF A FETAL EXAM

The emphasis in obstetrical scanning today is rightfully directed toward real time, preferably a linear array system. Improvements in real-time technology combine improved visualization of fetal structures with the capacity to constantly readjust the transducer as the fetus moves. The great variability in fetal position makes a rigid scanning format impossible, but a routine approach utilizing a check list is helpful in preventing oversights.

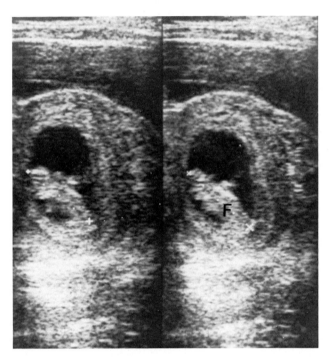

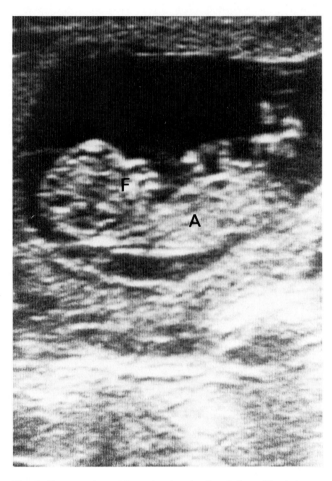

Fig. 1. A gestational sac showing a relatively young fetus of about 8 weeks. The head area, trunk (F), and limbs can be seen.

Fig. 2. Fetus at about 12 weeks showing head, face (F), abdomen (A), and limbs.

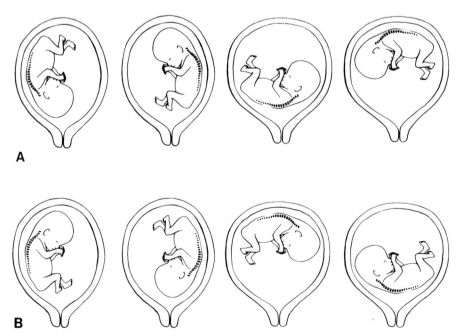

Fig. 3. Diagrammatic illustration indicating the method of determining fetal left side from right side. **A.** Fetus lying on right side. **B.** Fetus lying on left side.

Fetal Heart Motion

It is a good habit to always check for fetal heart motion first. Knowing the fetus is viable allows the sonographer to establish a rapport with the mother centered on the fetus.

Fetal Position

The assessment of fetal lie by ultrasound is critical in the recognition of fetal anatomy. In most instances the fetus is in a cephalic or vertex presentation. The term "cephalic" is useful because, unlike "vertex," it does not require recognition of the face when the fetus is in a head first position. When the fetus is in a cephalic presentation, the abdominal organs will line up in a clockwise fashion on a transverse view, so that the spine is followed by the stomach, umbilical vein, and liver, regardless whether the fetal back is to the left or right (Fig. 4). When the fetus is in a breech position, however, the structures are aligned in an anti-clockwise direction.

It is wise to look at the lower uterine segment in the midline early in the scan. This is helpful because:

1. If the patient's bladder is full, the cervix and its relationship to the placenta are shown.
2. If the bladder is *too* full, this area can be documented before the patient is allowed to void.
3. If the bladder is empty but the placenta is low-lying, a "post-void" film can be obtained, saving the patient at least one trip off and on the table. If the bladder is empty, return to this area at the end of the study; the bladder may have filled in the interim.

Especially if an entire sonogram is done with real-time it is difficult to determine fetal position from the

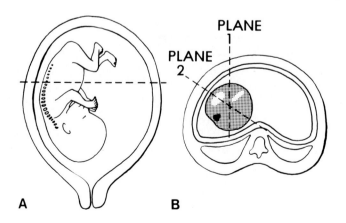

Fig. 4. Diagrammatic illustrations demonstrating the method for planning long axis ultrasonograms of the fetus.

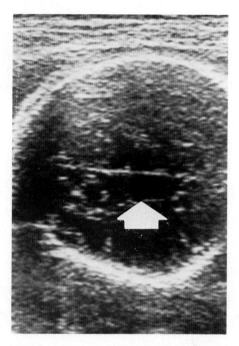

Fig. 5. Axial view of the skull. The lateral borders of the lateral ventricles can be seen (*arrow*). The medial borders are not seen because they shelve too obliquely to the ultrasonic beam. Notice the central line from the falx.

films in retrospect. A longitudinal section often cannot be distinguished from a transverse unless labeled. However, a midline cut showing the presenting fetal part in the same picture as the bladder, vagina, and cervix definitely establishes fetal position.

Biparietal Diameters

The next step is to try for head views. The opportunity may not exist later. Obtain a few good "biparietal diameters," making sure that at least one image shows the complete outline of the head so the circumference can be measured. Without removing the transducer from that axis, slide up the fetal skull and document the lateral ventricles (Fig. 5). If the fetus is not in the optimal position for these views, scan whatever is visible and keep returning to the head throughout the study. Getting the mother to walk around may encourage a change in fetal position.

Spine

Many views require knowledge of how the spine lies, for example, a transverse view as for a "trunk circumference" (Fig. 6). It is therefore best to localize the spine next, although it may be necessary to recheck the spinal position repeatedly as the baby moves (Fig. 7). Often it is impossible to line up the entire spine on a single cut if the fetus is curled, so several sequential views may be necessary (Fig. 8). The sacral

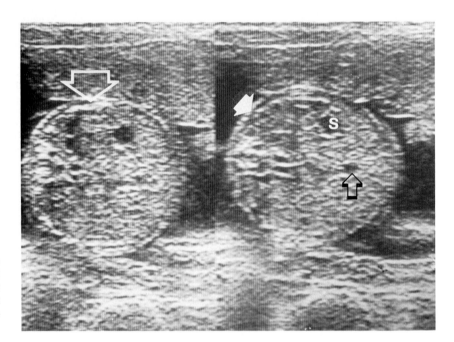

Fig. 6. A view at the appropriate level for a "trunk circumference" shows the stomach (S) and a portion of the portal vein (*arrow*). Note the pseudo ascites (*arrow*). There should be a rib (*open arrow*) visible on either side of an abdominal circumference.

region is often obscured by shadowing from the adjacent iliac wings and must be demonstrated from a more dorsal angle to the fetus (Fig. 7).

If the baby's spine is anterior, it is possible to obtain a fine view of the spine (Fig. 7), but the skin area may be lost in near field reverberations. The distance between spine and transducer should be increased by gently decreasing transducer pressure once the spine is lined up, or perhaps by angling from a distance slightly further away. If the spine is not in

an optimal position when you wish to photograph it (spine down), return later in the study.

Longitudinal views of the spine do not demonstrate the skin covering well and it is desirable to take transverse scans of the spine to show that there is no soft tissue defect (Fig. 7). Although spiral widening can be visualized longitudinally, it is often subtle or confusing if the fetus is curled. Transverse views depicting a normal relationship between the three ossification centers are usually more conclusive. Adjust the beam angle so that the skin covering is seen on each view. To ensure that each section has been seen adequately include enough fetal anatomy to show where the section was taken, that is, iliac wings should be seen on transverse sacral views, some heart on thoracic spine views, and so on. If the fetus is spine-down, turn the mother on her side, have her walk or empty her bladder, and then *wait*. Films taken in the spine down position are not adequate.

Once the spine is localized, scan transversely through the fetus, always remaining directly perpendicular to the spine. Start with the chest, then move along the spinal axis to the abdomen. After an "abdominal circumference" is taken with the beam as perpendicular to the proximal portal sinus as possible, slide the transducer slightly caudal to see the kidneys (Fig. 7). If possible, change the direction of the beam to come in from the posterior fetal aspect so that the spine will not shadow the kidney furthest from the beam. If this proves impossible, try scanning from the anterior approach to show both kidneys on the same scan.

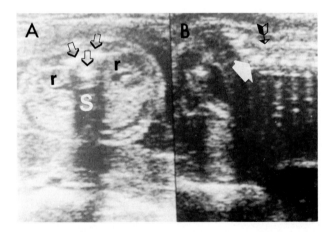

Fig. 7. A. Transverse view of the spine showing the three ossification centers (*arrows*). Lateral to the spine lie the kidneys (r). Both kidneys show a small degree of splaying of the pelvicalyceal system, a normal variant. Note the shadowing (S) from the spine. **B.** Longitudinal view of the spine. Echoes from the anterior and posterior ossification centers of the vertebral body (*solid arrow*) and from the lamina (*black arrow*) can be seen. Note that the skin can be seen covering the spine.

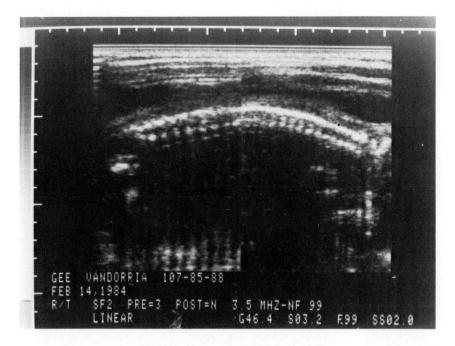

GEE VANDORRIA 107-85-88
FEB 14,1984
R/T SF2 PRE=3 POST=N 3.5 MHZ-NF 99
LINEAR   G46.4 S03.2 F.99 SS02.0

Fig. 8. Composite longitudinal view of the spine.

From there, continue moving caudally until the iliac wing comes in to view. It serves as a landmark for the head of the femur.

Limbs

Once the proximal femur is on the screen, the transducer can be rotated until the rest of the bone is lined up (Fig. 9). As with the biparietal diameter, it is best to take, if not photograph, more than one image to check your measurement.

When scanning fetal limbs, always start from a known landmark in the body and trace outward through the femur or humerus. Otherwise, the lower leg can be easily mistaken for the forearm, and vice versa. Label on the screen during the study, if possible, and use automatic calipers to avoid doubts over measurements in retrospect. Bones in the distal extremities are often more easily photographed separately; obtain the long axis of one, then rock the transducer slightly to see the other. Trace these bones past their distal ends to visualize digits.

Longitudinals

In addition to a view of the spine, at least one longitudinal should be taken through the fetal body that does not include the spine. This can be a composite shot that demonstrates (a) the diaphragm, (b) the stomach, and (c) the bladder (Figs. 10, 11). Views that show the aortic arch and fetal heart (Figs. 12, 13), and inferior and superior vena cava (Fig. 14) are useful to document the overall configuration of the fetus. If the stomach or bladder contains no fluid, return later in the study.

Neck

The neck is relatively short and presents a confusing ultrasonic pattern in the fetus, being dominated by the three major ossification areas of the spine—the vertebral body and the posterior elements. The spinal cord itself is a barely visible small structure in the center of the canal. Soft tissue organs such as the thyroid may be seen in the neck anterior to the cervical spine. The esophagus and tongue may be recognized when the fetus swallows (Fig. 15, 24).[5]

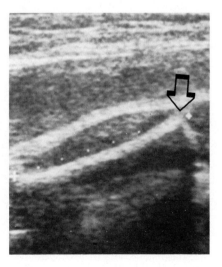

Fig. 9. Longitudinal view of the femur showing the greater trochanter (*arrow*)—the dots mark the usual site where femoral length measurements are obtained. Note the soft tissues anterior to the femur.

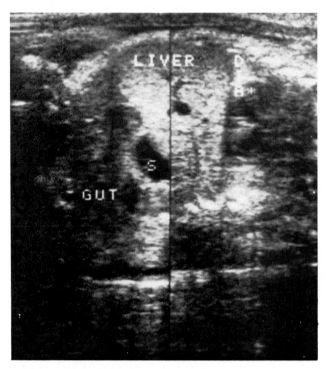

Fig. 10. A longitudinal view of the trunk showing the diaphragm (D), the heart (H), the liver, stomach (S), and gut.

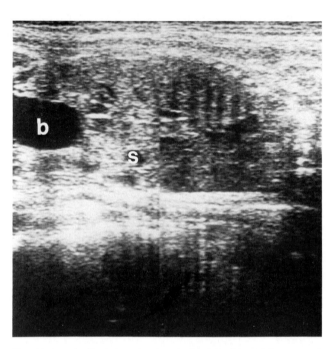

Fig. 11. Longitudinal view showing the bladder (b), and the stomach (S). The liver and the lungs are seen through rib shadows.

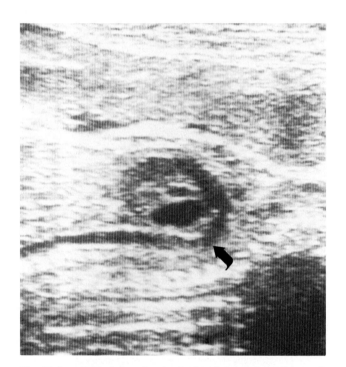

Fig. 12. Longitudinal view showing the heart and aortic arch (*arrow*).

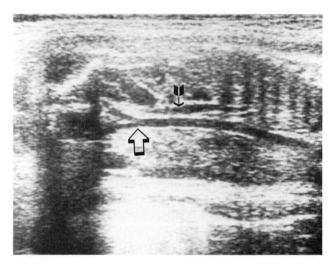

Fig. 13. Longitudinal view showing the aortic bifurcation (*large arrow*); the inferior vena cava (*black arrow*) is visible. Note the rib shadowing.

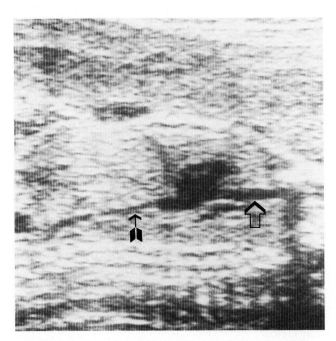

Fig. 14. Longitudinal view. The superior vena cava (*open arrow*) and inferior vena cava (*black arrow*) are seen entering the right atrium.

CENTRAL NERVOUS SYSTEM

Brain

Brain growth, which begins about the 18th day after conception, is rapid. The forebrain develops into the cerebrum with lateral ventricles and a third ventricle. By about 8 weeks of gestation there is free communication between the ventricles and by approximately the 12th week the lateral ventricles fill most of the cranial vault; little brain tissue is seen and the skull mostly contains fluid. The echogenic choroid plexus may be identified in the floor of the ventricle. The cortical mantle is poorly defined but becomes progressively more evident and wider with further growth.

The surface of the cerebral cortex at 13 weeks is smooth. There is progressive growth and development of sulci and gyri throughout fetal life, which is manifested by the appearance of curvilinear echogenic lines from these structures. The infolding of the hemisphere produces the Insula which can be ultrasonically identified as early as 16 weeks (Fig. 17).[5a]

The common carotid arteries arise from the third pair of the aortic arches between the sixth and eighth week of fetal life. By the second trimester the cerebral arterial circulation is well defined. With real-time instrumentation one can identify a number of intracerebral arteries such as the circle of Willis and the brain stem, the middle cerebral artery and the Sylvian fissure, the basilar artery and the brainstem, and so on.

The fetal intracranial structures have been ana-

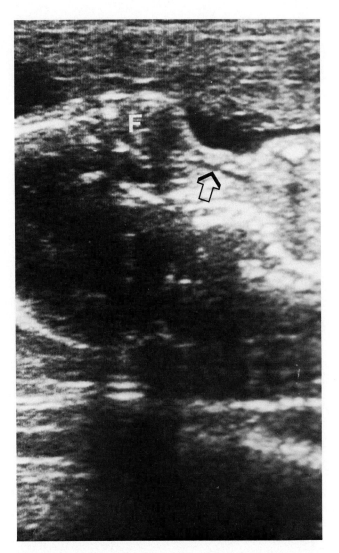

Fig. 15. View of the neck. The face (F) lies superior to the esophagus (*arrow*), which can be seen within the soft tissues of the neck.

lyzed in great detail by several authors.[6,7] An axial approach as for the biparietal diameter is the most convenient. Such an approach only shows the lateral borders of the lateral ventricles (Fig. 5) because of the oblique axis of the medial borders as they relate to the ultrasonic beam. The ventricles are relatively large in proportion to the cranium in the second trimester and may be mistaken for hydrocephalus.[8] There is a reduction in ventriculo–hemispheric ratio with time and by the 19th to 20th week the ratio is less than one third. Normal standards for ventricular size have been established.[9,10] The choroid plexus can fill most of the lateral ventricles including the temporal horn. The anterior extension of the choroid plexus extends to the level of the foramen of Monroe where it dips inferiorly to extend into the roof of the third ventricle. The choroid plexus appear as relatively large structures

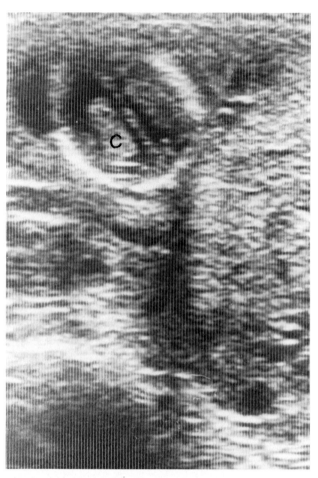

Fig. 16. View of the fetal head at approximately 16 weeks showing large choroid plexus (C).

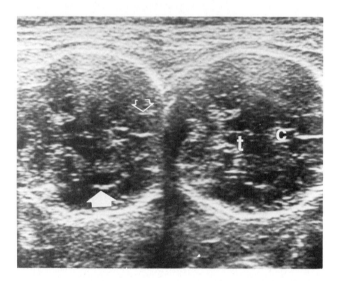

Fig. 17. View through the midbrain showing the two thalami (t), with the slit of third ventricle in between. The cavum septum pellucidum (c) is seen superiorly. The lateral borders of the frontal horns of the lateral ventricles (*open arrow*) are visible. The Insula can be seen (*closed arrow*).

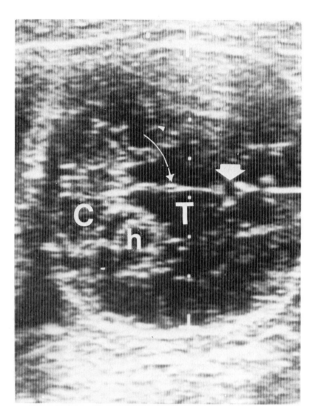

Fig. 18. View showing the thalamus (T), third ventricle (*curved arrow*), cavum septum pellucidum (*closed arrow*), frontal horns of the lateral ventricles, hippocampus (h), and cerebellum (C).

in the 12th to 16th week and may dominate the intracranial appearances (Fig. 16).[11] Whereas the ventricles continue to enlarge slightly throughout the rest of pregnancy, the choroid plexus appear to stay about the same size. Choroid plexus cysts are occasionally seen in the second trimester and are of no pathologic significance (see Chapter 18).

At a slightly lower transverse axial level, the dominant structure is the thalamus. This structure forms a relatively sonolucent diamond- to heart-shaped structure in the center of the head with a thin cavity, the third ventricle, in its center (Fig. 17). In the anterior part of the skull centrally lies the cavum septum pellucidum—a boxlike sonolucent recess or cistern that atrophies after birth but is still visible in most neonates (Fig. 17). Anterior to the cavum septum pellucidum are two linear echoes that lie parallel to the falx. These two echoes are derived from the lateral aspect of the frontal horns of the lateral ventricles. Posteriorly, if the axial section is taken at a line parallel to the orbitomeatal line, there will be a central line due to the falx; if it is taken at a more oblique level angling caudally, the echogenic line of the tentorium angles laterally

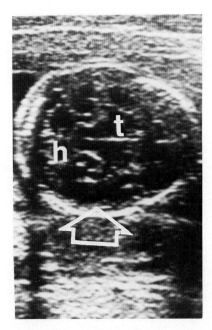

Fig. 19. View showing the cerebral peduncles as they merge with the thalamus (T). The hippocampus (h) can be seen. The sonolucent area around the insula can be seen (*arrow*).

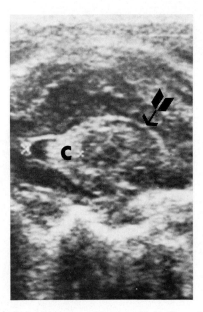

Fig. 21. Sagittal view showing a lateral ventricle. The anterior (*black arrow*), occipital, and temporal horns can be seen. The choroid plexus (C) is visible.

surrounding the echogenic vermis of the cerebellum (Fig. 18). Moving inferiorly, the thalamus merges with cerebral peduncles, which are also echopenic. They are about half the size of the thalamus. The basilar artery can be seen pulsating between the peduncles where the superior borders curve down and meet. Adjacent and lateral to the cerebral peduncles lie the circular

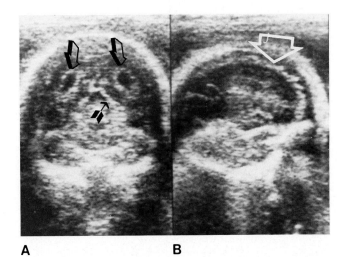

A   **B**

Fig. 20. A. Coronal view showing the lateral ventricles superior to the tentorium (*arrow*) and the echogenic vermis of the cerebellum. **B.** Sagittal view showing an apparent space between the brain and skull (*arrow*), a normal variant.

echopenic hippocampus; lateral to them are the trigone of the lateral ventricles (Fig. 19).[12]

Toward the periphery of the brain both on sections through the thalamus and the cerebral penduncle, one can see a linear structure parallel with the skull that contains a pulsatile vessel—the middle cerebral artery (Fig. 17). This artery can be traced from the circle of Willis and delineates the Insula. The Insula is surrounded by a sonolucent area of amniotic fluid.[5a] A finding seen commonly in young fetuses (under 30 weeks) is a line around the brain looking like an apparent subdural collection (Fig. 20). This is thought to represent the fetal subarachnoid space.[13] At a still lower level, an axial view shows three compartments separated by intervening areas of shadowing (due to bone) on each side of the brain; this section is through the anterior, middle, and posterior fossa. A small sonolucent area surrounded by vessels will be recognized as the pineal; within the posterior fossa the mildly echogenic cerebellar hemispheres will be seen. Sagittal coronal views (Figs. 21, 22) will show the brainstem and lateral ventricles.

As one examines the anterior portion of the skull at a low level, one sees the structures that compose the face, the orbits, maxilla, mandible, and so on (Figs. 23, 24). These structures are described in detail in chapter 9. In a more posterior location arising from the border of the skull will be the ears, which have a hemispherical shape with various ridges within (Fig. 25).[14]

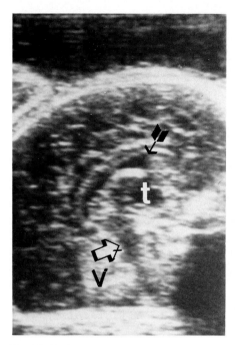

Fig. 22. Midline sagittal view showing the brainstem (*open arrow*), the vermis of the cerebellum (V), and the cavum septum pellucidum (*black arrow*). The gyri are visible within the brain substance.

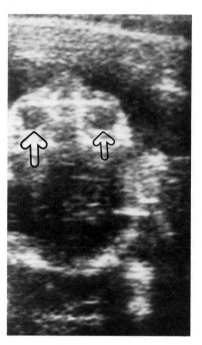

Fig. 23. View showing the orbits (*arrows*). Within the orbits the outline of the globes can be seen.

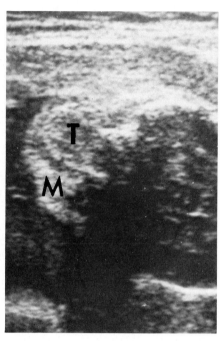

Fig. 24. View showing the tongue (T) surrounded by the mandible (M).

FETAL SKELETON

Limbs

Shortly after the fetal heart and trunk become visible, evidence of fetal limb formation is seen. At this early stage (8 to 9 weeks) distinct digits or segments of the limbs cannot be defined although considerable limb movement is seen. By about 9 to 10 weeks after the last menstrual period the proximal and distal limbs and digits become visible and by about 15 weeks detailed anatomy of the limbs can be made out. Not only can digits be counted but individual bones within the feet and hands can be made out (Fig. 26). The tibia, fibula, radius, and ulna can be seen as two separate bones in each limb. The humerus and femur become structures that can be measured as a standard of fetal age (Fig. 9).

Epiphyseal ossification is visible in the distal femur first and is good evidence that the fetus is at least 33 weeks of gestation.[15,16] Additional later ossification centers are seen at the proximal end of the femur and tibia and adjacent to the humerus.

Capturing this normal anatomy is sometimes difficult because the limbs may lie at virtually any axis in relationship to the fetal trunk. Real time is essential. Often a froglike position is assumed, with the knees brought up adjacent to the abdomen.

The skull is visible as a distinct curvilinear line around the head from about 10 weeks on.

Spine

The spine has a complex series of echoes associated with it. Early in pregnancy three echogenic areas are seen in the spine—the vertebral body and posterior elements. Later detailed sonographic correlation with anatomic dissection of the fetal spine shows that the echogenic areas within the spine on a longitudinal section are made up of the anterior vertebral body, a small ossification center, a large ossification center from the

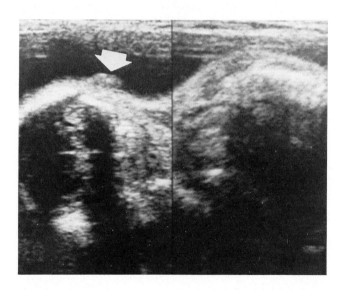

Fig. 25. The fetal ear (*arrow*) can be seen adjacent to the head.

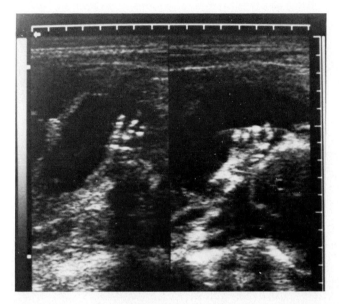

Fig. 26. View of the fetal hand showing metacarpals and digits.

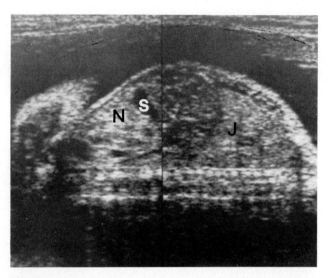

Fig. 27. Longitudinal view of the fetus. The lungs (J) in this case are slightly more echogenic than the liver. The stomach (S) lies between the liver and the gut (N). Most of the spine can be seen.

posterior segment of the vertebral body, echoes from the posterior lamina, and echoes from the spinous process (Fig. 27). Additional lines within the spinal canal are seen from a membrane that lines the spinal canal and a tiny line from the center of the spine that represents the spinal canal.[17] The sacral spine takes a rather marked anterior angulation so it lies at a slightly different axis to the remainder of the spine (Fig. 7). The ribs can be seen with acoustical shadowing beyond, lining the margins of the chest and upper abdomen (Fig. 28); the costochondral junctions are visible and sometimes confused with the spine.

Scapula and Iliac Wings
A linear echo from the scapula is seen on either side of the upper portion of the chest (Fig. 29). The iliac crests are visible as winglike structures from about 12 weeks on adjacent to the bladder (Fig. 30). Soft tissues are visible in the thigh, calf, and upper and lower arm. Thigh thickness is measurable and is a potential means of following fetal growth (Fig. 8).

Identifying the skin around the abdomen and the skull can assist in determining whether or not the fetus is suffering from fetal edema or diabetes mellitus. The skin thickness should not be more than about 2 to 3 mm.

BODY CAVITIES

The body cavities begin to form during the third week of gestation and are fairly complete by the end of the seventh week. The yolk sac and the fetal bowel within

the umbilical cord may remain after the embryonic period and be identified as late as 11 weeks after gestation.

Fetal Thorax
The ossification of the ribs begins early in the embryonic period; they are usually easily defined in the midsecond trimester. The relative position of the ribs and the vertebral bodies permits the sonographer to determine the position of the fetus in utero and to recognize the relative positions of the heart, diaphragm, and liver (Fig. 31). The lungs in utero contain no air and the most prominent intrathoracic structure is the fetal

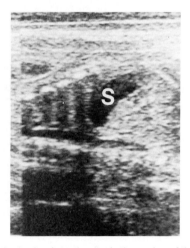

Fig. 28. Rib shadowing from the ribs in the region of the costochondral junctions is visible. The stomach (S) lies between the less echogenic lungs and the more echogenic gut. The large vessel is the aorta.

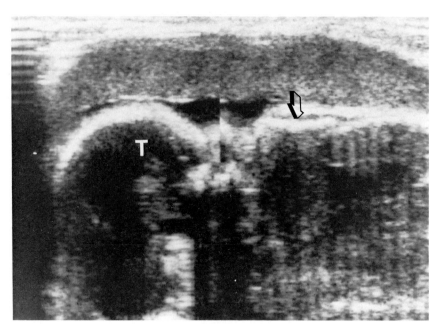

Fig. 29. The scapula (*arrow*) is seen lateral to the superior aspect of the chest. Rib shadowing is visible. T = head.

heart. The lungs are of an even echogenic structure and appear similar to the liver.

Heart

The heart begins to develop 18 to 19 days after conception with the formation of a pair of elongated cardiogenic cords that become canalized to form two thin-walled endocardial heart tubes. These rapidly fuse to form a single median endocardial heart tube. The tube undergoes a period of elongation with localized constriction and dilatation to form the bulbus cordis,

ventricle, atrium, the truncus arteriosus and the sinus venosus (20 to 25 days). At this time, cardiac contraction begins.

The heart by the beginning of the second trimester can be depicted as a pulsatile, fluid-filled structure within the thorax. The cardiac valves and the foramen ovale motion can be delineated with real-time by about 16 weeks.

The study of the fetal heart depends upon the recognition of its position within the thorax during the fetal period. The cardiac alignment can be estab-

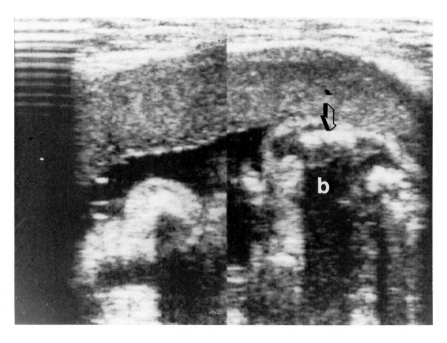

Fig. 30. Transverse views through the pelvis showing the iliac wing (*arrow*) with acoustic shadowing obscuring the bladder (b).

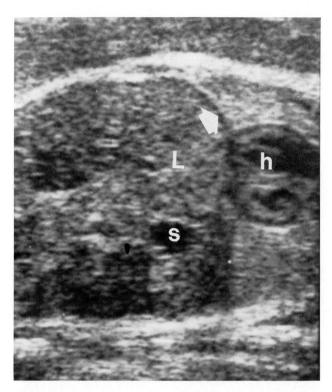

Fig. 31. Longitudinal view showing the diaphragm (*arrow*) between the less echogenic liver (L) and more echogenic lung. h = heart. S = stomach.

lished by identifying its relationship to the spine, thorax, liver, and stomach. The features that help identify the right from the left chambers in a normal heart include:

1. The relationship of the heart to the spine and stomach; the stomach will be close to the left ventricle. The spine will be close to the atria.
2. The identification of (a) the inferior and superior vena cava (Fig. 14) as they enter the right atrium, (b) the ascending aorta and the aortic valves as the aorta leaves the left ventricle (Figs. 12, 32), (c) foramen ovale motion into the left atrium, and (d) the pulmonary artery leaving the right ventricle.

The central fibrous trigone (the central fibrous body) surrounding the base of the aorta can be very echogenic and identifies the base of the aorta, which is the most superior part of the interventricular system. The mitral valve originates higher on the septum and closer to the central fibrous body whereas the tricuspid valve originates more toward the apex. This is best seen in the "four-chamber" view (Fig. 32). Ultrasound provides a means of evaluating the cardiac chamber size, valve functions, septal motion, and the pericardium.

The heart should be identified in a long axis and

four-chamber view (Fig. 32). The atrial septum is usually easily seen and the left atrium is identified by observing the direction of the excursion of the foramen ovale, which moves within the left atrium. The right ventricle is slightly larger than the left. The normal fetal heart beats at an average of 140 beats per minute (range 120 to 160).

The aortic arch and its major branches such as the carotid can be readily visualized within the thorax (Fig. 12). The aorta can be followed into the abdomen to at least the level of bifurcation and the iliac arteries (Fig. 13). The vena cava is easily identified (Fig. 14). A major branch that enters the inferior vena cava is the ductus venosus, which travels obliquely through the liver from the umbilical vein towards the fetal heart. Hepatic veins can also be seen entering the inferior vena cava.

Fetal and Neonatal Circulation

Oxygenated blood leaves the placenta via the umbilical vein, which enters the portal system in the left lobe of the liver (Fig. 33). A large branch of the portal vein supplies most of the liver; blood from this vessel subsequently passes through the hepatic veins to the inferior vena cava and right atrium. A smaller vessel, the ductus venosus, carries blood directly into the vena cava and from there to the right atrium.[18,19]

The blood from the vena cava enters the right atrium and passes through the foramen ovale into the

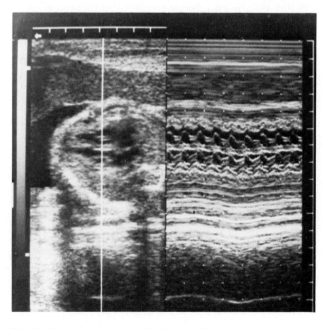

Fig. 32. Four-chamber view of the heart, with the line passing through the tricuspid and mitral valves. The ventricles can be seen to the left of the line. The M-mode study is taken through the site that the line passes through.

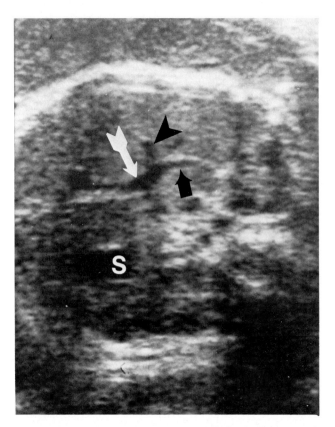

Fig. 33. Transverse view showing the umbilical vein (*large arrow*). S = stomach. The left portal vein (*arrowhead*) and ductus venosus (*black arrow*) can be seen.

left atrium. The blood then passes into the left ventricle and leaves via the ascending aorta. A small amount of blood remains in the right atrium and passes through the right ventricle and pulmonary artery into the lungs. Most of the blood, however, passes from the pulmonary artery through the patent ductus into the aorta. Much of the blood in the aorta returns to the placenta via the two umbilical arteries but some remains to circulate through the lower extremities.

Fetal Abdomen

The fetal abdomen lies between the diaphragm and the pelvis. The diaphragm can usually be identified in the second trimester as an echo-free line located between the mildly echogenic fetal lung and the usually slightly more echogenic fetal liver (Fig. 31). In the third trimester the echogenicity may be reversed, the lungs becoming more echogenic. The pelvis can be defined by the identification of the pelvic bones and the fluid-filled urinary bladder. Gut (usually echogenic) lies between the bladder and the liver (Fig. 11). The gallbladder is often identified from the second trimester as a somewhat ovoid fluid-filled structure, but care must be taken not to confuse it with the um-

bilical vein (Fig. 34). Tracking the vascular structures prior to gallbladder recognition is essential. The fetal stomach, duodenum, liver, and the biliary apparatus develop from the primitive foregut in the latter part of the embryonic life (fifth to eighth week). The fluid-filled fetal stomach can be seen and lies in the left upper quadrant (Figs. 10, 11). The stomach serves as a landmark for identifying adjacent organs such as the liver, spleen, and the left kidney. It has a shape similar to that seen in the adult. The liver, which is a relatively large structure, is identified as a mildly echogenic organ immediately beneath the curvilinear diaphragm. The left lobe is relatively larger in the fetus than in the adult.[20] The spleen can sometimes be seen lateral and posterior to the stomach.

The pancreas embryologically arises from the dorsal and ventral buds of the foregut and is primarily identified by its relationship to other organs such as

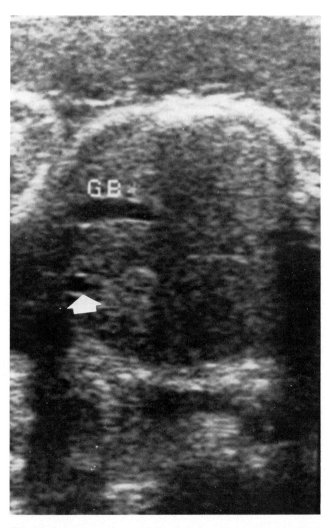

Fig. 34. Transverse view of fetal abdomen. The gallbladder (GB) is seen separate from the umbilical vein (*arrow*).

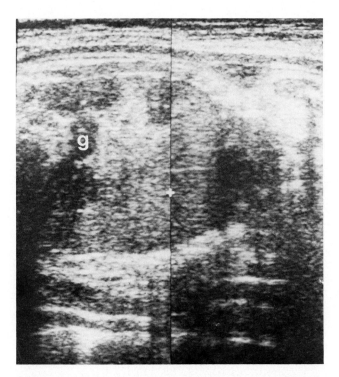

Fig. 35. Longitudinal view showing the liver and transverse colon (g). The colon at this late stage in pregnancy is relatively large and echogenic.

the stomach, spleen, and left adrenal and to vascular structures such as the splenic, left renal, and superior mesenteric veins. The fetal pancreas is slightly more echogenic than the liver and can be recognized with good quality systems when the fetus is examined in a spine posterior position.[21]

The fetal gut is normally more echogenic than the liver (Figs. 11, 27, 28). Actual fluid-filled segments apart from the stomach are not visible until the third trimester when normal colonic loops can achieve a relatively large dimension (over 2 cm).[22,23] The contents are usually more echogenic than those of the stomach. As pregnancy proceeds the fluid-filled loops become more obvious and cease to have the homogeneous echogenic appearance seen in early pregnancy (Fig. 35).[24]

Urinary and Genital Systems

The kidneys initially develop in the anatomic pelvis, but by the time they are visible they have already migrated to their final paraspinal position. The fetal kidneys may be identified as relatively sonolucent structures adjacent to the spine (Fig. 36) by 15 weeks.[25] Normal fetal renal size charts have been constructed (see Appendix).[26,27] Further development leads to the deposition of renal sinus and perirenal fat and the differentiation of the renal pyra-

mids and collecting system. These structures can be seen in the second and third trimester.

Bladder development is completed by about the 12th week. The bladder is a fluid-filled structure in the anterior midline pelvis which changes in size with urine formation (Fig. 11). It fills or partially empties over the course of approximately an hour.[28]

The urinary bladder serves as a predictable landmark for the visualization of the external genitalia, which can be identified as early as 14 weeks although only with consistency after 18 weeks. The genitalia are described in detail in Chapter 14; the scrotum with testicles and a penis will be seen in males and the labia will be seen in females.

The fetal adrenal glands are relatively large structures with a shape and echogenicity reminiscent of the kidneys (Figs. 37, 38). They can be seen most of the time after 26 weeks.[29] The fetal adrenals are pyramidal or triangular in shape. Although echogenic prior to 32 weeks, an echogenic core to each limb is seen beyond that stage.[30]

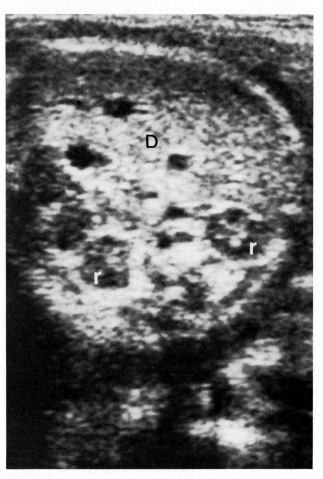

Fig. 36. Transverse view showing the kidneys (r) lying lateral to the spine. D = liver.

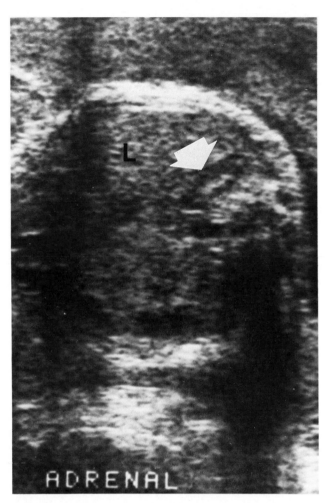

Fig. 37. Transverse view showing the adrenal (*arrow*) lateral to the spine. L = liver. Note the echogenic core to the adrenal. The left adrenal is obscured by shadowing from the spine.

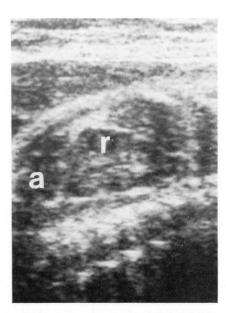

Fig. 38. Longitudinal view showing the adrenal (a) lying superior to the kidney (r). The adrenals in the third trimester are quite large.

CONCLUSION

The sonologist now has a method available to monitor the fetus almost from conception to delivery. Significant contributions have already been made but recent developments in instrumentation and correlation with clinical problems will undoubtedly lead to a greater elucidation of anatomic structures. The end result of any scan is the direct result of the interest and capability of the physician or sonographer perfoming the examination.

REFERENCES

1. Moore KL: The Developing Human, 2nd ed. Philadelphia, Saunders, 1977
2. Sauerbrei E, Cooperberg PL, Poland BJ: Ultrasound demonstration of the normal fetal yolk sac. J Clin Ultrasound 8:217, 1980
3. Mantoni M, Pedersen JF: Ultrasound visualization of the human yolk sac. J Clin Ultrasound 7:459, 1979
4. Crooij MJ, Westhuis M, Schoemaker J, Exalto N: Ultrasonographic measurement of the yolk sac. Br J Obstet Gynaecol 89:931, 1982
5. Bowie JD, Clair MR: Fetal swallowing and regurgitation: Observation of normal and abnormal activity. Radiology 144:877, 1982
5a. Jeanty P, Chervenate F, Romero R, et al: The sylvian fissure: A commonly mislabeled landmark. J Ultrasound Med 3:15, 1984
6. Hadlock FP, Deter RL, Park SK: Real-time sonography: Ventricular and vascular anatomy of the fetal brain in utero. Am J Roentgenol 136:133, 1981
7. Johnson ML, Dunne MG, Mack LA, Rashbaum CL: Evaluation of fetal intracranial anatomy by static and real-time ultrasound. J Clin Ultrasound 8:311, 1980
8. Chinn DH, Callen PW, Filly RA: The lateral cerebral ventricle in early second trimester. Radiology 148:529, 1983
9. Denkhaus H, Winsberg F: Ultrasonic measurement of the fetal ventricular system. Radiology 131:781, 1979
10. Jeanty P, Dramaix-Wilmet M, Delbeke D, et al: Ultrasonic evaluation of fetal ventricular growth. Neuroradiology 619:127, 1980
11. Crade M, Patel J, McQuown D: Sonographic imaging of the glycogen stage of the fetal choroid plexus. Am J Roentgenol 137:489, 1981
12. McGahan JP, Phillips HE: Ultrasonic evaluation of the size of the trigone of the fetal ventricle. J Ultrasound Med 2:315, 1983
13. Laing FC, Stamler CE, Jeffrey RB: Ultrasonography of the fetal subarachnoid space. J Ultrasound Med 2:29, 1983
14. Birnholtz JC: The fetal external ear. Radiology 147:819, 1983
15. Chinn DH, Bolding DB, Callen PW, Gross BH, Filly RA:

Ultrasonographic identification of fetal lower extremity epiphyseal ossification centers. Radiology 147:815, 1983

16. McLeary RD, Kuhns LR: Sonographic evaluation of the distal femoral eiphyseal ossification center. J Ultrasound Med 2:437, 1983

17. Graham D, Chezmar J, Sanders RC: CNS Anomalies in the Fetus: Ultrasound Annual. New York, Raven, 1983

18. Morin FR, Winsberg F: Ultrasonic and radiographic study of the vessels of the fetal liver. J Clin Ultrasound 6:377, 1978

19. Chinn DH, Filly RA, Callen PW: Ultrasonic evaluation of fetal umbilical and hepatic vascular anatomy. Radiology 144:153, 1982

20. Gross BH, Harter LP, Filly RA: Disproportionate left hepatic lobe size in the fetus. J Ultrasound Med 1:78, 1981

21. Cyr DR: Ultrasonic visualization of the fetal pancreas and hepatic venous circulation. Med Ultrasound 7:27, 1983

22. Skovbo P, Smith-Jensen S: Hyperdistended fluid-filled bowel loops mimicking gastrointestinal atresia. J Clin Ultrasound 9:463, 1981

23. Berkowitz RL, Hobbins JC: Echo-spared areas in fetal abdomen. Contemp Ob/Gyn 20:31, 1982

24. Zilianti M, Fernandez S: Correlation of ultrasonic images of fetal intestine with gestational age and fetal maturity. Obstet Gynecol 62:569, 1983

25. Bowie JD, Rosenberg ER, Andreotti RF, Fields SI: The changing sonographic appearance of fetal kidneys during pregnancy. J Ultrasound Med 2:505, 1983

26. Grannum P, Bracken M, Silverman R, Hobbins JC: Assessment of fetal kidney size in normal gestation by comparison of ratio of kidney circumference to abdominal circumference. Am J Obstet Gynecol 136:249, 1980

27. Lawson TL, Foley WD, Berland LL, Clark KE: Ultrasonic evaluation of fetal kidneys. Radiology 138:153, 1981

28. Wladimiroff JW, Campbell S: Fetal urine-production rates in normal and complicated pregnancy. Lancet 151, 1974

29. Lewis E, Kurtz AB, Dubbins PA, Wapner RJ, Goldberg BB: Real-time ultrasonographic evaluation of normal fetal adrenal glands. J Ultrasound Med 1:265, 1982

30. Rosenberg ER, Bowie JD, Andreotti RF, Fields SI: Sonographic evaluation of fetal adrenal glands. Am J Roentgenol 139:1145, 1982

9 | Dating Gestation in the First 20 Weeks

Gregory D. O'Brien
John T. Queenan

Perhaps the greatest impact of ultrasonography on obstetrics has been the provision of an accurate means of determining gestational age. If this is to be reasonably accurate and practically useful, it is best done in the first 20 weeks of pregnancy. Normal biologic variation of the fetus is minimal during this period. Accurately performed measurements will correctly estimate the true fetal age within 1 week in at least 95 percent of cases.

Various parameters have been measured to assess gestational age by diagnostic ultrasound. Gestational sac size,[1-4] crown–rump length,[5-8] biparietal diameter,[9-13] head circumference,[14,15] and femur length[16-19] are among the methods most popularly used. A gestational sac is confirmatory of an early pregnancy at 5 to 5½ weeks of gestation. Currently, high-resolution real-time equipment enables early visualization of the fetus, and hence estimation of the sac size or volume has been superceded by crown–rump length measurement. Head circumference measurements are time consuming and open to technical error; hence, the discussion of dating technique will be confined to crown–rump length measurement (CRL), biparietal diameter (BPD), and fetal femur length (FL).

CROWN–RUMP LENGTH

See Appendix 8. Fetal echoes can now be visualized from as early as 6 weeks following menstruation. However, accurate assessment of CRL is not possible until 6½ to 7 weeks' gestation. It is important to realize that this early visualization is dependent on the resolution of the equipment used, and these limitations should be established for each particular instrument. Moreover, patient obesity and occasionally a retroverted uterus may cause difficulty in visualizing early fetal echoes. Studies have shown there is no difference in the accuracy of measurements made by real-time or static scanners.[20] Most obstetrician-gynecologists use linear array real-time scanners.

The technique involves the measurement, between 6½ and 14 weeks' gestation, of fetal length from the tip of the cephalic pole to the tip of the caudal pole. Figures 1 and 2 are of typical CRL measurements at different gestations. The fetus should preferably be at rest and assuming its natural curvature. Unfortunately, there are many pitfalls in the technique of measurement. High resolution real-time scanners have helped to overcome many of these problems. Inclusion of the yolk sac or lower limbs in the measurement, excessive curling or extension of the fetus, and a tangential section of the trunk may all lead to errors. Excessive curvature of the fetus after 12 weeks' gestation can lead to erroneously shortened measurements.

A well-performed CRL measurement, however, is the most accurate method for the assessment of gestational age. The estimated fetal age will be accurate to within 3 to 5 days of the true age. Between 8 and 12 weeks' gestation, the fetus grows at approximately 10 mm per week. Consequently, this fast growth rate compensates for a degree of poor technique without a great loss of accuracy. After 12 weeks' gestation, the increased biologic variation and difficulty in obtaining good measurements with a curled fetus may lead to inaccuracies.

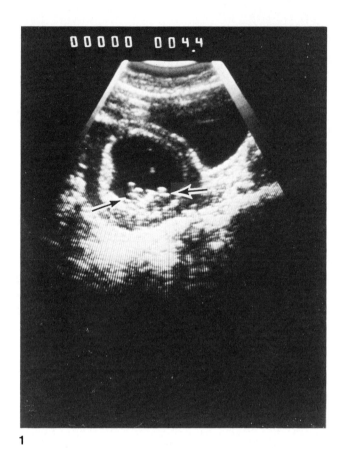

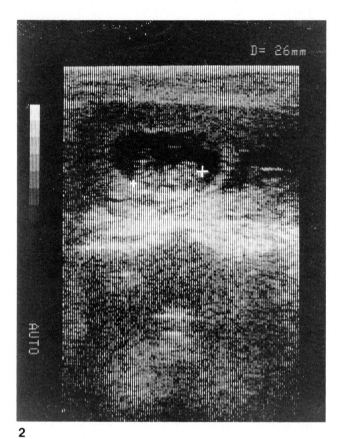

1   2

Figs. 1 and 2. Typical CRL measurements taken by real-time scanners. (*Reprinted with permission from Contemporary Ob/Gyn.*[28])

If accurate dating is of the utmost importance, a CRL measurement should be performed at approximately 8 to 12 weeks' gestation. This may be most important in the fetus at risk for congenital anomalies as subsequent abnormal measurements may be an indicator of the anomaly.

BIPARIETAL DIAMETER (BPD)

See Appendix 1. BPD has been the established and accepted method of gestational dating almost from the original application of diagnostic ultrasound to obstetrics. Unfortunately, its application to the assessment of gestational age has been too often throughout the whole of pregnancy. If the BPD is to be used for the accurate assessment of gestational age, then the best time for this is from 14 to 20 weeks' gestation. Figures 3, 4, and 5 are examples of typical sections used for measuring the BPD.

The technique for measuring BPD is well established and no significant difference has been found between the results from real-time or static scanners.[21-24] However, there are still problems with BPD mea-

surements. In up to 8 percent of patients, a BPD measurement may be unobtainable due to fetal head position such as direct occiput anterior or occiput posterior or when the head is deep in the pelvis below the symphisis.[17] Fortunately, before 20 weeks' gestation, with a mobile fetus, and utilizing the full bladder technique, it is rarely a problem. Dolichocephaly and brachycephaly may cause problems even at this early gestation. Although brachycephaly has been reported to have a comparatively high incidence in early pregnancy, it should not alter the measurements markedly.[15,25]

Moreover, there has not been worldwide uniformity in establishing a plane of section of the fetal skull at which the BPD is measured. The plane of section at the level of the thalamic nuclei as recommended by the American College of Obstetricians and Gynecologists[26] is not always applicable before 17 to 18 weeks' gestation. To add to the confusion, there are at least 25 BPD charts produced by investigators throughout the world.[13]

Before 20 weeks' gestation, the widest transverse diameter of the skull is easily found and measured. The rate of growth of BPD is uniform at 3 to 4 mm

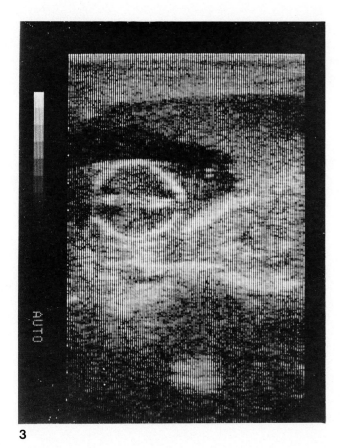

3

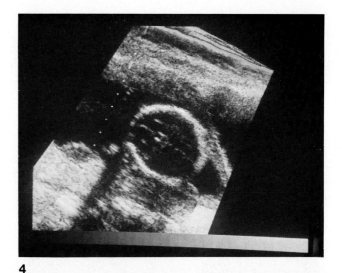

4

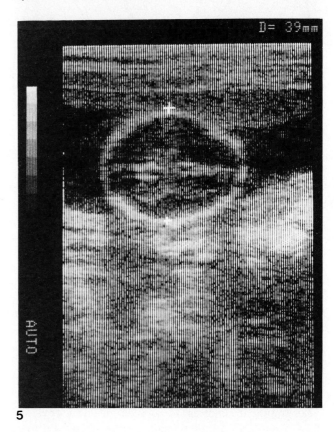

5

per week and reaches its maximum growth rate at this time. Regardless of which chart is used for assessing age, there is minimal difference between the values at this early gestation. There is still, however, a need for a new data based on current high resolution equipment as recommended by other investigators.[12,27]

The BPD from 14 to 20 weeks' gestation is still an accurate predictor of fetal age despite these pitfalls. The 95 percentile limits for correct estimation of age are within 1 week.

FETAL FEMUR LENGTH

See Appendices 2 and 5. Recently, another parameter, the femur length (FL) has been established as an accurate predictor of gestational age.[16,19] Because of the normal biologic variation, this measurement is again most accurate in the 14 to 20 weeks' gestational age group.

The technique for measuring FL has been described and the two methods of approach are illustrated in Figures 6 and 7. Examples of FL measurement can be seen in Figures 8,9, and 10.[2] As with the other parameters, there are pitfalls in performing an accurate measurement. Undermeasurement can be a problem if a tangential section of the calcified portion of the

Figs. 3,4, and 5. Level of the fetal skull at which the BPD has been measured.

femur is obtained. Artifactual bowing of the femur may occur depending on the view of the femur and this will give a shortened measurement. Altering the angulation of the transducer will alleviate this problem. If the bone is orthogonal to the incident sound beam or in the "near field," poor lateral resolution and beam width effect tend to increase the measurement. The distance of the femur from the transducer and hence,

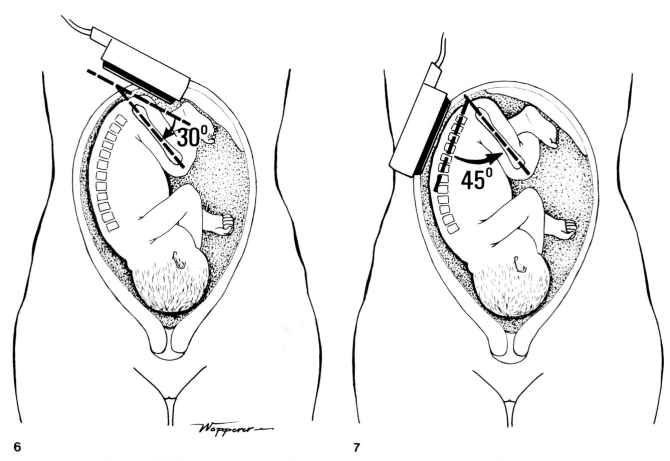

6   7

Figs. 6 and 7. Techniques for measuring fetal femur length. (*Reprinted with permission from Contemporary Ob/Gyn.* [28])

its position in the field of focus, may also alter the measurement. A persistently reproducible measurement should avoid these problems. The measurement of this parameter is very dependent on lateral resolution and the data charts for assessing fetal age should be suited to the particular equipment used. Its accuracy, as a predictor of fetal age is the same as that for the BPD measurement. It can be calculated by the formula:

$$\text{Gestation (days since LMP)} = 2.22 \times \text{femur length (in mm)} + 62.5 \quad [1]$$

The graphs in Figures 11 and 12 are the ones we have used and found to suit a number of different populations.

BPD AND FL

In assessing fetal age in the 14 to 20 weeks' gestation group, there are now two parameters to rely on and both have a high degree of accuracy. Ideally, both parameters should be measured. This will prevent any inaccuracies resulting from poor technique in the measurement of one parameter. It also provides a routine

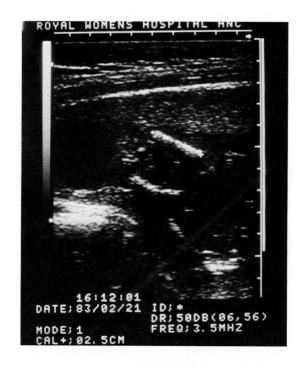

Fig. 8. Femur measurement at 17 weeks' gestation. Note the curvature and apparent shortening of the lower femur.

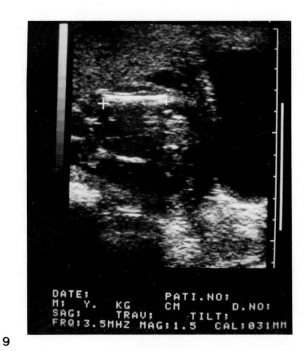

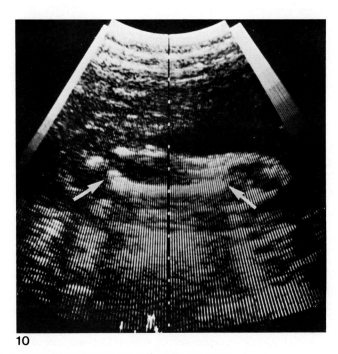

9   10

Figs. 9 and 10. Femur measurements at 19 weeks' gestation by linear array and sector scanners. (*Reprinted with permission from O'Brien, Queenan, et al, 1981.[16]*)

check of two areas of fetal anatomy and hence may be an indicator for some congential anomalies.

CONCLUSION

Accurate assessment of fetal gestational age is now available, and it is essential that it be done early in pregnancy. The problems of iatrogenic prematurity and the time-consuming and costly testing for apparent postdatism can be avoided in many situations.

It is important to learn and practice these techniques if the measurements of these parameters are to be done well. They should also be performed "blind" without knowledge of the menstrual age. Too often, measurements are "altered" to suit the menstrual age.

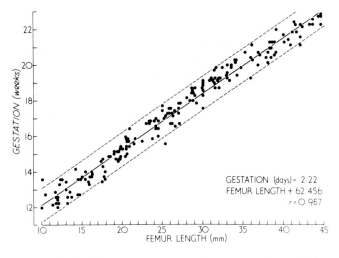

GESTATION (days)= 2.22 FEMUR LENGTH + 62.456
r = 0.987

Fig. 11. Graph of femur measurement—linear regression analysis for estimation of fetal age. (*Reprinted with permission from O'Brien, Queenan, et al, 1981.[16]*)

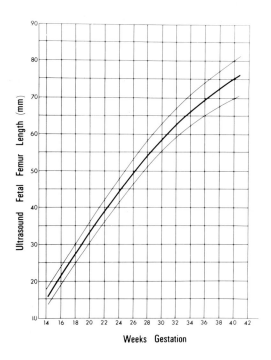

Weeks   Gestation

Fig. 12. Growth of femur throughout normal pregnancy. (*Reprinted with permission from O'Brien, Queenan, et al. 1981.[29]*)

The availability of two parameters after 14 weeks' gestation provides an inbuilt mechanism for cross-checking, and hence errors should be avoided. Accuracy is essential. It is also important to be aware of the pitfalls and limitations of these measurements. Pregnancy dating is an important function of diagnostic ultrasound and certainly, it will remain its most common application in the field of obstetrics.

REFERENCES

1. Hellman LM, Kobayashi M, et al: Growth and development of the human fetus prior to the twentieth week of gestation. Am J Obstet Gynecol 103:789, 1969
2. Jouppila P: Ultrasound in the diagnosis of early pregnancy and its complications. A comparative study of A, B, and Doppler methods. Acta Obstet Gynecol Scand 50 (Suppl 15), 1971
3. Kohorn EI, Kaufman M: Sonar in the first trimester of pregnancy. J Obstet Gynecol 44:473, 1974
4. Robinson HP: Gestation sac volumes as determined by sonar in first trimester of pregnancy. Br J Obstet Gynecol 82:100, 1975
5. Robinson HP: Sonar measurement of fetal crown–rump length as means of assessing maturity in first trimester of pregnancy. Br Med J 4:28, 1973
6. Robinson HP, Fleming JEE: A critical evaluation of sonar "crown–rump length" measurements. Br J Obstet Gynecol 82:702, 1975
7. Drumm JE, Clinch J, et al: The ultrasonic measurement of fetal crown–rump length as a method of assessing gestational age. Br J Obstet Gynecol 83:417, 1976
8. Kurjak A, Cecuk S, et al: Prediction of maturity in first trimester of pregnancy of ultrasonic measurement of fetal crown–rump length. J Clin Ultrasound 4:83, 1976
9. Campbell S: The prediction of fetal maturity by ultrasonic measurement of the biparietal diameter. J Obstet Gynecol Br Cwlth 76:603, 1969
10. Sabbagha RE, Turner H, et al: Sonar BPD and fetal age definition of the relationship. Obstet Gynecol 43:7, 1974
11. Hughey M, Sabbagha RE: Cephalometry by real-time imaging: A critical evaluation. Am J Obstet Gynecol 131:825, 1978
12. Hadlock FP, Deter RL, et al: Fetal biparietal diameter: A critical re-evaluation of the relation to menstrual age by means of real-time ultrasound. J Ultrasound Med 1:97, 1982
13. Kurtz, AB, Wapner RJ, et al: Analysis of biparietal diameter as an accurate indicator of gestational age. J Clin Ultrasound 8:319, 1980
14. Campbell S: Fetal head circumference against gestational age, in Sanders RC, James J Jr (eds): The Principles and Practice of Ultrasonography in Obstetrics and Gynecology, 2nd ed. New York, Appleton-Century-Crofts, 1980
15. Law RG, MacRae RD: Head circumference as an index of fetal age. J Ultrasound Med 1:281, 1982
16. O'Brien GD, Queenan JT, et al: Assessment of gestational age in the second trimester by real-time ultrasound measurement of the femur length. Am J Obstet Gynecol 139:544, 1981
17. O'Brien GD, Queenan JT: Growth of the ultrasound fetal femur length during normal pregnancy. Part 1. Am J Obstet Gynecol 141:833, 1981
18. Hohler CW, Quetel TA: A comparison of ultrasound fetal femur length and biparietal diameter in late pregnancy. Am J Obstet Gynecol 141:759, 1981
19. Yeh M, Bracero L, et al: Ultrasonic measurement of the femur length as an index of fetal gestational age. Am J Obstet Gynecol 144:519, 1982
20. Adam AH, Robinson HP, et al: A comparison of crown–rump length measurements using a real-time scanner in an antenatal clinic and a conventional B-scanner. Br J Obstet Gynecol 86:521, 1979
21. Docker MF, Settatree RS: Comparison between linear array real-time ultrasonic scanning and conventional compound scanning in the measurement of fetal biparietal diameter. Br J Obstet Gynecol 84:924, 1977
22. Cooperberg PL, Chow T, et al: Biparietal diameter: A comparison of real-time and conventional B-scan techniques. J Clin Ultrasound 4:421, 1976
23. Adamn AH, Robinson HP, et al: A comparison of biparietal diameter measurements using a real time scanner and conventional scanner equipped with a coded cephalometry system. Br J Obstet Gynecol 85:487, 1978
24. Wladimiroff JW, Eggink JH, et al: Clinical note. A comparative study between a linear-array real-time handheld scanner (minivisor) and a compound scanner (diasonograph) in the measurement of the fetal biparietal diameter. Ultrasound Med Biol 7:73, 1981
25. Hadlock FP, Deter RL, et al: The effect of head shape on the accuracy of BPD in estimating fetal gestational age. Am J Roentgenol 137:83, 1981
26. ACOG Technical Bulletin, Number 63, 1981
27. Johnson ML, Dunne MG, et al: Evaluation of the fetal intracranial anatomy by static and real-time ultrasound. J Clin Ultrasound 8:311, 1980
28. O'Brien GD: The booking exam for early fetal assessment. Contemporary Ob/Gyn 20:55, 1983
29. O'Brien GD, Queenan JT: Growth of ultrasound fetal femur length during normal pregnancy. Am J Obstet Gynecol 141:759, 1981

10 | Assessment of Gestational Age in the Second and Third Trimesters

David Graham
Roger C. Sanders

ESTIMATION OF GESTATIONAL AGE IN THE SECOND AND THIRD TRIMESTERS

Accurate determination of gestational age is of the upmost importance in the management of the pregnant patient. Knowledge of the gestational age allows diagnosis of normal or abnormal fetal growth patterns and is important in the timing of repeat cesarean section, preterm delivery, and prenatal intervention. Most commonly, gestational age is determined from the patient's recollection of the last menstrual period (LMP), the mean duration of pregnancy from the LMP being 280 days. However, in a significant percentage of patients the LMP is either uncertain or is incorrect, as judged by subsequent clinical outcome. Hertz et al.[1] reported that only 18 percent of patients could give an LMP that they regarded as reliable whereas Wenner et al.[2] reported that one-third of their group had a nonspecific LMP. Other clinical estimation techniques, such as physical examination in the first trimester, fundal height measurement in second and third trimester, and the detection of quickening of fetal heart tones with the head stethoscope, may be used but are subject to considerable error, up to ±4 weeks. The reliability of clinical estimators of gestational age has been reviewed by Bowie.[3] The most accurate clinical estimator of pregnancy duration was, not surprisingly, in the patient who has in vitro fertilization, followed by the patient who has ovulation induction. In the patient with noninduced pregnancy an LMP given from memory was found to have 95 percent confidence range of ±3 to 4 weeks, whereas from recorded dates the range was only ±2 to 3 weeks. Estimation of gestational

age from fetal heart recording, fundal height measurements were equally inaccurate with variations of 3 to 6 weeks. A single sonographic estimation from the crown–rump length (CRL) or from a biparietal diameter (BPD) measurement prior to 26 weeks was found to be more accurate than this clinical dating.

Ultrasound has been used extensively in the assessment of gestational age, usually by measurement of the size of the fetus or of some body part and assignment of a gestational age by assuming that the fetal size is at the 50th percentile. The sonographic assessment of gestational age in the first trimester is discussed in Chapter 9; this chapter focuses on sonographic assessment of gestational age in the second and third trimesters, when a number of fetal parameters are available for use, including biparietal diameter, head circumference, femur length, and abdominal circumference.

BIPARIETAL DIAMETER (BPD)

See Appendix 1. The BPD is the most commonly measured parameter of fetal size and is relatively easy to obtain, especially with real-time equipment. Sonographically the BPD may be rapidly and reproducibly measured by visualization of transverse sections of the head until one is obtained that shows the thalamus and cavum septum pellucidum (Fig. 1).[4] Although this level does not necessarily produce the widest transverse diameter of the head, it is one that may be consistently obtained on repeat examination. Although several techniques have been used for the actual mea-

147

surement (viz. measurements from leading edge to leading edge, leading edge to trailing edge and middle-to-middle measurements), it appears that because of the wide variation of normal measurements at any particular gestational age that the method of measurement does not materially affect the results obtained.[5] The most commonly accepted method and the one that would be expected to have the most precise end points for measurement is the leading edge to leading edge (outer-to-inner) measurement.

Errors in Measurement

A number of errors account for the variation of BPD with gestational age (GA) found throughout pregnancy.

Use of Different Techniques of Measurement. Although it had been thought that BPD measurements obtained with bistable, gray scale, or real-time techniques might be different, several studies have shown no statistical differences between these methods.[6-8] Real-time ultrasound technology certainly allows one to obtain a satisfactory plane for measurement more rapidly. Visualization of intracranial structures with gray scale technology provides a standard level for measurement and allows more accurate comparison of results obtained from different centers and different populations and also more reliably allows assessment of BPD growth from sequential studies in any particular individual.

Observer Error. Lawson et al.[8] have shown that the interobserver error in 14 percent of patients was statistically different and was on the order of ±1 mm compared to the overall mean. Two further studies yielded standard deviations at the 70 percent confidence limit of 1.74 and 2.64 mm, respectively.[7,9] The effect of this magnitude of error (±2 SD = 5.28 mm) would be dependent on gestational age. In the second trimester, when the fetal head is growing relatively rapidly, this degree of error would not affect gestational age by more than 1 to 2 weeks. Near term, however, with significant slowing of the fetal head growth a normal finding, the discrepancy would be much greater and approach as much as ±4 weeks.

Different Populations. In a study of 17 different BPD charts, Kurtz et al.[5] considered differences in patient populations as a possible factor in the differences seen between some of these charts. However, since no individual study was found to have either consistently higher or consistently lower BPD measurements, this was not considered to be significant factor. Sabbagha[10] in a study of measurements from four B-scan studies

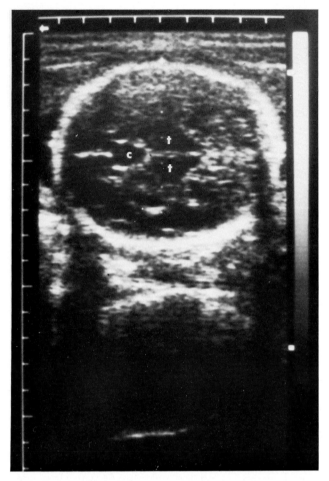

Fig. 1. Biparietal diameter. Transverse section at the level used for measurement of the BPD. The cavum septum pellucidum is seen anteriorly (c). Between the thalami (t) is seen the slit-like third ventricle.

showed that composite BPDs, derived from all four groups, did not differ significantly from the BPDs in each group. Similarly, no significant differences have been found in BPD measurements between whites and blacks.[11,12]

Intrinsic BPD Differences. Intrinsic differences in BPD at any given menstrual age may be a result of genetic variations in head size in fetuses of the same conceptional age or of differences in actual GA attributable to differences in the timing of fertilization or in the length of the preovulatory phase of the cycle.

Use of Different Nomograms. Although most nomograms show the same general relationship of BPD and GA there are often significant differences in gestational age assigned to any particular BPD measurement. For example, the mean GA assigned to a BPD of 8.0 cm in the Yale chart[13] is 33 weeks but is only 31 weeks in the Weiner chart, a composite chart derived from a number of studies.[14] When the normal variation of ±2 to 3 weeks at this stage of pregnancy is added to this, significant errors in assignment of GA may result.

Changes in Head Shape with Premature Rupture of Membranes (PROM) and with Prematurity. With PROM, especially with associated prematurity, there may be lateral flattening of the head resulting in a somewhat dolichocephalic slope.[15] Use of this section for BPD measurement will tend to underestimate the gestational age. Whether this effect is indeed significant may be determined by calculation of the cephalic index (q.v.).

Positional Problems. Although, in most examinations, a satisfactory BPD measurement may be obtained, in approximately 5 percent of examinations the fetus is in a position that makes measurement of the BPD inaccurate or impossible, i.e., face up, face down, or deeply engaged. In such instance other parameters such as femoral length or intraorbital distance must be used for dating.

The importance of fetal lie has been studied by Poll,[16] who found that BPD measurements of infants in breech position were frequently below the accepted norms, even with a normally growing fetus. This finding has not, however, been consistently seen with other investigators.

Use of Single Rather Than Repeated Measurements. Although small differences have been seen in the GA assigned to particular BPD measurements most studies show the same general relationship of BPD and GA, that is, there is a linear increase of BPD with GA until approximately 28 to 30 weeks, after which there is a slowing of BPD growth and a widening of confidence limits. When a BPD measurement is used for gestational age assessment, it is therefore important that the first study be done early in pregnancy to increase the accuracy of the assigned dates. An initial study obtained at 16 to 20 weeks allows one an opportunity not only to obtain an accurate gestational age assessment but also to examine major fetal organ systems. An initial examination at this time is preferable to one at 12 to 14 weeks since a measurement error of approximately ±1 mm is less significant with the larger measurement obtained at 16 to 20 weeks. In the last trimester overreliance on a single random measurement of BPD may result in inaccuracies in estimation of gestational age because of wider variation. Reliance on a single BPD measurement in the last 10 weeks of pregnancy may in fact be quite misleading, especially in the patient in whom there is symmetrical intrauterine growth retardation (IUGR) with a smaller

than expected head size. In such instances the GA may be significantly underestimated, leading to problems in clinical management.

Whether or not a second BPD estimation later in pregnancy in addition to the early screening is of any value in increasing the accuracy of assignment of gestational age has been a subject of some disagreement. O'Brien[17] evaluated the efficacy of a second BPD between 18 and 30 weeks of gestation in the prediction of the onset of labor, the accuracy of prediction being determined by analysis of the difference between the sonographically predicted EDC and the date of onset of spontaneous labor. Although it was found that the combined result of both examinations did not increase accuracy of the EDC prediction, the sample size of 50 patients was small.

In an attempt to avoid the errors inherent in extrapolation of GA from single measurements of BPD, Sabbagha et al. proposed the Growth Adjusted Sonographic Age (GASA).[18] This method is based on the observation that, when studied sequentially, fetuses may be classified into below average, average, or above average groups on the basis of BPD growth. Two separate BPDs are obtained in the usual manner, the first prior to 26 weeks of pregnancy and the second preferably in the period of 30 to 33 weeks. The incremental growth obtained is then compared to that which would be expected in each of the three groups and the fetus assigned to one of these groups. The GA assigned at the first BPD estimation is retained if the fetus shows oversize growth. If growth is above or below average the original GA is recalculated. With this method, an accuracy of prediction of GA of ±1 to 3 days (95 percent confidence limits) is claimed. Not only is the GASA thought to better define the duration of pregnancy, but it also allows placement of the fetus in a specific percentile growth bracket and may therefore aid in the earlier diagnosis of IUGR.

Use of Different Tissue Velocities for the Sound Beam. Although an assumed tissue velocity of ultrasound of 1540 m/sec is used as the reference in the United States, a number of the studies derived in Europe used a velocity of 1600 m/sec, resulting in an error of 4 percent. This error would assume greater significance in the last weeks of pregnancy.

Advantages of BPD

Despite the errors described above, the BPD remains the most commonly measured parameter in pregnancy and offers the following advantages:

1. A satisfactory measurement may be obtained in more than 95 percent of cases.

2. There are well-defined end points for measurement, and visualization of fixed intracranial landmarks allows one to obtain a reproducible level for measurement.

3. The relationship of BPD growth to gestational age has been extensively investigated and similar results obtained in a number of large scale studies.

Disadvantages of BPD

1. The accuracy of the measurement in predicting gestational age decreases as pregnancy advances. Because of this wide variation, a single BPD estimation obtained in the last weeks of pregnancy is therefore of very limited value in assigning gestational age.

2. Changes in head shape due to prematurity or to a relative decrease in the amount of amniotic fluid may cause an underestimation of true gestational age.

3. With a breech presentation and with multiple pregnancy (q.v.) the relationship of BPD to GA may be different from the singleton in cephalic presentation.

4. A deviation from normal growth may cause an underestimation of gestational age in growth-retarded infants or an overestimation of gestational age in infants large for their gestational age.

5. Where static scans are used to obtain BPD measurements, difficulty may be encountered in rapidly obtaining a satisfactory plane.

Effect of Head Shape and BPD

As described above, dolichocephaly secondary to prematurity or to a relative lack of amniotic fluid, e.g., with PROM or IUGR, may lead to an underestimation of gestational age (Fig. 2). Conversely, brachycephaly may lead to a larger than expected BPD and thus an overestimation of gestational age. This, however, is significantly less common than dolichocephaly. Such changes in head shape may also be seen transiently as a relatively common finding.

The degree to which head shape effects the BPD may be estimated by calculation of the cephalic index (CI) using the formula

$$CI = \frac{BPD}{OFD} \times 100\% \qquad [1]$$

where OFD is the occipitofrontal diameter. The normal range is 78.3% ± 4.4% (±1 SD).[15]

The occipitofrontal diameter is measured on the same image used for the BPD. Using these criteria Hadlock found that approximately 15 percent of BPD measurements were technically unsatisfactory.[15] In a study

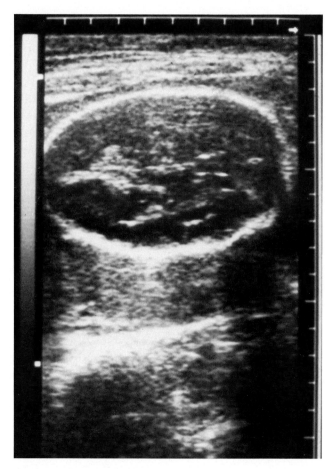

Fig. 2. Dolichocephaly. Transverse section of the head of a third trimester fetus with marked oligohydramnios shows lateral flattening of the head with a corresponding increase in OFD.

of 200 consecutive patients, Hohler[19] found that if these criteria were applied then an abnormal head shape would have made estimation of gestational age from BPD measurement invalid in 38.5 percent of cases even though the measurements of BPDs had been judged by an independent observer to be of good technical quality. Use of 79 ± 9 percent (±2 SD) to define a normal head shape still made the cephalic index abnormal in over 14 percent of cases. Because of the influence of change in head shape on BPD measurements GA should not be estimated from BPD unless the cephalic index is within the normal range. Where the cephalic index is outside this range then the head circumference should be used. Accuracy of the head circumference in prediction of gestational age in the third trimester (±2 to 3 weeks) is comparable to the accuracy of the BPD during this period. In a study by Hadlock, the head circumference measurements were within ±1 week of the true gestational age.[20]

The actual measurement of the head circumference may be obtained in one of several ways:

1. Use of an electronic caliper or light pen, either incorporated into the real-time equipment or with a separate commercial computer measurement system. This provides an easy, accurate method of measurement.
2. Use of a map measurer around the circumference of the outline. Although this technique gives relatively accurate results, it is tedious and there may be difficulty in obtaining a satisfactory map measurer outline.
3. Use of an average diameter gives an approximation of the head circumference (HC) that may be accurate enough for routine screening using the formula

$$HC = \frac{BPD + OFD}{2}\, \pi \qquad [2]$$

Biparietal Diameter Measurements in Multiple Pregnancy

The relationship of BPD and gestational age in the twin pregnancy has not been as well established as it has been in the singleton and a number of studies have resulted in conflicting conclusions. Although Divers[21] and Leveno[22] found that the BPDs in twins were smaller at all gestational ages, others have found mean BPD values corresponding to those of singletons until the third trimester, when gradual slowing is noted in twins. A major problem in the evaluation of BPD growth in twin-pairs has been the special problem of discordant growth with IUGR in one twin or with twin–twin transfusion, with one twin being LGA and the other SGA. Crane[23] corrected for this by studying only twin-pairs with normal growth and found normal twin BPD growth similar to that of singletons not only during the second trimester but throughout pregnancy.

Measured differences in the BPD between the members of a twin-pair may assume significant clinical importance, the significance increasing with the size of the difference. In Leveno's study[22] the risk of a twin infant being SGA was threefold greater when paired BPD differences were 5 mm or more compared to 4 mm or less. Other studies[21,24,25] produced similar findings, namely the smaller of a twin pair is at significantly increased risk of being SGA; with Crane's study the incidence of fetal death increased from 2 to 7 percent for twin pairs with 0 to 6 mm BPD differences to 20 percent when the difference was 7 mm or more.[23] Where a difference in BPD growth appears after 30 weeks it appears to be less important in predicting poor outcome than the same degree of difference occur-

ring earlier in pregnancy, which is more likely to indicate twin–twin transfusion. Where a BPD difference is measured sonographically, the HC should also be estimated to determine whether this BPD difference is real or is merely due to a change in head shape (e.g., dolichocephaly) in one of the pairs. With a real BPD difference the HC measurements between the two will also be different; if the HC of the twins is unchanged, however, the difference is due to a head shape change. Crane has found that an intrapair difference of more than 5 percent in HC was significant. In summary, with twin pregnancies the following hold:

1. There are significant discrepancies in the type of BPD growth pattern noted in a number of different studies.
2. In unselected series of twin-pairs BPD growth appears to be similar to that of singletons up to approximately 30 weeks, slowing thereafter.
3. There is evidence that where only twins with *normal* growth are examined the pattern of BPD growth is the same as singletons. It would therefore appear that GA assignments of twins should be appropriate from singleton charts.
4. Differences in BPD between members of a twin-pair may assume significant clinical significance. Where this difference is noted prior to 30 weeks and is more than 5 mm in BPD or greater than 5 percent in HC then twin-to-twin transfusion or a fetal anomaly of one infant is likely. After 30 weeks IUGR in one of the pair is more likely.
5. In patients with suspected multiple pregnancy an ultrasound examination should be performed as early as possible, preferably at the time that a CRL would be valid. Fetal growth may then be followed at sequential intervals dependent on the clinical course and the findings at any particular examination.

ABDOMINAL CIRCUMFERENCE (AC)

See Appendices 7 and 10. The circumference of the fetal abdomen is most conveniently and reproducibly measured through the liver, using a level that includes the horizontal portion of the portal sinus (Fig. 3). This level is at the same level as the stomach and slightly cephalad to the kidneys; therefore where the fetus is prone and shadowing from the spine prevents visualization of the portal sinus a section at the level of the stomach gives a good approximation.

The AC is obtained rapidly with real time by visualizing transverse sections of the fetus at right angles

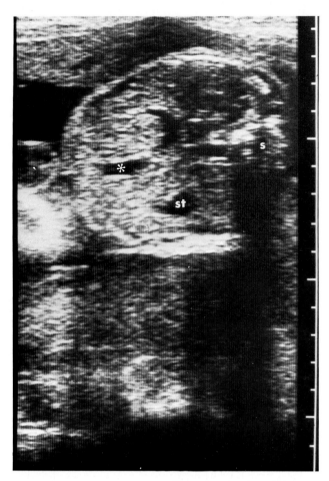

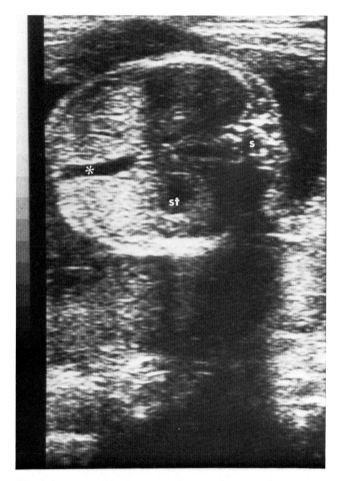

Fig. 3. Abdominal circumference. Transverse section of abdomen with correct orientation for measurement of the AC. The umbilical vein is clearly seen (*). s = spine, st = stomach.

Fig. 4. Incorrect abdominal circumference. Slight angulation of the transducer produced this section, which is not at right angles to the fetal spine. The section of the umbilical vein extends to the abdominal wall and the shape is ovoid rather than round.

to the spine. Since the umbilical vein enters the fetal abdomen and travels through the liver obliquely, in a cephaled and posterior direction, a scan that shows the umbilical vein extending to the anterior abdominal wall is probably an oblique rather than a true transverse scan (Fig. 4).

As with the head circumference, the actual measurement may employ a map measurer, electronic digitizer, or the average diameter method. This last method is quite practical for routine use since the image being measured is usually almost round. A suitable AC section is first obtained and then the widest and narrowest diameters of this scan are measured (using outer-to-outer technique). Multiplying this average diameter by π will give the circumference.

The abdominal circumference has a relationship to gestational age similar to that of the BPD, i.e., a fairly linear relationship until the last weeks of preg-

nancy when there is some flattening of the growth and a widening of the standard deviation.[26-28] This late flattening does not, however, appear to be as marked as with the BPD. However, because a reproducible AC is more difficult to obtain than a reproducible BPD or FL, this measurement should not be used as a sole estimator of gestational age unless other measurements cannot be obtained.

FEMORAL LENGTH

See Appendix 5. The femoral length (FL) is a relatively easy measurement to obtain and is, in fact, more consistently obtained than a satisfactory BPD. Although femoral length should be included as an additional parameter in the assessment of gestational age in all second and third trimester pregnancies it is especially

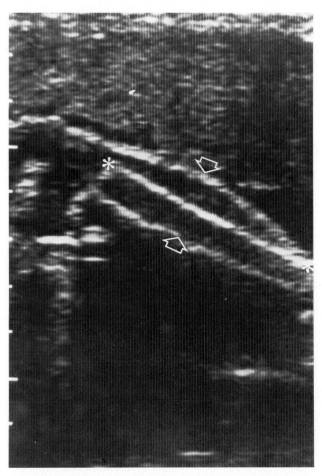

Fig. 5. Femur length. Measurement of the femur length is shown by the markers (*). The skin of the thigh is also visualized (*arrows*).

Errors in Measurement

1. Not visualizing the entire length of the shaft, thus underestimating the femoral length and the gestational age.
2. Using a sector scanner rather than a linear array, giving an inconsistent overestimate of length.
3. Using a chart that is not appropriate for the endpoints measured.

FEMORAL LENGTH AND BIPARIETAL DIAMETER

The femoral length has a linear relationship with the BPD up to term and therefore has a curve similar to the BPD when compared to gestational age, i.e., growth appears to slow in the third trimester.[29-31] Whether or not a reliable FL has been obtained may be determined by examining the femur length–biparietal diameter ratio (FL/BPD). When this ratio is measured, a relatively linear relationship is found throughout pregnancy. After 22 weeks Hohler has found that the ratio

$$\frac{FL}{BPD} \text{ is } 79 \pm 6 \text{ percent (90 percent confidence)}^{29} \quad [3]$$

This ratio is useful not only as an internal verification of the measurements obtained but may also be used to detect pathology of the head or limbs and as an aid in the classification of IUGR. An abnormal FL/BPD ratio may then be obtained in the following circumstances:

1. FL/BPD too high
   a. overestimation of femoral length
   b. underestimation of BPD, e.g., if there is dolichocephaly
   c. microcephaly
   d. craniosynostosis
2. FL/BPD too low
   a. underestimation of FL
   b. overestimation of BPD, e.g., if there is brachycephaly
   c. short-limb dysplasia or other skeletal dysplasia
   d. hydrocephalus or other intracranial pathology increasing head size

In a study of 1016 ultrasound femur measurements in patients with accurate menstrual dates, O'Brien[31] showed that the 95 percent confidence limits of a femur measurement at 14 to 20 weeks were ±6 days, from 20 to 30 weeks were ±12 days, and from 30 to 41 weeks were ±18 days. A combination of BPD, HC, and AC measurements and the femur length gives a three-

useful where it is difficult or impossible to obtain a reliable BPD, for example, where position or engagement of the head makes visualization difficult or where the head is pathologically large or small. Unfortunately, there is not yet a standardized way of measuring femur length and the visualized femoral neck may or may not be included in the measurement, which affects the validity of the results obtained. It appears that the most commonly reported series are using measurement of the visualized portion of the shaft, excluding the femoral neck (Fig. 5).

The measurement is best obtained with a linear array transducer since concern has been raised that images obtained with a sector scanner may overestimate the true length. The angle of the femur to the beam path does not, however, appear to significantly alter the measurement. Two or three pictures of the femur are obtained and the average length taken as the measurement, provided the measurements are within 2 mm of each other.

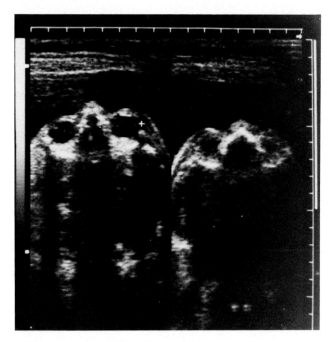

Fig. 6. Intraorbital diameter. In this face-up third-trimester fetus, measurement of the intraorbital distance is shown by the markers.

dimensional profile of the fetus, which may aid in the early diagnosis of IUGR.

INTERORBITAL DISTANCE

See Appendix 4. In those instances where a satisfactory BPD cannot be obtained, e.g., face-up, face-down position, or deeply engaged head, other parameters must be measured to estimate gestational age. One such parameter which has been proposed is that of the interorbital distance (Fig. 6). Mayden et al.[32] and Jeanty et al.[33] have produced charts of this measurement. This parameter is especially easy to obtain where the fetus is face up and simply represents the transverse distance between the lateral walls of the orbits. The values obtained may be used not only for assessing gestational age but also for diagnosis of malformations associated with hyper- or hypotelorism.

SUMMARY

Estimation of gestational age is the commonest indications for obtaining a sonogram in the pregnant patient. Although gestational age may be estimated from the LMP or a number of other clinical criteria these have been shown to be relatively inaccurate compared to a sonographic determination, properly timed. Although the CRL appears to be the single most accurate

sonographic estimator of gestational age, this measurement is only usable in the first trimester. In the second and third trimesters other variables, principally the BPD, HC, AC, and femur length, are more valid. They are, however, less accurate partially because of the techniques used and partially because of the greater variability of fetal size at any particular gestational age as pregnancy advances. Although traditionally a single BPD measurement has been relied upon for dating there is considerable evidence that such a limited approach leads to inaccurate dating in a significant percentage of patients. This is due to a number of factors, including head shape changes and positional changes. It is therefore more accurate to measure at least two, and preferably more, parameters in all second and third trimester pregnancies. Before the BPD and FL are used for dating, their validity should be assessed by calculation of the cephalic index and the BPD/FL ratio. Where these are abnormal, reliance should not be placed on these measurements and other parameters should be used.

Hadlock[34] has proposed a third trimester composite gestational age derived from the BPD, HC, AC, and FL. Between 30 and 36 weeks an average gestational age from BPD–AC–FL was found to be the best combination (mean error 0 to 4 weeks, SD 1 to 2 weeks) whereas from 36 to 42 weeks a combination of HC–AC–FL was a better combination (mean 0.2, SD 1 to 2).

REFERENCES

1. Hertz RH, Sokol RJ, Knoke JD, et al: Clinical estimation of gestational age: Rules for avoiding preterm delivery. Am J Obstet Gynecol 131:395, 1978
2. Wenner WM, Young EB: Nonspecific date of last menstrual period. An indication of poor reproductive outcome. Am J Obstet Gynecol 120:1071, 1974
3. Bowie JD, Andreotti RF: Estimating gestational age in utero in ultrasonography, in Callen P (ed), Obstetrics and Gynecology. Philadelphia, Saunders, 1983
4. Hadlock FP, Deter RL, Marrist RB, et al: Fetal biparietal diameter: Rational choice of plane of section for sonographic measurement. Am J Radiol 138:871, 1983
5. Kurtz AB, Wapner RJ, Kurtz RJ, et al: An analysis of biparietal diameter as an accurate indicator of gestational age. J Clin Ultrasound 8:319, 1980
6. Cooperberg PL, Chow T, Kite V, et al: Biparietal diameter. A comparison of real-time and conventional B-scan techniques. J Clin Ultrasound 6:421, 1976
7. Docker MF, Setatree RS: Comparison between linear array, real time ultrasonic scanning and conventional compound scanning in the measurement of the fetal biparietal diameter. Br J Obstet Gynaecol 84:924, 1977

8. Lawson TL, Albacelli JN, Greenhouse SW, et al: Gray scale measurement of the biparietal diameter. J Clin Ultrasound 5:17, 1976
9. Davidson JW, Lind T, Farr V, et al: The limitations of ultrasonic fetal cephalometry. J Obstet Gynaecol Br Commun 80:769, 1973
10. Sabbagha RE, Hughey M: Standardization of sonar cephalometry and gestational age. Obstet Gynecol 52:402, 1978
11. Sabbagha RE, Barton FB, Barton BA: Sonar biparietal diameter. I. Analysis of percentile growth differences in two normal populations using same methodology. Am J Obstet Gynecol 126:479, 1976
12. Hohler CW, Lea J, Collins H: Screening for IUGR using the ultrasound BPD. J Clin Ultrasound 4:187, 1977
13. Hobbins JC: Yale Nomogram, Siemens Corporation. Electromedical Division, 1979
14. Weiner SN, Flynn MJ, Kennedy AW, et al: A composite curve of ultrasonic biparietal diameters for estimating gestational age. Radiology 122:781, 1977
15. Hadlock FP, Deter RL, Carpenter RJ, et al: Estimating fetal age: Effect of head shape on BPD. Am J Roentgenol. 137:83, 1981
16. Poll V, Kasby CB: An improved method of fetal weight estimation using ultrasound measurements of fetal abdominal circumference. Br J Obstet Gynaecol 86:922, 1979
17. O'Brien WF, Coddington CC, Cefalo RC: Serial ultrasonographic biparietal diameters for prediction of estimated date of confinement. Am J Obstet Gynecol 138:467, 1980
18. Sabbagha RE, Hughey M, Depp R: Growth adjusted sonographic age: A simplified method. Obstet Gynecol 51:383, 1978
19. Hohler CW: Cross checking pregnancy landmarks by ultrasound. Contemp OB/GYN 20:169, 1982
20. Hadlock FP, Deter RL, Marrist RB, et al: Fetal head circumference: Relation to menstrual age. Am J Radiol 138:649, 1982
21. Divers WA, Hemsell DL: The use of ultrasound in multiple gestations. Obstet Gynecol 53:500, 1979
22. Leveno KS, Santos-Ramos R, Duenholler JM, et al: Sonar cephalometry in twin pregnancy: Discordancy of the biparietal diameter after 28 weeks. Am J Obstet Gynecol 138:615, 1980
23. Crane JP, Tonich PG, Kopta M: Ultrasonic growth patterns in normal and discordant twins. Obstet Gynecol 55, 678, 1980
24. Moulton MC: Divergent biparietal diameter growth rates in twin pregnancies. Obstet Gynecol 49:543, 1977
25. Haney AF, Crenshaw MC, Dempsey PJ: Significance of biparietal diameter differences between twins. Obstet Gynecol 51:609, 1978
26. Deter RL, Harrist RB, Hadlock FP, et al: Fetal head and abdominal circumferences. II. A critical reevaluation of the relationship to menstrual age. J Clin Ultrasound 10:365, 1982
27. Hadlock FP, Deter RL, Harrist RB, et al: Fetal abdominal circumference as a predictor of gestational age. Am J Roentgenol 139:367, 1982
28. Tamura RK, Sabbagha RE: Percentile ranks of sonar fetal AC measurements. Am J Obstet Gynecol 138:457, 1980
29. Hohler CW, Quetel TA: Fetal femur length: Equations for computer calculation of gestational age from ultrasound measurements. Am J Obstet Gynecol 143:479, 1982
30. Jeanty P, Kirkpatrick C, Dramaix-Wilmet MS, et al: Ultrasonic evaluations of fetal limb growth. Radiology 140:165, 1981
31. O'Brien GD, Queenan JT: Growth of the ultrasound fetal femur length during normal pregnancy. Am J Obstet Gynecol 141:833, 1981
32. Mayden KL, Tortora M, Berkowitz RL, et al: Orbital diameters: A new parameter for prenatal diagnosis and dating. Am J Obstet Gynecol 144:289, 1982
33. Jeanty P, Dramaix-Wilmet M, VanGansebke D, et al: Fetal ocular biometry by ultrasound. Radiology 143:513, 1982
34. Hadlock FP, Deter RL, Harrist RB, et al: Computer assisted analysis of fetal age in the third trimester using multiple fetal growth parameters. J Clin Ultrasound 11:313, 1983

11 | Ultrasound Diagnosis of Intrauterine Growth Retardation

Charles W. Hohler

One of the major applications of diagnostic ultrasound in pregnancy is the detection of intrauterine growth retardation. This is the case for several reasons. First, ever since Lubchenco and co-workers[1] presented the concept that there was clinical utility to knowledge of the percentage distribution of birthweights at any given gestational age, many other authors have demonstrated that those babies born small-for-gestational age (SGA) have a poorer prognosis than their more normally grown peers.[2-9] Westwood et al. have shown, however, that full-term, nonasphyxiated, SGA infants have an impaired potential for physical growth, but a good prognosis for neurologic and cognitive development. Previous findings of more severe cognitive deficits are attributed by the authors to a failure to distinguish the effects of isolated intrauterine growth retardation from those due to asphyxia and other potentially confounding factors.[10] Second, clinical methods fail to detect from one-third to one-half of all SGA fetuses[11-13]; and, third, gestational age cannot be accurately determined, clinically, in up to 40 percent of cases.[14-15]

McKeown and Record[16] were among the first investigators to plot weight by gestational age for single and multiple births. Greunwald[17-18] expanded the concept of a fetal "growth curve" of weight for gestational age and attributed growth problems to external influences that modify the intrauterine environment. From such analyses, the concept has developed that birth weight is a function of gestational age, but, as Wilcox has recently pointed out,[19] the "fetal growth curve," with its assumption that birth weight depends on gestational age, has tended to obscure the fact that the true direction of cause and effect is not known. In any large group of births, both birth weight and gestational age have a Gaussian or bell-shaped distribution. Thus, the three-dimensional approach of Wilcox is useful to describe the bivariate distribution problem faced by the ultrasonologist when trying to "fix" both weight and age estimates for any given fetus.

Despite the shortcomings of two-dimensional, weight for dates, fetal growth curves, the approach to analysis of change in fetal size using them is simple, coherent, and has become widely used due to its demonstrated clinical relevance to perinatal mortality and morbidity. We will use this approach in the remainder of our discussion.

THE CONCEPT OF THE SMALL-FOR-GESTATIONAL AGE (SGA) FETUS

From the above discussion, it is apparent that the SGA fetus is a statistical entity, not to be confused with the low-birth-weight (LBW) fetus born with a birth weight of less than 2500 g. SGA babies constitute a high-risk group, and make up approximately one-third of all LBW infants; they have a six- to eight-fold increased chance of dying in the perinatal period compared to infants of average weight for gestational age.[20-21] Neonatal mortality risk, in relation to birth weight and gestational age, has recently been reviewed by Koops et al.,[22] who found that SGA infants continue to exhibit a higher neonatal mortality rate than AGA infants at all gestational ages (Fig. 1).

There are three major, conventional, weight-for-

Neonatal Mortality Risk
by Birthweight and Gestational Age

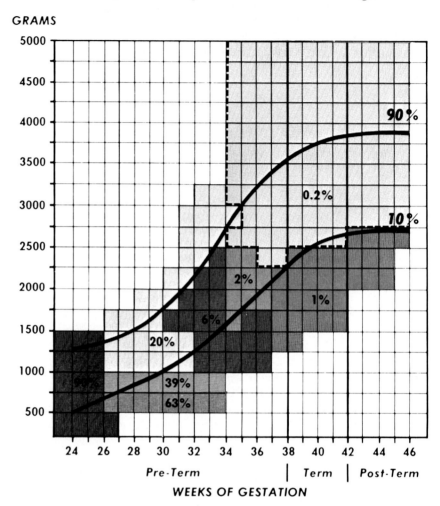

Fig. 1. Neonatal mortality risk calculated by birth weight and gestational age for the period 1974 through 1980, based on 14,413 live births at the University of Colorado Health Sciences Center, shows categorically that small for gestational age babies have a worse neonatal mortality risk than do their more normal grown peers. (*Reprinted with permission from Koops et al: Pediatriacs, 101:6, 1982.*)

1974-1980 BASED ON 14,413 LIVEBIRTHS AT UNIVERSITY OF COLORADO
HEALTH SCIENCES CENTER

dates categories: AGA, SGA, and LGA, representing appropriate, small, and large for gestational age, respectively. Typically, between the 10th and 90th percentiles is defined as the range specified as AGA. Below the 10th percentile is defined as SGA, and above the 90th percentile is defined as LGA. These growth curve demarcations, while convenient, are somewhat arbitrary. The babies growing under the 10th percentile for dates constitute a heterogeneous population of constitutionally small and growth-retarded babies. Additionally, not all babies that are growing above the 10th percentile are completely "normal." Miller et al.[23] have shown that in fetuses with the same gestational age and having the same external body dimensions, birth weights may differ by as much as 30 to 40 percent.

They further showed that birth weight by itself was frequently not a valid measure of fetal growth impairment. By including measurements of body length and head size, along with birth weight, four distinct patterns of fetal growth impairment were identified. The four patterns included infants who had abnormally short body lengths for dates, infants who had evidence of disproportionate growth when body length and head circumference were impaired, infants who accumulated excessive amounts of soft tissue mass, and infants who accumulated too little soft tissue mass. They further pointed out that the difference between normal and abnormal fetal growth is a zone and not a line. By concentrating their emphasis on weight for height, they were able to circumvent the problem of

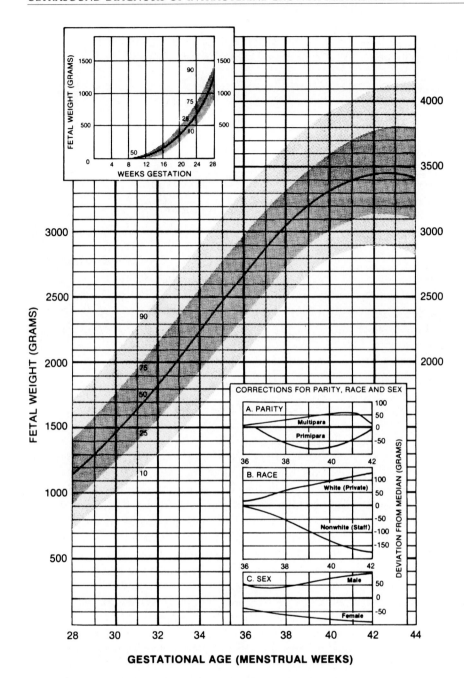

Fig. 2. The fetal weight versus gestational age nomogram indicating 10th, 25th, 50th, 75th, and 90th percentile confidence limits throughout pregnancy is shown. This is the nomogram used by the author in development of the fetal growth profile for laboratories at or near sea level. (*Reprinted with permission from Brenner: A Standard of Fetal Growth for the United States of America. Am J Obstet Gynecol 126, 1976.*)

the necessity of accurately dating the pregnancy in order to arrive at a conclusion as to the nutritional status of the fetus. Daikoku et al.,[24] using this same line of reasoning, found that only 47 percent of those fetuses showing other evidence of abnormal growth had birth weights below the 10th percentile. They included in their study calculation of the Ponderal Index (PI = weight/crown–heel length^3 × 100), measurement of the crown–heel length and the head circumference plus weight in order to identify fetuses with growth

abnormalities. As these studies show, an evaluation of weight alone is not adequate to fully assess the status of fetal intrauterine nutrition.

Comparison of weight for dates reference "standards" reveals clinically significant differences. Three of the commonly used growth curves of weight for dates are those of Lubchenco,[1] Usher and McLean,[25] and Brenner et al.,[26] which is the reference standard (Fig. 2) that is used by the author. After 30 weeks' gestation, the Lubchenco 90th, 50th, and 10th percentile weights are about 100 g less than those found by Brenner et al. at comparable percentiles at the same gestational ages. Racial mix of the study populations, as well as altitude, has been felt to account for the differences found; however, Cotton et al.[27] have recently reported the results of an analysis of the birth weights, lengths, and gestational ages of neonates from a very stable population living at 3100 m, which indicates that babies born of mothers who have lived at that altitude for at least 2 years have the same weights and the same gestational ages as those babies born in Denver and at sea level. The mean birth weight for the entire group of 215 babies delivered in that study was 3.18 kg ± 2.16 (1 standard deviation). Other obstetric factors may also contribute to differences in reference growth curves. The reference standard of Lubchenco and associates,[1] derived from deliveries at 24 to 42 menstrual weeks' gestation, was based on relatively few (5635) selected infants born to Caucasian mothers of low socioeconomic status at a high elevation (5280 feet). Furthermore, fetal growth standards for past generations, for other countries, and for specific United States groups, may not be representative of present day fetal growth standards in the United States.

ETIOLOGY

The etiologies of intrauterine growth retardation are numerous, but can be grouped into three main categories (Fig. 3). Maternal disease states, such as severe diabetes mellitus, chronic hypertension, chronic renal disease, and some collagen diseases such as systemic lupus erythematosus can cause vascular damage in the uteroplacental bed that can lead to reduced placental perfusion, which, in turn, leads to deprivation, in the fetus, of oxygen and/or vital nutrients, especially glucose. Such reduced placental support of the growing fetus is broadly termed, clinically, "uteroplacental insufficiency" or UPI.

Extensive, primary placental pathology, such as infarction, can also lead to UPI, but this is not as common as decreased placental perfusion secondary to maternal vascular disease. The changes seen in fetal growth depend on both the duration of reduced placental perfusion and the extent of the reduction. Naeye[28] found in an analysis of 11,082 term singleton pregnancies that birth weights progressively increased with increasing blood pressures until the hypertensive range was reached when maternal edema and proteinuria were absent. Birth weights leveled off or decreased when pressures reached the hypertensive range. The pressure threshold at which growth slowed increased the diastolics of 75 mm Hg in the lowest maternal

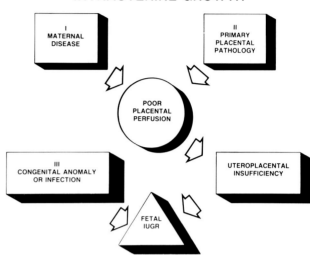

CAUSES OF SUB-OPTIMAL INTRAUTERINE GROWTH

Fig. 3. Categories of pathology that may lead to fetal intrauterine growth retardation are grouped into those that cause poor placental perfusion and those which cause primary anomalies, chromosomal abnormalities, or infection in the fetus.

pregnancy weight gain category to nearly 100 mm Hg in the highest weight gain category. Decreases in birth weight associated with hypertension were most severe when mothers were thin and had low pregnancy weight gains. In addition, diuretics reduced birth weights in low-maternal-weight-gain pregnancies, but not in high-weight-gain ones. Thus, it was found that fetal growth increased with increasing maternal blood pressures. This effect was thought to be mediated through uteroplacental blood flow. The relationship of blood pressure, blood volume, and maternal weight gain were also explored by the author. It was also shown that the body length and head circumferences of fetuses continued their pressure-associated increases when diastolic pressures exceeded 100 mm Hg. This is in keeping with the older data of Greunwald[29] that uteroplacental underperfusion has less effect on body lengths and head circumferences than on birth weights.

Primary fetal developmental abnormalities caused by such problems as congenital heart disease, a variety of congenital anomalies of the genitourinary and central nervous systems, as well as many chromosomal abnormalities, such as trisomy 21, 18, and 13, can all lead to intrauterine growth retardation. In addition, certain congenital viral infections such as rubella or cytomegalic virus can also cause a fetus to be underweight for gestational age.

Phenotypic expression of fetal growth problems in utero is dependent upon etiology, duration, and severity of the underlying pathology (Fig. 4). When there are intrinsic fetal abnormalities such as anomalies or

IUGR PHENOTYPES

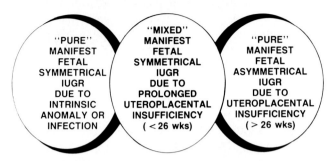

Fig. 4. The overlap between pure patterns of symmetrical IUGR and asymmetric IUGR is often found. The phenotypic expression of such patterns makes it difficult to determine the etiology of intrauterine growth retardation based solely on newborn physical examination.

infection, then growth of fetal head size, trunk size, body length, and all fetal organs is proportionately reduced to a certain similar percentage of normal expected values. Measurement of various parts of the fetus will, therefore, show no change in the symmetry of the fetal body. Hence, this type of IUGR is called symmetrical or "low profile" type IUGR.[30]

On the other hand, intrauterine growth retardation on the basis of uteroplacental insufficiency affects various fetal organs at different rates and to varying degrees. This leads to an asymmetry of organ sizes, which is only relative, not absolute[31]; hence, the equating of asymmetrical intrauterine growth retardation with uteroplacental insufficiency in the majority of cases. There is, in most cases, "overlap" of phenotypic expression, such that on the basis of physical examination of the newborn, it is impossible to determine whether the IUGR is of the symmetrical or asymmetrical type. This is usually the case when uteroplacental insufficiency has been long-standing (i.e., since prior to 26 weeks of gestation).[32]

MEASUREMENTS

Biparietal Diameter

From the above analysis, plus study of newborn infants, it is seen that intrauterine growth retardation can be manifest by a variety of combinations of decreased weight, crown–heel length, head and/or abdomen circumference, decreased subcutaneous fat deposition and/or muscle mass. From the ultrasonologist's point of view, this means that it is not likely to be sufficient to measure just one part of the fetal body to detect what are usually numerous and subtle, and even sometimes undetectable patterns of intrauterine growth retardation. BPD measurement, in particular, has been shown to be too insensitive a measurement,

by most authors, to use alone to detect intrauterine growth retardation. Queenan et al.[33] have reported an accuracy rate of 50 percent for the detection of intrauterine growth retardation when serial biparietal diameters were used as the sole indicator of the condition. Hohler et al.[34] came to a similar conclusion from an analysis of 43 SGA babies born in a population of 1500 patients scanned to predict fetal age and weight by BPD measurement. Intrauterine growth retardation was most accurately determined when an absolutely small BPD was found at the time of the last ultrasound examination in a woman with accurate gestational age assessment. However, a 50 percent false positive detection rate and poor sensitivity to intrauterine growth retardation were found using the BPD measurement as a screening test in this manner. Crane et al.[35] have made the point that arrest of biparietal diameter growth seems to occur several weeks prior to deterioration of placental function as evidenced by falls in estriols, the appearance of meconium in the amniotic fluid, or the presence of a positive contraction stress test and/or late decelerations in labor, and based a management policy upon this fact, not intervening on the basis of a third trimester biparietal diameter growth arrest pattern unless fetal distress was also documented by an ominous estriol pattern and/or a positive contraction stress test. Ellis and Bennett[36] have examined the possibility of using a single ultrasound measurement of the biparietal diameter at 32 to 34 weeks of gestation in order to detect intrauterine growth retardation. Only 4 of 40 SGA infants were below the fifth percentile for their gestational age according to head measurements, a 90 percent false negative rate. The authors state that a single head measurement of growth-retarded infants, whose size fell below the 10th percentile at 32 to 34 weeks, would have detected only 6 percent of these infants. Their conclusion was that most SGA fetuses have measurable reductions in growth only after 34 weeks. Sabbagha[37] has taken the approach that the probability of intrauterine growth retardation being present can be predicted on the basis of accurate estimation of gestational age and the determination of whether or not the biparietal diameter measurement falls below the 25th percentile for dates. He has shown that the fetus with a biparietal diameter growing above the 75th percentile for dates has only a 3.5 percent chance of being less than 2500 g at term, while a fetus growing at less than the 25th percentile has a 42.3 percent chance of being less than 2500 g at term.

Total Intrauterine Volume (TIUV)

Based on the disappointing results from measurement of biparietal diameter for the early detection of intrauterine growth retardation, the estimate of total intrauterine volume was developed by Gohari et al.[38] in 1977. It was the feeling of the authors that total intrauterine volume measurement (TIUV) was an accurate predictor of intrauterine growth retardation. TIUV was calculated from the longitudinal, transverse, and anteroposterior dimensions of the uterus measured with a static B-scanner. Using the TIUV and a simultaneous biparietal diameter for dating of the pregnancy, it was possible to diagnose 75 percent of the cases of IUGR with a single examination. If the total intrauterine volume fell within what the authors called the "gray zone" between the definitely normal and the definitely abnormal zones on their curve, there was a 32 percent chance (7 of 22 cases) that the fetus was growth retarded. It was the feeling of the authors that because all of these infants were symmetrically growth retarded, however, the BPDs were smaller than expected for their gestational ages. Correction for this fact would have led to estimation of total intrauterine volumes that would have all been in the abnormal zone. The measurement of the TIUV was proposed in that study as a screening method for patients at risk for intrauterine growth retardation. Chinn et al.[39] in contrast, found in a group of 252 patients that the total intrauterine volume measurement was sensitive in 70 percent, specific in 72 percent, and accurate in predicting IUGR in only 41 percent of cases. They concurred with Gohari et al., however, that the results of the use of the total intrauterine volume were least predictive when the BPD was employed as an indicator of gestational age. Despite this limitation, and even after correction for small biparietal diameters in the symmetrically undergrown babies, they did not find an improvement in the predictive value of the total intrauterine volume technique. Furthermore, they found that there is a considerable overlap of TIUV in the normal versus abnormal groups. Two other studies have elucidated some of the problems inherent in attempting to take accurate measurements of the uterus and the significance of bladder distension in determination of uterine volume.[40-41] Because of the limitations pointed out by these authors, Middleton and coworkers[42] developed a method of measurement of the maximal longitudinal and transverse uterine areas (LTUA). They found the measurement to be less prone to observer variability and more sensitive in diagnosing intrauterine growth retardation than the total intrauterine volume measurement. Intraobserver variability of measurement was reduced from 10 percent using the TIUV method to 3.7 percent using LTUA. Interobserver variability was found to be 6.5 percent of the LTUA method and 12.9 percent for the TIUV. Sensitivity for the LTUA measurement was 70 percent and for TIUV was 40 percent while the specificities were

94 and 96 percent, respectively. The LTUA method consists of adding the maximum longitudinal and transverse areas of the intrauterine contents. It does not represent a true volume measurement. No confirmation of these results by other authors has, as yet, been forthcoming.

Because of the difficulty of interpretation of the total intrauterine volume in the absence of certain clinical dates, and because of the necessity of use of a contact B-scanner, TIUV measurement has recently decreased in popularity. Rather, a more direct approach to observation of the amount of amniotic fluid and direct measurement of the fetus has developed.

The new concept of a "growth profile" includes measurement of the fetal biparietal diameter as well as head circumference, abdominal circumference, femur length, and, more recently, thigh diameters and circumference. From such measurements, an estimate of fetal weight for dates, as well as an estimate of body symmetry, can be made. Such growth profiling, intuitively, has some attraction, since it departs from the strict weight for dates concept, which does not detect all fetuses with growth impairment. A review of the basis for such a growth profile concept is provided from the work of Deter et al.[43] As yet, however, growth profiling has not been subjected to rigorous, published, prospective testing, so that judgment about this approach must remain, for now, suspended. Diagnostic ultrasound methods, therefore, are not perfect, and are capable of detecting the majority, but not all of the fetuses suffering mild growth impairment.

Ultrasound measurement of head size, abdomen size, body length, and thigh circumference shows the most promise for improvement for intrauterine growth retardation detection. The best use of these measurements can be made when the gestational age is well established on clinical and/or ultrasound grounds, early in pregnancy, i.e., before 20 weeks of gestation. Diagnostic ultrasound is much less reliable for the detection of intrauterine growth retardation when clinical dating is uncertain. Thus, it is axiomatic that ultrasound evaluation of fetal growth depends on accurate knowledge of menstrual age.

Amniotic Fluid Volume

The amount of amniotic fluid in the uterus has also been examined as a possible predictor of the presence of intrauterine growth retardation. Initial attempts to use a qualitative assessment of a smaller than 1 cm pocket of amniotic fluid using a dynamic-imaging, linear array scanner by Manning and co-workers[44] were found to be a fairly reliable indicator of the presence of intrauterine growth retardation. In 120 patients, qualitative amniotic fluid volume was normal in 91 patients, and 86 were delivered of a normal fetus (93.4

percent). In contrast, qualitative amniotic fluid volume was decreased in 29 patients, and 26 were delivered of a fetus with intrauterine retardation (89.9 percent). Perinatal morbidity was increased tenfold in patients with decreased amniotic fluid volume. Overall, 26 of 31 intrauterine growth retarded fetuses (83.4 percent) demonstrated decreased qualitative amniotic fluid volume. However, Philipson et al.[45] found that routine sonographic screening to detect oligohydramnios is probably not warranted. Consecutive ultrasound examinations were done in 2453 singleton pregnancies with intact membranes, with 3.9 percent found to be complicated by oligohydramnios. Forty percent of the infants from oligohydramnios-complicated pregnancies were SGA, compared with 8 percent of infants from pregnancies without oligohydramnios. Of 46 SGA births, 38 (83 percent) were preceded by sonographically diagnosed oligohydramnios. The authors found a 40 percent predictive value of the presence of oligohydramnios, but also found that only 16 percent of SGA births would be preceded by sonographically diagnosed oligohydramnios. Therefore, 84 percent of the cases would be missed. However, the criteria for diagnosis of oligohydramnios, the severity of the intrauterine growth retardation detected, and the populations under study are different in the Manning and Philipson groups. If, on the other hand, severe oligohydramnios has developed, then not only is the sensitivity and specificity of this ultrasonic parameter increased, but also the perinatal mortality and morbidity associated with intrauterine growth retardation that may be present.

The presence of a normal amount of amniotic fluid, together with a small biparietal diameter measurement from an average shaped head and the presence of phosphatidylglycerol in the amniotic fluid has been found to be capable of detecting 80 percent of all SGA fetuses.[46] In a study of 249 pregnancies, Gross et al. performed an ultrasound examination and amniocentesis at or beyond 34 weeks of gestation. A fetal biparietal diameter of 8.7 cm or less and the presence of phosphatidylglycerol in amniotic fluid were found to be capable of detecting 80 percent of all SGA fetuses. The limitation of this approach is that it will not be possible to detect the SGA infant in a preterm pregnancy. Since a majority of SGA infants develop IUGR during the third trimester, the use of this model for more complete detection of intrauterine growth retardation would be difficult.

Head Size

See Appendix 2. The same parameters that are used to estimate gestational age can be used to evaluate fetal growth. Head size is measured by BPD and circumference. These are indirect estimates of brain

HEAD CIRCUMFERENCE MEASUREMENT TECHNIQUE

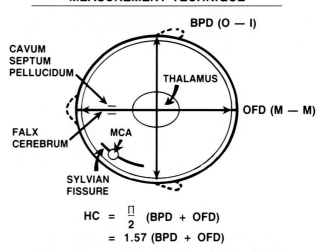

$$HC = \frac{\pi}{2} (BPD + OFD)$$
$$= 1.57 (BPD + OFD)$$

Fig. 5. Head circumference measurements technique using the two diameters method is shown above. The BPD measurement is an "outer-to-inner" measurement whereas the OFD measurement is a "middle-to-middle" measurement when using a linear array, dynamic-imaging instrument. Circumference is calculated using the general formula shown for the circumference of a circle.

weight, estimation of which has been approached more directly, but with more technical difficulty by Jordaan et al.[47,48] The proper plane for fetal BPD and/or head circumference measurement is shown in Figure 5. The BPD is measured using a leading edge technique (i.e., "outer-to-inner"), which is considered standard. Head circumference measurement can be carried out using any one of several methods—map reader, calculation from measurement of the major and minor axes of the elliptical head, or by direct tracing through use of a planimeter or computer light pen. These techniques have been shown to be comparable in clinical use.[49]

Head circumference measurements are becoming extremely important for the evaluation of not only gestational age but also intrauterine growth retardation.[50] Measurement of the fetal head circumference has been shown to be accurate with the use of dynamic-imaging ultrasound equipment.[51] Biparietal diameter measurement may not be useful for the detection of intrauterine growth retardation because of antenatal molding of the fetal head which can go on due to position of the fetus in utero, the presence of leiomyomata in the uterine wall, the presence of more than one fetus in the uterus, or to other unknown factors. The quantitative analysis of this phenomenon has been carried out by Hadlock et al.[52] The ultrasound measurement of the cephalic index is important when deciding whether or not the change in the biparietal diameter size from one examination to the next truthfully reflects a change in brain size. Head shape changes may cause the biparietal diameter to become smaller than would be anticipated on the basis of a normal growth curve, which may lead the clinician to conclude that intrauterine growth retardation was beginning to occur. However, a check of the head circumference would reveal that the circumference had grown appropriately and was truthfully reflecting brain size versus dates. It is for this reason that multiple fetal parameters should be evaluated when estimating fetal size, weight, and adequacy of growth between examinations. This variable change in head shape during the last half of pregnancy could also account for the large number of false positive diagnoses of intrauterine growth retardation of the "late flattening type" seen in previous studies. By calculation of the cephalic index and finding that the head shape is "average," the inclusion of the biparietal diameter into the growth profile is legitimized. Unless and until such a cephalic index calculation is performed on every patient, the use of the biparietal diameter to judge adequacy of fetal growth should not be accepted.

Abdomen Size

See Appendices 2, 7, and 10. Abdomen circumference measurement reflects fetal liver size. Liver size, in turn, is largely determined by the amount of stored glycogen present, which, in turn, is influenced very quickly by the factors that lead to intrauterine growth retardation, especially of the asymmetric type. Asymmetric intrauterine growth retardation is frequently related to a gradually increasing placental insufficiency of unknown etiology. The manifestations of this in the fetus appear consistent with diminished nutrient uptake and/or inadequate utilization. A notable feature of this condition is that while body weight is reduced, the brain size is disproportionately maintained, but not absolutely spared compared to other organs such as the liver. Animal models being developed to study this phenomenon more closely will permit detailed studies of many aspects of IUGR that are inaccessible through direct study of human gestation.[53]

A circumference measurement of a well-defined plane with standard landmarks is widely used to follow IUGR (Fig. 6). This was first suggested by Campbell and Wilkin,[54] and is the plane perpendicular to the long axis of the fetal spine, which contains a profile of a portion of the umbilical segment of the right portal vein (known more commonly as the "umbilical vein") as it enters into the substance of the fetal liver. Actual measurement techniques are very similar in principle to those used for head circumference. Two perpendicular diameters (the anterior–posterior abdominal diameter and the transverse abdominal diameter) or perimeter measurements can be used to estimate this measurement. It is important to avoid inclusion of the

ABDOMINAL CIRCUMFERENCE MEASUREMENT TECHNIQUE

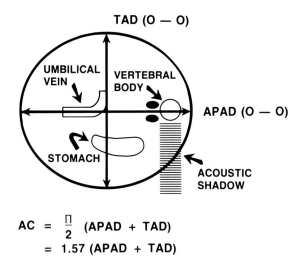

$$AC = \frac{\Pi}{2} (APAD + TAD)$$
$$= 1.57 (APAD + TAD)$$

Fig. 6. Abdominal circumference measurement technique is shown. All measurements are "outer-to-outer" measurements as the subcutaneous fat deposition should be included to accurately estimate fetal weight. The formula for the circumference of a circle, shown above, is used to calculate the circumference.

upper poles of the kidneys and/or the lower portion of the fetal heart. Abdomen shape is not constant and is influenced by fetal breathing so there is no comparable measurement to the cephalic index in the head which relates the anterior–posterior diameter of the abdomen to the transverse diameter. Studies by Deter et al.[55] have shown growth of the abdominal circumference to be almost linear throughout pregnancy, with a growth rate of 1 to 1.28 cm per week. Hadlock et al.[56] found that the variability in predicting menstrual age from abdominal circumference measurements is broader than that observed with the fetal biparietal diameter. Tamura and Sabbagha[57] have examined the abdominal circumference growth in a study of 200 low-risk pregnant women from 18 to 41 weeks of gestation. They divided abdominal circumference measurements into those that were growing at less than the 25th percentile, those that were average (i.e., between the 25th and 75th percentiles), and those growing above the 75th percentile. They found the reproducibility of abdominal circumference measurements using a digitizer pen fell within 2 percent of the mean. Furthermore, they found that the accuracy of the abdominal circumference measurement fell within 5.2 percent of the actual anatomic value. By combined use of the biparietal diameter measurements and abdominal circumference percentile ranks for their population, they were able to identify nine growth patterns, two of which are at high risk for asymmetric intrauterine growth retardation. Those are the patterns that have

27 THEORETICAL FETAL GROWTH PATTERNS DETECTABLE WITH ULTRASOUND

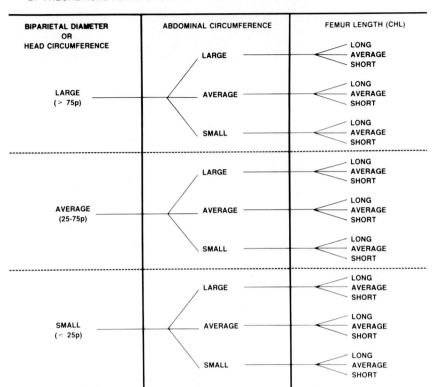

Fig. 7. By incorporation of fetal body length into the investigation of fetal growth, it should be possible to detect any one of 27 theoretical fetal growth patterns, shown above, with diagnostic ultrasound. The concept of fetal weight for height, in addition to fetal weight for dates, could then be approached using diagnostic ultrasound.

normal biparietal diameters but small abdominal circumferences. When the biparietal diameter and abdominal circumference were both small (i.e., less than the 25th percentile), the babies were at high risk for symmetric intrauterine growth retardation.

Body Length
Babies with the same head circumference and abdominal circumference measurements can have widely different body weight. Different body length can account for this normal weight variation. No direct measurement of fetal body length with ultrasound is yet possible clinically, although Wittmann et al.,[58] in a series of 255 patients, found that a simple combination of crown–rump length times area of the trunk allowed identification of an "at risk" group that comprised 11 percent of their population, almost half of which (45 percent) truly suffered from intrauterine growth retardation. There was a 10 percent false negative rate, with an overall false positive rate of approximately 6 percent in this study. It is also possible to measure body length indirectly using ultrasound measurement of the fetal femur length. Fazekas and Kosa[59] found from postmortem fetal examinations that there exists a linear relationship between femur length and actual crown–heel length. The formula has been found to be applicable

to ultrasound femur length measurements. The statistical accuracy of such measurements and body length calculations has been examined in a preliminary fashion in our laboratory. The formula for calculation of crown–heel length from ultrasound femur length is given as CHL = (6.61 × FL in cm) + 4.4. In an unpublished study from our laboratory on 12 patients scanned within 24 hours of delivery, a correlation coefficient (R) of 0.9199 was found (R^2 = 0.8464). The standard error was 2.438 ($p < 0.00002$). Using this formula allows an indirect calculation of fetal "height" in utero as well as weight. Thus, it may now be possible to begin to explore several hitherto undetectable growth patterns (Fig. 7), which not only reflect weight for dates, but also weight for height. This concept of weight for height measurement is not new. It has been studied by several investigators over the past two decades and quantified as the Rohrer Ponderal Index (RPI), which is calculated using the following formula: RPI = (crown-heel length³ ÷ the weight × 100) × 100. The pathologic studies of Miller and Hassanein,[60] as well as those of McLean and Usher,[61] have shown that intrauterine growth retardation can manifest itself as a loss of subcutaneous tissue, muscle mass, or both, as well as a decrease in body length. O'Brien and Queenan[62] have examined the relationship between

FEMUR LENGTH
MEASUREMENT TECHNIQUE

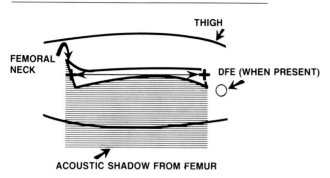

Fig. 8. The technique for femur length measurement is shown. It is important that caliper placement be such that a line connecting caliper dots at each end of the bone could be connected with a straight line that would bisect the shaft of the femur. The femoral neck should be excluded from the measurement; thus, the longest possible dimension of the femur is not always the correct one. Likewise, measurement of the femoral shadow might also be misleading.

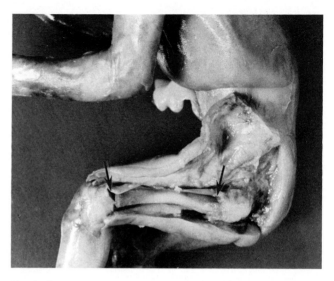

Fig. 9. Gross dissection of an 18-week fetus, aborted because of the presence of the Arnold–Chiari malformation, is shown. The arrows are placed at the ends of the central shaft of the femur, which is the actual part of the femur that is measured with diagnostic ultrasound.

femur length and the presence of intrauterine growth retardation. They, too, found that a reduced ultrasound fetal femur length correlated in all cases with a shortened crown–heel length in the neonate. Based upon the establishment of normal growth curves for ultrasound femur length during pregnancy, abnormal fetal growth and length can now begin to be identified.[63-67] Thigh circumference measurements have also been suggested by some authors to evaluate soft tissue mass, but no formal studies have shown how such ultrasound measurements relate to intrauterine growth retardation.[68]

The technique for femur length measurement by ultrasound is illustrated in Figure 8. Although the femur can appear somewhat curved on ultrasound, this is an optical illusion. The bone is straight, though the shape in some projections can approximate that of a parallelogram. It is important that the measurement of the femur be taken in such a manner that an imaginary line connecting the markers at each end of the femur would traverse the central shaft of the femur and not describe an angle that would connect the longest or shortest diagonals of the parallelogram. It is important to realize that it is not only the longest measurement of the femur that is the correct one, even though this has been recommended by other authors. The distal femoral epiphysis, if present, should not be included in the measurement of the femur length. Figure 9 shows the dissection of a fetal femur at 18 weeks of gestation from an abortus with the Arnold–Chiari malformation of the brain. The arrows denote the ends of the central calcified shaft or diaphysis of the femur. Figure 10 shows the proper measurements

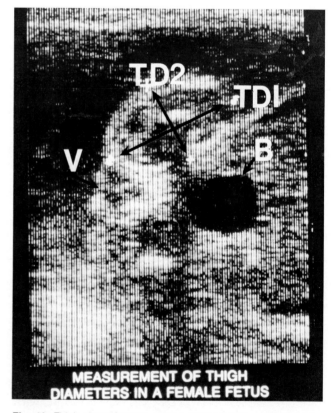

Fig. 10. Thigh circumference can be measured by calculating the circumference of the thigh using two diameters at right angle to each other (TD1 and TD2) and application of the formula for the circumference of a circle in similar fashion to the application for head circumference and abdominal circumference measurement. (B) Fetal bladder. (V) Vulva. All measurements of the thigh diameter should be outer-to-outer measurements.

of thigh diameters to be taken in order to calculate thigh circumference, using the same general formula as was used for head circumference and abdominal circumference described above.

WEIGHT FOR DATES

Campbell and Wilkin[54] found a close relationship between fetal abdominal circumference and fetal weight. They studied 140 fetuses within 48 hours of delivery and found 95 percent confidence limits of plus or minus 16 percent for weight prediction throughout the weight range of 1000 to 4000 g. Warsof et al.[69] developed a methodology based on measurement of biparietal diameter and abdominal circumference that reduced the standard error. This is currently the best method that has been developed for estimation of fetal weight regardless of whether or not the baby is of average, large, or small weight for gestational age. Warsof's original work was modified by Shepard and co-workers[70] to give the formula as follows (weight in kilograms, biparietal diameter and abdominal circumference in centimeters):

$$\log_0 \text{wt.} = -1.7492 + 0.166\,(\text{BPD}) + 0.046\,(\text{AC}) - 0.002646\,(\text{AC})\,(\text{BPD}).$$

Estimates obtained using this formula have been found to be relatively uniform over all weight classes. Deter et al.[71] have compared the results of Campbell and Wilkin and the original Warsof, plus Shepard modifications as previously discussed, in 125 patients using dynamic-image ultrasound. The Campbell–Wilkin and original Warsof methods systematically overestimated the weight by 5.3 percent and 1.6 percent, respectively, while the Shepard modification method gave systematic underestimates of about 3.2 percent. Variability of the two Warsof methods was similar and significantly smaller than that seen with the Campbell–Wilkin method. In the author's facility, the modification of the Warsof formula published by Shepard provides a systematic underestimate of actual fetal weight that is approximately 5 to 6 percent under the actual weight in all weight classes tested. Jordaan has recently looked at the use of head circumference, together with abdominal circumference, to estimate fetal weight and has found that it is a better brain size modulus than the biparietal diameter and avoids the errors of underestimation that occur when the biparietal diameter is unusually small in cases of dolichocephaly.[72] Alternatively, Thompson and Manning[73] have examined the relationship of volume and weight of the newborn. By developing a volume model representing trunk and limbs as cylinders with the dimensions related to mor-

phometric parameters, it was found that the deviation of neonatal weight estimates from actual weights 3 days postpartum was $\pm$ 4.1 percent (1 standard deviation). In 31 fetuses undergoing ultrasound examinations prior to delivery by cesarean section, the deviation of the weight estimate from the actual weight 3 days postpartum was $\pm$ 8.1 percent (1 standard deviation), or $\pm$ 7.4 percent (absolute mean error). This method compares favorably with other available methods.

The various methods that have been applied to estimation of fetal weight in utero require further testing. A method that is simple, quick, and reliable has yet to be found. The most useful method of calculating weight based on knowledge of the biparietal diameter and abdominal circumference requires solving a formula that is complex and most easily accomplished with use of a small handheld calculator or computer, although reference tables are available. Several authors have tested the reliability of this method and have found it quite satisfactory across all weight ranges tested.[74-76] Two separate groups have established formulas for estimation of weight for babies of less than 34 weeks' gestation and/or under 1500 g.[77,78] It can be anticipated that future work in this area will develop other formulas applicable by rapid calculation by computer or calculator for estimating fetal weight for clinical management decisions. What remains to be tested is whether or not clinical knowledge of an accurate estimate of fetal weight will improve obstetric management and improve reproductive outcome.

BODY SYMMETRY

Growth delay can often manifest itself as a change in the relationship of one organ size or body part to another. In normal pregnancy, the head and body dimensions grow at different rates and their mutual ratio changes as the pregnancy advances. The ratio of the head circumference to the abdominal circumference has been investigated as particularly useful in the detection of asymmetrical intrauterine growth retardation, usually due to uteroplacental insufficiency.[79-82] The ratio of the head circumference to abdominal circumference is greater than 1 until usually 36 to 37 weeks of gestation, at which time the abdominal circumference becomes larger than the head circumference, and the ratio declines to 1 or below throughout the remainder of the third trimester in a normal pregnancy. By calculation of a greater than normal head circumference to abdominal circumference ratio, it is possible to diagnose growth retardation earlier than is possible using measurement of the biparietal diameter alone. Therefore, the determination of this ratio is now considered an essential part of an adequate and complete standard antepartum obstetric ultrasound examination. When using this ratio, however, it is important to realize that it is not a constant value and, therefore, accurate knowledge of gestational age is crucial to proper interpretation. The mean, 5th percentile, and 95th percentile confidence limits for the head circumference to abdomen circumference ratio are shown in Table 1, while the various clinical interpretations of the ratio that should be considered are shown in Figure 11.

Campbell and Thoms[79] found in 31 small-for-dates fetuses that 22 (70 percent) had head circumference to abdominal circumference ratios above the 95th percentile. Two of these babies died, 53 percent developed intrapartum distress, and 36 percent were delivered by cesarean section. In addition, 17 showed a "late flattening" type of growth of the biparietal diameter. Nine had head circumference/abdominal circumference ratios within the normal range. Of these, two were delivered by cesarean section, one developed fetal distress in labor, and two had congenital abnormalities (cystic fibrosis and rubella). Six of these nine fetuses showed "low profile" growth of the biparietal diameter. This is in keeping with the data of Crane and Kopta,[82] who found that in 47 patients, all of ten small-for-dates fetuses were correctly predicted by a head circumference to abdominal circumference ratio more than two standard deviations above the mean for gestational age. Deter et al.[43] have also looked at the use of the head circumference to abdominal circumference ratio determined by the method of Campbell and Thoms, measured between 14 and 39 weeks. Only 23.1 percent of the fetuses having abnormal values were actually small for gestational age at delivery by current standard criteria of weight for dates below the tenth percentile. Crane and Kopta[32] and Crane et al.,[35] as well as Daikoku,[24] have pointed out the difficulty of clinically separating fetuses that are small for getational age into two clearly distinct patterns on the basis of symmetry of body growth. This is not unexpected because though the fetal liver is usually more severely affected than the brain in asymmetric fetal intrauterine growth retardation, the concept of absolute "brain sparing" does not appear to be valid. In fact, it was demonstrated by Crane and Kopta that the percentage decrease in head circumference was similar in a group of 33 consecutive small for gestational age infants, 20 of whom suffered from asymmetric intrauterine growth retardation due to uteroplacental insufficiency compared to 13 infants classified as symmetrically growth retarded due to causes other than uteroplacental insufficiency.

TABLE 1

Normal Values for the Head Circumference to Abdominal Circumference Ratio for Various Gestational Ages Is Shown with 5th and 95th Percentile Confidence Limits Also Given

Menstrual Age (weeks)	Number of Measurements	H:A Circumference Ratio		
		5th Centile	Mean	95th Centile
13–14	18	1.14	1.23	1.31
15–16	39	1.05	1.22	1.39
17–18	77	1.07	1.18	1.29
19–20	54	1.09	1.18	1.26
21–22	41	1.06	1.15	1.25
23–24	22	1.05	1.13	1.21
25–26	18	1.04	1.13	1.22
27–28	36	1.05	1.13	1.22
29–30	23	0.99	1.10	1.21
31–32	31	0.96	1.07	1.17
33–34	42	0.96	1.04	1.11
35–36	49	0.93	1.02	1.11
37–38	67	0.92	0.98	1.05
39–40	47	0.87	0.97	1.06
41–42	4	0.93	0.96	1.00

The findings from these ultrasound studies are entirely consistent with data from animal models[53] as well as previous clinical data derived from the study of outcome of human pregnancies. Winick[83] first quantified growth in terms of cellular and organ growth in several species, including the human, and described three distinct phases of growth that were identified as pure hyperplasia, hyperplasia and concomitant hypertrophy, followed by hypertrophy alone. Winick and Nobel[84] then demonstrated that undernutrition during hyperplastic growth curtailed the rate of cell division and could result, if the undernutrition was prolonged, in an organ with a permanently reduced cell number. The same degree of nutrition imposed during the hypertrophic phase retarded the expected increase in cell size, though this was reversible if proper nutrition could be maintained. Further studies in human infants with varying degrees of malnutrition revealed similar growth patterns in a variety of organs.[85-87] The effect of various factors on intrauterine growth retardation in the fetal rhesus monkey have been described in similar fashion by Cheek.[88] Naeye[89] and Miller,[90] in two separate studies, have found a similar effect in humans on development of proper muscle mass as well as architecture and biochemistry. An organ specific pattern of growth retardation has been demonstrated in humans by Naeye[89] and by Greunwald.[91] In summary, it has been shown in animals and humans that the head circumference to abdominal circumference ratio is helpful in the diagnosis of retarded growth, particularly when it is desirable to distinguish between the types of growth retardation described as symmetric

INTERPRETATION OF THE HC/AC RATIO

NORMAL   NORMALLY GROWING FETUS
          SYMMETRICALLY GROWTH-RETARDED
            FETUS

HIGH   ASYMMETRICAL GROWTH-RETARDED
            FETUS
          LARGE HEAD (E.G. HYDROCEPHALUS)

LOW   MACROSOMIA
          MICROCEPHALY
          CRANIOSYNOSTOSIS

Fig. 11. The differential diagnosis for the interpretation of the head circumference to abdominal circumference ratio is shown.

and asymmetric based on the disparity between liver size and brain size at any given gestational age. Further, it has been shown that it is probably unusual for these patterns of symmetric and asymmetric growth retardation to occur in their pure form. Finally, other methods of fetal evaluation, in addition to measurement of the head circumference to abdominal circumference ratio, are being looked at as alternative methods for the detection of intrauterine growth retardation. Ellis and Bennett[92] examined 434 patients with ultrasound measurements of the fetal head area and abdominal area. They found that only four out of a total of 40 SGA infants (10 percent) were below the 5th percentile, with a false negative rate of 90 percent. This was on the basis of a single ultrasound examination at 32 to 34 weeks of gestation. Of the growth-retarded infants that had been measured at that time interval, 5.9 percent would have been detected, according to the authors, by this measurement alone. Fetal abdominal area, measured alone, identified 19.5 percent of all of the SGA babies. The overall false negative rate was 80.5 percent, and the authors found that of those measured at 32 to 34 weeks, only 25 percent were detected. Examination of the fetal head area to abdominal area ratio showed an identification rate of 18.9 percent of all of the SGA infants, with an overall false negative rate of 81.1 percent. Again, of those scanned at 32 to 34 weeks of gestation, the authors found that only 25 percent would have been detected. From those results, it appears that a large proportion of growth-retarded infants cannot be identified by a single ultrasound examination of the fetal head and/or abdominal area at 32 to 34 weeks of gestation. However, measurement closer to delivery date might have changed these results considerably. It appears that measurement of head and abdominal cross-sectional areas has no distinct advantage over measurement of circumferences for the detection of intrauterine growth retardation.

Neilson et al.[93] scanned 474 women with singleton pregnancies twice during pregnancy. At the first examination in early pregnancy fetal crown–rump length or biparietal diameter was obtained to fix gestational age. The second examination was performed at 34 to 36 weeks of gestation, at which time seven fetal variables were measured. They found that fetal head measurements proved to be the least sensitive indicators of growth retardation, correctly identifying only 56 to 59 percent of cases. Measurements of abdomen area and circumference, however, correctly identified 81 and 83 percent of cases, respectively, but the most effective screening index was found to be the product of crown–rump length and trunk area—with this index, 34 out of 36 small-for-dates fetuses (94 percent) were correctly identified. Their results, at this time, have not been confirmed by others.

PRACTICAL METHODOLOGY

The diagnosis of intrauterine growth retardation is not usually suspected clinically prior to 12 weeks of gestation. Although it is possible for symmetric intrauterine growth retardation prior to 20 weeks, asymmetric intrauterine growth retardation is unusual prior to 24 weeks of gestation. Symmetric, "reduced growth potential" type intrauterine growth retardation can be seen in conjunction with the presence of structural congenital anomalies, including neural tube defects, as well as with chromosomal abnormalities and congenital viral infections. Thus, if the diagnosis of intrauterine growth retardation is suspected prior to 24 weeks of gestation, a careful evaluation of the fetus for the presence of these factors should be carried out. Amniotic fluid volume estimation is also extremely important. After 12 weeks of gestation, the growth profile of the fetus should include the following:

Measurement of:

- BPD (biparietal diameter) ⎫ used to
- OFD (occipito–frontal diameter) ⎬ calculate head
                                   circumference

- APAD (anterior–posterior abdominal diameter) ⎫ used to calcu-
- TAD (transverse abdominal diameter) ⎬ late abdominal
                                       circumference
- FL (femur length)
- Thigh diameters (used to calculate thigh circumference)

Calculation of:

- HC (head circumference)
- AC (abdominal circumference)

- TC (thigh circumference)
- CI (cephalic index)
- FL/BPD (femur length to biparietal diameter ratio)
- FL/AC ratio (femur length to abdominal circumference)
- HC/AC (head circumference to abdominal circumference ratio)
- EFW (fetal weight based on BPD and AC)
- EGA (age estimate based on BPD, HC, AC, and FL)

From these routine measurements and calculations, an analysis of all of the following can be carried out:

- Gestational age
- Weight for dates
- Weight for height
- FL/BPD ratio
- FL/AC ratio

Four images are required to document the reference planes of the BPD, AC, FL, and TC in order to permanently record the measurements taken during each examination. Placental grade may also require photographic documentation, though placental grading significance vis-à-vis IUGR remains unclear. Other photographs of pertinent anatomical landmarks or unusual areas of interest should also, of course, be recorded at the time of each examination. Observations about placental location, the amount of amniotic fluid, the presence or absence of related uterine or other pelvic pathology, and the recording of fetal activity patterns of the heart, chest wall, body, and limbs complete the assessment of fetal status. Increasingly, the use of a computer is becoming a necessity in order to perform all of these calculations rapidly enough to maintain productivity while expanding the scope of the fetal growth evaluation being carried out in the course of a standard antepartum obstetric ultrasound examination. The three-dimensional approach to estimation of intrauterine fetal nutrition (Fig. 12) afforded by this form of expanded growth profiling will, it is hoped, make possible new avenues of research into human fetal development while at the same time providing increased benefits directly related to patient care in medically complicated pregnancies, and those complicated by fetal abnormalities or illnesses acquired during development.

SUMMARY

Direct measurements of the fetus have a major and dominant role in the basic detection of intrauterine growth retardation and the recognition of its "pattern,"

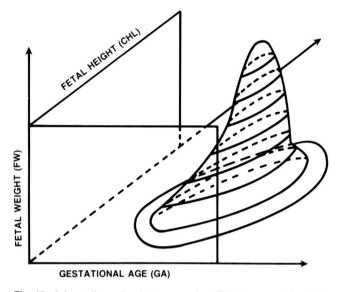

Fig. 12. A three-dimensional representation of the concepts of weight for dates, as well as weight for height, is demonstrated. In the future, calculation of fetal height in utero will allow the investigation of fetal growth in both dimensions and, thus, define a new concept of normal intrauterine fetal growth.

which can often point to specific etiologies. As a first step basic to accurate use of ultrasound to detect intrauterine growth retardation, exact estimation of gestational age is essential. It appears, however, even with potential screening strategies of implementation of diagnostic ultrasound in obstetric care that not all potential cases of intrauterine growth retardation will be detected with ultrasound. In a recent study by Persson and Kullander,[94] it was found that with two ultrasound examinations, one in the 17th week of pregnancy and one in the 33rd week of pregnancy, that if an ultrasound examination had been performed within 3 weeks of delivery, 92 percent of the fetuses with growth retardation were detected. Altogether, their program detected 60 percent of the growth-retarded fetuses. It was found that symmetric growth retardation occurred in more than 80 percent of all the instances of retarded growth. Based on a single examination in the 33rd week of pregnancy, they were able to detect 46 percent of all the cases of growth retardation in their population; with a further examination in the 37th week, 80 percent were detected. The authors also make the comment that if one examination is performed in the 38th week, several cases of growth retardation would escape detection before birth, since growth retardation was found to be five times more common in preterm than in term deliveries in Malmo, Sweden. The authors conclude that in order to detect 80 percent of the instances of growth retardation, all pregnancies would have had to be examined at least twice in the last trimester. The smallest 20 percent of fetuses found at the 33rd week examination were reexamined at 35 and 38 weeks. This procedure detected 60 percent of all of the SGA infants born during 1981. It is obvious that further work is required to determine the optimal strategy for use of ultrasound in the detection of intrauterine growth retardation.

Once IUGR is discovered, the clinical problem shifts from detection to evaluation of fetal well-being and to a search for the etiology of the growth delay. In cases of uteroplacental insufficiency, antepartum fetal heart rate testing, use of the fetal biophysical profile[95] to assess fetal well-being, and the use of maternal perception of fetal movements can also be used to assist in the evaluation of fetal adaptation. Once detection and assessment of well-being have been accomplished, then the search for possible correctable etiologies and/or the clinical correction of underlying maternal pathologic conditions may permit nonintervention until fetal lung maturity can be determined. If the lungs are mature, it appears that long-term outcome is improved by prompt delivery, rather than waiting until deterioration in fetal condition is detected through antepartum fetal heart rate testing and/or biochemical testing, such as use of plasma or urinary estriols. Nothing is to be gained by allowing a fetus known to be suffering from intrauterine growth retardation to remain in utero with mature lungs. The situation can only deteriorate with possible death of the fetus when placental reserve is outrun. When chronic uteroplacental insufficiency is the etiology, frequent antepartum fetal heart rate testing cannot universally prevent such a catastrophic outcome.[96]

Much work remains to be done to improve our ability to estimate fetal weight for dates accurately and precisely. New alternative weight estimation methods must be derived so that proper assessment of fetal growth can be achieved. More complete understanding of the interrelationship between fetal structure and function as it relates to fetal weight, mass, and length versus CNS function, must be achieved if we are to be in a position to appreciate the subtle changes in fetal nutrition that occur over short periods of time, when placental reserve is tenuous.[97]

New technologic advances in diagnostic ultrasound, dynamic-imaging equipment, resolution and display capacity, together with the increased use of computer-assisted evaluation of fetal growth patterns will make that job considerably more successful in the future. Doppler techniques assessing pressure in the umbilical vein may be of considerable value.[98]

Thus, we will be in a position to ask, not the routine questions about gestational age and weight, but rather the more fundamental questions concerning functional lung maturity, fetal adaptation to the altered abnormal intrauterine environment when uteroplacental insufficiency exists, and about the status of intrauterine fetal nutrition.

REFERENCES

1. Lubchenco LO, Hansman C, et al: Intrauterine growth as estimated from liveborn birthweight data at 24–42 weeks of gestation. Pediatrics 32:793, 1963
2. Jones MD, Battaglia FC: Intrauterine growth retardation. Am J Obstet Gynecol 127:540, 1977
3. Bard H: Neonatal problems of infants with intrauterine growth retardation. J Reprod Med 21:359, 1978
4. Koops BL: Neurologic sequelae in infants with intrauterine growth retardation. J Reprod Med 21:343, 1978
5. Harvey D, Prince J, et al: Abilities of children who were small for gestational age babies. Pediatrics 69:296, 1982
6. Davies DP: Growth of "small for dates" babies. Early Hum Dev 5:95, 1981
7. Parkinson CE, Wallis S, et al: School achievement and behavior of children who were small for dates at birth. Dev Med Child Neurol 23:41, 1981
8. Winer EK, Tejani NA, et al: Four to seven year evaluation in two groups of small for gestational age infants. Am J Obstet Gynecol 143:425, 1982
9. Tejani N, Mann LI: Diagnosis and management for the small for gestational age fetus. Clin Obstet Gynecol 20:943, 1977
10. Westwood M, Kramer MS, et al: Growth and development of full-term, nonasphyxiated, small for gestational age newborns: Follow-up through adolescence. Pediatrics 71:376, 1983
11. Wittmann BK, Robinson HP, et al: The value of diagnostic ultrasound as a screening test for intrauterine growth retardation: Comparison of five parameters. Am J Obstet Gynecol 134:30, 1979
12. Beazley JM, Underhill RA: Fallacy of the fundal height. Br Med J 4:404, 1970
13. Tejani N, Mann WI, et al: Antenatal diagnosis and management of the small for dates fetus. Obstet Gynecol 47:31, 1976
14. Dewhurst CJ, Beazley JM, et al: Assessment of fetal maturity and dysmaturity. Am J Obstet Gynecol 113:141, 1972
15. Campbell S: The assessment of fetal development by diagnostic ultrasound. Clin Perinatol 1:507, 1974
16. McKeown T, Record RG: Observations on fetal growth in multiple pregnancy in man. J Endocrinol 8:386, 1952
17. Greunwald P: Growth of the human fetus. I. Normal growth and its variation. Am J Obstet Gynecol 94:1112, 1966
18. Greunwald P: Introduction—the supply line of the fetus; definitions relating to fetal growth, in Greunwald P (ed), The Placenta. Baltimore, University Park Press, 1975, p 1
19. Wilcox AJ: Birthweight, gestation, and the fetal growth curve. Am J Obstet Gynecol 139:863, 1981
20. Butler NR, Alberman ED: Perinatal problems: The sec-

ond report of the 1958 British Perinatal Mortality Survey. New York, Churchill-Livingstone, 1969

21. Usher RH: Clinical and therapeutic aspects of fetal malnutrition. Pediatr Clin N Am 17:199, 1970
22. Koops BL, Morgan LJ, et al: Neonatal mortality risk in relation to birthweight and gestational age: Update. J Pediatr 101:969, 1982
23. Miller HC, Hassanein K: Diagnosis of impaired fetal growth in newborn infants. Pediatrics 48:511, 1971
24. Daikoku NH, Johnson JWC, et al: Patterns of intrauterine growth retardation. Obstet Gynecol 54:211, 1979
25. Usher R, McLean F: Intrauterine growth of liveborn caucasian infants at sea level: Standards obtained from measurements in seven dimensions of infants born between 25 and 44 weeks of gestation. Pediatrics 74:901, 1969
26. Brenner WE, Edelman DA, et al: A standard of fetal growth for the United States of America. Am J Obstet Gynecol 126:555, 1976
27. Cotton EK, Hiestand M, et al: Re-evaluation of birthweights at high altitude. Am J Obstet Gynecol 138:220, 1980
28. Naeye RL: Maternal blood pressure and fetal growth. Am J Obstet Gynecol 141:780, 1981
29. Greunwald P: Chronic fetal distress and placental insufficiency. Biol Neonate 5:215, 1963
30. Campbell S, Dewhurst CJ: Diagnosis of the small for dates fetus by serial ultrasound cephalometry. Lancet 2:1002, 1971
31. Greunwald P: The relation of deprivation to perinatal pathology and late sequels, in Greunwald P (ed), The Placenta. Baltimore, University Park Press, 1975, pp 338–341
32. Crane JP, Kopta MM: Comparative newborn anthropometric data in symmetric versus asymmetric intrauterine growth retardation. Am J Obstet Gynecol 138:518, 1980
33. Queenan JT, Kubarych SF, et al: Diagnostic ultrasound for detection of intrauterine growth retardation. Am J Obstet Gynecol 124:865, 1976
34. Hohler CW, Lea J, et al: Screening for intrauterine growth retardation using the ultrasound biparietal diameter. J Clin Ultrasound 4:187, 1977
35. Crane JP, Kopta MM, et al: Abnormal fetal growth patterns—Ultrasonic diagnosis and management. Obstet Gynecol 50:205, 1977
36. Ellis C, Bennett MJ: J R Soc Med 74:739, 1981
37. Sabbagha RE: Intrauterine growth retardation—Antenatal diagnosis by ultrasound. Obstet Gynecol 52:252, 1978
38. Gohari P, Berkowitz RL, et al: Prediction of intrauterine growth retardation by determination of total intrauterine volume. Am J Obstet Gynecol 127:255, 1977
39. Chinn DH, Filly RA, et al: Prediction of intrauterine growth retardation by sonographic estimation of total intrauterine volume. J Clin Ultrasound 9:175, 1981
40. Grossman M, Flynn J, et al: Pitfalls in ultrasonic determination of total intrauterine volume. J Clin Ultrasound 10:17, 1982
41. Grossman M: Significance of bladder distension in uterine volume determination. Perinatol-Neonatal, Sept/Oct, 1982, p 45
42. Middleton WD, Bowie JD, et al: LTUA—a new and more

reproducible method of estimating intrauterine size. J Ultrasound Med 1:123, 1982
43. Deter RL, Harrist RB, et al: The use of ultrasound in the detection of intrauterine growth retardation: A review. J Clin Ultrasound 10:9, 1982
44. Manning FA, Hill LM, et al: Antepartum detection of IUGR: Use of qualitative amniotic fluid volume. Am J Obstet Gynecol 139:254, 1981
45. Philipson EH, Sokol RJ, et al: Oligohydramnios: Clinical associations and predictive value for intrauterine growth retardation. Am J Obstet Gynecol 146:271, 1983
46. Gross TL, Sokol RJ, et al: Using ultrasound and amniotic fluid determinations to diagnose intrauterine growth retardation before birth: A clinical model. Am J Obstet Gynecol 143:265, 1982
47. Jordaan HVF, Dunn LJ: A new method of evaluating fetal growth. Obstet Gynecol 51:659, 1978
48. Jordaan HVF, Clark WB: Prenatal determination of fetal brain and somatic weight by ultrasound. Am J Obstet Gynecol 136:54, 1980
49. Hadlock FP, Kent WR, et al: An evaluation of two methods for measuring fetal head and body circumferences. J Ultrasound Med 1:359, 1982
50. Deter RL, Harrist RB, et al: The use of ultrasound in the assessment of normal fetal growth: A review. J Clin Ultrasound 9:481, 1981
51. Hadlock FP, Deter RL, et al: Fetal head circumference accuracy of real-time ultrasound measurements at term. Perinatol-Neonatol, Sept/Oct, 1982, p 97
52. Hadlock FP, Deter RL, et al: The effect of head shape on the accuracy of BPD in estimating fetal gestational age. Am J Roentgenol 137:83, 1981
53. Evans MI, Mukherjee AB, Schulman JD: et al: Animal models of intrauterine growth retardation. Obstet Gynecol Sur 38:183, 1983
54. Campbell S, Wilkin D: Ultrasonic measurement of fetal abdomen circumference in the estimation of fetal weight. Br J Obstet Gynaecol 82:689, 1975
55. Deter RL, Harrist RB, et al: Longitudinal studies of fetal growth with dynamic-image ultrasonography. Am J Obstet Gynecol 143:545, 1982
56. Hadlock FP, Deter RL, et al: Fetal abdominal circumference as a predictor of menstrual age. Am J Roentgenol 139:367, 1982
57. Tamura RK, Sabbagha RE: Percentile ranks of sonar fetal abdominal circumference measurements. Am J Obstet Gynecol 138:475, 1980
58. Wittmann BK, Robinson HP, et al: The value of diagnostic ultrasound as a screening test for intrauterine growth retardation: Comparison of nine parameters. Am J Obstet Gynecol 134:30, 1979
59. Fazekas IG, Kosa F: Forensic Fetal Osteology. Budapest, Akademiai Kiado, 1978, p 264
60. Miller HC, Hassanein K: Diagnosis of impaired fetal growth in newborn infants. Pediatrics 48:511, 1971
61. McLean F, Usher R: Measurements of liveborn fetal malnutrition infants compared with similar gestation and with similar birth-weight normal controls. Biol Neonate 16:215, 1970
62. O'Brien GD, Queenan JT: Ultrasound fetal femur length

in relation to intrauterine growth retardation. Am J Obstet Gynecol 144:35, 1982

63. Hohler CW, Quetel TA: Fetal femur length: Equations for computer calculation of gestational age from ultrasound measurements. Am J Obstet Gynecol 143:479, 1982
64. O'Brien GD, Queenan JT: Growth of the ultrasound fetal femur length during normal pregnancy. Am J Obstet Gynecol 141:833, 1981
65. Quinlan RW, Brumfield C, et al: Ultrasonic measurement of femur length as a predictor of fetal gestational age. J Reprod Med 27:392, 1982
66. Hadlock FP, Harrist RB, et al: Ultrasonically measured fetal femur length as a predictor of menstrual age. Am J Roentgenol 138:875, 1982
67. Jeanty P, Kirkpatrick C, et al: Ultrasonic evaluation of fetal limb growth. Radiology 140:165, 1981
68. Deter RL, Hadlock FP, et al: Evaluation of normal fetal growth and the detection of IUGR, in Callen PW (ed), Ultrasonography in Obstetrics and Gynecology. Philadelphia, Saunders, pp 128–131
69. Warsof SL, Gohari P, et al: The estimation of fetal weight by computer-assisted analysis. Am J Obstet Gynecol 128:881, 1977
70. Shepard MJ, Richards VA, et al: An evaluation of two equations for predicting fetal weight by ultrasound. Am J Obstet Gynecol 142:47, 1982
71. Deter RL, Hadlock FP, et al: Evaluation of three methods for obtaining fetal weight estimates using dynamic-image ultrasound. J Clin Ultrasound 9:421, 1981
72. Jordaan HVF: Estimation of fetal weight by ultrasound. J Clin Ultrasound 11:59, 1983
73. Thompson TR, Manning FA: Estimation of volume and weight of the perinate: Relationship to morphometric measurement by ultrasonography. J Ultrasound Med 2:113, 1983
74. Sampson MB, Thomason JL, et al: Prediction of intrauterine fetal weight using real-time ultrasound. Am J Obstet Gynecol 142:554, 1982
75. Ott WJ, Doyle S: Normal ultrasonic fetal weight curve. Obstet Gynecol 59:603, 1982
76. Timor-Tritsch IE, Itskovitz J, et al: Estimation of fetal weight by real-time sonography. Obstet Gynecol 57:653, 1981
77. Thurnau GR, Tamura RK, et al: A simple estimated fetal weight equation based on real-time ultrasound measurements of fetuses less than 34 weeks gestation. Am J Obstet Gynecol 145:557, 1983
78. Key TC, Dattel BJ, et al: The ultrasonographic estimation of fetal weight in the very low birthweight infant. Am J Obstet Gynecol 145:574, 1983
79. Campbell S, Thoms A: Ultrasound measurement of the fetal head to abdomen circumference ratio in the assessment of growth retardation. Br J Obstet Gynaecol 84:165, 1977

80. Kurjak A, Latin V, et al: Ultrasonic recognition of two types of growth retardation by measurement of four fetal dimensions. J Perinatal Med 6:102, 1978
81. Wladimiroff JW, Bloemsa CA, et al: Ultrasonic assessment of fetal head and body sizes in relation to normal and retarded fetal growth. Am J Obstet Gynecol 131:857, 1978
82. Crane J, Kopta M: Prediction of IUGR via ultrasonically measured head/abdominal circumference ratios. Obstet Gynecol 54:597, 1979
83. Winick M: Cellular changes during placental and fetal growth. Am J Obstet Gynecol 109:166, 1971
84. Winick M, Noble A: Cellular response in rats during malnutrition at various ages. J Nutrition 89:300, 1966
85. Brasel J, Winick M: Differential cellular growth in the organs of hypothyroid rats. Growth 34:197, 1970
86. Winick M, Rosso P, et al: Cellular growth of cerebrum, cerebellum and brainstem in normal and marasmic children. Exp Neurol 26:393, 1970
87. Winick M, Rosso P: The effect of severe early malnutrition on cellular growth of human brain. Pediatr Res 3:181, 1969
88. Cheek D: Fetal and Postnatal Cellular Growth. New York, Wiley, 1975, p 209
89. Naeye RL: Malnutrition, probable cause of fetal growth retardation. Arch Pathol 79:284, 1965
90. Miller HC: Fetal growth and neonatal mortality. Pediatrics 49:392, 1972
91. Greunwald P: Pathology of the deprived fetus and its supply line, in Elliott K (ed), Size at Birth. CIBA Found Symp 27:3, 1974
92. Ellis C, Bennett MJ: Detection of intrauterine growth retardation by ultrasound: Preliminary communication. J R Soc Med 74:739, 1981
93. Neilson JP, Whitfield CR, et al: Screening for the small for dates fetus: A two-stage ultrasonic examination schedule. Br Med J 280:1203, 1980
94. Persson PH, Kullander S: Long-term experience of general ultrasound screening in pregnancy. Am J Obstet Gynecol 146:942, 1983
95. Vintzileos AM, Campbell WA, et al: The fetal biophysical profile and its predictive value. Obstet Gynecol 62:271, 1983
96. Evertson LR, Gauthier RJ, et al: Fetal demise following negative contraction stress tests. Obstet Gynecol 51:671, 1978
97. Luther ER, Gray JH, et al: The effect of maternal glucose infusion on breathing movements in human fetuses with intrauterine growth retardation. Am J Obstet Gynecol 142:600, 1982
98. Trudinger BJ, Giles WB, et al: Feto-placental blood flow resistance and placental microvascular anatomy: A Doppler ultrasound-pathological correlation. Paper presented at the American Institute of Ultrasound in Medicine in New York, 1983

12 | Ultrasound: Fetal Movements and Fetal Condition

Paul F. Chamberlain
Frank A. Manning

The occurrence of fetal movements in utero has been recognized since biblical times—"from the moment your greeting reached my ears the child in my womb leapt for joy."[1] Despite this long recognition, the pattern and significance of these fetal biophysical functions as a means of monitoring fetal condition has remained unexplored until the recent past. For many years the major clinical significance ascribed to fetal movements has been in the confirmation of pregnancy ("quickening") in the mid-trimester, and as a warning of possible fetal demise in the third trimester should a decrease or cessation of fetal movements be noted by the pregnant patient.

Over the last 10 to 20 years, the significance of fetal movements as an indicator of fetal condition has received increasing amounts of attention. Many authors have reported an association between fetal movements as perceived and recorded by the gravida and perinatal outcome.[2-8] "Fetal movement charts" are now a standard part of obstetrical care in many institutions and act as an additional simple way to monitor fetal condition.[8]

With the advent of diagnostic real-time obstetric ultrasound, a new era in the study of fetal movements started. For the first time the practicing obstetrician could view his previously "unseen second patient" within its natural environment. This has allowed confirmation of the pioneering kymographic observations on human fetal breathing movements that Ahfeld reported almost 80 years ago and an appreciation of the spectrum of fetal movements.[9-11]

Further application of real-time ultrasound to early gestation has also confirmed the occurrence of embryonic and fetal movements in utero previously studied only in in vitro preparations of early spontaneous or therapeutic terminations of pregnancy.[12,13]

It is the aim of this chapter:

1. To review the role of diagnostic real-time ultrasound in the assessment of fetal movements and of the intrauterine environment.
2. To outline a program of fetal well-being assessment based upon these observations.

Towards this end, the role of diagnostic real-time ultrasound in the assessment of embryonic and fetal movements in early pregnancy is first outlined. Then fetal breathing movements, gross and fine fetal body movements, fetal tone, and qualitative amniotic fluid volume evaluation by real-time ultrasound are reviewed. Finally a program of fetal well-being assessment based on composite biophysical profile scoring (BPS) is outlined. The results of this method of fetal assessment to a large, high-risk obstetric population are reported and future trends in this method of fetal assessment suggested.

EARLY PREGNANCY ULTRASOUND STUDIES ON EMBRYONIC AND FETAL MOVEMENTS

The ultrasound appearance of early normal intrauterine pregnancy at the end of the fifth week from the last menstrual period (the third week of conceptual age) reveals itself as a group of echoes located within the uterine cavity.[14] Between the fifth and sixth weeks of gestational age the gestational sac becomes evident as a well demarcated circular, sonolucent structure within the uterus. Embryonic heart motion is evident between the fifth and sixth gestational weeks (around the 26th day conceptual age) and the embryonic movements noted as changes in embryonic tissue echo positions ("fibrillations") are evident between the seventh and eighth week of gestation.[15-18] With advancing gestational age, especially after the end of the embryonic period and with the commencement of the fetal period, fetal movements as observed by real-time ultrasound become progressively more frequent, complex, and coordinated. Differentiation between fetal trunk and limb movements is evident between the eighth and ninth week of gestation.[16,19] By the tenth week of gestation fetal movements in normal healthy intrauterine pregnancies can be identified with 100 percent reliability.[20]

Many methods for the classification of embryonic and fetal movements in early pregnancy have been proposed.[15,17,19-24] Of these, that described by Reinhold is the most widely referenced and is summarized in Table 1. Strong and brisk fetal movements are by far the most frequent type seen in early normal pregnancy. They have a characteristic "Moro reflex" appearance and have been termed "startle-type" fetal movements by some authors.[24,25] This type of movement causes displacement of the fetus from its original position in the uterine cavity into the amniotic fluid and is followed by a period of time during which the fetus slowly drifts back to a dependent portion of the uterine cavity. These movements may be self-stimulated by the fetus (i.e., by hand–face, hand–genital, or other self-contact) or may result from contact between the fetal skin and uterine wall or externally or internally induced stimulations (i.e., external pressure applied to the maternal abdomen or internal maternal visceral peristalsis).[25] They may be repetitive, and occur alone or interspersed with other types of fetal movements.

Slow and sluggish type fetal movements are less frequent than the previously outlined strong and brisk reflexes. They are isolated to individual fetal parts and cause little or no change in fetal location within the amniotic cavity. Birnholz has described this type of fetal movement under several headings, including independent limb (asymmetric or unilateral extensor movements of the arms or legs) and isolated head (extension or flexion of the fetal head without associated trunk or limb) movements.[24] This type of fetal motor activity is clearly evident by the tenth to twelfth week of gestation and, with the newer ultrasound technology and its higher resolution capabilities now available, probably even earlier.

TABLE 1
Classification of Fetal Movements in Early Pregnancy

1. Strong and brisk
   Forceful initial motor impulse
   Movement involves entire fetal body
   Movement results in a change in location and posture
   "Startle or Moro" type movement
   Frequency of between 3–8 per minute
   May be associated slow movements interspersed
2. Slow and sluggish
   No initial motor impulse
   Movement confined to fetal parts, i.e. limbs
   Frequency of 1–3 per minute
   Occur in absence of strong and brisk movements
3. Absence of spontaneous fetal movements
4. Induced movements
   "Motor Provocation Test"—brisk and strong "Moro" type fetal movement or sequence of movements following fetal stimulation, i.e., external or internal in response to uterine contractions, etc.

Adapted from Reinhold E: Identification and differentiation of fetal movements, in Keller PJ (ed), Contributions to Gynaecology and Obstetrics. Basel, Karger, 1979, vol 6, pp 29–32.

The "motor provocation test," easily induced by manipulation of the ultrasound transducer on the maternal abdomen, characteristically in early normal intrauterine pregnancy causes a brisk and strong Moro-type reflex fetal response. This test has clinical usefulness when the absence of spontaneous fetal motion is encountered during early pregnancy real-time ultrasound examination (see below).

Both Mulz,[26] and Henner, Haller, and Kubli[27] have attempted quantification of early fetal movements in utero. They report that fetal movements progressively increase during the first half of pregnancy, peaking around the seventeenth week of gestation and decrease from then until term. They also report that the course covered by the normal healthy fetus within the amniotic cavity and the amplitude and velocity of early fetal movements increase during the first half of pregnancy.

The effects of maternally administered drugs on fetal movement early in pregnancy has been reported by Reinhold.[22] He found rapid cessation of all types of spontaneous fetal movements and a negative response to the "motor provocation test" after the induction of general anesthesia. The duration of the drug effect was very variable and the first type of early fetal movements to recur following maternal drug administration was of the slow and sluggish variety. Once these movements were demonstrable, the "motor provocation test" again became positive. Diazepam was noted to have a significant suppressant effect on all types of early fetal movements whereas Ritodrine had no demonstrable effect. The effect of cigarette smoking and alcohol on fetal movements at this stage of pregnancy has not been studied, as they have in later gestation, but it seems reasonable to presume that their effects in early pregnancy are no different to those observed in later gestation (see Fetal Breathing Movements and Gross and Fine Fetal Body Movements).

The failure to identify spontaneous fetal movements in early pregnancy is of ominous prognostic significance.[15,19,22,23,27-29] The occurrence of strong and brisk early fetal movements in cases of threatened abortion with vaginal bleeding bodes well for successful pregnancy outcome. Anderson noted a successful course for pregnancy in 72 of 74 cases where this type of fetal movement was noted in cases referred because of first trimester bleeding[19,28]; conversely, Reinhold reported a 25 percent pregnancy failure rate where this type of fetal movement was not observed in patients referred for the same clinical indication.[23] Henner, Haller, and Kubli noted a decrease in both the course covered by the fetus during movement and in the amplitude and velocity of these fetal movements in pathologic pregnancies.[26] Failure to identify early fetal movements should lead one to suspect the diagnosis of either missed abortion or anembryonic pregnancy, especially if these ultrasound findings are associated with signs and symptoms of early pregnancy loss. The presence of fetal heart motion in the absence of spontaneous brisk and strong fetal movements or only slow and sluggish fetal movements is an ominous finding especially if associated with a negative "motor provocation test." However, a positive "motor provocation test" under these circumstances allows a more optimistic outlook for pregnancy success.

The relationships between early fetal movements and pregnancy hormone assay [human placental lactogen (hPL) and human chorionic gonadotropin (hCG)] is inexact.[23] In general, a higher hPL level is associated with vigorous fetal motor activity and a lower level with predominantly slow and sluggish type fetal movements. Much overlap, however, was noted, though consistently low hPL levels were associated with the absence of any type of spontaneous fetal movements but the presence of fetal heart motion. No correlation between hCG levels and early fetal movements was recorded. Serum estradiol and progesterone levels have also been assessed as indicators of pregnancy outcome in cases of threatened abortion.[30] In general, normal levels of both these hormones was associated with successful pregnancy outcome (i.e., a low false positive rate) but the converse of abnormal hormone levels with poor outcome was associated with a high incidence of false positive results. These authors concluded that ultrasound was a better predictor of pregnancy outcome than either of these hormone assays.

GROSS AND FINE FETAL BODY MOVEMENTS AND FETAL TONE

The investigation of gross and fine fetal body movements has not been as extensive in either the animal or human fetus as has the investigation of fetal breathing movements. Moreover, methods of classification of fetal body movements into gross and fine categories is not generally established. In the following discussion the term gross fetal movements is used to describe (1) fetal stretching movements, as detected with real-time ultrasound by extension or flexion of echoes from the region of the fetal chest and abdomen, and (2) fetal rolling movements, again as detected with real-time ultrasound and observed about a longitudinal axis of the fetus and best described as a "pitch and yaw" type movement. All other types of fetal movements, i.e., isolated limb movements, small joint movements (i.e., hand-finger), hand-face contact, facial movements, tongue protrusion, sucking, and eye movements, are included in the category of fine fetal movements.

Fetal tone, as in the immediate neonatal period when Apgar scoring is performed, is a subjective measure of the length of time required for a fetal part to return to its original position following the initiation of a fetal movement. This is most easily judged by observation during isolated limb or small joint (i.e., hand) movements and the time required for extension with return to flexion to occur.[31] It is a subjective, nonquantitative measurement.

THE RELATIONSHIP OF FETAL MOVEMENTS TO SLEEP STATE, HYPOXEMIA, AND LABOR

Animal studies would suggest that isolated fetal limb movements occur in all sleep states but that they are significantly less frequent in low voltage, rapid-eye movement sleep.[32] A diurnal pattern in isolated limb movements does not exist and hypoxemia has a profound depressant effect on both their number and length of time that they are present. Uterine activity also has a significant depressant effect on the incidence of isolated limb movements and this effect is most evident in low voltage REM sleep. During labor the limb movements that do occur tend to be associated with uterine contractions.

HUMAN EMBRYONIC AND FETAL MOVEMENTS IN SPONTANEOUS AND THERAPEUTIC TERMINATIONS OF PREGNANCY

The response of the human embryo and fetus to cutaneous stimulation at various menstrual ages has been reported by a variety of authors.[12,13] The first embryonic reflexes that can be elicited are from the perioral area of the face supplied by the maxillary and mandibular divisions of the trigeminal nerve; they are evident at a menstrual age of 7.5 weeks. This reflex involves contraction of the neck muscles on the contralateral side to stimulation resulting in withdrawal of the stimulated area from the stimulating agent and has been referred to as an "avoidance" reflex. Caudal extension of the reflex to involve trunk flexion is seen by 8 weeks; by 8.5 weeks extension of both arms at the shoulders and rotation of the pelvis have been added. At this menstrual age this "avoidance" reflex is termed a "total pattern" reflex, as it is a generalized fetal body neuromuscular response and probably corresponds to the strong and brisk early fetal movements described by Reinhold and outlined earlier (see: Early Pregnancy Ultrasound Studies on Embryonic and Fetal Movements).

Fetal reflex responses towards the stimulating agent ("feeding reflexes") can again initially be elicited from the perioral area and appear approximately half a week later than the "avoiding" type. They are initially of the "total pattern" type and are stereotyped and jerky in appearance.

By 9.5 weeks' menstrual age local reflexes from the perioral area are identifiable, consisting of a "squint" or "scowl" type response. Upper and lower limb reflexes appear around 10.5 weeks' menstrual age. Initially palmar stimulation results in a quick partial finger closure movement in which the thumb does not participate. Wrist rotation, elbow flexion, medial rotation, and pronation accompany the same stimulus by 11 weeks. Finger extension is evident by 12 weeks and thumb opposition with a true grasp by 15 weeks. Plantar flexion in response to stimulation of the sole of the foot appears at the same menstrual age as partial finger closure. By 11.5 weeks a Babinski-type reflex with dorsiflexion of the great toe and fanning of the other toes in association with knee and hip flexion and extension is evident in response to plantar stimulation. Genital and anal stimulation cause bilateral flexion of the thighs with pelvic rotation at this menstrual age also.

Between 11 and 14 weeks' menstrual age, local reflexes either singly or in combinations dominate the fetal reflex function and with advancing menstrual age become increasingly graceful, flowing, and adopt functional sequences that will be present in the postnatal period. It is of interest to note in Humphrey's original reports that with advancing anoxia the pattern of fetal reflex response to cutaneous stimulation changed, with those reflexes most recently attained (i.e., local reflexes) being the first to be lost and a continued regression back to the most primitive "total pattern" type responses occurring before death. Birnholz et al., using phased array ultrasonography, have reported on the sequence of appearance of fetal movements from early pregnancy up to term.[24] Comparison of their data reveals striking similarities with that of both Fitzgerald and Windle's and Humphrey's though the ultrasound appearance of fetal movements is somewhat later than that documented in response to cutaneous stimulation.

PATTERNS OF GROSS FETAL BODY MOVEMENTS DURING THE LAST THIRD OF PREGNANCY

Several real-time ultrasound studies on gross fetal body movement over the last third of human pregnancy have been reported.[33-40] Gross fetal body movements occur 10 percent of the time during this period of gestation, with a range of 0 to 50 percent of any one given hour being occupied by this fetal biophysical function. On an average 30 gross fetal body movements occur per hour (range: 0 to 130). At all gestational ages through the last third of pregnancy an increase in the number of gross body movements was noted in the late evening and early morning. Absence of gross body movements were observed for up to 75 minutes and only 1 percent of 45-minute intervals showed total absence of this fetal function. In contrast to human fetal breathing movements (FBMs) no relationship between maternal food intake or plasma glucose concentrations was noted (see Fetal Breathing Movements).

Latent phase labor had no effect on gross body movement incidence; however, a significant reduction in these occurred in association with active phase labor. Periodic increases in gross body movements during active phase labor occurring every 1 to 1.5 hours and lasting for between 20 to 60 minutes were noted despite the overall reduction in gross body movement incidence. Heart rate variability was noted to increase with these episodes of increased fetal motor function. External physical stimulation has been reported to have no effect on the incidence of gross fetal body movements although our own observations suggest that this may not apply to fine body movements.[41]

Both central nervous system (CNS) depressants and stimulants would appear to have similar effects on fetal body movements as on FBM activity. The major difference in control of these two respective fetal biophysical functions involves glucose-hyperglycemia promoting increased FBM activity, and hyperglycemia stimulating increased fetal body movements.[42] (See Fetal Breathing Movements.)

FETAL MOVEMENTS AND PREGNANCY OUTCOME

Manning, Platt, and Sipos have reported on the relationship between fetal movements (defined as flexion and/or extension of the fetal trunk or limbs, or both) as documented by real-time ultrasound and pregnancy outcome.[39] All patients were delivered within 1 week of the last examination. These authors found a mean incidence of fetal movements of 10 to 16 in a 20-minute observation period and that this incidence was the same in normal and complicated pregnancies except Rh isoimmunization with an affected fetus, where the incidence of fetal movements was significantly reduced. Forty-six of 50 patients had at least one documented fetal movement on the last examination before delivery and within this group two intrauterine deaths occurred related to maternal diabetic ketoacidosis and decompression of a hydrocephalic infant, respectively. Three other fetuses with fetal movements present on the last examination before delivery were delivered with low 5-minute Apgar scores; two of these cases were related to intrapartum fetal distress and the third to severe congenital heart disease. Two neonatal deaths occurred among these latter three fetuses. Four of 50 patients had absent fetal movements on the last examination preceding delivery and 3 intrapartum deaths occurred among these. The fourth patient with absent fetal movements in this subgroup also had a positive oxytocin challenge test but was eventually delivered of a normal fetus. A strong positive correlation between the presence of the other fetal biophysical variables (i.e., FBMs) and the number of fetal movements was noted, as was a similar relationship with fetal movements and a reactive nonstress test. These authors concluded that the presence of fetal movements was a reassuring sign of a normal fetus provided no acute changes in maternal or fetal status or intrapartum fetal distress occurred but that the converse of poor pregnancy outcome with absence of fetal movements might either reflect a physiologic or pathophysiologic fetal state requiring multiple biophysical variable analysis to further clarify fetal well-being.

The subjective nature of fetal tone assessment virtually always implies that if fetal movements are present fetal tone is normal, as the differentiation between normal and decreased tone is subject to much observer variation in interpretation.

Finally, the absence of fetal movements should lead one to suspect the possibility of congenital neuromuscular disease, especially if observed over extensive periods. Myotonia congenita and Wernig–Hoffman syndromes are associated with total absence of all types of fetal movements.[43,44] Maternal blunt abdominal trauma may have a similar effect for prolonged periods of time reflecting fetal concussion.[31] Hyperkinetic generalized fetal motor activity indicative of grand mal type seizures in utero have also been observed.[45,46] We have seen this last phenomenon twice, with one infant actually convulsing at the time of delivery by cesarean section.

FETAL BREATHING MOVEMENTS

Despite Ahlfeld's observations on human fetal breathing movements in the late 1880s it was not until the early 1970s that the occurrence of this fetal biophysical function as a normal part of intrauterine development became widely accepted. Initial reports from the Nuffield Institute in Oxford, England, in 1970 by Dawes and colleagues and subsequent reports in 1972 and 1974 by the same authors on both acute and chronically catheterized fetal lamb preparations provided much insight into the physiology and pathophysiology of FBMs.[47-49] Studies in both the fetal lamb and the fetal monkey subsequently confirmed these initial findings.[50,51] The significance of these animal studies lies in the fact that they provided the stimulus for the more recent real-time ultrasound investigations of FBMs in human pregnancies; because of this, they are now briefly reviewed.

ANIMAL STUDIES OF FETAL BREATHING MOVEMENTS

In their initial report in 1970, Dawes et al. documented the occurrence of FBMs in the fetal lamb from 0.3 to 0.95 of gestation (term in fetal lamb is 147 days). In early gestation experiments, FBMs were noted visually as paradoxical movements of the chest and abdomen (indrawing of the chest wall with distension of the abdomen with inspiration) in saline bath preparations. In the more advanced gestational age experiments (0.68 to 0.95 of gestation) catheters were placed in the fetal carotid artery to record heart rate, blood pressure, and to allow for intermittent arterial blood gas sampling. Catheters were also placed in the fetal trachea to record changes in intrathoracic pressures and in some cases tracheal flow meters were used. Electrocorticogram (ECOG) activity was recorded using electrodes placed biparietally.

These experiments revealed the presence of two types of discontinuous respiratory activity:

1. Gasping type movements—single, brief, relatively deep respiratory efforts which recurred irregularly at a slow rate of 1 to 3 per minute.
2. Rapid irregular fetal breathing movements—bursts of irregular respiratory activity of a very much higher frequency (1 to 4 Hz) lasting for variable lengths of time (seconds to 1 hour or more).

Intratracheal pressure changes associated with both these types of FBMs were small (−2 to −10 mm Hg, occasionally to −40 mm Hg) and were associated with a small forward–backward flow of tracheal fluid. Peak tracheal flow rates of up to 6 ml/sec were recorded but the duration of the respiratory movements was so short (0.2 seconds) that net change in fluid volume rarely exceeded 0.5 ml. FBMs were present for up to 40 percent of the time over the last third of gestation and with advancing gestation their frequency and amplitude increased.

Two types of ECOG activity were also found:

1. *REM sleep.* Fast wave (10 to 20 Hz), low voltage (<25 mV peaks) was recorded for 54 to 69 percent of the time. This was associated with rapid eye movements, and rapid irregular FBMs always occurred during this ECOG pattern.
2. *Non-REM sleep.* Slow wave (3 to 12 Hz), high voltage (40 to 100 mV peaks) was recorded for 31 to 46 percent of the time. No particular pattern of FBMs was associated with this sleep state.

Changes in sleep state from non-REM to REM activity always preceded the onset of rapid irregular FBMs and the latter always ceased before the ECOG activity reverted to non-REM type patterns.

The presence or absence of FBMs was unrelated to arterial blood gas tensions and pH over a wide range of spontaneous variation except when fetal Pao_2 was very low (<10 mm Hg), at which point FBMs became markedly reduced. Fetal hypoglycemia was also noted to be associated with a decrease in FBMs. Further investigations were reported in 1974 into the effects of hypoxia, hypocapnea, hyperoxia, and hypercapnea on FBMs. Fetal hypoxia was invariably associated with the cessation of rapid, irregular FBMs and also with a significant reduction in the percentage of time fast-wave, low-voltage ECOG activity was recorded. Fetal hypercapnea had the directly opposite effects on both FBMs and ECOG activity. Fetal hypocapnea was also associated with a reduction in the incidence of FBMs

while fetal hyperoxia had no demonstrable effects. Tracheal flow rates (or liquid ventilation rates), which are the fetal equivalent of minute volume ventilation rates postnatally, were noted to vary in accordance with the incidence of FBMs. The effects of asphyxia induced by intermittent cord occlusion was also studied and noted to cause cessation of all normal FBMs with the onset of gasping type FBMs of long duration (>1 second) and large amplitude (up to −75 mm Hg). These were associated with inhalation of large volumes of amniotic fluid and debris (up to 10 ml) despite the fact that the density and viscosity of amniotic fluid is 1000 times that of air.[52]

Abnormal patterns of FMBs have been reported before intrauterine death in both the sheep and monkey fetus.[53,54] In both these animal studies an almost uniform finding was the occurrence of prolonged periods of apnea accompanied by intermittent episodes of gasping type FBMs for varying lengths of time prior to fetal demise. Tracheal pressure catheter readings showed these gasping type FBMs to be of long duration, large amplitude, and low frequency as described by Dawes et al. in association with cord occlusion and fetal asphyxia. Simultaneous real-time ultrasound examination at the time of fetal gasping was unable to distinguish this abnormal FBM activity from normal patterns. In some animal experiments a "picket fence" pattern of FBM activity of constant frequency and fixed amplitude was also noted to precede intrauterine death for variable time periods.

The response of FBMs to drug administration has revealed in general a decrease or complete cessation in this biophysical function following CNS depressant administration. "Catch-up" in FBM activity may occur with reversal of the normal circadian pattern of FBMs in the chronic fetal sheep model in response to long-term intermittent diazepam administration.[55] Some drugs may have different effects, depending on the route of administration, as has been clearly demonstrated with nicotine.[52] This drug causes suppression of FBMs if given to the ewe whereas an increase in FBMs occurs if it is administered directly to the fetus.

CNS stimulants may increase FBM incidence, but by far the most important agent in the induction of FBM activity is maternal (and hence fetal) glucose intake (see Ultrasound Studies of Human FBMs).

Dawes et al. suggested normal FBMs occur in the presence of a partially closed glottis and that asphyxia causes loss of this reflex function, allowing inhalation into the tracheobronchial tree to occur. The appearance of markers of fetal lung maturity of alveolar origin in the amniotic fluid with advancing gestation supports at least partial patency of this anatomic structure in normal, nonasphyxiated pregnancy during the expiratory phase of fetal breathing.

TABLE 2
Classification of Human Fetal Breathing Movements

Pattern	Rate	Amplitude	Character	Fetal Movements	Comments
Type I	40–90	Variable	Regular, progressive increase in both rate and amplitude, then movements cease or decline	Commonly associated with rolling trunk and limb movements	Usually seen before 36 weeks
Type II	60–90	Mixed low and high	Rapid, irregular movements with intermittent slow deep fetal breaths	Commonly associated with startle-like trunk movements	May occur at any gestational age
Type III	30–60	Relatively fixed	Regular, slower movements, constant in both rate and amplitude	Associated with trunk and/or limb movements	Usually observed after 36 weeks' gestation
Type IV	10–15	Large	Regular exceedingly rapid large movements	Unusual	Usually palpable commonly interpreted as fetal hiccups by the mother; may occur at any gestational age
Type V	5–20	Variable	Usually regular, isolated movements distinctive in the slow respiratory component not associated with any rapid movements	Unusual	Associated with prolonged apnea, may occur at any gestational age and may represent fetal gasping movements

Reproduced with permission from Manning FA: Antepartum assessment of human fetal breathing movement, in Chiswick M (ed), Laboratory Investigation of Fetal Disease. Edinburgh, Churchill Livingstone, 1982, pp 71–76.

ULTRASOUND STUDIES ON HUMAN FBMS

In 1971, Boddy and Robinson reported on the occurrence of FBMs in human pregnancies using gated-A-mode ultrasound.[11] This was the first direct evidence of this fetal biophysical function in human pregnancy and subsequent studies confirmed these original findings.[56] The role of A-mode ultrasound in the documentation of human FBMs is now of historic interest only because of the many inaccuracies of this technique and because of recent advances in real-time B-mode ultrasound technology.[57] Human FBMs are detectable from 11 weeks' gestational age onwards.[58] Early in pregnancy they are very irregular, both in rate, incidence, and amplitude, but with advancing gestation through the mid-trimester their character becomes more regular in all these parameters.[59] Table 2 outlines a method for classification of human FBMs as documented by real-time ultrasound examination.[52] Five types of human FBMs have been described. Chest wall and abdominal wall components of human FBMs coexist in a paradoxical fashion, with inward displacement of the rib cage (2 to 5 mm) and outward displacement of the abdominal wall (4 to 8 mm) during inspiration.[35,60] Expiration is associated with the opposite chest and abdominal wall movements. The ratio of inspiratory to expiratory times is between 2:1 to

5:1.[52] On longitudinal scanning, displacement of the liver, kidneys, and stomach caudally with inspiration attests to a significant diaphragmatic component in this fetal movement. Comparisons between human FBMs and that of the neonate with hyaline membrane disease reveal striking similarities, with rib retraction and abdominal distension occurring with inspiration in the latter condition as well. Both the fetus in utero and the newborn with hyaline membrane disease "ventilate" in the face of markedly increased airways resistance.

In the last third of normal gestation human FBMs are discontinuous and have a significant circadian rhythm.[33-35] They are present on an average 31 percent of the time and can occupy from 0 to 86 percent of any 1-hour observation period. Any half-hour observation period is associated with an 8 percent chance of encountering an apneic interval spanning the whole observation period. Figures from our own laboratories would put this chance at 18 percent in high-risk obstetric patients submitted for biophysical profile scoring during the same period of pregnancy.

The rate of human FBMs decreases with advancing gestation (58 per minute at 30 to 31 weeks; 47 per minute at 38 to 39 weeks) and their character becomes increasingly regular. Apneic intervals between successive episodes of FBMs of up to 122 minutes duration have been recorded; however, 97 percent of breath to breath intervals are less than 6 seconds in duration.[61] The absence of FBMs for periods greater than this has been suggested as the appropriate definition of fetal apnea during this stage of pregnancy. The distribution of fetal apneic intervals is similar throughout the last third of pregnancy though their length tends to increase as term approaches (longest documented apneic interval at 30 to 31 weeks: 65 minutes, longest documented apneic interval at 38 to 39 weeks: 122 minutes). Apneic intervals are shorter during the second and third hours following maternal food ingestion (longest documented apneic interval: 45 minutes), suggesting that this may be the ideal time to look for this fetal biophysical function.

A circadian pattern in human FBMs through the last third of pregnancy has been noted. Increases in FBMs occur after maternal meals, starting in the second and third hours after food intake and are preceded by peak maternal plasma glucose concentrations. Early in the third trimester these postprandial peaks in FBMs are preceded by troughs in FBM activity, but this pattern of preprandial troughs in FBM activity does not persist as term approaches. Throughout the third trimester troughs in FBM incidence occur in the late evening, with a signficant peak again noted in the early morning. This nocturnal cyclicity probably reflects a fetal circadian rhythm in breathing activity as maternal plasma glucose concentrations steadily decrease to low values in the early morning but may be related to maternal sleep state as they occur during periods of maternal REM sleep.[62]

The relationship between human FBM activity and maternal food intake has been further investigated using the 50-g oral glucose tolerance test.[36] Again, significant increases in FBM activity were noted in the second and third hours following maternal glucose loading; these increases in FBMs were again preceded by peak maternal plasma glucose concentrations. FBMs were observed in 97 percent of the 15-minute intervals during the second and third hours following glucose loading. The reason for this increase in FBM activity following both maternal meals and maternal oral glucose loading is unknown but may be related to fetal cerebral glucose metabolism with carbon dioxide production and a resultant stimulation of central chemosensitive areas in the ventral surface of the medulla.[36]

Fetal hiccoughing occurs intermittently at all gestational ages during the last third of pregnancy. Its occurrence has no relationship to the time of day or maternal food intake. It is present approximately 2 percent of the time. Hiccoughing has a characteristic real-time ultrasound appearance, with rapid inward and outward movement of the fetal chest wall echoes.[35]

The fetal body tends to tremor or shake with hiccoughing but not with other types of FBMs. Chest wall movement is of larger amplitude with hiccoughing (5 to 10 mm) and the cycle time is more rapid (0.1 to 0.2 seconds) than with other types of FBMs.[35,60] It is thought that hiccoughing may reflect fetal stomach distension and thereby be an index of fetal swallowing.

Human FBMs decrease during labor (prelabor control; 25.6 percent latent phase labor; 8.3 percent active phase labor, 0.8 percent).[37] In some patients a periodic pattern of increased FBM activity associated with increased gross fetal body movements and increased fetal heart rate variability occurs in the latent phase of labor, but with the onset of active phase of labor fetal apnea predominates. These changes are unrelated to changes in maternal plasma glucose concentrations or maternal venous pH or Pco_2 values. Artificial rupture of the membranes, epidural anesthesia, and Syntocinon induction have no appreciable effects on the incidence of FBMs. The etiology of reduced FBM activity in labor may be due to a decrease in fetal Po_2 related to increasing uterine activity or to external stimulation of the fetus by either the uterine musculature or during descent through the pelvis. An association between tactile or thermal stimulation of the facial areas of the fetal rhesus monkey and fetal apnea has been reported.[63]

Real-time B-mode ultrasonography has failed to identify gasping type FBMs in either the human or animal fetus, although these types of FBMs have been reported using A-mode technology.[52,55,58,64]

The predominant effect of pharmacologic agents on FBM activity in human pregnancies has been with CNS depressants. Alcohol, general anesthetics, sedatives, and narcotic analgesics all markedly decrease the incidence of human FBMs.[65] Cigarette smoking by the gravida has a similar effect, and this is related to increases in maternal plasma nicotine levels.[66] The duration of this effect lasts for 1 hour after the last cigarette is smoked. The effects of CNS stimulants on human FBMs is less clear, although adrenaline and other catecholamines have been associated with an increase in FBM activity.[59,67] It appears that the fetal CNS is less sensitive to the effects of CNS stimulants than it is to CNS depressants in terms of FBM activity.

Amniocentesis has no immediate effects on FBMs, although a significant decrease in their incidence has been reported at 24 and 48 hours following the procedure.[68,69] This decrease in FBM activity may be related to uterine activity initiated by or following the procedure.

From the preceding animal and human studies it is evident that a wide variety of factors—physiologic, pathophysiologic, and iatrogenic—affect the changes of detecting human FBMs at any given time. The most important of these is the inherent cyclicity of human FBM activity and this represents the most frequent reason for failure to detect this fetal biophysical parameter. In terms of using the presence or absence of this fetal function as a method of antenatal well-being assessment, absence of human FBMs due to normal physiologic reasons represents the most common cause of false positive test results (i.e., delivery of a normal healthy fetus in the face of a positive biophysical variable test result of fetal compromise). This same principle of inherent cyclicity probably applies to other biophysical variables, as has been shown by Patrick et al. in long-term studies on fetal heart rate reactivity.[38]

Bearing these limitations in mind, single biophysical variable analysis using the presence or absence of human FBMs as a predictor of pregnancy outcome has been reported.[58,70] Boddy and Dawes in 1975, using an A-scan model reported poor pregnancy outcome in terms of a high incidence of fetal distress in labor (15 of 17 cases) and antenatal unexpected intrauterine death (10 of 11 cases) if human FBM activity could not be detected for 50 percent or more of the period of observation (not stated) or if fetal gasping was noted.

Platt et al.,[70] using an arbitrary observation interval of 30 minutes duration, with a definition of normal human FBM activity if present for 60 seconds or longer during this time period, noted a significant relationship between the presence of normal human FBMs and successful pregnancy outcome, as judged by the absence of fetal distress in labor and 5-minute Apgar scores of greater than 7. When FBMs were present the false negative rate was 4.3 percent (5 of 116 cases), and in four of these cases an acute intrapartum cause of fetal distress was identified (i.e., abruptio placenta, cord prolapse, etc). In contrast, 50 percent (10 of 20 cases) with absent human FBM activity at the last examination before delivery had 5-minute Apgars of less than 7 and 60 percent (12 of 20 cases) developed intrapartum fetal distress, as evidenced by fetal heart rate monitoring and/or scalp pH evaluation.

Manning et al., using the same criteria for poor outcome and for normal human FBM activity as Platt et al.,[70] compared human FBM monitoring to the nonstress test (NST) as a method of predicting pregnancy outcome.[71] When both tests were normal, predictive accuracy of normal outcome was similar to each individual test, and combining the two normal tests did not significantly reduce the false negative test rate (the false negative rates: human FBMs-present, 4 percent; NST-reactive, 4.8 percent; human FBMs-present/NST-reactive, 3.2 percent). Conversely, the predictive accuracy of a single positive test of poor pregnancy outcome (true positive result) was 16.7 percent for the

nonreactive NST and 25 percent for human FBM absent. Combination of the two positive tests gave the highest true positive rate (44.5 percent). Combinations of normal and abnormal tests gave a similar predictive accuracy of good outcome as a single normal test alone, but had a significantly lower false positive rate than a single abnormal test alone.

Using the same endpoints for judging pregnancy outcome the role of human FBM monitoring in the evaluation of the abnormal contraction stress test (CST) has been reported.[72] The finding of normal human FBMs, as described previously in a 30-minute observation interval, was associated with 100 and 87 percent false positive test rates in patients with equivocal and positive CST results, respectively. Conversely, the absence of human FBM activity in a 30-minute observation interval in a patient with a positive CST was uniformly associated with fetal distress in labor.

Intrauterine fetal tachypnea, with rates of up to 200 per minute have been reported in association with diabetic pregnancy.[58,73] The significance of this finding in terms of fetal well-being is unclear at this time.

From the above data it is evident that single biophysical variable monitoring, if normal, is a very good predictor of normal pregnancy outcome, but that combinations of abnormal variables are required to predict poor outcome.

ULTRASOUND: THE EVALUATION OF AMNIOTIC FLUID VOLUME

The association between alterations in amniotic fluid volume (AFV) and abnormal fetal status is well recognized by the clinical relationship between oligohydramnios and congenital urinary tract abnormalities, intrauterine growth retardation (IUGR) and postterm pregnancy.[74-76] Conversely, polyhydramnios may be associated with open neural tube defects, congenital upper gastrointestinal tract obstruction or malformation, and both immunologic and nonimmunologic hydrops fetalis.

Since the advent of diagnostic obstetric ultrasound a means has become available for the assessment of AFV. As yet there are no generally accepted criteria for the diagnosis by ultrasound of either oligohydramnios or polyhydramnios. Several groups of authors have suggested criteria for the ultrasonic diagnosis of both these conditions.[76-79] Of these, only the description of qualitative AFV (qAFV) for the diagnosis of oligohydramnios described by Manning and Platt[77] allows for easy reproducibility and standardization. These authors have suggested that AFV should be considered normal if at the time of ultrasound scanning

TABLE 3
Suggested Ultrasound Criteria for Classification of Qualitative Amniotic Fluid Volume

	Column Height*	Number of Patients (%)
Normal	>2.0 cm	7356 (96.8)
Marginal	2.0 to 1.0 cm	160 (2.25)
Decreased	<1.0 cm	64 (0.925)

* Measured in two perpendicular planes.

a pocket of fluid of 1 cm or greater in two perpendicular planes is identified. Failure to fulfill these criteria suggests a diagnosis of oligohydramnios (decreased qAFV). Further reports from these same authors have identified a high association between decreased qAFV and IUGR (89.4 percent) and this finding has been suggested as a possible screening test for IUGR.[75,77]

Further data from our laboratories support the clinical significance of qAFV assessment.[80] In a retrospective chart review of 7580 high-risk referred obstetric patients relating qAFV as measured at the time of the last biophysical profile score evaluation to perinatal outcome using the criteria for qAFV assessment outlined in Table 3, we found significant increases in both gross and corrected perinatal mortality and in the incidence of lethal congenital anomalies (Table 4). The incidences of IUGR and fetal distress (both ante- and intrapartum) were also significantly related to qAFV determination, as shown in Table 5.

From these data it is evident that qAFV estimation if marginal or decreased is associated with 23.8-fold and 59.5-fold increases, respectively, in corrected perinatal mortality as compared to normal qAFV. An 8.2-fold increase in the incidence of lethal congenital anomalies occurred in association with decreased qAFV.

The association between decreased qAFV and IUGR in this much larger study did not confirm the previously reported extremely high association with IUGR. However, a 3.3-fold and 6.5-fold increase in the incidence of this condition was found in the marginal and decreased qAFV groups, respectively, when compared to normal qAFV.

The relationship between fetal distress in labor with both IUGR and congenital anomaly is well

TABLE 5
Incidence of IUGR* and Fetal Distress† Related to qAFV

	IUGR	Fetal Distress
Normal	6%	2.8%
Marginal	20%	21%
Decreased	39%	31%

* Both weight < 10th percentile weight for gestational age and sex.
† Defined as:
  i. Emergency termination of pregnancy due to a positive oxytocin challenge test, nonreactive nonstress test showing either repetitive variable or late decelerations or persistent bradycardia, and/or a BPS of ≤2 prior to the onset of labor.
  ii. Intrapartum occurrence of repetitive variable or late decelerations and/or fetal scalp pH of <7.20 and/or cord venous pH of <7.20.
  iii. 5-minute Apgar of <7.

recognized.[75,81] Our results suggest a significant role for qAFV assessment in the prediction of this occurrence, with 7- and 11-fold increases being noted with marginal and decreased qAFVs, respectively. This may well represent cord compromise associated with reduced amniotic fluid volumes.

In summary, this easily obtained ultrasound parameter has significant prognostic value in terms of pregnancy outcome and appears to have a real role in antenatal fetal monitoring.

COMPOSITE FETAL ACTIVITY ASSESSMENT: FETAL BIOPHYSICAL PROFILE SCORING

The introduction of high-resolution dynamic ultrasound methods in clinical obstetrics now permits accurate and specific examination of the fetus at risk for death or damage in utero. Chronic asphyxia, the single most common cause of perinatal death, is recognizable in utero by application of dynamic ultrasound techniques. Fetal biophysical activities such as gross body movement, tone, breathing movements, and reflex and reactive responses are not random events, but rather highly specific movements regulated by complex central neurologic pathways. Since central nervous system tissue is exquisitely oxygen sensitive, it follows that if such activities are observed to be present then functioning and therefore well-oxygenated neurologic

TABLE 4
Perinatal Outcome Related to Qualitative Amniotic Fluid Volume

	Normal qAFV	Marginal qAFV	Decreased qAFV
Gross perinatal mortality	4.65	56/1000	187/1000
Corrected perinatal mortality	2.1/1000	50/1000	125/1000
Percent of major anomalies	1.15	1.87	9.4

TABLE 6
Technique of Biophysical Profile Scoring

Biophysical Variable	Normal (Score = 2)	Abnormal (Score = 0)
1. Fetal breathing movements	At least one episode of at least 30 seconds' duration in 30 minutes' observation	Absent or no episode of ≥30 seconds in 30 minutes
2. Gross body movement	At least three discrete body/limb movements in 30 minutes (episodes of active continuous movements considered as a single movement)	Two or fewer episodes of body/limb movements in 30 minutes
3. Fetal tone	At least one episode of active extension with return to flexion of fetal limb(s) or trunk. Opening and closing of hand considered normal tone.	Either slow extension with return to partial flexion or movement of limb in full extension or absent fetal movement.
4. Reactive fetal heart rate	At least two episodes of acceleration of ≥15 bpm and at least 15 seconds' duration associated with fetal movement in 30 minutes	Less than two accelerations or acceleration <15 bpm in 30 minutes
5. Qualitative amniotic fluid volume	At least one pocket of amniotic fluid that measures at least 1 cm in two perpendicular planes	Either no amniotic fluid pockets or a pocket <1 cm in two perpendicular planes

pathways are operant. Thus, the presence of a normal activity is a powerful predictor of a normal and intact central nervous system. The absence of a given activity is considerably more difficult to interpret, since in the normal fetus periodicity is a characteristic of biophysical activities. These activities and their periodicity are markedly influenced by sleep–wake cycles in the fetus, and the absence of a given activity (e.g., fetal breathing movements) for short periods of time is often observed during quiet sleep. Since CNS depression due to asphyxia will also abolish such activity it may be exceedingly difficult to differentiate the normal fetus in quiet sleep from the asphyxiated fetus if only a single variable is considered. However, by observing a variety of fetal activities over an extended period of time it becomes possible to differentiate the normal fetus in quiet sleep from the asphyxiated fetus.

During an observation period with a dynamic ultrasound method several fetal biophysical activities may be observed simultaneously. Such activities may include breathing movements, gross and fine body movements, purposeful and reflex movements, and flexor tone. Fetal biophysical profile scoring is an attempt to categorize some of these activities in order to differentiate the normal fetus from the fetus at risk.[31] The biophysical profile score is derived from observation of five discrete variables: fetal movement, tone, breathing, reactivity (NST), and qualitative amniotic fluid volume (Table 6). The first four of these five variables are indirect measures of immediate central nervous system function. The fifth variable, qualitative amniotic fluid volume, is best viewed as a long-term indication of fetal asphyxia. The latter occurs because prolonged or repeated episodes of fetal asphyxia cause

TABLE 7
Biophysical Profile Scoring: Comparative Perinatal Mortality Statistics

	Number of Patients	Percent High Risk	Perinatal Mortality	Corrected Perinatal Mortality*	False-Negative Perinatal Mortality†
Unselected general population†	16,000	20%	13.5	10.2	—
High-risk general population‡	3,200	100%	68	51.0	—
Prospective blinded	216	100%	50.9	32.4	10.1
Prospective not blinded	1,184	75%	11.7	5.09	0.8
Prospective not expanded	3,100	75%	11.2	3.52	0.9
Prospective expanded	7,400	75%	10.4	2.1	0.6

* Corrected for lethal congenital anomalies.
† Deaths of a normal fetus within 7 days after a normal test result (biophysical profile score 8 to 10).
‡ Untested population.

a dramatic decrease in fetal urine production due to redistribution of fetal cardiac output. Oligohydramnios, in the presence of functioning fetal kidneys, is associated with an extremely high incidence of perinatal morbidity and mortality.[80]

The fetal variables comprising the profile score are observed simultaneously and assigned an arbitrary score of 2 when normal and 0 when abnormal. Each observation period is continued until either all variables are observed as normal or 30 minutes elapses (Table 6). In our experience, which includes in excess of 15,000 observations, the average time to derive a profile score is 10 to 12 minutes and in only 2 percent of cases is a full 30 minutes observation required.

The relationship between the composite score of fetal activities and amniotic fluid volume and outcome is striking (Table 7). In a tested population with results blinded, an abnormal score (<4) was associated with a 50- to 100-fold increase in perinatal mortality.[31] Fetal biophysical profile scoring has been integrated extensively in our management of the pregnancy at risk. In general, fetal biophysical profile scoring is begun at 30 weeks' gestation and repeated at weekly intervals. The frequency of testing is increased to twice weekly in pregnancies complicated by diabetes or that have gone past the forty-second completed week of gestation. In total, in excess of 15,000 fetal biophysical profile scores have been recorded in more than 7400 referred high-risk pregnancies. The outcomes of these pregnancies have been encouraging. Overall the perinatal mortality has been reduced and in particular the death rate among fetuses who are structurally normal has fallen (Table 7). The false negative rate, defined as death of a normal fetus within 1 week of a normal test is extremely low, ranging from 1.4 to 2.1 per 1000 patients and 0.6 to 0.8 per 1000 tests.

As a result of these observations, we have entirely abandoned the use of nonspecific biochemical markers of fetal condition such as plasma estriols and human placental lactogen, and the use of single biophysical tests such as fetal movement or heart rate testing alone.

CONCLUSION AND FUTURE TRENDS

The role of real-time ultrasound in the assessment of FBMs, gross and fine fetal body movements, fetal tone, and qualitative AFV has been reviewed. The physiologic, pathophysiologic, and iatrogenic factors that affect these biophysical variables has been summarized and a method of fetal well-being assessment based on composite biophysical profile scoring outlined. The results of this method of fetal assessment to a large, high-risk obstetric population has been presented.

Review of the preceding data reveals the importance of fetal rest/activity cycles and circadian rhythm in determining whether or not a specific fetal biophysical function will be present at any given time of observation. Our present inability to identify with any degree of certainty human fetal sleep state severely limits our ability to decide whether or not the absence of any given biophysical variable is physiologic or pathologic. Future research into eye movement patterns as detected by real-time ultrasound may help clarify this situation and thereby reduce the false positive rates associated with BPS assessment.

The observation of regression in fetal reflex responses in response to anoxia may allow in the future a more sensitive method for the detection of fetal compromise if normal patterns of these reflexes through the latter half of pregnancy can be obtained and confirmed. It is conceivable that loss of small joint function may precede a loss of fetal trunk or limb movements in response to hypoxia and this may be an earlier warning of impending fetal compromise.

Fetal tone is the most useful indicator of antenatal asphyxia when used in Apgar scoring in the neonatal period. At present our assessment of this fetal parameter is subjective and hence open to observer variation in interpretation. An objective method for quantification of this fetal function would allow for a more precise definition of normalcy and might thereby improve testing reproducibility.

Finally, qAFV assessment is a static measurement of a parameter that is not solely under fetal control. Estimation of fetal urine production might provide a better indication of fetal status as it is a direct fetal measurement and may vary in association with the cardiac output redistribution that occurs in association with hypoxemia.

REFERENCES

1. Luke: Chapter 1, Verses 44–45
2. Sadovsky E, Yaffe H: Daily fetal movement recording and fetal prognosis. Obstet Gynecol 41:6, 1973
3. Sadovsky E, Yaffe H, Pilishuk WL: Fetal movements monitoring in normal and pathologic pregnancy. Int J Gynaecol Obstet 12:75, 1974
4. Sadovsky E, Polishuk WZ: Fetal movements in utero. Obstet Gynecol 50:49, 1977
5. Sadovsky E: What do movements of the fetus tell about its well-being? Contemp Obstet Gynecol 12:59, 1978
6. Timor-Tritsch IE, Dierker LJ, Hertz RH, et al: Fetal movements: A brief review. Clin Obstet Gynecol 22:583, 1979
7. Timor-Tritsch IE, Zador E, Hertz RH: Classification of human fetal movement. Am J Obstet Gynecol 126:70, 1976

8. Rayburn WF: Antepartum fetal assessment: Monitoring fetal activity. Clin Perinatol 9(2):231, 1982
9. Ahlfeld F: Die intrauterine taetigkeit der thorax-und Zwerchtfell-Muskulatur. Intrauterine Atmung Monatsschr 21:142, 1905. Quoted by Goodlin RC: History of fetal monitoring. Am J Obstet Gynecol 133:323, 1979
10. Duenhoelter JH, Pritchard JA: Fetal respiration: A review. Am J Obstet Gynecol 129:326, 1977
11. Boddy K, Robinson JS: External method for the detection of fetal breathing in utero. Lancet 2:1231, 1971
12. Humphrey T: Some correlations between the appearance of human fetal reflexes and the development of the nervous system. Prog Brain Res 4:93, 1964
13. Fitzgerald GE, Windle W: Some observations on early human fetal movements. J Comp Neurol 76:159, 1942
14. Robinson HR: The diagnosis of early pregnancy failure by sonar. Br J Obstet Gynaecol 82:849, 1975
15. Van Dongen LGR, Goudie EG: Fetal movement patterns in the first trimester of pregnancy. Br J Obstet Gynaecol 87:191, 1980
16. Shawker TH, Schuette WH, Whitehouse W, et al: Early fetal movements—A real-time ultrasound study. Obstet Gynecol 55:194, 1980
17. Reinhold E: Clinical value of fetal spontaneous movements in early pregnancy. J Perinat Med 1:65, 1973
18. Manning FA: Unpublished observations
19. Anderson SG: Real-time sonography in obstetrics. Obstet Gynecol 51:284, 1978
20. Jouppila P: Fetal movements diagnosed by ultrasound in early pregnancy. Acta Obstet Gynaecol Scand 55:131, 1976
21. Reinhold E: Identification and differentiation of fetal movements, in Keller PJ (ed), Contributions to Gynaecology and Obstetrics. Basel, Karger, 1979, vol 6, pp 29–32
22. Reinhold E: New trends in real-time ultrasound in early pregnancy, in Keller PJ (ed), Contributions to Gynaecology and Obstetrics. Basel, Karger, 1979, vol 6, pp 123–128
23. Reinhold E: Fetal movements and fetal behaviour: Ultrasonics in early pregnancy—Diagnostic scanning and fetal motor behaviour, in Keller PJ (ed), Contributions to Gynaecology and Obstetrics. Basel, Karger, 1976, vol 1, pp 102–127
24. Birnholz JC, Stephens JC, Faria M: Fetal movement patterns: A possible means of defining neurologic developmental milestones in utero. Am J Roentgenol 130:537, 1978
25. Hollander HJ: Historical review and clinical relevance of real-time observations of fetal movements, in Keller PJ (ed), Contributions to Gynaecology and Obstetrics. Basel, Karger, 1979, vol 6, pp 26–28
26. Mulz D: Fetal behaviour during pregnancy, in Keller PJ (ed), Contributions to Gynaecology and Obstetrics. Basel, Karger, 1979, vol 6, pp 57–60
27. Henner UD, Haller N, Kubli F: Quantification of active fetal body movements in the first half of pregnancy, in Keller PJ (ed), Contributions to Gynaecology and Obstetrics. Basel, Karger, 1979, vol 6, pp 33–41
28. Anderson SG: Management of threatened abortion with real-time sonography. Obstet Gynecol 55:259, 1980
29. Levine SC, Filly RA: Accuracy of real-time sonography in the determination of fetal viability. Obstet Gynecol 49:475, 1977
30. Eriksen PS, Phillipsin T: Prognosis in threatened abortion evaluated by hormone assays and ultrasound scanning. Obstet Gynecol 55:435, 1980
31. Manning FA, Morrison I, Lange IR, et al: Antepartum determination of fetal health: Composite biophysical profile scoring. Clin Perinatol 9:285, 1982
32. Natale R, Clewlow F, Dawes GS: Measurement of fetal forelimb movements in the lamb in utero. Am J Obstet Gynecol 140:545, 1981
33. Patrick J, Campbell K, Carmichael L, et al: Patterns of human fetal breathing during the last 10 weeks of pregnancy. Obstet Gynecol 56:24, 1980
34. Patrick J, Natale R, Richardson B: Patterns of human fetal breathing activity at 34 to 35 weeks' gestational age. Am J Obstet Gynecol 132:507, 1978
35. Patrick J, Fetherston W, Vick H, et al: Human fetal breathing movements and gross fetal body movements at weeks 34–35 of gestation. Am J Obstet Gynecol 130:693, 1978
36. Natale R, Patrick J, Richardson B: Effects of human maternal venous plasma glucose concentrations on human fetal breathing movements. Am J Obstet Gynecol 132:36, 1978
37. Richardson B, Natale R, Patrick J: Human fetal breathing activity during electively induced labor and term. Am J Obstet Gynecol 133:247, 1979
38. Brown R, Patrick J: The non-stress test: How long is enough? Am J Obstet Gynecol 141:646, 1981
39. Manning FA, Platt LD, Sipos L: Fetal movements in human pregnancies in the third trimester. Am J Obstet Gynecol 54:699, 1979
40. Patrick J, Campbell K, Carmicheal L, et al: Patterns of gross fetal body movements of 24-hour observation intervals during the last 10 weeks of pregnancy. Am J Obstet Gynecol 142:363, 1982
41. Richardson B, Campbell K, Carmichael L, et al: Effects of external physical stimulation on fetuses near term. Am J Obstet Gynecol 139:344, 1981
42. Holden JP, Jovanovic L, Druzin M, et al: Maternal hyperglycemia is not associated with increased fetal activity in diabetic pregnancy. Scientific Abstracts, 28th Annual Meeting of the Society for Gynecologic Investigation, St. Louis, MO, March 18–21, 1981 (Abstract 44)
43. Patrick J: Personal communication
44. Harman CR: Personal communication
45. Manning FA: Unpublished observation
46. Platt L: Personal communication
47. Dawes GS, Fox HE, Leduc BM, et al: Respiratory movements and paradoxical sleep in the fetal lamb. J Physiol 210:47, 1970
48. Dawes GS, Fox HE, Leduc BM, et al: Respiratory movements and rapid eye movement sleep in the fetal lamb. J Physiol 220:119, 1972
49. Boddy K, Dawes GS, Fisher R, et al: Fetal respiratory

movements, electrocortical and cardiovascular responses to hypoxemia and hypercapnia. J Physiol 243:599, 1974

50. Merlet C, Hoerter J, Devilleneuve C, et al: Mise en evidence de movements respiratoires, chez le foetus d'agneau in utero au cours du dernier mois de la gestation. C R Acad Sci D Paris 270:2462, 1970

51. Martin CB, Murata Y, Petrie RH, et al: Respiratory movements in fetal rhesus monkeys. Am J Obstet Gynecol 119:939, 1974

52. Manning FA: Antepartum assessment of human fetal breathing movements, in Chiswick M, (ed), Laboratory Investigation of Fetal Disease. Edinburgh, Churchill Livingstone, 1982, pp 71–76

53. Patrick JE, Dalton JJ, Dawes GS: Breathing patterns before death in fetal lambs. Am J Obstet Gynecol 125:73, 1976

54. Manning FA, Martin CB, Murata Y, et al: Breathing patterns before death in the primate fetus. Am J Obstet Gynecol 135:71, 1979

55. Worthinton D, Piercy WN, Smith BT: Modification of ovine fetal respiratory-like activity by chronic diazepam administration. Am J Obstet Gynecol 131:749, 1978

56. Boddy K, Mantell CD: Observation on fetal breathing movements transmitted through the maternal abdominal wall. Lancet 2:1219, 1972

57. Boddy K: Fetal circulation and breathing movements, in Beard RW, Nathanielsz PW (eds), Fetal Physiology and Medicine, the Basis of Perinatology. London, Saunders, 1976, p 302

58. Boddy K, Dawes GS: Fetal breathing. Br Med Bull 31:3, 1975

59. Tamura RK, Manning FA: Fetal breathing movements, in Sciarra JJ (ed), Gynecology and Obstetrics. Hagerstown, MD, Harper and Row, 1981, vol 3, pp 1–11

60. Mantell CD: Breathing movements in the human fetus. Am J Obstet Gynecol 125:550, 1976

61. Patrick J, Campbell K, Carmichael L, et al: A definition of human fetal apnoea and the distribution of fetal apneic intervals during the last 10 weeks of pregnancy. Am J Obstet Gynecol 136:471, 1980

62. Sterman MB, Hoppenbrouwers T: in Sterman MB, McGinty DJ, Adinolfi AM (eds), Brain Development and Behavior. New York, Academic, 1971, p 203

63. Manning FA: Fetal breathing movements as a reflection of fetal status. Postgrad Med 61:116, 1977

64. Manning FA, Platt LD: Human fetal breathing monitoring—Clinical considerations. Semin Perinatol 4:311, 1980

65. Goodin RC: History of fetal monitoring. Am J Obstet Gynecol 133:323, 1979

66. Manning F, Wyn Pugh E, Boddy K: Effect of cigarette smoking on fetal breathing movements in normal pregnancies. Br Med J 1:552, 1975

67. Fox HE, Persel D, Angel E: Fetal Breathing Movements, in Saunders R, James E (eds), The Principles and Practice of Ultrasonography in Obstetrics and Gynecology, Norwalk, Appleton-Century-Crofts, 1980, chap 12

68. Manning FA, Platt LD, Lemay L: Effect of amniocentesis on fetal breathing movements. Br Med J 2:1582, 1977

69. Hill LM, Platt LD, Manning FA: Immediate effect of amniocentesis on fetal breathing and gross body movements. Am J Obstet Gynecol 135:689, 1979

70. Platt LD, Manning FA, Lemay M, et al: Human fetal breathing: Relationship to fetal condition. Am J Obstet Gynecol 132:514, 1978

71. Manning FA, Platt LD, Sipos L, et al: Fetal breathing movements and the non-stress test in high risk pregnancies. Am J Obstet Gynecol 135:511, 1979

72. Manning FA, Platt LD: Fetal breathing movements and the abnormal contraction stress test. Am J Obstet Gynecol 133:590, 1979

73. Manning FA, Heaman M, Boyce D, et al: Intrauterine fetal tachypnoea. Obstet Gynecol 58:398, 1981

74. Seeds AE: Current concepts of amniotic fluid dynamics. Am J Obstet Gynecol 138:575, 1980

75. Manning FA, Hill RM, Platt LD: Qualitative amniotic fluid volume determination by ultrasound: Antepartum detection of intra-uterine growth retardation. Am J Obstet Gynecol 139:254, 1981

76. Zamah NM, Gillieson MS, Walters JH, et al: Sonographic detection of polyhydramnios: A five-year experience. Am J Obstet Gynecol 143:523, 1982

77. Manning FA, Platt LD: Qualitative assessment of amniotic fluid volume: A rapid screen for detecting the small for gestational age fetus, in Scientific Abstracts, 26th Annual Meeting of the Society for Gynecologic Investigation, San Diego, California, March 21–24, 1979

78. Crowley P: Non-quantitative estimation of amniotic fluid volume in suspected prolonged pregnancy. J Perinat Med 8:249, 1980

79. Rayburn WF, Motley ME, Sempel LE, et al: Antepartum prediction of the post-mature infant. Obstet Gynecol 60:148, 1982

80. Chamberlain PF, Manning FA: Qualitative amniotic fluid volume and perinatal outcome: The significance of marginal and decreased amniotic fluid volumes. Amer J Obstet Gynecol (in press)

81. Powell-Phillips WD, Towell ME: Abnormal fetal heart rate associated with congenital abnormalities. Br J Obstet Gynaecol 87:270, 1980

13 The Impact of Ultrasound on Prenatal Diagnosis

Virginia L. Corson
Haig H. Kazazian, Jr.

The incorporation of ultrasound into prenatal diagnostic testing has evolved over a period of time in which an appreciation for the medical applications of human genetics has led to the expansion of genetic counseling services. The development of second trimester amniocentesis to monitor high-risk pregnancies in the late 1960s was followed by the establishment of prenatal diagnostic centers at both academic institutions and community hospitals.[1,2] Cooperation among genetic counselors, obstetricians, cytogeneticists, biochemical geneticists, and sonographers provides information and testing for prospective parents. In addition to its traditional use as a guide for the obstetrician performing an amniocentesis, ultrasound has expanded to include diagnosis of fetal anomalies. Increased sophistication of the ultrasound technology has enabled the prenatal detection (or suspicion) of abnormalities at early stages of pregnancy, and ethical dilemmas have arisen when quality of life questions are difficult to answer and a couple considers pregnancy termination. These dilemmas should be anticipated and confronted as greater experience with and understanding of the second trimester fetus is accumulated.

AMNIOCENTESIS AND FETOSCOPY

The majority of patients seen for counseling through a prenatal diagnostic center will undergo mid-trimester amniocentesis. An obstetric sonogram prior to the tap will confirm the gestational age of the fetus, localize the placenta, check for multiple gestation, and demonstrate fetal viability. An assessment of fetal age is important for several reasons. First, the threshold value used for determining whether a particular amniotic fluid or serum α-fetoprotein (AFP) value is elevated varies with gestational age. Second, should pregnancy termination be considered, ultrasound assessment of fetal age is the best available means of determining the length of gestation.

Ultrasound guidance to determine an insertion site enables the obstetrician to assess an appropriate depth and to avoid the umbilical cord and areas of wide placental surface. Visualization of an uterine contraction allows the obstetrician to delay the procedure for a short period of time. When amniocentesis was first performed, it was often carried out in clinical areas such as Labor and Delivery. The sonogram provided valuable obstetric information but did not assist in localization of the site of needle insertion. In many centers, amniocentesis is now scheduled in the ultrasound section, facilitating greater communication between the sonographer and the obstetrician.

Ultrasound provides similar information prior to fetoscopy, a higher risk, more invasive technique. Fetoscopy is used when visualization through a fiberoptic scope is necessary to scrutinize the fetus for the presence of an anomaly such as a syndactyly or polydactyly as one feature of a major malformation syndrome.[3] Because the field of vision seen through a fetoscope is limited, the sonographer must help orient the obstetrician to the fetal position so that a promising location for viewing the anatomy of concern can be selected. In addition, fetoscopy is used when a fetal blood sample is obtained for the diagnosis of hemoglobinopathies and clotting disorders, and ultrasound assists in the localization of fetal blood vessels on the placental surface or the umbilical cord.[4]

190

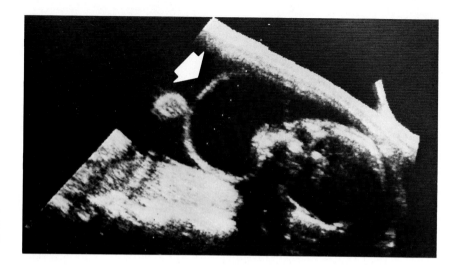

Fig. 1. Ultrasound diagnosis of an anterior encephalocele in a pregnancy with a family history positive for neural tube defects. Serum AFP was normal.

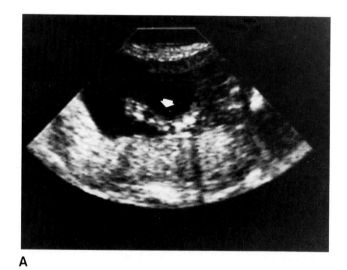

A

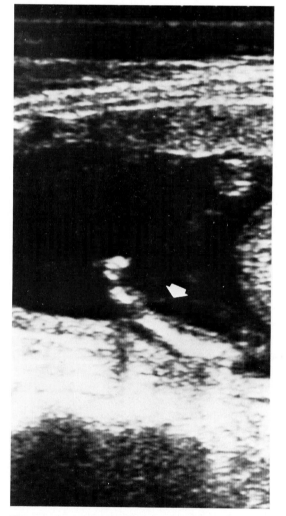

Fig. 2. A. Fetal limb at 17 weeks' gestation showing multiple fractures indicative of osteogenesis imperfecta. **B.** Normal limb at 19 weeks' gestation in a subsequent pregnancy to the same patient.

B

FETAL ANOMALIES AND MALFORMATION SYNDROMES

Many congenital abnormalities are not yet associated with chromosomal or biochemical defects and therefore cannot be diagnosed by amniotic fluid cell culture. Some of these problems involve fetal organs that can be studied by ultrasound during pregnancy, and couples at risk may elect to undergo sonographic examinations to rule out a particular anomaly.

Since the early 1970s, ultrasound has been used to examine the fetal spine and head for diagnosis of neural tube defects. A detailed sonogram is performed in conjunction with serum or amniotic fluid AFPs for couples who have had a previously affected offspring or a positive family history.[5,6] In such high-risk couples an elevation of AFP is less likely to occur in the event of a closed defect such as an encephalocele, and an ultrasound diagnosis is especially valuable (Fig. 1).

Some couples who have given birth to an infant with a form of short-limbed dwarfism will have a 25 percent risk of recurrence because the condition is known to be inherited as an autosomal recessive disorder. These couples will seek ultrasound assessment of fetal limb lengths in subsequent pregnancies. Serial sonograms during the second trimester have documented severe shortening of the limbs in pregnancies at risk for achondrogenesis[7] and the severe form of osteogenesis imperfecta[8] (Fig. 2). Although many of these dysmorphic syndromes are lethal at birth or shortly thereafter, some couples would consider prenatal diagnosis and elective pregnancy termination a preferable option.

Visualization of the fetal kidneys and bladder has made possible the prenatal diagnosis of a number of urinary tract anomalies.[9] The infantile form of polycystic kidney disease, an autosomal recessive disorder, can be detected during the second trimester. The development of hydronephrosis or obstruction of the bladder neck during the second or the third trimester can, in some cases, be managed by insertion of a catheter into the fetal bladder. Prenatal recognition of bilateral renal agenesis (Potter syndrome) and its associated anomalies, including peculiar facies, pulmonary hypoplasia, and limb abnormalities, can be helpful in planning obstetric management and in parental preparation.[10]

The diagnosis of hydrocephalus by measurement of ventricular ratios may also raise the questions of pregnancy termination, in utero therapy, and risk of associated anomalies. In some centers fetal echocardiography has become an option for couples who have had a previous child with a congenital heart defect.

The application of ultrasound to this area of fetal monitoring has lengthened the list of genetic disorders and sporadic anomalies that can be diagnosed during the prenatal period.

THE UNEXPECTED FINDING

The widespread use of obstetric sonograms prior to amniocentesis will on occasion lead to the diagnosis of an unsuspected complication. Some diagnostic problems will have a clear-cut interpretation, and the ultrasound findings will facilitate optimal obstetric management.

The diagnosis of a multiple gestation will be made in approximately 1 of 90 pregnancies and have implications for amniocentesis. With ultrasound guidance, separate amniotic sacs can be tapped. Fetal death in utero or, rarely, the presence of a hydatidiform mole will be documented. Follow-up studies may be recommended for some findings such as placenta previa or uterine fibroids. Each of these situations will require additional counseling for the parents, but the implications of the ultrasound diagnosis are straightforward.

In other pregnancies, the suspicion of a fetal anomaly like hydrocephalus or hydronephrosis may be raised during the course of a routine study. Counseling difficulties then arise if the presence of a defect is uncertain or if the long-term prognosis is not known. Repeat sonograms may be scheduled to assess any change in a suspected defect, and the couple will experience anxiety for the health of the fetus. The diagnosis of polyhydramnios or oligohydramnios will raise suspicion about a fetal abnormality. At times a variant will be seen on several occasions, and its significance will still be uncertain. For example, implications of the second trimester diagnosis of calcified areas within the fetal liver are unknown.[11]

While this technology develops, very little natural history information is available for counseling purposes when an unexpected structural anomaly is diagnosed during the second trimester. Documentation of fetal hydrocephalus or hydronephrosis can result in deliberations over pregnancy termination or fetal surgery. Couples are faced with decisions for which counselors cannot supply adequate information.[12] The limitations of available technology and its interpretations should be shared with the prospective parents.

OTHER TECHNIQUES

Ultrasound assessments can be used in conjunction with other techniques to address the question of fetal health. Its routine use to augment AFP screening for the diagnosis of neural tube defects in high-risk pregnancies has been discussed. Institution of AFP maternal screening programs in some states requires ultrasound back-up to assess fetal age and to identify multiple gestations when serum AFP values are elevated.[13] If no explanation for the elevation is evident, a detailed sonogram and an amniotic fluid AFP are considered. Historically, amniography has also been employed to visualize the fetal spine. However, this technique has become less useful as the resolution of ultrasound has improved.

The diagnosis of fetal limb defects was first undertaken by both ultrasound and radiology. A pregnancy at risk for lethal osteogenesis imperfecta could be monitored by both techniques. However, x-ray documentation of limb structure proved to be difficult during the second trimester, and again sonography became the visualization tool of choice. In addition, concern over an association between an increased risk for childhood malignancies and prenatal diagnostic radiation resulted in a reluctance to expose the fetus to x-rays for any reason.[14]

In some situations, defects seen on ultrasound raise the suspicion of a chromosome anomaly, and amniocentesis is considered. The diagnosis of fetal microcephaly at 19 weeks' gestation in a pregnancy of a 6/22 balanced translocation carrier persuaded a hesitant patient to request a fetal karyotype. Chromosome analysis confirmed the presence of a trisomy for part of the long arm of chromosome 6, and the pregnancy was terminated. This rearrangement had been documented in a previous pregnancy in an infant who expired shortly after birth with multiple anomalies including microcephaly, encephalocele, and omphalocele.[15]

The sonographic observation of in utero growth retardation from the second to third trimesters (see Chapter 11) may present another opportunity to consider a fetal karyotype.[16] The diagnosis of a chromosomal abnormality that is incompatible with life may influence subsequent obstetric management of the pregnancy. Cesarean section and heroic measures on behalf of the newborn can be avoided, and the parents will have some opportunity for their own psychologic preparation.

In special circumstances, sonography may be utilized to provide information on fetal sex.[17] For example, when a cytogenetic analysis for advanced maternal age demonstrates the unusual occurrence of 45X/46XY sex chromosome mosaicism, an in vitro event of cell culture or true fetal mosaicism must be considered. Indication of male genitalia by ultrasound would provide additional information for counseling.

Ultrasound can be used to support results obtained by other techniques, or it can alert the obstetrician or genetic counselor that other tests should be initiated. For some anomalies, no completely diagnostic test exists, and sonographic studies will be used in conjunction with other methods to assess fetal health.

THE TERTIARY CARE CENTER

The increased utilization of sonograms to monitor low-risk pregnancies and the availability of ultrasound equipment in obstetricians' offices and small community hospitals has resulted in the increased diagnosis of congenital anomalies in pregnancy. Referral to a tertiary medical center for confirmation of a suspected problem has become more frequent. In some cases, reassurance can be offered the patient and in other situations more precise characterization of a defect can be offered.

Cooperation between the ultrasound section and the prenatal diagnostic group in the tertiary care center is essential for the provision of optimal care to the patient. For purposes of genetic counseling and consideration of pregnancy options, input from the genetics group can be helpful when a defect has been diagnosed through an ultrasound referral.

The availability of ultrasound on a widespread basis could lead to potential pitfalls, however. The identification of fetal anomalies such as neural tube defects is difficult in the most experienced hands (see Chapter 18). The temptation for novice sonographers to monitor high-risk pregnancies themselves instead of referring such patients to tertiary centers could result in increased numbers of false positive and false negative diagnoses. Pregnancies at risk for anomalies should be followed through a center that provides genetic counseling, ultrasound, laboratory, and obstetric services.

FUTURE DILEMMAS

The sophistication of sonographic scanning may lead to new areas of decision making as more anomalies become amenable to prenatal diagnosis. Fetal echocardiography for pregnancies at increased risk of a cardiac defect is available, but until more experience is gained, the limits of the procedure as a diagnostic tool remain undefined. Quality of life questions will arise should second trimester diagnoses of minor cardiac defects, cleft lips, polydactyly, or other isolated birth defects become possible.

The role of ultrasound as a tool for prenatal diagnostic investigations has expanded over the past decade and will continue to grow. Advances in diagnostic capabilities will be accompanied by issues of in utero treatment, diagnostic uncertainty, and an increased incidence of problems in decision making.

REFERENCES

1. Golbus MS, Loughman WD, Epstein CJ, et al: Prenatal genetic diagnosis in 3000 amniocenteses. N Engl J Med 300:157, 1979
2. NICHD National Registry for Amniocentesis Study Group. Midtrimester amniocentesis for prenatal diagnosis. JAMA 236:1471, 1976
3. Mahoney MJ, Hobbins JC: Fetoscopy in the prenatal diagnosis of skeletal abnormalities. Birth Def: Orig Art Series XV:63, 1979
4. MacKenzie IZ, Maclean DA: Pure fetal blood from the umbilical cord obtained at fetoscopy: Experience with 125 consecutive cases. Am J Obstet Gynecol 138:1214, 1980
5. Milunsky A. Prenatal detection of neural tube defects. JAMA 244:2731, 1980
6. Haddow JE. Screening for spinal defects. Hosp Prac 17:128, 1982
7. Graham D, Tracey J, Winn K, et al: Early second trimester diagnosis of achondrogenesis. J Clin Ultra 11:336, 1983
8. Shapiro JE, Phillips JA, Byers PH, et al: Prenatal diagnosis of lethal perinatal osteogenesis imperfecta (OI Type II). J Pediatr 100:127, 1982
9. Hobbins JC, Grannum PAT, Berkowitz RL, et al: Ultrasound in the diagnosis of congenital anomalies. Am J Obstet Gynecol 134:331, 1979
10. Allen RW, Rehm NE, Scott JR, et al: Antepartum diagnosis and intrapartum management of lethal renal defects. Obstet Gynecol 58:379, 1981
11. Corson VL, Sanders RC, Johnson TRB, et al: Mid-trimester fetal ultrasound: Diagnostic dilemmas. Prenat Diag 3:47, 1983
12. Barclay WR, McCormick RA, Sidbury JB, et al: The ethics of in utero surgery. JAMA 246:1550, 1981
13. Macri JN, Weiss RR: Prenatal serum α-fetoprotein screening for neural tube defects. Obstet Gynecol 59:633, 1982
14. Schussman LC, Lutz LJ: Hazards and uses of prenatal diagnostic X-radiation. J Fam Pract 14:473, 1982
15. Stamberg J, Shapiro J, Valle D, et al: Partial trisomy 6q, due to a balanced maternal translocation (6;22)(q21;p13) or (q21;pter). Clin Gen 19:122, 1981
16. Johnson TRB, Corson VL, Payne PA, et al: Late prenatal diagnosis of fetal trisomy 18 associated with severe intrauterine growth retardation. Johns Hopkins Med J 151:242, 1982
17. Shalev E, Weiner E, Zuckerman H: Ultrasound determination of fetal sex. Am J Obstet Gynecol 141:582, 1981

14 | Ultrasonic Assessment of Genitourinary Anomalies In Utero

Roger C. Sanders

The greatest yield of fetal anomalies discovered in utero by ultrasound has occurred in the genitourinary system. This is not surprising since most mass lesions in the neonate are of renal origin. About two renal anomalies are found per 1,000 pregnancies.[1]

NORMAL FETAL GENITOURINARY ANATOMY

Normal fetal genitourinary anatomy is now well recognized. With current high-resolution, real-time ultrasonic systems, the kidneys can be seen from about 14 weeks after the last menstrual period. They lie on either side of the spine inferior to the stomach and the main portion of the liver at a level slightly inferior to the entrance of the ductus venosus (Fig. 1). A longitudinal paraspinous sonogram will show their long axis well (Fig. 2). As in the adult there is a relatively hypoechoic renal cortex and parenchyma with a more echogenic renal sinus. The sinus is a term used to describe the major vascular structures, the pelvis, calyx, fibrous tissue, and fat that lie in the center of the kidney. However, the fetal renal sinus echoes are relatively trivial and may not be easy to see. The capsular echoes around the kidneys are also relatively ill-defined, presumably due to the absence of fat. As in adults, it is not uncommon to see a minor degree of separation of the sinus echoes as a normal variant (Fig. 3). Differentiation between pyramids and cortex is usually not possible. The fetal bladder is detectable in the pelvis between high-level echoes derived from the bones of

the iliac crests and the ischial tuberosoties from about the 14-week period on (Fig. 4). In the normal fetus the bladder is rarely, if ever, empty; however, it normally empties incompletely and fills over a period of about an hour.

Normal standards for fetal renal length and volume[2-4] and for the ratio of kidney to abdominal circumference[5,6] have been developed (see Appendix 3). Tables have also been constructed for the size of the bladder versus gestational age and the rapidity with which the bladder fills and partially empties.[7,8] In the last few weeks of pregnancy the fetal adrenals become large and can be seen with ultrasound (Fig. 5). Indeed they can be so sizable that in the presence of renal agenesis they are mistaken for the kidneys.[9]

FETAL GENITALIA

One can frequently determine fetal sex as early as 16 to 17 weeks, with consistent distinction after approximately 24 weeks.[10] Definitive evidence that the fetus is a male is obtained by seeing the penis as well as the scrotum (Fig. 6A,6B,6C). If there is fluid present within the scrotum (a hydrocele),[11,12] the testicles can be outlined and an equally strong diagnosis of masculinity can be made in the absence of a visualization of a penis (Fig. 7). Isolated hydrocele in utero is generally without pathologic significance. Noncommunicating hydrocele may occur in which the fluid is not in communication with the peritoneum.[13]

There is a theoretical possibility of confusion be-

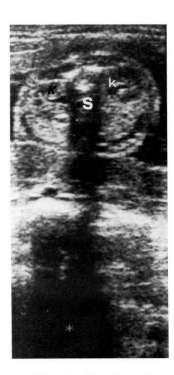

Fig. 1. Transverse section of fetal trunk with the fetus in the prone position. The fetal spine (S) lies between the normal fetal kidneys (K).

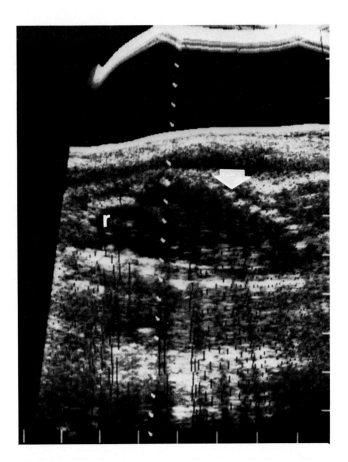

Fig. 2. Longitudinal section of fetal trunk. The fetal kidney (r) can be identified lying below the chest alongside the spine. Ribs (*arrow*) can be seen.

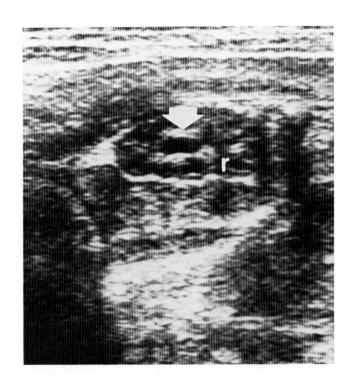

Fig. 3. Longitudinal section of fetal kidney (r) showing slight dilatation of the sinus echoes (*arrow*), a normal variant, which disappeared when the fetus voided.

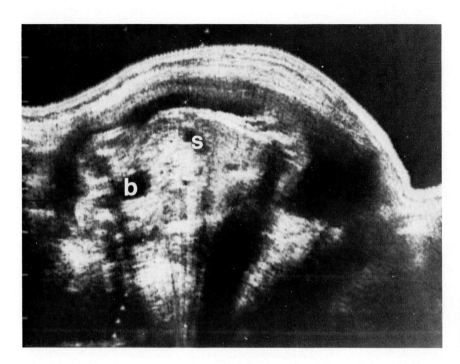

Fig. 4. Longitudinal section of fetus showing the fetal bladder (b) and stomach (S). The bladder partially empties and fills over about an hour in utero.

tween the scrotum and edematous labia. However, the normal labia generally have a recognizable ultrasonic pattern[14] (Fig. 8). Indeed, accuracy in sex prediction in the late second and third trimester is between 95 and 100 percent.[10,14]

AMNIOTIC FLUID VOLUME

It is now clear that fetal urine excretion is mainly or entirely responsible for amniotic fluid production[15,16]

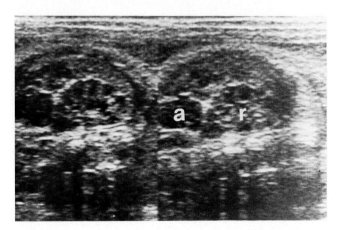

Fig. 5. Oblique section of a term fetus showing a fetal adrenal gland (a) superior to the kidney (r). The fetal adrenal grows to a large size in the third trimester.

from at least 18 to 20 weeks on and that in the presence of urethral obstruction, oligohydramnios, and eventually a total absence of amniotic fluid will occur with consequent pulmonary hypoplasia. When oligohydramnios occurs, the following possibilities exist: (a) ruptured membranes, (b) intrauterine growth retardation, (c) a renal anomaly, (d) postmaturity, and (e) fetal death. In order for oligohydramnios of renal origin to occur, the renal anomaly must be at a urethral level or affect both kidneys or ureters. Bilateral renal obstruction in utero can be associated with hydramnios.[17]

Some renal anomalies are invariably fatal. It is worthwhile attempting to recognize such gross anomalies prior to 22 weeks' fetal age so that a therapeutic abortion can be performed. However, the discovery of anomalies later in pregnancy can also influence management. In utero catheter techniques to drain bilaterally obstructed kidneys are now possible (see Chapter 22). With unilateral ureteropelvic junction obstruction early neonatal surgery may well be desirable so that further renal damage does not take place, and some advocate the percutaneous decompression of such anomalies in utero, fearing that abdominal distension could lead to pulmonary hypoplasia. Neonatal palpation as a screening method to detect renal enlargement cannot be relied on to detect the abnormal kidney.[17] Examples of ureteropelvic junction obstruction severe enough to necessitate surgery have been overlooked by competent neonatologists.

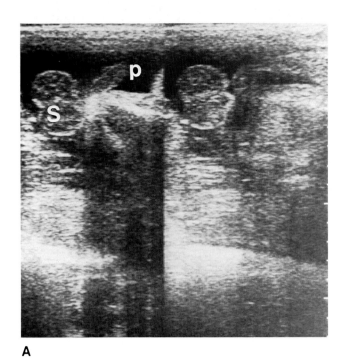

A

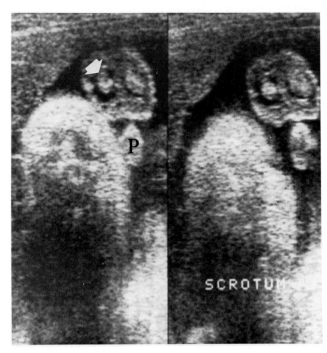

B

RENAL AGENESIS

The most devastating congenital renal anomaly is renal agenesis. In this condition there is no amniotic fluid and it is therefore often difficult to delineate fetal anatomy because of the absence of the good perifetal acoustical window normally provided by amniotic fluid. Nevertheless, a thorough examination will fail to reveal sonographic evidence of kidneys or bladder[9,18] (Fig. 9). In the last few weeks of pregnancy fetal kidneys can be thought to be present when they are really absent because the adrenal glands grow to a large size and have a reniform shape. It appears that when a kidney is not present, the adrenals assume an oval discoid shape.[9] Bilateral renal agenesis occurs about once in 3000 births. It is sometimes termed Potter syndrome, but this term has also been used for any renal condition associated with severe oligohydramnios. Potter syndrome consists of a "peculiar facies with wide-set eyes, parrot beak nose, pliable low-set ears and receding chin." Spade-like hands, wrinkled skin, pulmonary hypoplasia or dysplasia, limb anomalies, and ovoid adrenal glands are usually present.[19]

Hypoplastic kidneys can occasionally be seen and recognized, providing that comparison with normal in utero renal length tables is made.[2] Hypoplastic kidneys are associated with the fetal alcohol syndrome.[20]

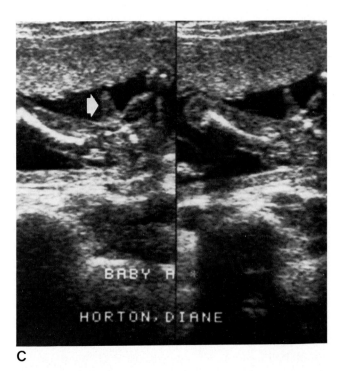

C

Fig. 6. A. Localized view of male genitalia showing scrotum (s) and penis (p). **B.** View of the male genitalia showing the penis (P) and the scrotum. The testicles (*arrow*) can be identified. They are surrounded by small hydroceles. **C.** The penis (*arrow*) is seen in the crotch between the femurs. Visualization of the penis was helpful in this case of fetal chromosomal mosaicism.

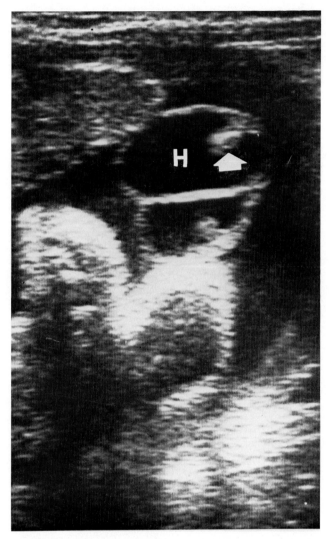

Fig. 7. Large hydrocele in utero (H). No other anomaly was found. The testicles (*arrow*) can be seen.

UNILATERAL HYDRONEPHROSIS

The commonest fetal renal anomaly is hydronephrosis. Unilateral hydronephrosis is usually due to ureteropelvic junction obstruction. A cystic sonolucent space located medially (the pelvis) can been seen in the center of the kidney with further smaller cysts (the calyces) budding from it (Fig. 10). As a rule one can visualize the thickness of the fetal renal parenchyma around the dilated system and deduce potential for renal salvage. The parenchyma varies in thickness with fetal age but should be visible as an hypoechoic area if the kidney is worth salvaging.

Distinguishing renal from gastrointestinal fluid-filled anomalies in utero can be a challenge. The kidneys are located lateral to the spine and any renal

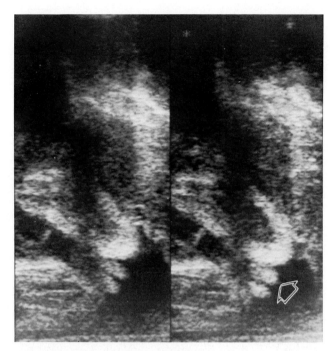

Fig. 8. The labia (*arrows*) can be seen in the female fetus between the femurs.

anomaly will involve the paraspinous area. Gastrointestinal anomalies may lie in contact with the spine but will not extend into a paraspinous location unless there is renal agenesis (Fig. 11).

A transient unilateral distention of the renal pelvis, possibly persisting over more than one examina-

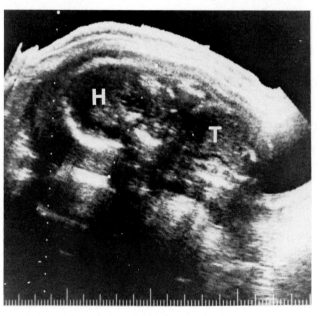

Fig. 9. Renal agenesis. There is oligohydramnios and fetal structures are difficult to discern. The head (H) and trunk (T) can be seen. No kidneys were visible on prolonged examination.

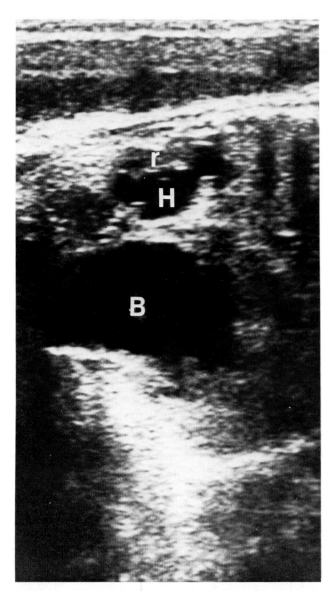

Fig. 10. Hydronephrosis in utero. The dilated pelvicalycele system (H) can be seen. Some renal parenchyma (r) is still present. The bladder (B) is quite large but not obstructed.

tion, has been observed. Such transient renal pelvic distention is more common bilaterally (Fig. 14), a phenomenon described later in the chapter. Apparent fetal hydronephrosis, even when unilateral, may be due to overdistension of the fetal bladder.[21] It is worthwhile reexamining the patient after the fetal bladder has emptied or repeating the sonogram at another time to confirm that hydronephrosis is persistent. Unilateral renal anomalies are not associated with oligohydramnios since one normal kidney provides adequate renal function and amniotic fluid; in fact, hydramnios may be present.[17,22,23]

The detection of unilateral hydronephrosis should

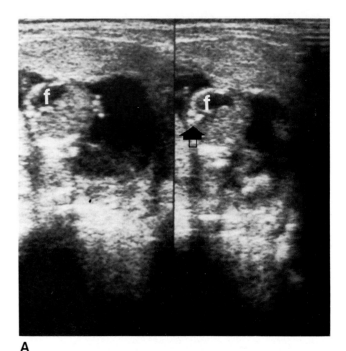

A

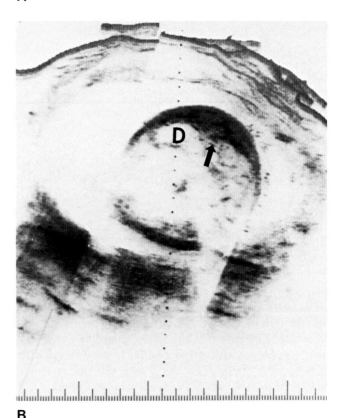

B

Fig. 11. A. The fluid-filled structure within the fetal trunk (f) suggested hydronephrosis but repeat examination showed the cystic mass to be the stomach even though it lies adjacent to the spine (*arrow*). **B.** Dilated obstructed kidney (D) lying adjacent to the spine (*arrow*). The problem was initially thought to be a duodenal atresia. Even though there was hydramnios, the position of the lesion makes it likely to be genitourinary in origin.

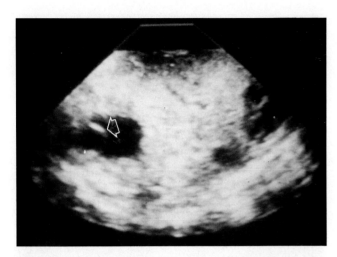

Fig. 12. The fetal bladder contains a curvilinear structure (*arrow*) which represents a ureterocele associated with an obstructed kidney.

stimulate an effort to look for the ureter. Although most unilateral hydronephrosis is due to ureteropelvic junction obstruction, a minority develop as a consequence of an ectopic ureterocele. Careful observation of the bladder may well show evidence of the curvilinear borders of the ureterocele (Fig. 12). Alternatively a bladder diverticulum may be seen.[21] Observation with real time may allow visualization of bladder contraction with simultaneous distension of the bladder diverticulum. The bladder diverticulum may prevent reflux into one ureter.

BILATERAL HYDRONEPHROSIS

Bilateral hydronephrosis is usually, although not invariably, associated with oligohydramnios. A few examples of bilateral ureteropelvic junction obstruction and the "prune belly" syndrome have been associated with hydramnios.[17] With severe bilateral renal obstruction the "prune belly" syndrome (otherwise known as the Eagle Barrett syndrome or agenesis of the abdominal wall) occurs. The prune belly syndrome consists of a dilated urinary bladder and posterior urethra, grossly enlarged ureters, distension of the renal pelves, a massively enlarged abdomen with little or no muscle in the abdominal wall, cryptorchidism (thought to be the result of a massively distended bladder preventing testicular descent), a small thorax with flared ribs, and persistent urachal anomalies (this represents another route by which the fetus attempts to decompress the bladder). Most of these features are thought to be secondary to urinary tract obstruction causing abdominal distension.[24,25] Gut anomalies such as malrotation and imperforate anus may occur and may be related to

the large bladder and ureters.[26] The dilated ureters are almost always visible and can be very large and dominate the ultrasonic appearance. They are coiled and tortuous and therefore difficult to follow. Prune belly syndrome may occur in the absence of urethral obstruction, gross fetal ascites, or sizable abdominal mass.[27] It is not uncommon in the "prune belly" syndrome for the kidneys to be rather small with a relatively mild degree of hydronephrosis even though the ureters are massively dilated[28] (Fig. 13). In some examples of urethral obstruction, particularly with urethral valves, the bladder may be grossly distended at a time when the ureters and kidneys demonstrate mild or no changes. Sometimes a dilated posterior urethra extending from the bladder towards the penis can be observed (all patients with the "prune belly" syndrome or urethral obstruction have so far been male). The abdominal wall may be lax and may be seen to undulate if the maternal abdomen is tapped.[28] It is suggested that only forms of cystic masses would cause a tense abdomen. The urachal cyst commonly associated with "prune belly" syndrome has been recognized in utero.[26] Although urethral atresia and urethral valves are commonly seen with the "prune belly" syndrome, occasional cases are seen in which no obstructing lesion is found at birth. The fetal ascites may not persist. It seems likely that the abdominal wall muscle deficiency in these cases results from transient fetal ascites in utero, with consequent weakening of the abdominal wall, cryptorchidism, and urachal anomalies.[27]

With very severe or complete urethral obstruction, the resultant oligohydramnios produces the already mentioned secondary phenomena—Potter's facies, limb contractions and hypoplastic lungs. As detailed in Chapter 22, providing adequate drainage may avoid the secondary problem, although renal function is often severely and irreversibly damaged.[29] Fetal ascites due to perforation of an obstructed urinary tract may occur in the third trimester and may actually be beneficial in preventing more severe damage due to obstruction.[30] The condition, however, carries such a poor prognosis even with catheter treatment that elective abortion prior to 22 weeks is probably desirable if a severe case is detected sufficiently early.[31,32]

Bilateral ureteropelvic junction obstruction occurs less frequently than the "prune belly" syndrome and is usually worse on one side than the other. The shape of the dilated renal pelvis in ureteropelvic junction obstruction is rounder than with obstruction at a lower level. No dilated ureters are seen. One should make an attempt to assess the amount of remaining renal parenchyma surrounding the kidney. If only a shell of parenchyma persists, it is likely but not certain that the kidney is not salvageable. If a substantial amount

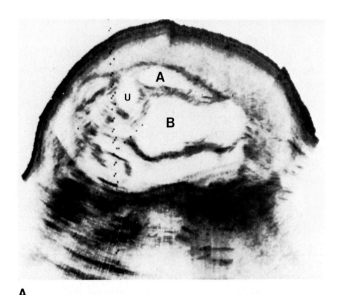

A

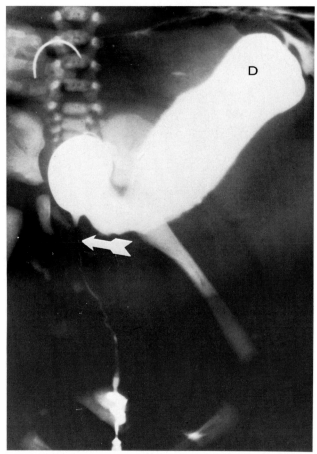

B

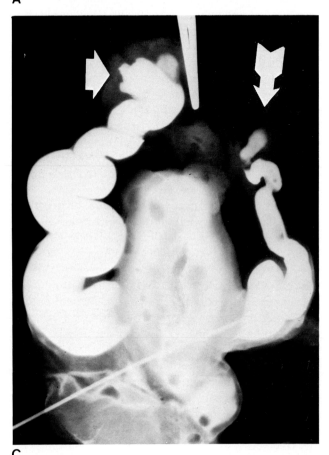

C

Fig. 13. A. Prune belly syndrome. The fetal abdomen is greatly distended and there is fetal ascites (A). The fetal bladder is markedly enlarged (B). The cystic structures posterior to the bladder were shown by percutaneous puncture to be dilated ureters (U). **B.** An autopsy cystogram shows urethral atresia (*arrow*). The bladder is greatly distended; it is partially a urachal diverticulum (D). **C.** Injection of the distended bladder and bilateral tortuous dilated ureters. The kidneys (*arrows*) were barely affected and were only slightly enlarged.

of renal parenchyma can be seen and one can be firm in the diagnosis of hydronephrosis, assessment of the degree of echogenicity of the renal parenchyma will give one a clue as to whether or not there has been permanent damage to the kidney in utero.[28] Dysplastic changes, secondary to hydronephrosis, are known to occur in utero if the obstruction occurred in the first trimester. The more echogenic the renal parenchyma, the more likely it is that there are dysplastic changes present. Cortical dysplasia is associated with lower urinary tract obstruction.[28]

The bladder may be greatly distended and yet the ureters and pelvis not dilated.[33] Such absence of hydronephrosis is generally the result of dysplastic changes within the kidneys. In such cases, there is almost always oligohydramnios, in addition to the large cystic structure (the bladder) within the fetal abdomen that could otherwise be mistaken for an ovarian cyst. A moderate degree of hydronephrosis bilaterally may well be a temporary phenomenon. We have observed several fetuses in which hydronephrosis persisted over several examinations and eventually disappeared spontaneously (Fig. 14). In one instance the hydronephrosis was still present after birth, but during the course of

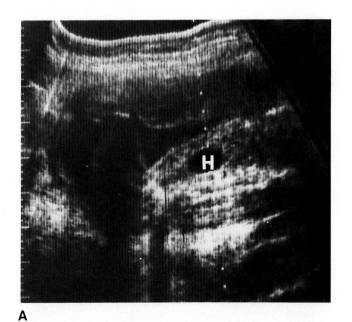
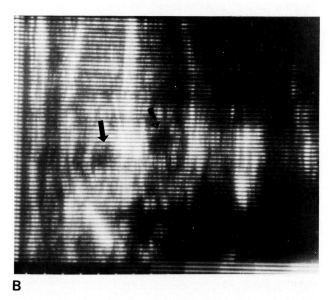

A   B

Fig. 14. A. Serial sonograms performed on this fetus in utero showed a dilated renal pelvis (H) compatable with an obstructed kidney. The condition was bilateral. **B.** Later sonograms again showed both kidneys to be obstructed (*arrows*). The sonogram after birth showed disappearance of the obstruction which was presumably related to an overdistended bladder. The bladder did not appear large in utero.

an ultrasonic examination one day after birth the neonate voided and the hydronephrosis disappeared. Presumably the hydronephrosis was related to overdistension of the bladder although repeated observation in utero had not shown a correlation with bladder size.[17] Smyth et al.[34] report obstructed kidneys in utero which resolved, but at birth the neonate had the "prune belly" malformation. However, there was no evidence of urinary tract obstruction or decreased renal function 1 year after delivery. Since hydronephrosis can be transient, before contemplating interventional procedures in utero, one should make sure that hydronephrosis is persistent and that there is a genuine reduction in amniotic fluid quantity. Monitoring bladder size is helpful in determining the severity of urethral obstruction.

Primary megaureter in which only the ureters are dilated has been recognized in utero.[35] We have seen a case with fairly severe hydronephrosis and dilated ureters but a bladder that emptied and filled normally with normal amniotic fluid due to idiopathic megaureter at birth.

MULTICYSTIC KIDNEY

Multicystic or dysplastic kidney, confusingly termed fetal polycystic kidney by some,[36,37] is now considered to be a stage in the evolution of hydro-

nephrosis.[14,38,39] Typically in this condition there are cysts which vary in size, which do not connect, and which are scattered throughout the kidney[40,41] (Fig. 15). Renal parenchyma may appear to be present, but it will not be in a peripheral location and will usually be more echogenic than normal renal parenchyma. What one is actually seeing are multiple small cysts below the threshold for sonographic resolution but large enough to cause echoes. There is considerable variation in the sonographic appearances of multicystic kidney and in one variant a single large cystic structure can occupy the entire kidney area. In another variant there are relatively few cystic structures present and the predominant picture is one of echogenic tissue secondary to many small cysts.[42] Dysplastic kidney may rarely be bilateral and closely resemble bilateral hydronephrosis ultrasonically. Administration of 20 mg Furosomide to the mother will cause a change in bladder size in bilateral fetal hydronephrosis but not in bilateral multicystic kidney and thus a distinction may sometimes be made.[37] It is nevertheless possible to have bilateral multicystic kidney and distension of the fetal bladder.[43] This is a consequence of previous ureteric communication with the bladder before the obstruction became complete. In addition to bilateral atretic ureters, hypoplastic renal arteries, and absence of functioning renal glomeruli, these fetuses may have urethral atresia.

Multicystic kidney may be localized to one seg-

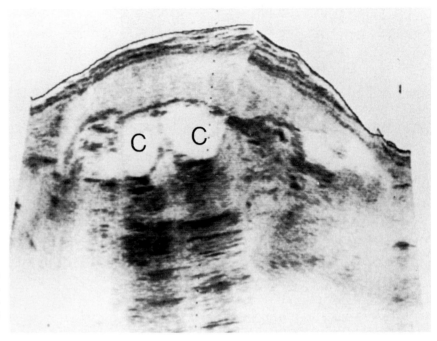

Fig. 15. Multicystic kidney. A large bilocular cystic structure (C) is present within the fetal abdomen. The position of the cysts made the condition unlikely to be hydronephrosis since the largest cyst was not centrally located.

ment of the kidney, presumably as a result of a local infundibular stenosis or atresia. This variant so far has not been recognized in utero.

FAMILIAL HYDRONEPHROSIS

Most conditions that affect the kidney in utero do not have a genetic basis. However, a rare form of dominant congenital hydronephrosis with ureteropelvic junction obstruction has been reported.[44] Urethral valves with secondary obstruction of both kidneys have occurred in several family members.[45] A mildly increased incidence of renal obstruction and neurologic anomalies are seen in spina bifida and diabetes mellitus with the VATER complex, secondary to the neurologic problems.

POLYCYSTIC KIDNEY DISEASE

Adult and infantile polycystic kidney represent two genetic anomalies in which renal screening is worthwhile.

Infantile polycystic kidney can be diagnosed prior to birth in the progeny of families with a previous history of infantile polycystic kidney. The condition is bilateral. The kidneys are much enlarged and have a relatively large echogenic sinus echo complex (Fig. 16). No discrete cysts are visible sonographically because individual cysts are too small to be seen, but

they are large enough to cause echoes.[46] Oligohydramnios occurs because urine excretion is poor. The condition has been recognized prior to 22 to 24 weeks, allowing a termination to be performed.[47] Use of the fetal kidney size tables such as the kidney/abdominal cir-

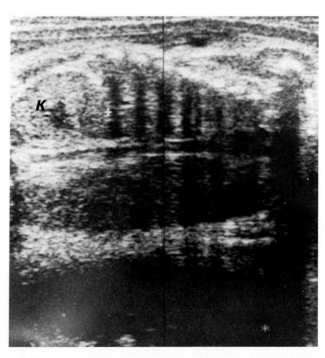

Fig. 16. Longitudinal view of fetal trunk showing infantile polycystic kidney. The kidneys (K) are enlarged (5.5 cm) and more echogenic than usual. There is a small amount of dilatation of the renal sinus.

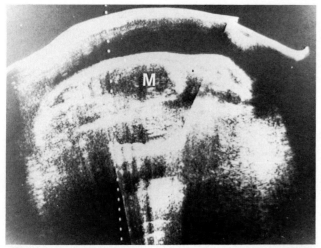

A

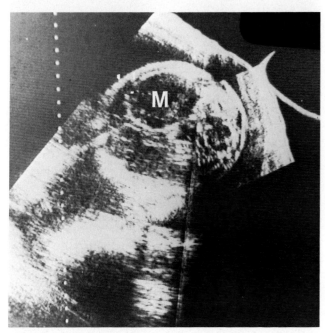

B

Fig. 17. A. Mesoblastic nephroma in utero. A mass (M) can be seen within the fetal abdomen. (*Courtesy of Dr. M. Toxopeus, Winchester, W. Va.*) **B.** Transverse section showing the fetal mass (M).

cumference ratio[5] substantiates the diagnosis. The much enlarged kidneys may be somewhat difficult to distinguish from the liver, which lies adjacent to them.

Infantile polycystic kidney occurs in Meckel syndrome. The other principal components of Meckel syndrome are encephalocele and polydactaly.[48] At least two components should be present to make the diagnosis. Other associated malformations are microcephaly, cleft palate, and ambiguous genitalia. This autosomal recessive syndrome is quite common and is alleged

to be responsible for 5 percent of neural defects. Oligohydramnios usually prevents one from obtaining amniotic fluid for α-fetoprotein estimation so the diagnosis is made with sonography. Robert syndrome is another rare familial recessive syndrome in which cystic kidneys occur. Other features of this syndrome are congenital heart disease, phocomelia, cleft palate, and lenticular opacities.[49]

Adult polycystic kidney has been diagnosed in utero at 20 weeks.[47] Bilateral large echogenic kidneys are found. The cysts are more likely to be visible than those in infantile polycystic kidney.

MEGACYSTIS MICROGUT SYNDROME

Megacystis microgut syndrome is a rare entity generally affecting females in which there is a giant bladder with secondary hydronephrosis and the colon is hypoplastic and demonstrates little or no peristalsis. The colon does not contain ganglion cells.[34,50,51] Polyhydramnios is common. Survival has not been recorded. Distinction from other causes of hydronephrosis is not easy, but the presence of polyhydramnios with a very large bladder supports the possibility. The gut changes cannot be recognized by ultrasound.

GENITOURINARY MASSES

A few focal masses within the kidney have been discovered in utero but not yet reported (Fig. 17). These masses have so far been mesoblastic nephroma. Experience in neonates suggests that these masses may contain cystic components but are generally solid with internal echoes. Masses in the vicinity of the kidney, mainly neuroblastoma, have also been discovered in utero (Fig. 18). Neuroblastoma are of mixed echogenicity and generally occur in an adrenal or less commonly a paraspinous location medial to the kidney.[52] In one instance, in utero discovery of a mass that changed in configuration with time led to a provisional diagnosis of adrenal hematoma but at subsequent operation it was discovered that there was an underlying neuroblastoma associated with a significant bleed.

HYDROMETROCOLPUS

Anomalies of other segments of the genitourinary system can be discovered in utero. Under the influence of maternal hormones the uterus and vagina can enlarge and be filled with fluid with the creation of a hydrometrocolpus. This condition has not yet been

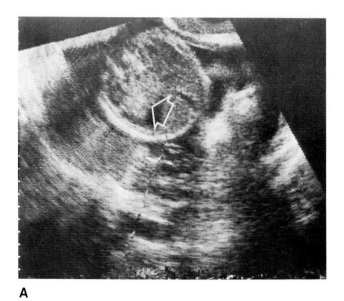

A

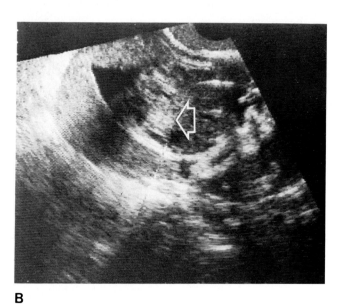

B

Fig. 18. A. Neuroblastoma in utero, transverse section. The echogenic mass (*arrow*) within the fetal abdomen was shown at birth to be a neuroblastoma. **B.** Longitudinal section showing the echogenic mass (*arrow*).

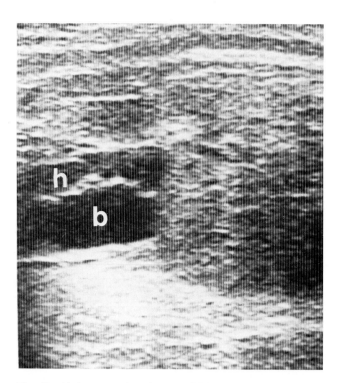

Fig. 19. Hydrometrocolpus in utero. Within the fetal trunk a cystic structure (h) is seen posterior to the bladder (b). This was still visible for a few days after birth but disappeared spontaneously and presumably represented hydrometrocolpus.

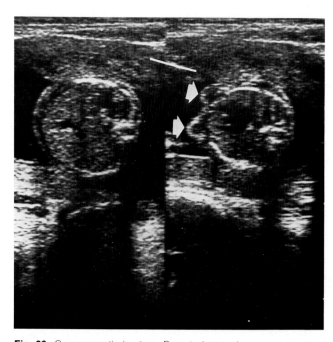

Fig. 20. Gynecomastia in utero. Breasts (*arrows*) were seen on two sonograms in utero but the breasts were not visualized just prior to delivery.

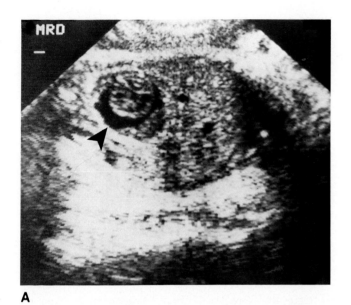
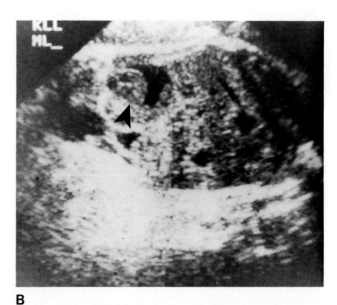

A   B

Fig. 21. A. Hemorrhagic ovarian cyst in utero. A cystic structure (*arrowhead*) containing an echogenic ball (B) is present within the fetal abdomen. At surgery, after delivery, it proved to be a hemorrhagic ovarian cyst. **B.** Another view of the hemorrhagic ovarian cyst (*arrowhead*).

diagnosed in utero and confirmed pathologically at birth; however, we believe we have found such a case (Fig. 19). The sonographic findings disappeared spontaneously within 2 days once the fetus was delivered so that surgical confirmation was not possible. In another unusual case transient fetal gynecomastia was observed (Fig. 20).

GENITAL TUMORS

Sacrococcygeal teratoma and ovarian cysts have been seen in utero on a number of occasions. Both can be associated with hydramnios. Sacrococcygeal teratoma arising from the region of the coccyx is the commonest form of in utero tumor.[53-55] These tumors are usually echogenic but may contain cystic areas. They may protrude exophytically from the coccyx or may involve the lower pelvis and abdomen. Hydrops may occur and is said to be due to high-output heart failure.[56] Theoretically a fluid-filled meningocele could be confused with a sacrococcygeal teratoma. Teratoma can achieve such a large size that delivery may be difficult; dystocia is said to be present in 13 percent.[57] The prognosis is relatively good and recognition facilitates management by dicatating the type of delivery; cesarian section is desirable. The diagnosis may be made prior to 24 weeks thus allowing elective abortion.[53]

Ovarian cysts not uncommonly occur in the fetus and neonate due to the influence of the maternal hormones. Most are simple cysts or serous cystade-

noma.[58-61] These cysts frequently tort and develop hemorrhage within them so they may not appear cystic and may contain internal echoes (Fig. 21). Their position can be surprisingly variable; it is not uncommon to see such cysts in the region of the liver because the broad ligament is much more pliable in the fetus and neonate than it is in older children and adults. Bilateral ovarian cysts have been seen in utero.[62] Confusion with bilateral hydronephrosis is avoided by seeing the kidneys cephalic to the cyst adjacent to the spine.

REFERENCES

1. Schulman CC, Elkhazen N, Picard C: Diagnostic chez le foetus des malformations urinaires par l'echographie. J d'Urologie 87:431, 1981
2. Jeanty P, Dramaix-Wilmet M, Elkhazen N, et al: Measurement of fetal kidney growth on ultrasound. Radiology 144:159, 1982
3. Bertagnolie L, Lalatta F, Gallicchio R, et al: Quantitative characterization of the growth of the fetal kidney. J Clin Ultrasound 11:349, 1983
4. Lawson TL, Foley WD, Berland LL, et al: Ultrasonic evaluation of fetal kidneys. Radiology 138:153, 1981
5. Grannum P, Bracken M, Silverman R, et al: Assessment of fetal kidney size in normal gestation by comparison of ratio of kidney circumference to abdominal circumference. Am J Obstet Gynecol 136:249, 1980
6. Awoust JT, Keuwez JT, Levi S: Limitations of fetal kidney biometry. Paper presented at the World Federation

of Ultrasound in Medicine and Biology in Brighton, England, 1982

7. Campbell S, Wladimiroff JW: The antenatal measurement of fetal urine production. J Obstet Gynaecol BC 80:680, 1973

8. Kurjak A, Kirkinen P, Latin V, et al: Ultrasonic assessment of fetal kidney function in normal and complicated pregnancies. Am J Obstet Gynecol 141:266, 1981

9. Dubbins PA, Kurtz AB, Wapner RJ, et al: Renal agenesis: Spectrum of in utero findings. J Clin Ultrasound 9:189, 1981

10. Shalev E, Weiner E, Zuckerman H: Ultrasound determination of fetal sex. Am J Obstet Gynecol 141:582, 1981

11. Vanesian R, Grossman M, Metherell A, et al: Antepartum ultrasonic diagnosis of congenital hydrocele. Radiology 126:765, 1978

12. Miller EI, Thomas RH: Fetal hydrocele detected in utero by ultrasound. Br J Radiol 52:624, 1979

13. Meizner I, Katz M, Zmora E, et al: In utero diagnosis of congenital hydrocele. J Clin Ultrasound 11:449, 1983

14. Schotten A, Giese C: The "female echo": Prenatal determination of the female fetus by ultrasound. Am J Obstet Gynecol 138:463, 1980

15. Smith FG, Adams FH, Borden M, et al: Fetus and newborn: Studies of renal function in the intact fetal lamb. Am J Obstet Gynecol 96:240, 1966

16. Harrison MR, Nakayama DK, Noall R, et al: Correction of congenital hydronephrosis in utero II: Decompression reverses the effects of obstruction on the fetal lung and urinary tract. J Pediatr Surg 17:965, 1982

17. Sanders RC, Graham D: Twelve cases of hydronephrosis in utero diagnosed by ultrasonography. J Ultrasound Med 1:341, 1982

18. Kierse M, Meerman R: Antenatal diagnosis of Potter syndrome. Obstet Gynecol 52:64, 1978

19. Allen RW, Rehm NE, Scott JR, et al: Antepartum diagnosis and intrapartum management of lethal renal defects. Obstet Gynecol 58:379, 1981

20. Quazi Q, Masakawa A, Milman D, et al: The genitourinary system: Renal anomalies in fetal alcohol syndrome. Pediatrics 63:886, 1979

21. Shalev J, Itzchak Y, Blau H, et al: The prenatal ultrasonic diagnosis of urethral obstruction and diverticulum of the urinary bladder. Pediatr Radiol 12:48, 1982

22. Henderson SC, Van Kolken RJ, Rahatzad M: Multicystic kidney with hydramnios. J Clin Ultrasound 8:249, 1980

23. Ray D, Berger N, Ensor R: Hydramnios in association with unilateral fetal hydronephrosis. J Clin Ultrasound 10:82, 1982

24. Glazer GM, Filly RA, Callen PW: The varied sonographic appearance of the urinary tract in the fetus and newborn with urethral obstruction. Radiology 144:563, 1982

25. Pagon RA, Smith DW, Shepard TH: Urethral obstruction malformation complex: A cause of abdominal muscle deficiency and the "prune-belly." J Pediatr 94:900, 1979

26. Woodard JR: The prune belly syndrome. Urol Clin N Am 5:75, 1978

27. Mueller-Heubach E, Mazer J: Sonographically documented disappearance of fetal ascites. Obstet Gynecol 61:253, 1983

28. Christopher CR, Spinelli A, Severt D: Ultrasonic diagnosis of prune-belly syndrome. Obstet Gynecol 59(3):391, 1982

29. Harrison MR, Filly RA, Parer JT, et al: Management of the fetus with a urinary tract malformation. JAMA 246:635, 1981

30. Cass AS, Khan AU, Smith S, et al: Neonatal perirenal urinary extravasation with posterior urethral valves. Urology 18:258, 1981

31. Farrant P: Early ultrasound diagnosis of fetal bladder neck obstruction. Br J Radiol 53:506, 1980

32. Cooperberg PL, Romalis G, Wright V: Megacystis (prune-belly syndrome): Sonographic demonstration in utero. J Canad Radiol 30:121, 1979

33. Oesch I, Jann X, Bettex M: Ultrasonographic antenatal detection of obstructed bladder. Eur Urol 8:78, 1982

34. Smyth AR II: Ultrasonic detection of fetal ascites and bladder dilation with resulting prune belly. J Pediatr 98:978, 1981

35. Deter RL, Gonzales ET, Wait RB: Prenatal detection of primary megaureter using dynamic image ultrasonography. Obstet Gynecol 56:759, 1980

36. Garrett WJ, Grunwald G, Robinson DE: Prenatal diagnosis of fetal polycystic kidney by ultrasound. Aust N Z H Obstet Gynaec 10:7, 1970

37. Shawker L, Anderson C: Intrauterine diagnosis and management of fetal polycystic kidney disease. Obstet Gynecol 59:385, 1982

38. Cussen LJ: Cystic kidneys in children with congenital urethral obstruction. J Urol 106:939, 1971

39. Perrin EV: Renal dysplasia in anomalies of the urinary tract and in chronic pyelonephritis. Am J Pathol 43:18A, 1963

40. Older RA, Crane LM, Morgan CL: In utero diagnosis of multicystic kidney by gray scale ultrasonography. Am J. Radiol 133:130, 1979

41. Legarth J, Verder H, Gronvall S: Prenatal diagnosis of multicystic kidney by ultrasound. Acta Obstet Gynaecol Scand 60:523, 1981

42. Nelson LH, Resnick MI, Sumner TE: Sonolucencies in fetal and infant abdomen: Implications for management. Urology 15:528, 1980

43. Bartley JA, Golbus MS, Filly RA, et al: Prenatal diagnosis of dysplastic kidney disease. Clin Genet 11:375, 1977

44. McKusick VA: Mendelian Inheritance in Man. Catalog of Autosomal Dominant, Autosomal Recessive and X-linked Phenotypes, 5th ed. Baltimore, MD, Johns Hopkins University Press, 1978

45. McCormick MK: Prenatal detection of the autosomal dominant type of congenital hydronephrosis by ultrasonography. Prenat Diag 2:157, 1982

46. Habif DV Jr, Berdon WE, Yeh MN: Infantile polycystic kidney disease: In utero sonographic diagnosis. Radiology 142:475, 1982

47. Weiss H, Zerres K, Hansmann M: Prenatal diagnosis of cystic renal changes by ultrasonography. Ultraschall 2:244, 1981

48. Wapner RJ, Ross RD, Jackson LG: Ultrasonographic parameters in the prenatal diagnosis of Meckel' syndrome. Obstet Gynecol 57:388, 1981

49. Jaffe S, Rose JS, Godmilow L, et al: Prenatal diagnosis of renal anomalies. Am J Med Genet 1:241, 1977
50. Vezina WC, Morin FR, Winsberg F: Megacystis-microcolon-intestinal hypoperistalsis syndrome: Antenatal ultrasound appearance. Am J Roentgenol 133:749, 1979
51. Nelson LH, Reiff RH: Megacystis-microcolon-hypoperistalsis syndrome and anechoic areas in the fetal abdomen. Am J Obstet Gynecol 144:464, 1982
52. Janetschek G, Weitzel D, Stein W, et al: Prenatal diagnosis of a neuroblastoma by sonography: J Urol (in press).
53. Seeds JW, Mittelstaedt CA, Cefalo RC: Prenatal diagnosis of sacrococcygeal teratoma. J Clin Ultrasound 10:193, 1982
54. Stauffer RA: Sacrococcygeal teratoma. Med Ultrasound 5:119, 1981
55. Zaleski AM, Cooperberg PL, Kliman MR: Ultrasonic diagnosis of extrafetal masses. J Can Assoc Radiol 30:55, 1979
56. Cousins L, Benirschke K, Porreco R, et al: Placentomegaly due to fetal congestive failure in a pregnancy with a sacrococcygeal teratoma. J Reprod Med 25:142, 1980
57. Gergely RZ, Eden R, Schifrin BS, et al: Antenatal diagnosis of congenital sacral teratoma. J Reprod Med 24:229, 1980
58. Lee TG, Blake S: Prenatal fetal abdominal ultrasonography and diagnosis. Radiology 124:475, 1977
59. Crade M, Gillooly L, Taylor KJW: In utero demonstration of an ovarian cystic mass by ultrasound. J Clin Ultrasound 8:251, 1980
60. Rankin RS: Case of the winter season. Semin Ultrasound 1:233, 1980
61. Mortag TW, Auletta FJ, Gibson M: Neonatal ovarian cyst: Prenatal diagnosis and analysis of the cyst fluid. Obstet Gynecol 61:38S, 1983
62. Jouppila P, Kirkinen P, Tuononen S: Ultrasonic detection of bilateral ovarian cysts in the fetus. Eur J Obstet Gynec Reprod Biol 13:87, 1982

15 | Fetal Cardiac Ultrasound

Lindsey D. Allan

INTRODUCTION

Although fetal heart pulsation has been detected ultrasonically for many years it is only very recently that the anatomic details of fetal heart structure have been studied.[1,2] The study of the fetal heart has been neglected for several reasons, despite the fact that congenital heart disease is the commonest form of congenital anomaly.

Firstly, until recently imaging techniques were not of sufficient quality to study the heart in detail. Secondly, the heart appears anatomically complex on first sight. Thirdly, the almost endless permutations and complexity of congenital heart malformations have seemed daunting to noncardiologists. However, the last few years have seen the introduction of real-time cross-sectional imaging techniques that allow the fetal heart to be seen in superb anatomic detail. This, coupled with a logical segmental approach to cardiac anatomy, means that the fetal heart can be included in screening the fetus for abnormality. Once experience is gained a 2- to 3-minute appraisal looking for specific intracardiac structures will exclude the vast majority of major cardiac defects and can readily be accomplished by a good obstetric ultrasonographer. Nonetheless congenital heart malformations are very diverse and complex. The correct evaluation of an anatomic defect is essential if an accurate prognosis is to be given. A relatively minor difference in the anatomic defect can considerably influence the likely morbidity, mortality, or surgical operability for an individual child. It is for these reasons that suspected abnormalities should be referred for evaluation to a center with wide experience in pediatric echocardiography.

METHOD OF STUDYING THE NORMAL FETAL HEART

It is possible to visualize fetal cardiac anatomy between 16 weeks' gestation and term. The optimum image quality is achieved between 18 and 28 weeks' gestation and it is in this gestational age range that the fetal heart can be seen in finest detail. Image quality, and therefore diagnostic accuracy, in this age range is at least as good, if not better, than in postnatal life. Fetal orientation is first of all discovered by scanning the maternal abdomen. A cross-sectional view of the fetal thorax is then sought. This will display the four chambers of the fetal heart. The following features should be noted in this plane of section:

1. The heart lies with the apex pointing to the left of the midline.
2. The heart occupies about one-third of the fetal thorax.
3. There are two atrial chambers of approximately equal size.
4. There are two ventricular chambers of approximately equal size and thickness, the right ventricle lying closer to the anterior chest wall, opposite to the spine, than the left ventricle. The right ventricle is usually slightly larger than the left ventricle.
5. The atria are connected to their respective ventricu-

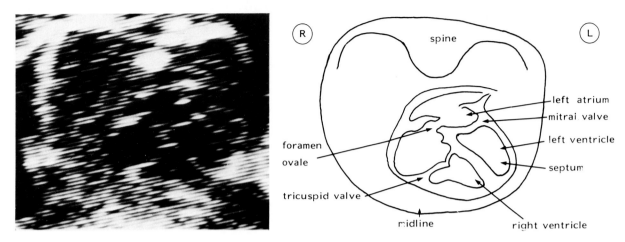

Fig. 1. The four chambers of the fetal heart are seen in a cross section of the fetal thorax. The apex points to the left of the midline; the right ventricle lies closer to the anterior chest wall than the left. The atria and the ventricles are of approximately equal size on the right and left sides of the heart.

lar chambers via a valve that can be seen to open.

6. The atrial septum has a defect in it that represents the normal foramen ovale.

7. The ventricular septum appears intact.

These features can all be noted in Figure 1. By angling the transducer cranially from this section the

origin of an artery from the left ventricle can be seen (Fig. 2). In the normal heart this should be the aorta, but until the transducer has been further swiveled to show that this artery connects to the arch of the aorta this cannot be assumed. The origin of the head and neck vessels from the arch must be identified (Fig. 3). The pulmonary artery must then be sought arising

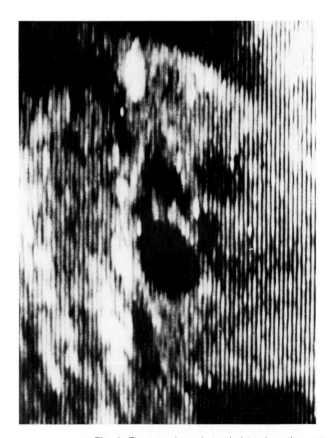

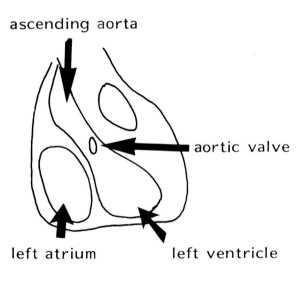

Fig. 2. The transducer is angled to show the aorta, containing the aortic valve, arising from the left ventricle in the normal heart.

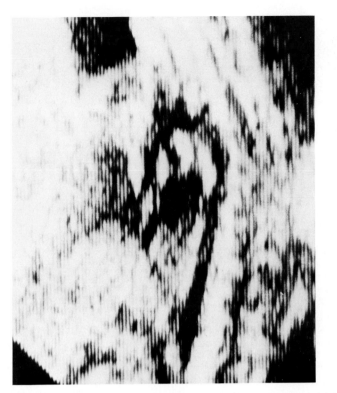

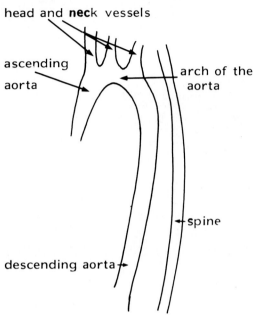

Fig. 3. The aorta must be followed from the left ventricle to the arch of the aorta, from which arises the head and neck vessels.

from the right ventricle. The connection of the main pulmonary artery to the descending aorta, via the ductus arteriosus, must be identified (Fig. 4). It is possible and important to differentiate between the two great arteries by noting several features:

1. The aorta arises in the center of the heart, from the left ventricle, and sweeps to the right before turning cranially.
2. The pulmonary artery arises from the top of the right ventricle and courses posteriorly towards the spine.
3. The pulmonary valve lies closer to the chest wall and more cranial than the aortic valve.
4. The ductus arteriosus lies below the aortic arch and in a slightly different plane of section.

The ease of swiveling the transducer should allow these planes of section to be identified without losing continuity. If all these normal features have been noted the vast majority of major congenital cardiac abnormalities are thereby excluded. There are some limitations in accuracy that will not be overcome without more specialized knowledge, or without improved resolution of imaging equipment. The defects that would be overlooked without more specialized knowledge than that described are numerically small. Those overlooked because of limitations in resolution are probably unimportant in terms of severity. For example, a defect in the ventricular septum of 2 to 3 mm would be overlooked with present day equipment,[3] and it is possible that a defect of this size in a fetal heart of 20 weeks' gestation could become functionally important in infancy if the defect grew at the same rate as the heart. It should be remembered, however, that the natural history of ventricular septal defects is to become smaller and close as the heart grows during childhood.[4]

We have used M-mode echocardiography to acquire all our measurement data for growth characteristics of intracardiac structures.[5] This is a specialized technique that requires more expensive equipment than is available in most obstetric departments. Detailed measurement is not necessary for routine study, however. The right and left ventricular walls should be of equal thickness and as thick as the ventricular septum. Similarly, both ventricles should be of approximately equal size, as should the aorta and pulmonary artery. Any divergence from these patterns should be appreciable on a cross-sectional study and the case referred for more specialized investigation and measurements.

FETAL ARRHYTHMIAS

Variations in fetal heart rate and rhythm are common in the normal fetus.[6] These include runs of sinus brady-

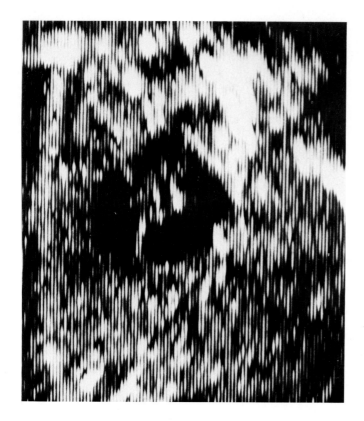
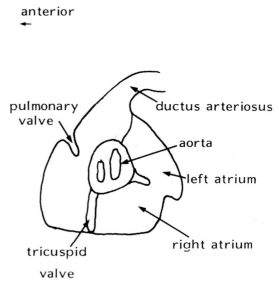

anterior

pulmonary
valve

ductus arteriosus

aorta

left atrium

right atrium

tricuspid
valve

Fig. 4. The main pulmonary artery, arising from the right ventricle, can be seen to connect to the ductus arteriosus. The pulmonary valve should be noted to be anterior and cranial to the aortic valve.

cardia, particularly in the mid-trimester, runs of sinus tachycardia mostly in the third trimester, and frequent premature contractions causing an irregular rhythm. It is only sustained bradycardias of less than 100 beats per minute or tachycardias of more than 200 beats per minute that should be considered abnormal. These require specialized investigation.

Evaluation of an arrhythmia is by recording atrial and ventricular contraction on M-mode echocardiography and comparing their relationship to each other. Figure 5 shows the atria to be contracting at an approximately normal rate of 140 beats per minute whereas the aortic valve is opening only about 60 times per minute. The aortic valve opening represents ventricular contraction. This tracing shows complete heart block. It is important to diagnose complete heart block for several reasons:

1. It is associated with structural cardiac abnormality in about one-third of cases.
2. It can cause intrauterine cardiac failure.
3. It is associated with maternal connective tissue disease in approximately half the cases.[7]

The maternal connective tissue disease may be subclinical but discovered serologically. Similarly

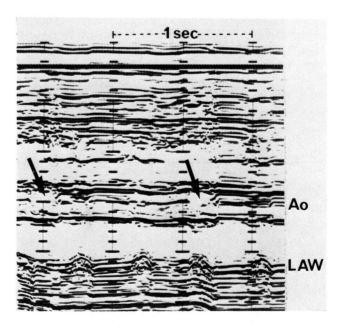

Fig. 5. The M-mode echocardiogram is recorded through the aorta and left atrium. The left atrial wall (LAW) can be seen to contract much more frequently than the aortic valve opens (*arrows*). Atrial contraction is around 140 beats per minute whereas ventricular contraction is around 60 times per minute.

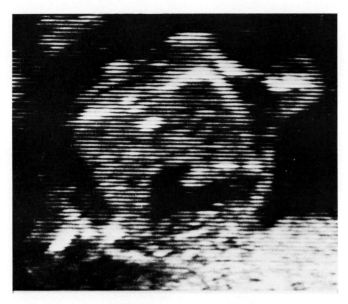
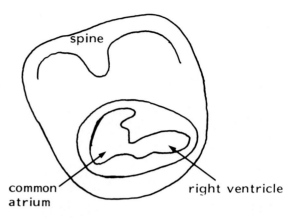

Fig. 6. A cross section of the fetal thorax can only demonstrate one ventricular chamber. There was mitral atresia. The left ventricle was thus only a slitlike posterior chamber.

tachycardias must be accurately evaluated. They are rarely associated with structural abnormality, but not infrequently cause nonimmune hydrops fetalis. Fetal tachycardias may respond to maternal drug therapy and this should be aggressively tried in preference to delivery of a premature hydropic fetus.[8,9] It should be stressed that drug therapy should not be started without proper evaluation of the type of arrhythmia present and appropriate maternal and fetal monitoring.

FETAL ABNORMALITIES

In a series of over 800 pregnancies, over half of which have had an indication for study, we have reliably detected 18 anomalies, 9 prior to, and 9 after, 26 weeks' gestation. All have had anatomic, or postnatal echocardiographic confirmation of the diagnosis made prenatally. The high-risk pregnancies selected for study included:

1. Family history of congenital heart disease.
2. Fetal arrhythmias (as defined above).
3. Nonimmune hydrops fetalis.
4. Fetal abnormality detected in a system other than the cardiovascular system.
5. Structural cardiac abnormality suspected by referring obstetrician.

Mothers with a previously affected child have approximately a 1 in 50 chance of recurrence of congenital heart disease in a sibling.[10] If the mother herself has or has had congenital heart disease the risk is of the

order of 14 percent of an affected offspring.[11] Nonimmune hydrops fetalis has a known association with structural congenital heart disease, both from autopsy[12] and echocardiographic studies.[13,14] It is important to look for a cardiac abnormality if the fetus has an extracardiac anomaly detected, as this may influence the prognosis and management of an individual case. A syndrome diagnosis or chromosomal abnormality may be suggested by the combination of anomalies in more than one system. Increasingly, suspected anomalies have been referred for evaluation by an obstetric ultrasonographer who has thought the cardiac appearance to be unusual on a routine antenatal scan. This will hopefully be an increasing source of referrals, allowing detection of "first-time affected" mothers. Three examples of the abnormalities detected are illustrated in Figures 6, 7, and 8. Figure 6 shows only one ventricular chamber because the left atrioventricular, or mitral valve, was atretic. Figure 7 shows only one artery arising from the heart. The pulmonary artery then arises from the posterior aspect of this single artery. There was only therefore one arterial valve found. Figure 8 shows a large tumor arising in the left atrium and obstructing the mitral valve. In two cases so far examined the cardiac abnormality was thought severe enough to merit termination of pregnancy. One was a case of ostium primum atrial septal defect with interrupted aortic arch and left atrial isomerism; in the second, a case of multiple cardiac tumors, the father was known to be affected by tuberose sclerosis. Detection of abnormalities in late pregnancy is still of importance as delivery can be arranged in a center with pediatric cardiac

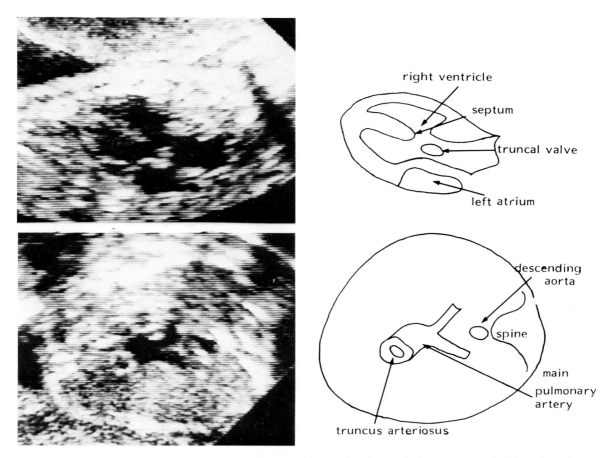

Fig. 7. Only one great artery is seen arising astride the ventricular septum (*top*). Arising from the back of this single arterial trunk was the main pulmonary artery with right and left branches.

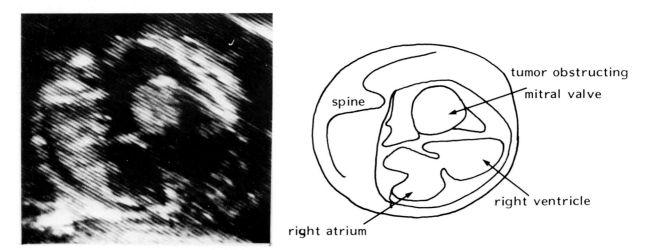

Fig. 8. A large intracardiac tumor is seen obstructing the mitral valve causing cardiac enlargement and fetal hydrops.

facilities. Immediate investigation and care of the affected infant can then take place, allowing the optimum chance of survival.

SUMMARY

The detection of congenital cardiac abnormalities is an important new addition to the growing list of defects that can be reliably predicted in prenatal life. Using the method described above it is relatively easy to predict structural normality of the heart. To elucidate all the components of an abnormality or accurately interpret and treat arrhythmias is much more difficult and experience should be concentrated in specialized centers. Interruption of a pregnancy in which an inoperable defect is found is probably justifiable. More importantly, reorganization of antenatal care to avoid delay in diagnosis, which contributes significantly to infant mortality in congenital heart disease, will maximize the chance of survival.

REFERENCES

1. Sahn DJ, Lange LW, Allen HD, et al: Quantitative real-time cross-sectional echocardiography in the developing normal human fetus and newborn. Circulation 62:588, 1980
2. Allan LD, Tynan MJ, Campbell S, et al: Echocardiographic and anatomical correlates in the fetus. Br Heart J 44:444, 1980
3. Latson LA, Cheatham JP, Gutgesell HP: Resolution and accuracy in two-dimensional echocardiography. Am J Cardiol 48:106, 1981
4. Alpert BS, Mellits ED, Rowe RD: Spontaneous closure of small ventricular septal defects. Am J Dis Child 125:194, 1973
5. Allan, LD, Joseph MC, Boyd EGCA, et al: M-mode echocardiography in the developing human fetus. Br Heart J 47:573, 1982
6. Wheeler T, Murrills A: Patterns of fetal heart rate during normal pregnancy. Br J Obstet Gynaec 85:18, 1978
7. McCue CM, Mantaleas ME, Tingelstad JB, et al: Congenital heart block in newborns of mothers with connective tissue disease. Circulation 56:82, 1977
8. Harrigan JT, Kangos JJ, Sikka A: Successful treatment of fetal congestive heart failure secondary to tachycardia. N Engl J Med 304:1527, 1981
9. Dumesic DA, Silverman NH, Tobias S, et al: Transplacental cardioversion of fetal supraventricular tachycardia with procainamide. N Engl J Med 307:1128, 1982
10. Nora JJ: Multifactorial inheritance hypothesis for the aetiology of congenital heart diseases. Circulation 38:604, 1968
11. Whittemore R, Hobbins JC, Engle MA: Pregnancy and its outcome in women with and without surgical treatment of congenital heart disease. Am J Cardiol 50:641, 1982
12. Beischer NA, Fortune DW, Macafee J: Non-immunologic hydrops fetalis and congenital abnormalities. Obstet Gynec 38:86, 1971
13. Allan LD, Little D, Campbell S, et al: Fetal ascites associated with congenital heart disease. Br J Obstet Gynaecol 88:453, 1981
14. Kleinman CS, Donnerstein RL, Devore GR, et al: Fetal echocardiography for evaluation of in utero congestive heart failure. N Engl J Med 306:568, 1982

16 | Sonographic Evaluation of the Fetal Chest

David Graham
Roger C. Sanders

The sonographic diagnosis of intrathoracic abnormalities has received little attention to date, partly because of the rarity of the conditions and partly because rib shadowing in the chest makes visualization of intrathoracic structures somewhat more difficult than visualization of intraabdominal structures. Thoracic and intrathoracic abnormalities may occur as primary lesions or may be secondary to more generalized conditions.

NORMAL ANATOMY

Examination of the chest in both longitudinal and transverse sections allows visualization of normal lungs, heart, rib cage, and chest wall.

Lungs
The normal lungs appear as relatively homogenous structures with ultrasound (Fig. 1). On a coronal view, the diaphragm may be seen (Fig. 1) as a line of decreased echogenicity between the lungs and liver. The echogenicity of the lungs is similar to that of the liver. In the third trimester the lung becomes more echogenic than the liver.

Rib Cage and Spine
The rib cage (Fig. 2) and spine are readily seen. Spina bifida lesions are evaluated by a series of longitudinal and transverse scans. Skeletal malformations may involve the rib cage secondarily usually causing hypoplasia of the chest. The scapula may also be visualized

as a linear echogenicity adjacent to the posterolateral chest wall (Fig. 2).

Occasionally, one may see a lucent stripe at the periphery of the chest inside the rib cage that mimics a small pleural effusion and appears to be analogous to the pseudoascites seen in the abdomen.[1]

Soft Tissues
The soft tissues of the chest wall may not be well differentiated sonographically because they are normally quite thin but do become more prominent as term approaches. However, significant thickening of these tissues may be seen in fetal anasarca where there is generalized body wall edema[2] or where there is increased subcutaneous fat deposition, as in the infant of a diabetic mother.

Occasionally what subsequently is presumed to be normal breast tissue is seen as soft tissue densities anteriorly (Fig. 3).

Heart
The heart is seen in cross section as an anterior structure in the midline and extending to the left side in which individual chambers are readily identified (Fig. 4). The heart may be evaluated by

1. M-mode echocardiography for evaluation of cardiac dysrhythmia, and for measurement of certain cardiac parameters such as left ventricular emptying and end diastolic volume.
2. Two-dimensional study: real-time recording of the fetal heart will allow diagnosis of structural cardiac

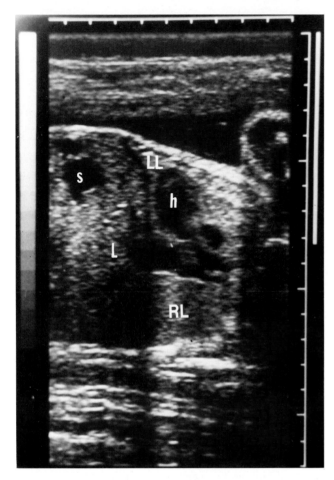

Fig. 1. Coronal view of normal chest. Coronal section through the chest and upper abdomen in a third trimester fetus which shows the heart (H), right lung (RL), left lung (LL), liver (L), and stomach (S).

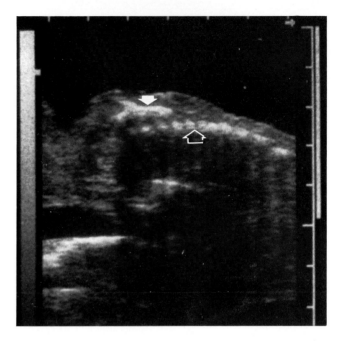

Fig. 2. Scapula and chest wall. A real-time coronal section of a mid-trimester fetus shows the scapula (*closed arrow*) lying adjacent to the rib cage (*open arrow*).

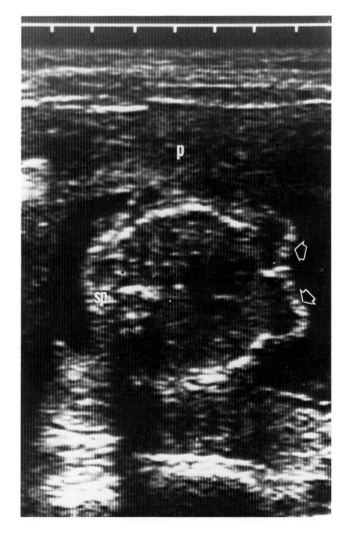

Fig. 3. Breast tissue. Soft tissue masses (*arrows*) anterior to the chest wall which appear to represent normal breast tissue. Spine, sp, placenta, p.

220

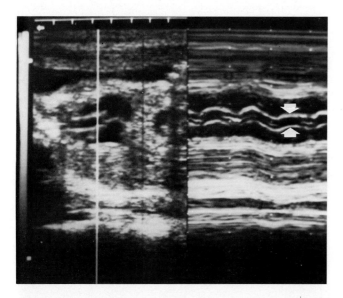

Fig. 4. Heart: three-dimensional and echocardiogram. A combined two-dimensional and M-mode echocardiogram in a midtrimester fetus shows the cursor passing through the aortic root. To the right, the corresponding M-mode tracing shows movements of the walls of the aortic root (*arrows*). Between the echoes from the wall movement can be seen the movement of the aortic valve.

defects such as obstructive lesions (Fig. 5) and ventriculoatrial defects.

Demonstration of Lung Maturity

Attempts have been made to correlate the sonographic appearances of the lungs with lung maturity, a finding that, if reliable, could be of immense clinical significance. This has been attempted by correlating the sonographic appearances of the lungs with the appearance of another organ such as the liver. Garrett et al.[3] found that where the lungs appeared more echogenic than the liver, there was evidence of lung maturity. In clinical practice, however, this has proven to be of little value since the lungs may appear more echogenic than the liver even in mid-trimester.

Fetal Breathing

Fetal breathing may be recognized with real-time ultrasound. The normal rate of Fetal Breathing Movements (FBM) ranges from 12 to 60 breaths per minute.[4] Assessment of FBM may be used as part of the fetal biophysical profile and has a good correlation with fetal well-being (see Chapter 12).[5] Two cases of intrauterine fetal tachypnea, both occurring in diabetics, have been described.[6,7] In the first case, recognition of the fetal tachypnea prompted early intervention and delivery of a normal fetus. Fetal breathing is more completely discussed in Chapter 12.

PULMONARY AND THORACIC LESIONS

Although congenital abnormalities of the lungs and intrathoracic structures are uncommon in the prenatal and immediate postnatal periods, a number of such anomalies have been recognized prenatally.

Cystic Adenomatoid Malformation (CAM)

This is a relatively uncommon lesion in which normal pulmonary tissue is replaced by cysts of varying sizes. There are three pathologic types based on the gross and microscopic features.[8] Type I has single or multiple large cysts (>2 cm diameter) and has a good prognosis after resection of the affected portion of lung. Type II has multiple small cysts (<1 cm diameter) and has a high incidence of anomalies of other organ systems, the most frequent being renal and gastrointestinal. In Type III malformation, there is a large non-cystic lesion producing a mediastinal shift. The prognosis for this type is poor.

In utero, CAM, which is generally a unilateral process, may appear to be bilateral due to herniation of affected lung to the opposite site with subsequent compression of normal pulmonary tissue. CAM may be associated with a nonimmune hydrops picture and

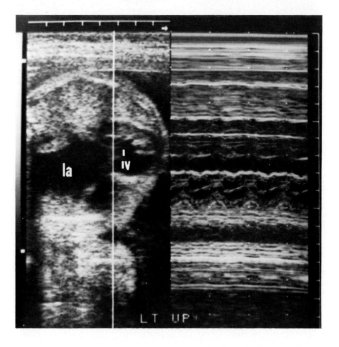

Fig. 5. Left ventricular outlet obstruction. A transverse section through the chest of a third trimester fetus shows a left ventricle (IV) that is enlarged and has evidence of myometrial thickening. The left atrium (IA) is markedly enlarged. At delivery, aortic valve hypoplasia was found.

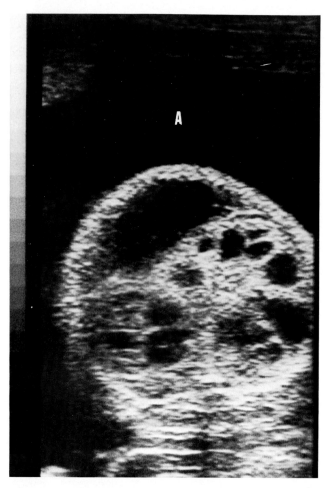

Fig. 6. Cystic adenomatoid malformation. A transverse section of the fetal chest shows replacement of normal pulmonary tissue by cysts of varying sizes. The amount of amniotic fluid (A) is increased.

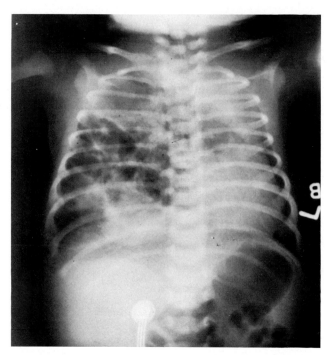

Fig. 7. Cystic adenomatoid malformation: radiograph. An AP radiograph of the chest of an above affected infant shows cystic masses, representing affected lung, in the right hemithorax. The heart is deviated to the left side.

polyhydramnios, presumably due to interference with venous return to the heart.[9-12]

The importance of the prenatal recognition of CAM is in excluding other organ system anomalies that potentially may be more life threatening and in allowing referral for delivery in a tertiary center where facilities for immediate postnatal surgery are available.

Sonographically one will see numerous cystic masses of varying size in the chest, usually bilaterally (Figs. 6, 7). There may also be sonographic evidence of fetal ascites, skin thickening and polyhydramnios.

Pleural Effusions

Pleural effusions occurring prenatally may be serous or chylous and may occur as primary lesions or as part of the spectrum of other conditions, e.g., immune or nonimmune hydrops or congestive heart failure.[13]

1. *Serous pleural effusions.* These may be seen:
   a. as an isolated finding of unknown etiology;

   b. secondary to immune or nonimmune hydrops[2];
   c. with chromosomal anomalies such as Turner syndrome (XO) or Down syndrome (trisomy 21); or
   d. secondary to cardiac lesions
2. *Chylous effusions.* Chylous effusions are a not uncommon cause of pleural effusions diagnosed at birth.[14,15] Chylous effusions have a male predominance of 2:1 and may be associated with maternal polyhydramnios. Although no definite etiology has been discovered, an underlying abnormality of the lymphatic system has been implicated.[16] Sonographically, the features of chylothorax are identical to those of the isolated pleural effusion, the definitive diagnosis being made by postnatal aspiration.[17]

Sonographically, pleural effusions will be visualized as cystic collections in each hemithorax (Fig. 8). The lungs may be seen as small echogenic masses displaced towards the midline. Other features depend on the cause of the pleural effusion, e.g., where pleural effusions are seen secondary to hydrops, immune or nonimmune, then skin thickening or peritoneal accumulations of fluid may also be visualized (Fig. 9).

The management of patients with a prenatal diagnosis of large pleural effusions remains uncertain. The

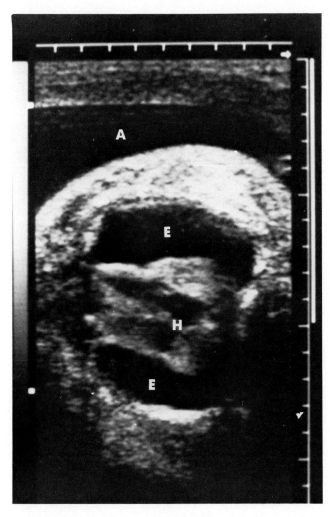

Fig. 8. Pleural effusion. A transverse section of the chest of a third trimester fetus with idiopathic hydrops shows large bilateral pleural effusions (E). The heart (H) is seen centrally. There is thickening of the soft tissues of the chest wall (*arrows*). Amniotic fluid (A).

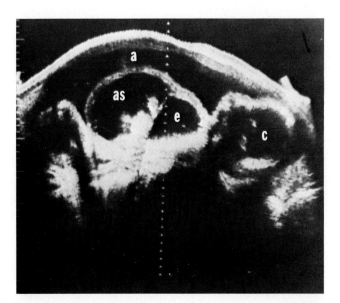

Fig. 9. Hydrops with pleural effusion. A longitudinal section of a fetus with nonimmune hydrops shows a vertex presentation. The cranium (c) is seen to the right. The hemithorax is filled by a massive pleural effusion (e). Ascites (as) surround the liver and bowel. The amount of amniotic fluid (a) is increased.

major problem associated with large effusions is the development of pulmonary hypoplasia, leading to respiratory distress in the immediate neonatal period.[13,18] It is technically possible to place intrathoracic catheters prenatally to shunt fluid from the thorax to the amniotic space and hence decrease the possibility of pulmonary hypoplasia. In the last trimester of pregnancy, premature delivery would be a serious consideration.

Pulmonary Sequestration

Pulmonary sequestration is characterized by the presence of nonfunctioning pulmonary tissue that usually does not have a communication with the bronchial tree and receives its blood supply from an anomalous artery from the aorta rather than a pulmonary arterial branch.[19,20] There are two major types:

1. *Intralobar sequestration:* the abnormal tissues lie within the normal lung, usually in a posterior segment of a lower lobe.

2. *Extralobar sequestration:* found between the lower lobe and the diaphragm or in the upper abdomen.

Pulmonary sequestration has been recognized prenatally by the presence of a nonpulsatile echogenic mass in the hemithorax.[21,22]

Intrathoracic Cysts

Cysts of neural or enteric origin occur in the mediastinum and appear sonographically as cystic masses that may be recognized prenatally.[23] Knochel et al. have reported prenatal diagnosis of a mediastinal meningocele.[22]

Diaphragmatic Hernia

While the embryology of the formation of the diaphragm is not completely understood, it does appear that return of the intestines to the abdominal cavity prior to closure of the lumbocostal trigone and pleuroperitoneal canal will result in a posterolateral hernia. The size of this defect varies from a tiny opening to complete absence of the hemidiaphragm. The size of the actual hernia has no direct relationship to the size of the defect.[24]

Diaphragmatic hernia most commonly occur posteriorly on the left side, (foramen of Bochdalek hernia) but may also occur anteriorly through the foramen of Morgagni. The hernia may involve intestine, stomach, and liver. Foramen of Bochdalek hernia may also occur, less frequently, on the right side. It is of interest that even in the presence of massive herniation, respiratory distress is rarely of the life-threatening severity in patients with left diaphragmatic hernia.[25]

Where the hernia is large, pulmonary hypoplasia is almost always present and affects both the bronchial tree and the alveoli.[26,27] The presence of pulmonary hypoplasia plus intestine in the hemithorax usually results in significant respiratory distress immediately after birth.[28]

Although stillborns with diaphragmatic herniation may have a 95 percent incidence of other anomalies, those infants born alive have a low incidence of such anomalies.[24]

The importance of prenatal diagnosis of diaphragmatic hernia is to allow delivery of the patient at a tertiary care center where facilities for immediate neonatal surgery are available. With the development of newer techniques of prenatal intervention, it is possible that prenatal correction of diaphragmatic hernia will become a viable possibility.[29]

Diaphragmatic herniation may be very difficult to recognize sonographically, especially where the herniated bowel does not contain swallowed amniotic fluid. Sonographically, two patterns may be seen:

1. non-fluid-containing bowel may simulate a solid tumor in the chest or may be impossible to visualize
2. fluid-containing bowel, usually the stomach, will be seen as one or more cystic masses in the chest, separate from the heart (Fig. 10)

In both instances, there will be a lack of visualized bowel in the fetal abdomen, which will have a small abdominal circumference. Polyhydamnios is present in a large percentage of cases.

Multiple cystic masses in the chest must be distinguished from CAM, but in the latter instance, normal fluid-filled bowel will be seen in its normal location in the abdomen. Single cystic masses as are seen in Fig. 10 may be caused by

• diaphragmatic hernia,
• pulmonary sequestration,[21,22]
• mediastinal cysts of neural or enteric origin,[23] or
• mediastinal meningocele.[22]

ABNORMALITIES OF CHEST WALL SHAPE

Several systemic conditions have as a feature, a narrow chest diameter or an unusual chest shape such as a long, narrow, or a bell-shaped chest. Fetal thoracic size may be measured sonographically and several such

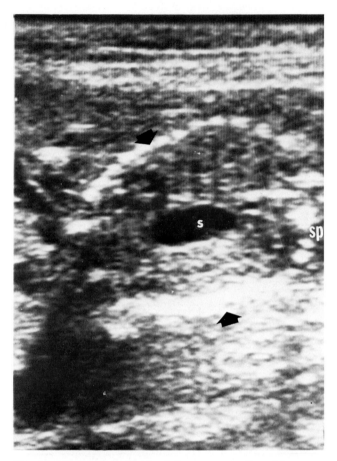

Fig. 10. Diaphragmatic hernia. A transverse section of the upper chest of a 19-week fetus shows a cystic structure (s) representing stomach herniated into the chest. Spine, sp. Ribs (*arrows*). At this stage, polyhydramnios was not present.

charts are available[30] (Fig. 11). Thoracic deformity is a feature of a number of dwarfism syndromes[31]:

1. Chondroectodermal dysplasia (Ellis–van Creveld syndrome) is an autosomal recessive condition, which has among its features a long narrow chest, symmetric limb shortening, and polydactyly, and has been diagnosed prior to 20 weeks.[32] Associated congenital cardiac lesions are not uncommon.
2. Thanatophoric dwarfism is an autosomal form of short-limbed dwarfism associated with a narrow chest.[33,34] Although the micromelia is marked, the length of the trunk may be normal. Marked narrowing of the thorax is almost always seen (Fig. 11). Thickening of the soft tissues of the limbs may help distinguish this from achondroplasia. As with many lethal forms of dwarfism, maternal polyhydramnios is a frequent association.
3. Achondrogenesis, a lethal, autosomal recessive, severe form of chondrodystrophy having marked limb shortening together with marked chest narrowing,[35]

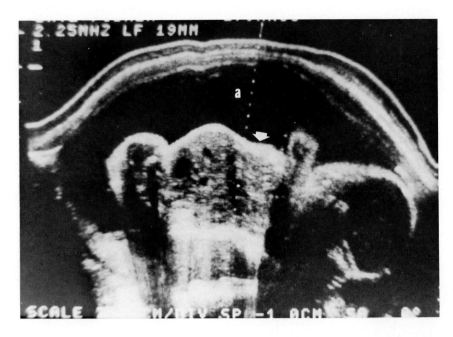

Fig. 11. Chest narrowing in thanatophoric dwarfism. A longitudinal section of the uterus shows a fetus in cephalic presentation. The chest (*arrows*) is narrow compared to the abdomen. Polyhydramnios (*a*) is present.

has been recognized early in the second trimester.[36] Again, maternal polyhydramnios is frequently associated.

4. Asphyxiating thoracic dystrophy (Jeune disease) is characterized by a narrow rigid thorax with multiple cartilaginous anomalies.[31] This disease, which usually progresses through respiratory insufficiency to death in early childhood, has been recognized prenatally.[37]

5. Achondroplasia, which involves a reduction in chest size, has been reported in a fetus with homozygous achondroplasia.[38]

6. Other types of short-limbed dwarfism, e.g. Saldino-Noonan, are also associated with abnormal chest shape.[31]

Prolonged oligohydramnios may also be associated with pulmonary hypoplasia.[39-41] Although the exact etiology is unknown, this may be related to restriction of fetal chest motion in utero. Abnormalities of chest shape, secondary to pulmonary hypoplasia may be recognized sonographically as in Figure 12.

Abnormalities in Chest Wall Fusion
During embryonic life at approximately the tenth week, the midgut, which had been in an extraabdominal location, returns to that cavity and undergoes rotation and fixation. The final integrity of the abdominal wall then becomes dependent on the fusion of five body folds after return of the intestines to the abdominal cavity. These folds (cephalic, caudal, and two lateral) come together at the base of the umbilical cord.

Failure of growth and fusion of the cephalic fold

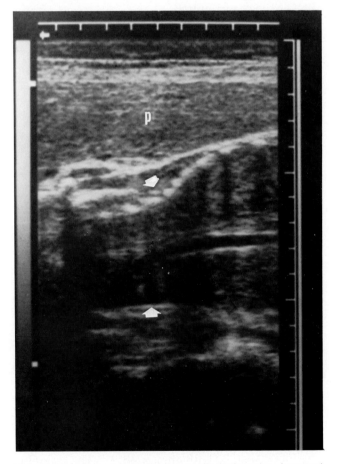

Fig. 12. Chest hypoplasia secondary to oligohydramnios. A coronal section of the chest of a 35-week fetus with prolonged oligohydramnios secondary to bladder outlet obstruction shows evidence of a bell-shaped chest with significant narrowing of the upper thorax (*arrows*). Placenta, p.

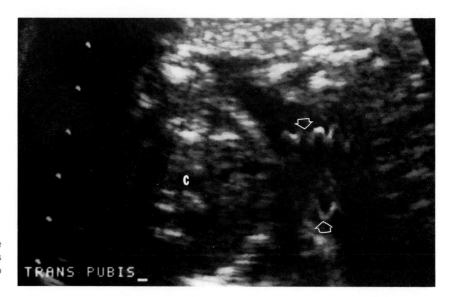

Fig. 13. Ectopia cordis. A static scan transverse section of the chest in a midtrimester fetus shows evidence of cardiac motion (*arrows*) anterior to the chest (c).

results in either ectopia cordis or a pentalogy of defects, the Pentalogy of Cantrell.

Ectopia Cordis. With ectopia cordis, a defect of anterior chest wall fusion results in exteriorization of the heart. This is easily recognized sonographically by the presence of a mass anterior to the chest wall that shows characteristic cardiac pulsations (Fig. 13).

Pentalogy of Cantrell. There is a pentalogy of defects:

1. Cleft or absent lower sternum.
2. Absence of diaphragmatic septum transversus.
3. Absence of diaphragmatic pericardium.
4. Congenital cardiac anomalies.
5. Omphalocele in the epigastric portion of the abdominal wall.

   The heart will protrude through the chest wall defect into the hernia sac to a varying degree. Sonographically, there will also be evidence of liver and bowel in the hernia sac.

Thoracopagus Conjoined Twins
In the thoracopagus type of conjoined twin, the most common of the types of fusion, there is fusion of the anterior thoracic and upper abdominal midline. There is a common pericardium in 90 and in 75 percent, the hearts are joined.[42] Hepatic and gastrointestinal fusions are also common. Thoracopagus twins have been recognized prenatally with ultrasound.[43-45] The major importance of prenatal diagnosis is in giving a prognosis—where a fused heart is demonstrated, there is little chance of survival—and in planning the mode of delivery.[42]

Sonography in such malformations will show the fusion of the chest and abdomen to a varying extent (Fig. 14).

Tumors of the Chest Wall
Occasionally, cystic hygroma, because of its size, will appear to be in a location adjacent to the chest wall.[46,47]

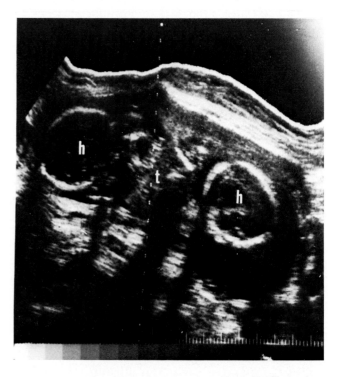

Fig. 14. Thoracopagus Twins. A longitudinal uterine section at 18 weeks' pregnancy shows separate fetal heads (h) and a fused thorax (t) compatible with thoracopagus twins. These twins shared a common heart on echocardiographic study.

Such masses, which usually have a multiseptated cystic appearance, are described in Chapter 19. Similarly, large solid masses, such as teratomas arising from the neck, may be adjacent to the anterior chest and appear as thoracic masses.[48,49]

Although not reported as being diagnosed prenatally, chest wall tumors such as hemangiomas or lymphangiectasia might be expected to be recognizable prenatally as complex soft tissue masses adjacent to the rib cage.

REFERENCES

1. Rosenthal SJ, Filly RA, Callen PW, et al: Fetal pseudoascites. Radiology 131:195, 1979

2. Fleischer AC, Killam AP, Boehm FH, et al: Hydrops fetalis: Sonographic evaluations of clinical implications. Radiology 141:163, 1981

3. Garrett WJ, Warren PS, Picker RH, et al: Maturation of the fetal lung, liver and bowel. Presented at Annual Meeting AIUM, San Francisco, 1981

4. Manning RA: Monitoring fetal breathing using real-time ultrasound. Hosp Prac 19:72, 1979

5. Manning RA, Platt DL, Sipos L: Antepartum fetal evaluation: Development of fetal biophysical profile. Am J Obstet Gynecol 136:787, 1980

6. Boddy K, Dawes GS: Fetal breathing. Br Med Bull 31:1, 1975

7. Manning FA, Heaman M. Boyce D, et al: Intrauterine fetal tachypnea. Obstet Gynecol 58:398, 1981

8. Stocher JT, Madewell JE, Drake RM: Congenital cystic adenomatoid malformation of the lung. Classification and morphologic spectrum. Hum Pathol 8:155, 1977

9. Graham D, Winn K, Dex W, et al: Prenatal diagnosis of cystic adenomatoid malformation of the lung. J Ultrasound Med 1:9, 1982

10. Kohler, HG, Rymer BA: Congenital cystic malformation of the lung and its relation to hydramnios. J Obstet Gynecol Br Commonw 80:130, 1973

11. Donn SM, Martin JN, White SJ: Antenatal ultrasound findings in cystic malformation. Pediatr Radiol 10:180, 1981

12. Aslam RA, Korones SB, Richardson RL, et al: Congenital cystic adenomatoid malformation with anasarca. JAMA 212:622, 1970

13. Lange, IR, Manning FA: Antenatal diagnosis of congenital pleural effusions. Am J Obstet Gynecol 140:839, 1981

14. Chernick V, Reed MH: Pneumothorax and chylothorax in the neonatal period. J Pediatr 76:624, 1970

15. Brodman RF: Congenital chylothorax. NY State J Med 553, March 1975

16. Randolph JG, Gross RE: Congenital chylothorax. Arch Surg 74:405, 1957

17. Defoort P, Thiery M: Antenatal diagnosis of congenital chylothorax by gray-scale sonography. J Clin Ultrasound 6:47, 1978

18. Boricelli L, Rizzo N, Orsini LF, et al: Ultrasonic real-time diagnosis of fetal hydrothorax and lung hypoplasia. J Clin Ultrasound 9:253, 1981

19. Felson B: The many faces of pulmonary sequestration. Semin Roentgenol 7:3, 1972

20. Gerle RD, Jaretzki A, Ashley CA, et al: Congenital bronchopulmonary foregut malformations. N Engl J Med 278:1413, 1968

21. Romero R, Chervenak FA, Kotzen J, et al: Antenatal sonographic findings in extralobar pulmonary sequestration. J Ultrasound Med 1:131, 1982

22. Knochel JQ, Lee TG, Melendez MG, et al: Fetal anomalies involving the thorax and abdomen. Radiol Clin N Am 20:297, 1982

23. Hobbins JC, Grannum PAT, Berkowitz RL, et al: Ultrasound in the diagnosis of congenital anomalies. Am J Obstet Gynecol 134:331, 1979

24. Calling DL: Diaphragmatic surgery, in Holder TM, Ashcroft KW (eds), Pediatric Surgery. Philadelphia, Saunders, 1980

25. Campbell DN, Lilly JR: The clinical spectrum of right Bochdalek's hernia. Arch Surg 117:341, 1982

26. Harrison MR, Jester JA, Ross NA: Correction of congenital diaphragmatic hernia in utero I. The model: intrathoracic balloon produces fetal pulmonary hypoplasia. Surgery 88:174, 1980

27. Haller JA, Signer RD, Golladay AE, et al: Pulmonary and ductal hemodynamics in studies of simulated diaphragmatic hernia of fetal and newborn lambs. J Pediatr Surg 11:675, 1976

28. Dibbins AW, Wiener LS: Mortality from congenital diaphragmatic hernia. J Pediatr Surg 9:653, 1974

29. Harrison MR, Bressack MA, Churg AM, et al: Correction of congenital diaphragmatic hernia in utero II. Simulated correction permits fetal lung growth with survival at birth. Surgery 88:260, 1980

30. Levi S, Erbsman F: Antenatal fetal growth from the 19th week. Am J Obstet Gynecol 121:262, 1975

31. Sillence DO, Rimoin DL, Lachman R: Neonatal dwarfism. Pediatr Clin N Am: 25, 453, 1978

32. Mahoney MJ, Hobbins JC: Prenatal diagnosis of chondroectodermal dysplasia (Ellis–van Creveld syndrome) with fetoscopy and ultrasound. N Engl J Med 297:258, 1977

33. Schaff MI, Fleischer AC, Battino R, et al: Antenatal sonographic diagnosis of thanatophoric dysplasia. J Clin Ultrasound 8:363, 1980

34. Colmin BJ, Schaff MI: Ultrasonic diagnosis of thanatophoric dwarfism in utero. Radiology 124:479, 1977

35. Smith WL, Breitweisser TD, Dinno N: In utero diagnosis of achondrogenesis, type 1. Clin Genet 19:51, 1981

36. Graham D, Tracey J, Winn K, et al: Early second trimester sonographic diagnosis of achondrogenesis. J Clin Ultrasound 11:336, 1983

37. Miskin M, Rothberg R: Prenatal detection of congenital anomalies by ultrasound. Semin Ultrasound 4:278, 1980

38. Bowie JD: Real time ultrasonography in the diagnosis of fetal anomalies. Clin Diag Ultrasound 10:227, 1982

39. Bain AD, Scott JS: Renal agenesis and severe urinary

tract dysplasia, a review of 50 cases with particular reference to the associated anomalies. Br Med J 1:841, 546, 1960

40. Renert WA, Berdon EW, Baker DH, et al: Obstructive urologic manifestations of the fetus and infant-relation to neonatal pneumomediastinum and pneumothorax (air-block). Radiology 105:97, 1972

41. Thomas IT, Smith DW: Oligohydramnios, cause of the non-renal features of Potter's syndrome, including pulmonary hypoplasia. J Pediatr 84:811, 1974

42. Edwards WD, Hagel DR, Thompson J, et al: Conjoined thoracopagas twins. Circulation 56:491, 1977

43. Gore RM, Filly RA, Parer JT: Sonographic antepartum diagnosis of conjoined twins. JAMA 247:3351, 1982

44. Wilson RL, Cetrulo CL, Shaub MS: The prepartum diagnosis of conjoined twins by the use of ultrasound. Am J Obstet Gynecol 126:737, 1978

45. Fagan C: Antepartum diagnosis of conjoined twins by ultrasonography. Am J Roentgenol 129:921, 1977

46. Shaub M, Wilson R, Collea J: Fetal cystic lymphangiona (cystic hygroma) prepartum ultrasonic findings. Radiology 121:449, 1976

47. Morgan C, Haney A, Christakos A, et al: Antenatal detection of fetal structural defects with ultrasound. J Clin Ultrasound 314:287, 1978

48. Shoenfeld A, Edelstein T, Dip O, et al: Prenatal ultrasonic diagnosis of fetal teratoma of the neck. Br J Radiol 51:742, 1978

49. Kang K, Hisseng L: Prenatal ultrasonic diagnosis of epignathus. J Clin Ultrasound 6:295, 1978

17 | Sonography of Fetal Abdominal Abnormalities

James D. Bowie

Although in some cases the presence of fetal abnormalities can be suspected because of the patient's history, these are often found incidentally during routine ultrasound examination. The majority of structural defects encountered will involve the central nervous system. Genitourinary (GU) abnormalities will be the second most common, with the gastrointestinal tract and abdominal wall a very close third. The majority of this last group as seen by sonography are abdominal wall defects and atresias of the esophagus or obstruction of the duodenum.[1] Sonography may also demonstrate diaphragmatic hernia, ascites, meconium pseudocysts, choledochal cyst, and anal atresia. Our approach is a practical one dealing with the technical problems of studying each area, the ultrasound appearance of these abnormalities, what must be included in the differential diagnosis, and what is known about sonograpic studies of these abnormalities from the available literature.

Each examination of the fetus must begin with a general survey or orientation of the entire uterus. This is true whether it is done with a static scanner or with real time. Our preference is to use real time. With these instruments there is a temptation to study whatever first comes into view and is of interest; the examiner must have the discipline to first look systematically at all the uterus, uterine wall, placenta, amount of amniotic fluid, and then carefully examine every part of the fetus. Too much attention to one area to the exclusion of others is a mistake.

The amount of fluid present is one part of the general survey that often provides a clue to look for other abnormalities. Unfortunately, this author does not know of any simple way to tell if there is too much or too little amniotic fluid. Our standard of judgment varies with the duration of the pregnancy. It is normal to have enough fluid for the fetus to move freely, even end over end, at 15 weeks of pregnancy while at 39 weeks this would be polyhydramnios (Fig. 1). At that time we expect to find only isolated pockets of fluid alongside the fetus and separating the limbs, but it is easy near term to overdiagnose oligohydramnios. Despite the difficulty in making this judgment the impression of oligo- or polyhydramnios is useful. Oligohydramnios (Fig. 2) is almost always associated with premature rupture of membranes (PROM) , intrauterine growth retardation (IUGR), or restricted fetal urine output from a structural abnormality.

Polyhydramnios is frequently unexplained. An easy to remember (but slightly inaccurate) approximation is that polyhydramnios is idiopathic in 60 percent of cases, has maternal causes (diabetes, Rh incompatibility, etc.) in 20 percent, and fetal causes in 20 percent.[2] Neural tube defects (NTD) account for 45 percent of fetal causes, and 80 percent of these NTD associated with polyhydramnios are cases of anencephaly. Gastrointestinal abnormalities are the cause for about 30 percent of polyhydramnios when there is a fetal abnormality, and cardiac problems about 7 percent.[3] Other miscellaneous fetal causes of polyhydramnios include mesoblastic nephroma, congenital chylothorax, congenital pancreatic cyst, asphyxiating thoracic dystrophy, sacrococcygeal and cervical teratoma, multicystic dysplastic kidneys, cystic hygroma,

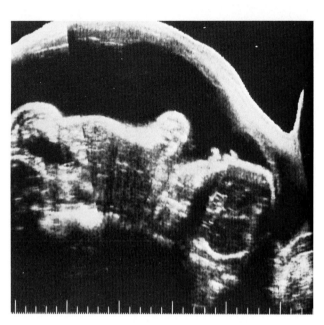

Fig. 1. Polyhydramnios as seen at term. The placenta is compressed anteriorly. The child was eventually shown to have a large diaphragmatic hernia and hypoplastic lungs.

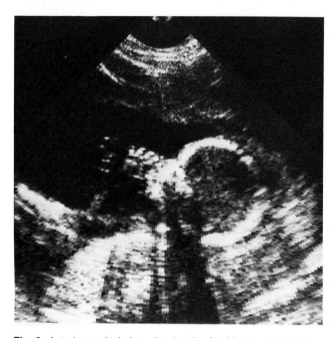

Fig. 3. Anterior sagittal view showing the fetal hand near the face. Fetal swallowing can be seen by observing opening of the mandible and elevation of the area of the pharynx.

trisomy 18, primary pulmonary hypoplasia, thanatophoric dwarfism, and miscellaneous other limb-shortening conditions.

Our approach has been to study the fetus in a systematic fashion beginning with the head, spine, and extremities and then going to the chest, heart, abdo-

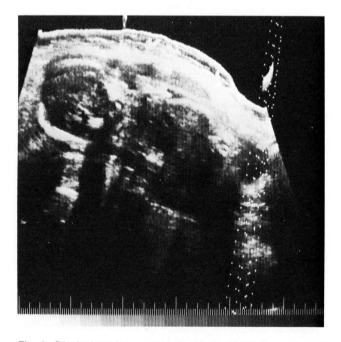

Fig. 2. Oligohydramnios as seen near term. There is crowding of fetal parts and no "pockets" of amniotic fluid could be found. This fetus had a severe form of sacrocaudal dysgenesis.

men, pelvis, and genitalia. We use the real-time sector scanner for this because we attempt in every case to obtain specific images in standardized scan planes. To produce consistently the same view in all fetuses is not possible but can be achieved in a high percentage of times by skilled examiners. During the initial study of the fetal head, a portion of the gastrointestinal (GI) system is examined when we obtain our routine sagittal and coronal views of the fetal face. In the anterior sagittal view fetal swallowing motion can be seen (Fig. 3). This is an intermittent phenomenon that occurs more frequently when polyhydramnios is present.[4] What appears to be fetal vomiting is rarely seen; two reported cases were associated with gastrointestinal obstructions. One of these was an esophageal atresia with tracheoesophageal (TE) fistula and the other a case of duodenal atresia.[4,5] The coronal view can show the lips and nose and has been used to demonstrate cleft lip abnormalities in utero (see Chapter 19 and Fig. 4).[6] After studying the heart and chest we then try to visualize the fetal diaphragm in coronal section and if this is not successful then a sagittal view is used (Fig. 5). Demonstration of the fetal diaphragm is more difficult early in pregnancy than in the third trimester. The rest of the abdominal anatomy is then usually viewed by axial and sagittal sections. An attempt is made to photograph and to explain every echofree area within the fetal abdomen. A special effort is made to show in either of these planes the site of insertion of the umbilical cord into the body wall (Fig. 6).

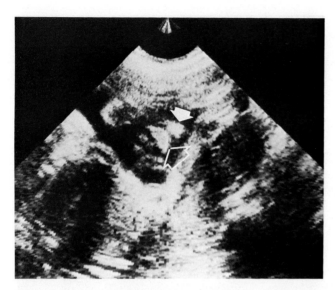

Fig. 4. Coronal view showing the tip of the fetal nose (*closed arrow*) and the upper lip of the fetus (*open arrow*).

Another important clue to the diagnosis of abdominal abnormalities is elevation of the serum α-fetoprotein (AFP). Serum screening programs are now available and result in an increased opportunity to diagnose fetal abnormalities. Although this test was originally advanced as a method of detecting neural tube defects it has a greater utility. When the serum AFP is above 2.5 times the median on two occasions, 18 percent of cases are explained by more advanced dates, 14 percent by multiple gestation, and 7 percent by fetal death.[7] The remainder are either false positive studies or associated with fetal abnormalities, including NTD, congenital nephrosis, omphalocele, gastroschesis, sacro-coccygeal teratoma, and cystic hygroma. As a result, the current recommendation when serum AFP is above 2.5 times the median on repeated studies is to perform an ultrasound examination. If this does not demonstrate an abnormality to explain the elevated AFP, then amniocentesis should be performed. In about 14 percent of these cases the amniotic fluid AFP (AFAFP) will be elevated.[7] The use of amniography when the ultrasound study is negative has not been established but has been reported to be of value for detection of both neural tube defects and body wall defects. Fetoscopy has also been recommended following a negative ultrasound study but is not widely available. When the imaging procedures are negative and AFAFP is elevated, there is a strong possibility of an occult fetal abnormality being present,[7] but false positive AFAFP studies occur. In one series limited to fetuses with a normal ultrasound study, 4 of 16 fetuses were normal when the AFAFP was above 5 SD, 3 of 5 were normal when it was between 4 and 5 SD, and 5 of 7 were normal when it was 3 to 4 SD.[8]

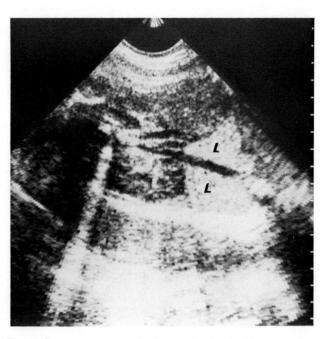

Fig. 5. Coronal view along the fetal aorta showing the separation of the fetal lungs (L) from the abdominal cavity.

TRACHEOESOPHAGEAL FISTULA AND ESOPHAGEAL ATRESIA

In 90 percent of cases of esophageal atresia there is an associated TE fistula. Usually this fistula is from the trachea to the distal esophagus.[9] This abnormality occurs sporadically as an isolated lesion and has no

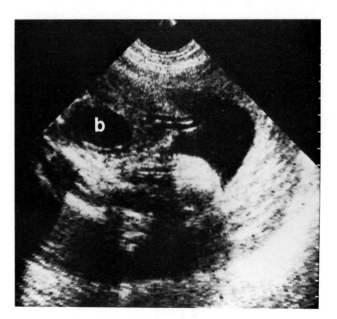

Fig. 6. Normal appearance of the insertion of the umbilical cord. In many cases it is possible to also show one or both umbilical arteries in proximity to the fetal bladder (b).

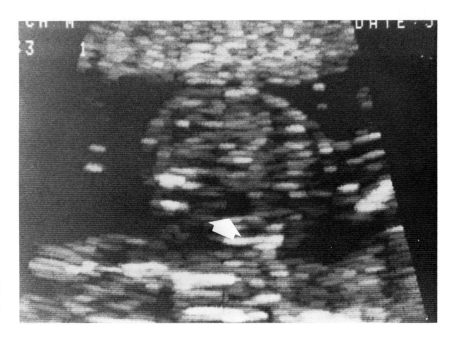

Fig. 7. A small amount of fluid is seen in the stomach (*arrow*) of this fetus, who subsequently proved to have an esophageal atresia with TE fistula.

known pattern of inheritance. It may be seen in about 30 percent of cases in combination with cardiovascular anomalies (PDA, VSD, and others), but other abnormalities of the VATER group are common. These include vertebral body and radial ray abnormalities, and anal and duodenal atresias. Associated genitourinary abnormalities are not as common. The most frequent of these is unilateral renal agenesis. Finally in about 3 to 5 percent there may be associated hydrocephalus or Down syndrome.

Esophageal atresia with TE fistula is rarely recognized by sonography. Frequently the only clue is a polyhydramnios, often mild, that is otherwise unexplained. Generally, when TE fistula is present there is fluid in the fetal stomach (Fig. 7), but in two reports of three patients persistent inability to demonstrate fluid in the fetal stomach over the course of the pregnancy led to the correct diagnosis of esophageal atresia, probably because of absence of a connecting TE fistula.[1,10] In each of these cases polyhydramnios was present and the earliest one was recognized at 26 weeks' gestational age. As mentioned above, fetal vomiting has rarely been seen in association with TE fistula. Amniography has also failed to diagnose TE fistula because ingested contrast could pass through the fistula into the fetal stomach.[11]

DUODENAL ATRESIA

The ultrasound findings in duodenal atresia are similar to the "double bubble" seen by plain film radiography in newborn children.[1,12-14] The stomach is distended with fluid and located in the left upper quadrant slightly posterior to the distended duodenal bulb with which it connects (Fig. 8). Since the stomach can normally be distended in the fetus, especially near term, the enlarged duodenum should be demonstrated and continuity between the two fluid structures should be proven to help confirm this diagnosis. Abnormalities of the left kidney, horseshoe kidney with a dilated renal pelvis, ectopic kidneys with cystic masses, as well as mesenteric or ovarian cyst, can produce confusing findings.[15] Generally, renal abnormalities are much nearer the spine than is the fetal stomach but the kidneys may have an abnormal position. In addition, duodenal atresia has been associated with polyhydramnios in all the reported cases and there may be elevation of amniotic fluid AFP levels. The earliest case recognized sonographically has been 32 weeks even though one patient had an earlier study at 22 weeks' gestation.

The "double bubble" finding in newborns is not always a result of duodenal atresia although this accounts for 40 to 60 percent of cases, but can be seen with duodenal web, in annular pancreas, duodenal stenosis, obstructing bands (Ladd's bands), volvulus, and obstruction from intestinal duplications. Nevertheless, when this finding is seen in utero the fetal heart should be examined as well since half of the patients have associated abnormalities, the most common of which is Down syndrome, which is found in 25 to 30 percent of cases. Common associated findings other than congenital heart disease include esophageal atresia, renal anomalies, imperforate anus, small bowel, and biliary atresias.

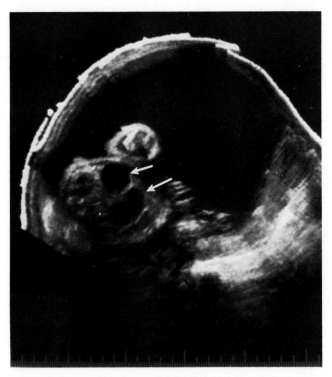

Fig. 8. Two fluid-filled structures (*arrows*) in the upper abdomen are seen as a result of duodenal atresia. These are the distended duodenum and stomach. (*Example provided by William Scheible, M.D., University of California, San Diego.*)

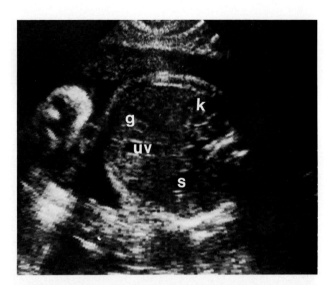

Fig. 9. Transverse view of the fetal abdomen showing normal structures, uv = umbilical vein, g = gallbladder, k = kidney, s = stomach.

CHOLEDOCHAL CYST

Two cases have been reported of a cystic mass near the gallbladder which proved to be a choledochal cyst.[16,17] One was observed at 25 weeks' gestation and the other at 36 weeks' gestation. In both cases this was the most common type of choledochal cyst, which is cystic dilatation of the common bile duct. In neither case was any other abnormality seen; amniotic fluid volume was not remarked on. Both infants appeared normal at birth and in one case [99m]TcPIPIDA was helpful in confirming the diagnosis postnatally.[16] When the dilated bile duct is seen as a fluid space next to the gallbladder, this should not be mistaken for duodenal atresia if the examiner is familiar with the anterior location of the normal fetal gallbladder (Fig. 9).

MECONIUM PERITONITIS

Bowel perforations resulting in meconium peritonitis, sometimes with formation of meconium pseudocyst, can be recognized in utero by sonography.[18,19] The cases thus far reported have all been associated with atresia of either jejunum or ileum. The abnormalities

have been seen at 30 to 32 weeks and may or may not be associated with polyhydramnios. A highly echogenic surface is seen by sonography in the approximate location of the peritoneum (Fig. 10). This may occur in any part of the peritoneal cavity, overlay the liver, or extend into the scrotum. In the cases we have reviewed one was in the right upper quadrant, one anterior in the left upper abdomen, and another in the left midabdomen. Recognition is easier when there is an associated mass. Typically these masses are adjacent to a peritoneal surface and have irregular, strongly reflective walls. The differential diagnosis of this finding includes cystic renal abnormalities, a dilated stomach, and mesenteric or ovarian cyst. The appearance of a meconium pseudocyst is generally distinct from abnormalities of the stomach or kidneys, but demonstration of these structures separate from the pseudocyst helps confirm this. Mesenteric and ovarian cyst may be the most difficult to distinguish from meconium pseudocyst. The former are usually rounder and smoother walled, and the latter have strongly echogenic margins (one of which is peripheral) typical of the calcific reaction stimulated by meconium. Since ovarian cysts have been associated with polyhydramnios for unknown reasons, this is not a distinguishing feature.[15] Small bowel atresias may also be recognized by the presence of multiple distended loops of bowel (Fig. 11) and has been recognized at 32 weeks' gestation.[20] Late in pregnancy, fetal bowel can be very prominent and a meconium-filled colon should not be mistaken for an abnormality. Using the real-time scanner, the colon can be distinguished by tracing its normal distribution; in some cases segmental peristaltic movements will be

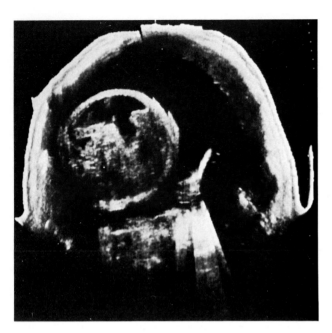

Fig. 10. Axial view of the fetal abdomen showing an irregular echo-free space with strongly echogenic borders. This was a meconium pseudocyst resulting from ileal atresia. Also note the polyhydramnios present. (*Reprinted with permission from Winsberg and Cooperberg* (*eds*), *Clinics in Diagnostic Ultrasound. New York, Churchill Livingston, vol 10, p 259.*)

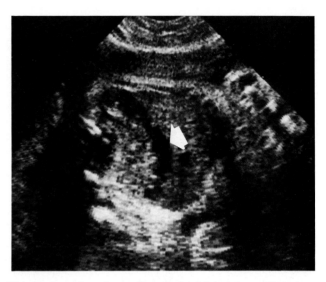

Fig. 12. An oblique image through the fetal abdomen that shows the typical appearance and distribution of the fetal colon (*arrow*).

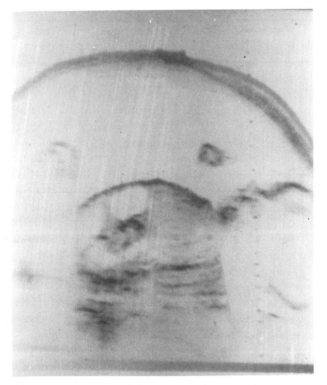

Fig. 11. Note the large echofree areas in the fetal abdomen as a result of multiple distended loops of bowel. This fetus had an ileal atresia. (*This example was provided by Roy A. Filly, M.D., University of California, San Francisco.*)

seen (Fig. 12). Less commonly distended loops of bowel may be seen at 32 to 33 weeks and may simulate small bowel obstruction when in fact none is present.[21]

ANAL ATRESIA

Anal atresia occurs in the spectrum of caudal dysgenesis and as such there may be associated anomalies of the GU tract and lumbosacral spine. Sacral abnormalities range from dysplasia to agenesis and spinal ones from narrowing of the disc space to block vertebrae. When the internal bowel terminates below the pelvic sling in males there is generally an orifice on the perineum and in females inside the posterior fourchette. With higher terminations a fistula may join the urinary system in males and the genital tract in females. There are associated urinary tract abnormalities in 25 percent of low terminations and 40 percent of high terminations. The most common are horseshoe kidney, absence of a kidney, hydronephrosis, or hypoplasia of a kidney. In 10 percent of cases associated cardiac abnormalities are seen. Fistulas have not been shown by ultrasound studies but large septated fluid structures separate from the bladder in the pelvis have correctly suggested the diagnosis of anal atresia.[22] However, in this case studied at 34 weeks it was thought that the absence of a fistulous tract contributed to the distended bowel observed in the pelvis. Dilated ureters should not be mistaken for abnormal bowel and examination of the kidneys should help make this distinction.

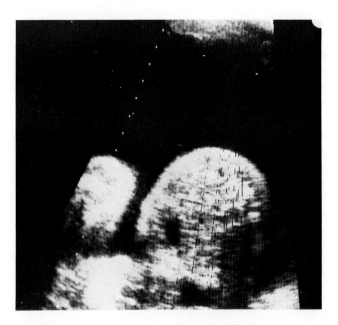

Fig. 13. Cross section of fetal abdomen below the level of the heart and chest. The circumference measured below two standard deviations for gestational age and the child was shown to have a large diaphragmatic hernia at birth.

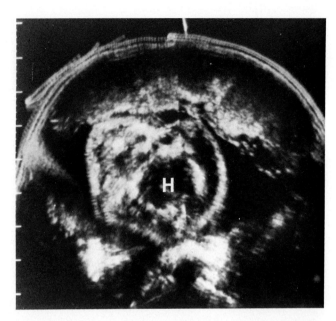

Fig. 14. A transverse section of the fetal chest at the level of the heart (H) shows a pleural effusion and irregular mass in the fetal chest. Fetal ascites was also present in this child with cystic adenomatoid malformation of the lung.

DIAPHRAGMATIC HERNIA

Most diaphragmatic hernias seen in newborn infants are a result of large defects in the posterior lateral part of the diaphragm, on the left side in 85 to 90 percent of cases, resulting in herniation of abdominal contents into the chest and associated with hypoplasia of the lung. Ninety percent of hernias involve the small bowel and the liver is included in 50 percent of cases.[23] The stomach is often included as well. In about one-half of cases there is a membrane containing the herniated abdominal contents. Intestinal malrotation is usually present and occasionally other congenital abnormalities are seen. Rarely large defects may be seen in the anterior medial diaphragm. These may be associated with other congenital anomalies and if large may also cause respiratory compromise.

The sonographic recognition of diaphragmatic hernia depends on finding distended loops of bowel in the thoracic cavity. Generally these are not recognized until later in pregnancy, when the bowel becomes more distended and is more easily identified. In one case when herniated bowel could not be shown, the abdominal circumference was abnormally low and there was associated polyhydramnios (Fig. 13). In one reported case there was polyhydramnios and the fetal bowel was seen next to the fetal heart.[24] Diaphragmatic hernia has also been identified by amniography, in which contrast-filled loops of small bowel were seen

in the chest cavity.[25] There is very little reported experience with the antenatal diagnosis of diaphragmatic hernia, which is unfortunate since early recognition is crucial in management of these infants.

A multicystic mass in the chest may also be seen as a result of cystic adenomatoid malformations of the lung.[26,27] In all prenatally diagnosed patients, fetal hydrops has been observed in association with this condition (Fig. 14). We have seen one fetus in which there was ascites and fluid in the chest as a result of diaphragmatic hernia, which might be confused with the pleural effusions and ascites seen with cystic adenomatoid malformation of the lung. Probably the most direct way to distinguish between these two possibilities is direct demonstration of the fetal diaphragm. This can be done in coronal views, which are our preference, as well as sagittal views. To our knowledge this approach has not actually been used in a case.

BODY WALL DEFECTS

Defects in the midline of the abdominal wall can occur in a low position and are referred to as cloacal extrophy. This condition consists of an omphalocele, extrophy of the bladder with prolapsed terminal ileum or colon, and a second opening for the blind end of the colon. Although no ultrasound reports of this condition could be found in the English literature, because this combi-

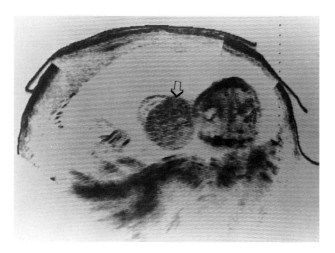

Fig. 15. Transverse section showing a large omphalocele (*arrows*) which contains largely liver. (*Reprinted with permission from Am J Roentgenol 138:1178, 1982.*)

nation of abnormalities occurs, investigation of the pelvis and bladder should be attempted when an omphalocele is found.

Defects of the midabdominal wall are usually a result of omphalocele or gastroschisis. Distinction between these two conditions can be made in utero. With an omphalocele the umbilical cord inserts into the base of the herniated mass that typically has a covering membrane. In most cases we have been able to review, the liver has been involved in the herniation although small bowel may be included as the only element seen in the mass (Fig. 15).[28-31] Unless the omphalocele is ruptured, the bowel may be difficult to recognize because of its solid appearance.[28] Although from the reported cases diagnosis usually occurs at 30 to 34 weeks, earlier recognition in the second trimester is possible.[1,30] Polyhydramnios is often present but not always severe. Complex defects have been reported that involve the upper abdominal wall, producing a large omphalocele, with defects in the lower sternum, anterior diaphragm in the diaphragmatic pericardium, and intracardiac defects (Fig. 16).[32]

In the case of gastroschisis the umbilicus is not involved and the opening is in the abdominal wall usually to the right of the umbilicus.[1,33] This condition has been recognized as early as 20 weeks' gestation, and later may have associated polyhydramnios. Some cases of unusually low or lateral positions of a gastroschisis have been described, but these represent variations of the amniotic band syndrome.[34] In one such case seen by ultrasound it was difficult to recognize the nature of the mass prenatally and even postnatally classification of the fetal abnormality was not easy.[35] With gastroschisis there is no covering membrane and almost always loops of bowel can be seen outside the

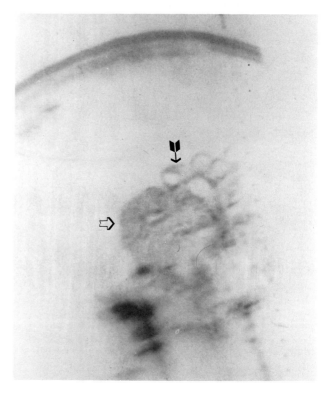

Fig. 16. A large defect involving the lower sternum and abdominal wall permits both liver (open arrow) and bowel (closed arrow) to herniate. (*Reprinted with permission from Winsberg and Copperberg (eds), Clinics in Diagnostic Ultrasound. New York, Churchill Livingston, vol 10, p 257.*)

fetal body. These may vary in appearance from ribbonlike structures to dilated loops with thick walls. This latter appearance is often associated with long-standing herniation and may indicate potential difficulty in reducing the bowel into the abdominal cavity because of thickening and fibrosis within the bowel wall and reduced capacity of the abdominal cavity. With gastroschisis there is usually a short fixation of the midgut that may lead to volvulus and Meckel's diverticulum may be present, but other anomalies are uncommon.

Distinction between gastroschisis and omphalocele can be made if an intact membrane is seen covering the herniated abdominal contents. However, distinction between a ruptured omphalocele and gastroschisis is not always possible (Fig. 17). When the liver is involved an omphalocele should be suspected and can be confirmed by seeing the umbilical cord insert into the base of the abnormality. Whenever bowel alone is seen herniated outside the abdomen then a gastroschisis should be the first choice. In many cases this distinction is unimportant since both require delivery by cesarean section with a pediatric surgeon in attendance. However, if omphalocele is suspected then a greater effort should be made to look for associated

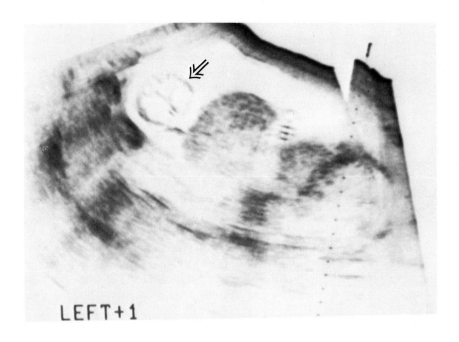

LEFT+1

Fig. 17. In this ruptured omphalocele distended loops of bowel are seen (*arrows*) outside the fetal abdomen. This condition is very difficult to distinguish from gastroschisis. (*Case provided by Roger C. Sanders, B.M.*)

anomalies, including intestinal atresias, stenoses, and renal abnormalities, cardiac anomalies, and cystichygroma.[36]

Omphalomesenteric duct anomalies are a spectrum of conditions that are the result of failure of the fetal vitelline duct to atrophy somewhere between the yolk sac and bowel lumen. The range of abnormalities produced range from umbilical polyps to omphalomesenteric sinuses. When this structure persists at its junction with the terminal ileum, it is referred to as Meckel's diverticulum. We are unaware of any case descriptions of these conditions diagnosed by ultrasound in utero.

MEGACYSTIS–MICROCOLON–INTESTINAL HYPOPERISTALSIS SYNDROME

This rare condition affects primarily female infants although a few cases involving males have been reported.[37,38] The most striking ultrasound finding in utero is the greatly distended fetal urinary bladder associated with hydronephrosis.[38,39] In some cases the bladder distension has been so great as to clinically and sonographically resemble polyhydraminios. This condition should be distinguished from Eagle–Barrett (prunebelly) syndrome, which is almost always found in males and does not involve the gastrointestinal tract (see Chapter 14). The distinction can be suspected in utero if a normal or increased amount of amniotic fluid is present which would be unusual for Eagle–Barrett syndrome or if the fetus is demonstrated to be female. However, often a distinction is not possible until the

neonatal period, when the gastrointestinal problems begin to appear. These cases are usually refractory to treatment and the prognosis is a grave one.

FETAL ASCITES

The normal echo-free area just inside the outer margin of the fetal abdominal wall should not be mistaken for ascites. Although the basis for this echo-free area is unclear it has been termed the "pseudoascites" sign (Fig. 18).[40] This phenomena can usually be distin-

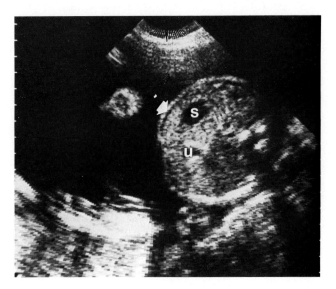

Fig. 18. Transverse section of the fetal abdomen showing the thin echo-free area (arrows) often referred to as "pseudoascites." Note the normal fetal stomach (S) and umbilical vein (Uv).

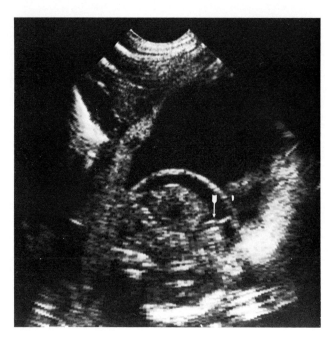

Fig. 19. Transverse section of a fetus with ascites shwoing the falciform ligament (arrow) that transverses the echo-free zone at the periphery of the abdomen.

guished from even small amounts of ascites by observing the nonuniform distribution of the ascites, the tendency of ascitic fluid to surround other abdominal organs, and the ability to visualize parts of the falciform ligament or the umbilical vein when ascites is present (Fig. 19).

Fetal ascites is commonly seen in association with hydrops.[41] This latter term often is used to indicate any edematous condition of the fetus but should be reserved for those cases showing some combination of pleural effusions, pericardial effusion, ascites, and skin edema when the underlying cause is heart failure, anemia, and hypoalbuminemia of the fetus. Thus hydrops is the typical abnormality seen in Rh (see Chapter 21) or other blood incompatibilities as well as large arteriovenous shunts or placental tumors. Morphologic abnormalities that can be found are listed in Table 1. In hydrops the umbilical vein is often enlarged and the fetal liver may be big. The placenta may be very large and may undergo trophoblastic hypertrophy, producing elevated human chronic gonadotrophin (hCG) levels, which in turn may produce theca lutein cysts in the mother.[42] It is unclear what the earliest

TABLE 1
Structural Anomalies Associated with Hydrops Fetalis That May Have Sonographic Manifestations

Fetus	Sonographic Manifestation	Abnormality
Head	Intracranial mass, associated with congestive heart failure and microcephaly	Arteriovenous malformation, vein of Galen aneurysm, cytomegalic inclusion virus, toxoplasmosis
Neck	Cystic neck masses	Lymphatic dysplasias
Thorax	Poorly contracting heart	Congestive heart failure
	Pericardial effusion, Tachycardia	Cardiac anomaly
	Asystole	Demise
	Mediastinal mass	Tumor
	Chest mass	Cystic adenomatoid malformation
	Small thorax	Dwarfism
	Cystic masses crossing diaphragm	Diaphragmatic hernias
Abdomen	Tubular anechoic structures	Gastrointestinal obstruction, atresias, or volvulus
	Abdominal masses	Tumors, neurofibromatosis
Retroperitoneum	Retroperitoneal mass	Neurogenic mass
	Hydronephrotic kidney	Hydronephrosis, posterior urethral valves
Extremities	Short arms, legs	Dwarfism
	Contractures	Arthrogryposis
	Fractures	Osteogenesis imperfecta
Placenta	Thick	Intrauterine infection, extramedullary hematopoiesis, anemia
	Mass	Chorioangioma
Amniotic Cavity	Number of fetuses, relative size, amniotic membrane	Twin–twin transfusion
	Umbilical cord anomalies	Single umbilical artery, umbilical cord torsion

Reprinted with permission from Fleischer AC, Killan AP, Bvehn FH, Hutchison AA, Jones TB, et al: Hydrops fetalis: Sonographic evaluation and clinical implications. Radiology 141:163, 1981.

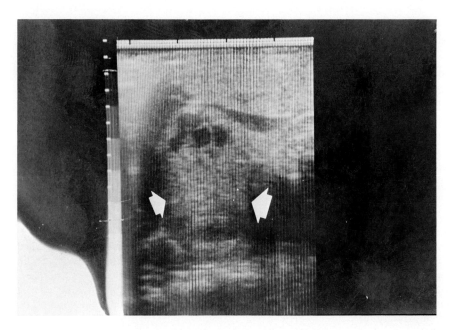

Fig. 20. A large mass (*arrows*) is seen at the caudal aspect of this fetus. Portions of the mass are fluid containing and this proved to be a sacrococcygeal teratoma. (*Case courtesy of Terry Silver, M. D., University of Michigan.*)

sonographic sign of hydrops is. This may be enlargement of the umbilical vein[43] or enlargement of the placenta.[44] Polyhydraminos may also be found with hydrops.

Cardiac causes of fetal ascites other than high-output heart failure are rare. Most common are abnormalities of cardiac rhythm, usually supraventricular tachycardia. Other causes include coarctation of the aorta, interruption of the aorta, and myocardial disorders. Fetal ascites may result from infections, bowel perforation, tumors, and twin–twin transfusions. In only one-quarter to one-half of fetuses with either ascites or hydrops will the abnormality be demonstrable by sonography.

OTHER CONDITIONS INVOLVING THE BODY WALL

Teratomas involve the cervical area, presacral area, and sacrococcygeal region. Those described in the literature have been primarily solid or mixed cystic and solid masses seen extending off the sacrum posteriorly (Fig. 20).[29,45,46] These masses have been detected as early as 16 weeks[46] and appear to enlarge with the pregnancy. These tumors are usually benign, but may be malignant in 10 to 30 percent of cases. Cystic portions and the presence of calcification suggest a benign tumor whereas elevation of AFP suggests a malignant one. Polyhydramnios is often found in conjunction with these masses and rarely hydrops of the fetus may result presumably from vascular shunting. Because these masses are highly vascular, extensive bleeding may oc-

cur; along with obstruction of labor, this is the major complication if these patients are permitted to be delivered vaginally. When a sacrococcygeal teratoma is suspected by ultrasound study a careful search should be made for other anomalies; these are present in about 20 percent of cases.

The Kleppel–Trenauney–Weber syndrome is a rare condition that consists of large cutaneous hemangiomas and asymmetric limb hypertrophy.[47] Since these masses may be located on the abdomen, buttocks, or legs, it is possible that they may be mistaken for either a teratoma or a gastroschisis as well as myelomeningocele. In the one reported case there was polyhydramnios with a normal amniotic fluid AFP. Since this condition does not require cesarean section and frequently spontaneously regresses, an effort should be made to distinguish these from other body wall masses. Comparison of limb lengths and identification of the multicentric distribution of the masses should help in this distinction.

CONCLUSION

In putting together the information for this chapter, the author is aware of many limitations that exist. First, there is actually little information available in the ultrasound literature dealing with examinations or discovery of abdominal abnormalities prenatally. Often only one or two case reports can be found. Second, there is a great deal of variation in the information presented in these reports, including differing uses of terminology and classifications. Finally, there is also a wide range of potential expressions of these conditions, and this alone produces some uncertainty that prior descriptions will be of benefit to readers when they are faced with the problem of prenatal diagnosis of a fetal abdominal abnormality. Some final suggestions are to look carefully and not focus on a study of only one area, to seek a second opinion whenever possible or when any uncertainty exists, to carefully document all observations, and to present your conclusions in the appropriate context of uncertainty that must surround a new and developing field.

REFERENCES

1. Jassani MN, Gauderer MWL, Fanaroff AA, et al: A perinatal approach to the diagnosis and management of gastrointestinal malformation. Obstet Gynecol 59:33, 1982
2. Alexander ES, Spitz HB, Clark RA: Sonography of polyhydramnios. Am J Roentgenol 138:343, 1982
3. Jacoly HE, Charles D: Clinical conditions associated with hydramnios. Am J Obstet Gynecol 94:910, 1966
4. Bowie JD, Clair MR: Fetal swallowing and regurgitation. Observation of normal and abnormal activity. Radiology 144:877, 1982
5. Dunne ME, Johnson ML: The ultrasonic demonstration of fetal abnormalities in utero. J Reprod Med 23:195, 1979
6. Christ JE, Meininger MG: Ultrasound diagnosis of cleft lip and cleft palate before birth. Plast Reconstr Surg 68:854, 1981
7. Gardner S, Burton BK, Johnson AM: Maternal serum alpha-fetoprotein screening: A report of the Forsyth County Project. Am J Obstet Gynecol 140:250, 1981
8. Hobbins JC, Venus I, Tortora M, et al: Stage II ultrasound examination for the diagnosis of fetal abnormalities with an elevated amniotic fluid alpha-fetoprotein concentration. Am J Obstet Gynecol 142:1026, 1982
9. Haught C: Congenital esophageal atresia and tracheoesophageal fistula, in Mustard WT, Ravitch MM, Synder WH, et al (eds), Pediatric Surgery. Chicago, Year Book, 1969, pp 357–379
10. Farrant P: The antenatal diagnosis of esophageal atresia by ultrasound. Br J Radiol 53:1202, 1980
11. Rao SB, Slovis TL, Cradock TV, et al: Visualization of the intestinal tract by amniography in a fetus with esophageal atresia. Pediatr Radiol 7:241, 1978
12. Lees RF, Alford BA, Brenbridge NAG, et al: Sonographic appearance of duodenal atresia in utero. Am J Roentgenol 131:701, 1978
13. Loveday BJ, Ban JA, Artkin J: The intrauterine demonstration of duodenal atresia by ultrasound. Br J Radiol 48:1031, 1975
14. Boychvek RB, Lyon EA, Goodhand TK: Duodenal atresia diagnosed by ultrasound. Radiology 127:500, 1978
15. Tabsh KMA: Antenatal sonographic appearance of a fetal ovarian cyst. J Ultrasound Med 1:329, 1982
16. Dewbery KC, Aluwihare M, Birch SJ, et al: Prenatal ultrasound demonstration of a choledochal cyst. Br J Radiol 53:906, 1982
17. Frank JL, Hill MC, Chirathivat S, et al: Antenatal observations of a choledochal cyst by sonography. Am J Roentgenol 137:166, 1981
18. Brugman SM, Bjelland JJ, Thomasson JE, et al: Sonographic findings with radiologic correlation in meconium peritonitis. J Clin Ultrasound 7:305, 1979
19. Lauer JD, Cradock TV: Meconium pseudocyst: Prenatal sonographic and antenatal radiologic correlation. J Ultrasound Med 1:333, 1982
20. Nikapota VLB, Lomann C: Gray scale sonographic demonstration of fetal small bowel atresia. J Clin Ultrasound 7:307, 1979
21. Skovb P, Smith-Jensen S: Hyperdistended fluid-filled bowel loops mimicking gastrointestinal atresia. J Clin Ultrasound 9:463, 1981
22. Bean WJ, Calonje MA, Aprill CN, et al: Anal atresia: A prenatal ultrasound diagnosis. J Clin Ultrasound 6:111, 1978
23. Bloss RS, Aranda JV, Beardmore HE: Congenital diaphragmatic hernia: Pathophysiology pharmacologic support. Surgery 89:518, 1981
24. Garrett WJ, Kossoff G: Gray scale examination of the fetus, in Sanders RC, James AE (eds.), Ultrasonography in Obstetrics and Gynecology. New York, Appleton-Century-Crofts, 1977, p 174
25. Marwood RP, Dawson OW: Antenatal diagnosis of diaphragmatic hernia. Br J Obstet Gynecol 88:71, 1981
26. Garrett WJ, Kossoff G, Lawrence R: Gray scale echography in the diagnosis of hydrops due to fetal lung tumor. J Clin Ultrasound 3:45, 1975
27. Graham D, Winn K, Dex W, et al: Prenatal diagnosis of cystic adenomatoid malformation of the lung. J Clin Ultrasound 1:9, 1982
28. Roberts C: Intrauterine diagnosis of omphalocele. Radiology 127:762, 1978
29. Zaleski AM, Cooperberg PL, Kliman MK: Ultrasonic diagnosis of extrafetal masses. J Can Assoc Radiol 30:55, 1979
30. Yaghoobian J, Chauday R, Pinck RL: Ante natal diagnosis of omphalocele by ultrasound. J Reprod Med 26:274, 1981
31. Nelson PA, Bowie JE, Filston HC, et al: Sonographic diagnosis of omphalocele in utero. Am J Roentgenol 138:1178, 1982
32. Wicks JD, Levine MD, Mettler FA: Intrauterine sonography of thoracic ectopic cordis. Am J Roentgenol 137:619, 1981
33. Giulian BB, Alvear DT: Prenatal ultrasonic diagnosis of fetal gastroschisis. Radiology 129:473, 1978
34. Neri A, Ovadia Y, Merlov P, et al: Amniotic band syndrome. Isr J Med Sci 18:505, 1981
35. Fried AM, Wooding JH, Shier RW, et al: Omphalocele in limb/body wall deficiency syndrome: Atypical sonographic appearance. J Clin Ultrasound 10:400, 1982
36. Mahour GH, Weitzman JS, Rosenkrantz JG: Omphalocele and gastroschisis. Ann Surg 117:478, 1973

37. Young LW, Yumis EJ, Girdany BR, et al: Megacystis-microcolon-intestinal hypoperistalsis syndrome: Additional clinical, radiologic, surgical, and histopathologic aspects. Am J Roentgenol 136:649, 1981
38. Krook PM: Megacysts-microcolon-intestinal hypoperistalsis syndrome in a male infant. Radiology 136:649, 1980
39. Vezina WC, Morin FR, Winsberg F: Megacystis-microcolon-intestinal hypoperistalsis syndrome: Antenatal ultrasound appearance. Am J Roentgenol 133:749, 1979
40. Rosenthal SJ, Filly RA, Callen PW, et al: Fetal pseudoascites. Radiology 131:195, 1979
41. Fleischer AC, Killam AP, Boehm FH, et al: Hydrops fetalis: Sonographic evaluation and clinical implications. Radiology 141:163, 1981
42. Fleming P, McLeary RD: Nonimmunologic fetal hydrops with theca lutin cysts. Radiology 141:169, 1981
43. Mayden KL: The umbilical vein diameter in Rh isoimmunization. Med Ultrasound 4:119, 1980
44. Kassner EG, Cromb E: Sonographic diagnosis of fetal hydrops. Radiology 115:399, 1975
45. Lees KF, Williamson BRJ, Brenbudge NAG, et al: Sonography of benign sacral teratoma in utero. Radiology 134:717, 1980
46. Seeds JW, Mittelstaedt CA, Cefola RC, et al: Prenatal diagnosis of sacrococcygeal teratoma: An anechoic caudal mass. J Clin Ultrasound 10:193, 1982
47. Hatjis CG, Philip AE, Anderson GG, et al. The in utero ultrasonographic appearance of Klippel–Treneauney–Weber syndrome. Am J Obstet Gynecol 139:972, 1981

18 | The Diagnosis of Abnormalities of the Fetal Central Nervous System

J. Malcolm Pearce
David Little
Stuart Campbell

In the 3 years since the last edition of this book there has been a marked improvement in ultrasound equipment together with a wider use of ultrasound in early pregnancy to confirm gestational age and exclude multiple gestation. This, and an expansion of screening by means of maternal serum α-fetoprotein (MSAFP), has increased our work load from referrals. Table 1 illustrates the change in reasons for referral. There has been a substantial increase in patients referred because of a raised MSAFP and an increase in patients referred because of suspicious ultrasound findings. We hope that this chapter will demonstrate that high resolution ultrasound (often called level II scanning) is the most accurate way to diagnose structural anomalies in the fetus. At present, limited resources only allow patients at high risk of a structural abnormality to have a high-resolution ultrasound performed by an obstetric ultrasonographer, but in the foreseeable future this facility will be offered to every pregnant woman. Table 2 illustrates the results that can be obtained from a routine ultrasound clinic in which although the majority of the ultrasound examinations were performed by nonmedical personnel, the training and supervision of such personnel is performed by obstetric sonologists.

This chapter will emphasize the diagnosis of abnormalities before the 26th week of gestation when the option of termination of pregnancy may be offered to the parents. We shall attempt to indicate the present role of an ultrasound examination in the diagnosis of abnormalities and hopefully give some indication of the future use of ultrasound in this area. Most of the conclusions will be based upon the results from our clinic at King's College Hospital (KCH), where between 1978 and June 1983 we have examined 2372 patients carrying a fetus at a high risk of a structural abnormality.

PRENATAL DIAGNOSIS OF NEURAL TUBE DEFECTS

The incidence of neural tube defects (NTD) varies from 1.2 per 1000 births in Japan to 8.1 per 1000 births in South Wales (Table 3). Caucasians, particularly those of Celtic origin, are at increased risk. Although the incidence of NTD is lower in the United States than in the United Kingdom it is higher on the Atlantic coast than on the Pacific coast.

The cause of NTD is unknown but has produced many ingenious theories. The present theory is that it is due to a relative deficiency of vitamins. Smithells and colleagues[1] have shown that the incidence of recurrent NTD may be reduced by giving periconceptional vitamin supplements. This is now the subject of a double-blind prospective trial but both the original study and the trial have been open to controversy.[2]

Prenatal diagnosis of NTD is desirable because anencephaly is invariably fatal and the outlook for babies with spina bifida is far from good. In a study of open spina bifida children carried out in a center designed to provide maximum support and treatment for these children two-thirds died in the first 5 years of life and of the remainder only 15 percent were free from major handicap.[3] Although NTD are recurrent (Table 4) more than 90 percent occur in patients that are not at risk. Fortunately, a screening test is available in the form of MSAFP.

TABLE 1
Reasons for Referral for High-Resolution Ultrasound
Examination to Exclude NTD
(1974–June 1983)

Reason for Referral	1974–1978	1978–June 1983	Total
Previously affected infant with:			
NTD	249	240	489
Isolated hydrocephaly	21	83	104
Microcephaly	5	45	50
Family history of NTD	16	121	137
Raised MSAFP	5	477	482
Raised AFAFP	15	100	115
Suspicious ultrasound	1	127	128
Total	312	1193	1505

α-Fetoprotein

α-Fetoprotein (AFP) is an oncofetal protein that is produced from the yolk sac in the embryo and from the liver in the fetus. Normally, it is virtually undetectable in the serum of the normal, nonpregnant female. AFP reaches the amniotic fluid via excretion from the fetal kidneys. Transfer of AFP from amniotic fluid to maternal serum appears to be by direct transfer across the placenta.[4] Fetal serum and amniotic fluid AFP reach a peak at about 16 to 18 weeks' gestation but the level in maternal serum continues to rise until about 32 weeks' gestation. This has been attributed to increasing placental permeability. Conditions such as NTD and omphalocele, in which there is a breakdown in the barriers between the fetal circulation and the amniotic fluid will lead to increased levels of amniotic fluid AFP which will be reflected in MSAFP. Impaired fetal swallowing or increased permeability in the fetal kidneys will also increase the amniotic fluid AFP. Increased placental permeability will increase the MSAFP without increasing the level in the amniotic fluid.

The first report of the UK Collaborative Study[7] recommended that MSAFP levels should be expressed in multiples of the median (MOM) rather than centiles, as MOM are less dependent upon laboratory precision than centiles. The upper level of normal recommended by the study was 2.5 MOM.[7] Using this level one can expect to detect 88 percent of anencephalics and 79 percent of open spina bifida if the MSAFP is estimated between 16 and 18 weeks' gestation.[7]

Not all patients with a MSAFP value above 2.5 MOM will be carrying a fetus with a neural tube defect. Table 5 lists some of the other important causes of a raised MSAFP, but it should be remembered that approximately 2 percent of an apparently normal population will have a raised MSAFP. MSAFP levels are very dependent upon gestational age so it is necessary to have a routine ultrasound service to confirm gestational age if a MSAFP screening program is offered. Simple ultrasound examination will also exclude multiple pregnancy and anencephaly (see below) as causes of a raised MSAFP. In areas with an incidence of NTD of 3 per 1000 births two consecutive raised MSAFP values suggests a 1 in 20 chance of the patient carrying a fetus with a neural tube defect.[7] In order to determine the cause of the raised MSAFP it is usual to proceed to amniocentesis to estimate amniotic fluid AFP (AFAFP) and acetylcholinesterase.

TABLE 2
Ultrasound Prenatal Diagnosis before 26 Weeks
from the Routine Clinic at KCH
(1978–June 1983; 11,664 deliveries)

Abnormality	Antenatal Clinic Detected	Antenatal Clinic Missed	Pregnancy Diabetic Clinic Detected	Pregnancy Diabetic Clinic Missed
Anencephaly	5	0	1	0
Spina bifida	7	0	0	0
Hydrocephaly	4	0	2	0
Encephalocele	1	0	0	0
Holoprosencephaly	0	0	1	0
Microcephaly	0	1	1	0
Duodenal atresia	1	0	0	0
Omphalocele	3	0	0	0
Renal anomalies	3	1	0	0
Fetal tumours	4	0	0	0
Cystic hygroma	1	0	0	0
Cardiac anomalies	0	0	0	3
Sacral agenesis	0	0	0	1
Total	29	2	5	4

TABLE 3
Incidence of NTD in Various Populations
(per 1000 Births)

Population	Spina Bifida	Anencephaly	Hydrocephaly	Total
South Wales	4.1	3.5	0.5	8.1
Charleston USA				
Caucasian	1.5	1.2	0.8	3.5
Negro	0.6	0.2	1.1	1.9
Japan	0.3	0.6	0.3	1.2

Amniocentesis

This is best performed under ultrasound guidance (see Chapter 28). A raised AFAFP will detect 98 percent of all NTD but carries a 1 in 200 false positive rate.[8] This figure can be reduced considerably by also performing an electrophoresis for acetylcholinesterase on the amniotic fluid.[9]

The procedure of amniocentesis carries a risk to a potentially ongoing normal pregnancy. A British study on the hazards of amniocentesis[10] suggested that the risk of fetal loss before 28 weeks' gestation was increased by 1 to 1.5 percent in patients undergoing amniocentesis. The study also showed late sequelae in the form of an unexpected increase in the incidence of respiratory distress syndrome and in major postural deformities. This study is in contrast to American[11] and Canadian[12] studies in which almost no effect was shown from amniocentesis. The studies are summarized in Table 6. All are open to criticism, especially over the selection of controls. For example, the British study[10] had an excess of older mothers and a deficiency of primigravidae in the group undergoing amniocentesis. Although it is difficult to draw conclusions from such discordant results we feel that there is probably an increased risk of pregnancy loss in patients undergoing amniocentesis but that it is only a very small increase.

Although the use of amniocentesis to resolve the problem of a raised MSAFP has a very low false positive rate if both AFAFP and acetylcholinesterase are

estimated these methods cannot give an accurate diagnosis of the severity and site of the neural tube defect. Not all patients carrying fetuses with a NTD will wish to undergo a termination of pregnancy if the defect is low and is not associated with hydrocephaly. The alternative to amniocentesis is a high-resolution ultrasound examination.

ANENCEPHALY

In 1972, Campbell et al.[13] reported the first termination of an anencephalic fetus diagnosed ultrasonically at 17 weeks' postmenstrual age. The absence of the cranial vault is readily appreciated on ultrasound examination from 12 weeks' gestation (Fig. 1). It may, with real-time apparatus, be evident before that time, although the decision to terminate the pregnancy is probably best left to 14 weeks' gestation to reduce the chance of error.

Table 7 includes the positive diagnosis of anencephaly in our unit. There have been no false positive diagnoses. Six of the cases were diagnosed from our

TABLE 4
Risks of Recurrence of NTD

History	Recurrence Risk
One previously affected infant	1 in 20
Two previously affected infants	1 in 10
Three previously affected infants	1 in 4
One parent affected	1 in 30

Reprinted with permission from Smith C: Computer programme to estimate recurrence risks for multifactorial familial disease. Br Med J 1:495, 1972.

TABLE 5
Cause of Raised MSAFP

Cause	Means of Resolution
Laboratory error	Repeat sample Use MOM (see text)
Incorrect gestational age Multiple gestation Hydatidiform mole Anencephaly	Simple ultrasound examination
Spina bifida Encephalocele Omphalocele Gastroschisis Renal dysplasia Infantile polycystic kidneys Obstructive uropathy	High-resolution ultrasound examination
Congenital Finnish nephrosis	Fetal bladder puncture (very high AFP in fetal urine)

TABLE 6
Fetal Loss as a Result of Mid-trimester
Amniocentesis for Prenatal Diagnosis

Study	MRC[a]		NICHD		Canadian
	A	C	A	C	A
No. of Cases	2428	2428	1040	992	1020
Fetal loss (%)	4.8	2.3	3.5	3.2	5.2

[a] A = amniocentesis subjects; C = controls.

routine ultrasound screening clinic (Table 2). All the cases were diagnosed before the MSAFP result was available and we have had no false positive and no missed cases of anencephaly. Ultrasound is the ideal method of detecting this condition, and confirmation by AFAFP is unnecessary.

Acrania is a similar anomaly in which there is absence of the cranium but with complete but abnormal development of brain tissue. The outlines of the brain structures are distorted and not surrounded by the well-defined echogenic line seen when a skull is present.[14]

SPINA BIFIDA

Campbell et al.[15] originally described the method for detecting spina bifida by performing a series of scans

with the static B-mode scanner along the entire length of the fetal spine at right angles to the long axis. The examination is quicker and easier with real-time apparatus. The normal spine with its intact neural arch appears as a closed circle whereas the incomplete neural arch appears as a saucer or U-shaped complex (Fig. 4). Care is needed, however, as this appearance can be produced artifactually by failing to keep the transducer exactly at right angles to the long axis of the spine. Having examined each vertebrae in the transverse plane the transducer should then be rotated until the fetal spine appears anteriorly on the screen. A longitudinal scan will then demonstrate the entire length of the fetal spine with the skin covering and the characteristic sacral curve (Fig. 2).

In practice we use a combination of both transverse and longitudinal views. The longitudinal view can be deceiving especially for low sacral lesions. Figure 3 illustrates a longitudinal section of a spine that ap-

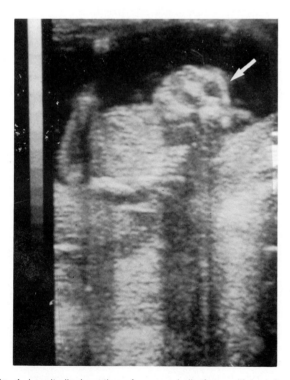

Fig. 1. Longitudinal section of anencephalic fetus with an absent cranial vault (*arrow*).

TABLE 7
Structural Abnormalities of the Fetal Central Nervous System Diagnosed Before 26 Weeks' Gestation (1978–June 1983)

Abnormality	Detected	Not Detected
Anencephaly	48	0
Spina bifida (open)	92	7
Spina bifida (closed)	5	0
Encephalocele	20	1
Isolated hydrocephaly	26	2
Microcephaly	9	0
Iniencephaly	3	0
Holoprosencephaly	1	0
Hydranencephaly	4	0
Macrocephaly	1	0
Porencephalic cyst	1	0
Sacral agenesis	0	1
Absent cerebellum	1	0
Dandy–Walker malformation	3	0
Joubert syndrome	1	0
Choroid plexus cysts	7	0
Scaphocephaly	1	0
Total	234	11

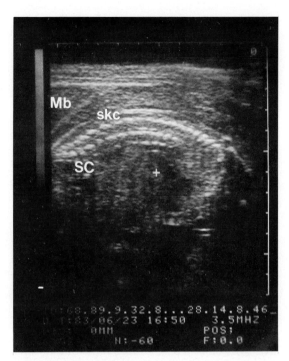

Fig. 2. Longitudinal section to show an intact fetal spine. The characteristic sacral curve (SC) and the skin covering (Skc) are also demonstrated. Mb = Maternal Bladder.

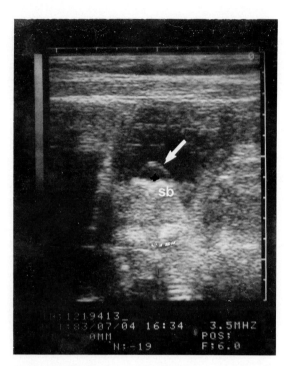

Fig. 4. A transverse section at sacral level demonstrating the bony defect of spina bifida (Sb) together with the sac of a meningocele (*arrow*).

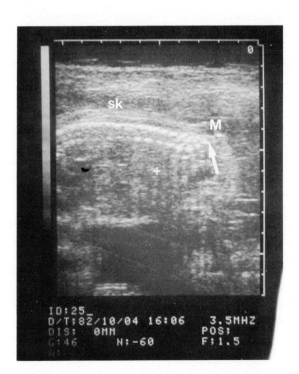

Fig. 3. A real-time picture of the longitudinal view of a spine with a sacral spina bifida. The arrow indicates an apparently intact sacrum. The echoes from the ossification centers in the spine appear normal but the transverse section at sacral level (Fig. 4) shows the meningocele. There is a suggestion of a bulge in the skin over the sacrum. Sk = skin covering, M = suggestion of a meningocele.

pears to be intact except perhaps for a bulge in the skin covering the sacrum, but as Figure 4 demonstrates this fetus has an obvious meningocele on transverse section at sacral level.

A high-resolution real-time apparatus not only allows a diagnosis of spina bifida to be made with ease but also will allow the site and the extent of the lesion to be predicted with a high degree of accuracy. The type of lesion may also be determined. A closed lesion will show the bony defect of spina bifida with skin covering. The bulge of a meningocele (Fig. 5) can be visualized and the presence of strands of nervous tissue within that bulge will allow the diagnosis of meningomyelocele to be made. The accurate identification of the site, extent, and type of lesion together with the presence of absence of hydrocephaly (see below) will allow a realistic prognosis to be given to the parents. If they choose to let the pregnancy continue the degree of hydrocephaly should be carefully monitored; if marked deterioration occurs in the third trimester then preterm delivery or draining of the cerebral ventricles in utero should be considered (see also the section on Hydrocephaly and Chapter 22).

In our unit at KCH, 92 cases of spina bifida have been correctly diagnosed (Table 7). We have missed seven cases of spina bifida, but five of these were low sacral lesions and were early in our experience. In the

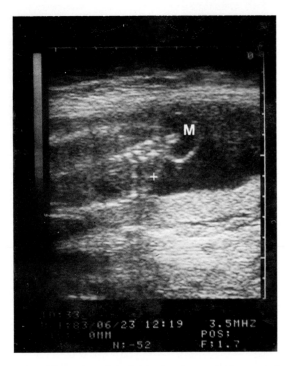

Fig. 5. An oblique view of the fetal spine demonstrating a meningocele (M). The absence of echoes within the sac excludes the diagnosis of meningomyelocele.

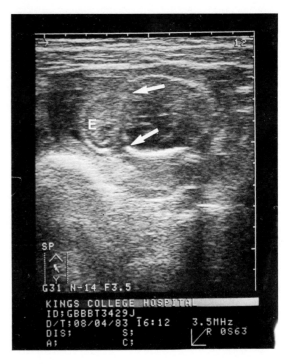

Fig. 6. A real-time picture of an encephalocele (E). Brain tissue occupies the encephalocele. The arrows point to bony defects in vault.

past 3 years our experience has increased and the resolution of the equipment has now improved such that we have only missed two cases in these years. We have had two false positive cases in which the presence of hydrocephaly was correctly diagnosed but in which the presence of associated spina bifida was incorrectly diagnosed. These are the results we have obtained from more than 1500 referrals of patients at risk of a neural tube defect. Since 1979 we have evaluated all our cases of raised MSAFP by high-resolution ultrasound examination and have not resorted to amniocentesis.

It should be noted that the exclusion of the diagnosis of spina bifida is made from the finding of a structurally normal fetal spine and not from observations of normal fetal leg movements or bladder emptying. We have observed apparently normal limb movements in cases of both spina bifida and anencephaly. We have only observed one case of spina bifida in which there was an obviously enlarged fetal bladder.

The majority of fetuses with spina bifida with or without coexisting hydrocephaly have a small biparietal diameter[16] and head circumference[17] for gestational age whereas measurements of the abdominal circumference and femur length are appropriate for gestational age. Caution should be observed in correcting the gestational age when this discrepancy is noticed and a diligent search should be made for spina bifida.

ENCEPHALOCELE

Encephalocele is recognized as a defect in the cranial vault, most commonly in the occiput. The defect may range from a simple bulging occipital meningocele containing no or minimal brain tissue to a major vault defect with large quantities of fetal brain in the sac—exencephaly. Figure 6 illustrates an encephalocele.

The diagnosis is usually apparent but small lesions may be missed if the cranial vault is not examined in detail. We have diagnosed 20 of the 21 cases we have had referred to our unit (Table 7). The missed lesion was an occipital meningocele with a bony defect that measured 1 cm at birth. The defect has been closed and the child has no residual neurologic impairment.

An encephalocele may form part of Meckel syndrome together with polycystic, kidneys and polydactyly. The diagnosis is important because Meckel syndrome has an autosomal recessive mode of inheritance whereas isolated hydrocephaly shows a multifactorial mode of inheritance.

HYDROCEPHALY (VENTRICULOMEGALY)

Lorber[18] observed that nearly all neonates with spina bifida have pathologically dilated ventricles. In our ex-

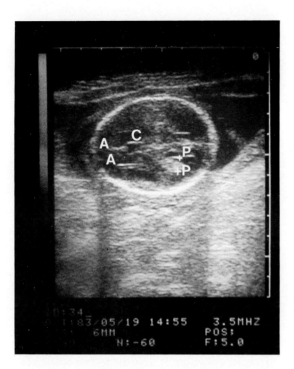

Fig. 7. A transverse section of a normal fetal head to demonstrate the anterior (A) and posterior (P) horns of the lateral cerebral ventricle. The midline echo broken in its anterior third by the cavum septii pellucidii (C) is also demonstrated.

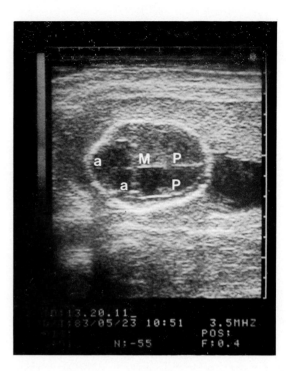

Fig. 8. A transverse section of a fetal head demonstrating ventriculomegaly. M = Midline, a = dilated anterior horn, P = dilated posterior horn.

perience about 80 percent of fetuses diagnosed as having spina bifida before 24 weeks' gestation also have dilated ventricles. Figure 7 illustrates a transverse section of the fetal head demonstrating the anterior and posterior horns of the cerebral ventricles. The ovoid fetal head is bisected by a central line that represents the echo from the medial aspects of the two cerebral hemispheres. The line is broken in its anterior third by the cavum septi pellucidi. Anterior to the cavum and parallel with the midline lie the echoes from the lateral border of the anterior horn of the lateral cerebral ventricle. The medial border of the ventricle is lost in the echo from the septum pellucidum. Posteriorly, the echoes from both the medial and lateral borders of the posterior horn of the lateral cerebral ventricle may be seen. Within the body and in the posterior horn of the lateral ventricle the choroid plexus is visible.

The diagnosis of ventriculomegaly is usually apparent (Fig. 8) but is best made by measurement of the anterior horn ventricular-hemisphere ratio (AVHR). This, as it was originally described[19] involved measurement of the lateral border of the distal anterior horn to the midline and then expressing this as a ratio of the distal cerebral hemisphere (midline to inner table of the skull). It should then be compared with the chart (Fig. 9). In practice a AVHR of more than 0.5

after 18 weeks' gestational age is pathologic. As can be seen from Figure 9 all but one of the pathologically proven cases of ventriculomegaly that we have diagnosed before 26 weeks' gestation have had an AVHR well above the upper limits of the normal range. In general, cases of isolated hydrocephaly have a higher AVHR than those associated with spina bifida.

Recently we have recognized several cases of ventriculomegaly in which the AVHR was borderline (or, in one case normal) where there was dilatation of the posterior horn of the lateral cerebral ventricle.[20] Our nomogram of posterior horn ventricular-hemisphere ratio (PHVR) has been published[21] and is illustrated in Figure 10 together with cases of pathologically proven hydrocephaly. In Figure 11, the case had a normal AHVR at 23 weeks' gestation but the PHVR was pathologic. This prompted detailed scanning of the spine, which revealed a meningomyelocele extending from the fourth lumber vertebrae to the fourth sacral vertebrae. The lesion and the pathologic dilatation of the posterior horn of the cerebral ventricle were confirmed at postmortem.

Ventriculomegaly associated with spina bifida usually prompts the parents to request a termination. In isolated ventriculomegaly, attempts have been made to drain the ventricle into the amniotic cavity and they have been reviewed in the report from the Kroc

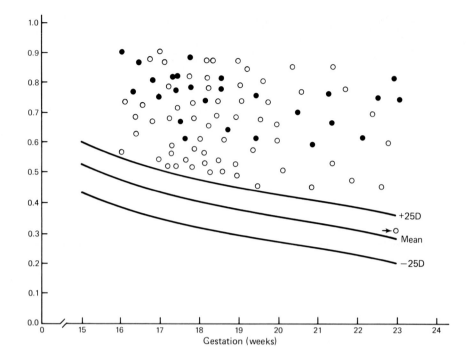

Fig. 9. The nomogram of the anterior horn to hemisphere ratio (AVHR). Pathologically proven cases of hydrocephaly are plotted and most are well above the normal range (closed circles are isolated hydrocephaly). (See text for discussion of arrowed case.)

Foundation.[22] Eight fetuses have undergone ventriculoamniotic shunt for isolated ventriculomegaly and in seven a decrease in ventricular size has been obtained. Six fetuses have survived the procedure and all received conventional shunts after birth. We await the long-term neurologic follow-up on these patients with interest. Until this is known we shall continue to offer

termination of pregnancy to our patients in whom ventriculomegaly is diagnosed before 26 weeks. We justify this in that, in general, infants that require to have a shunt inserted for ventriculomegaly in the first year of their lives have a poorer prognosis than those requiring shunt after the first year of life.[23]

We have included isolated ventriculomegaly with

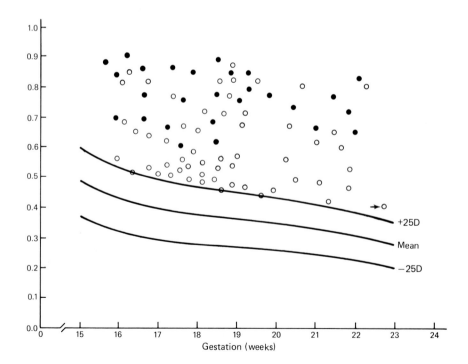

Fig. 10. The nomogram of the posterior horn to hemisphere ratio (PVHR). Again, pathologically proven cases are well above the normal range. The case arrowed showed a normal AVHR but a high PHVR and was associated with a large meningomyelocele.

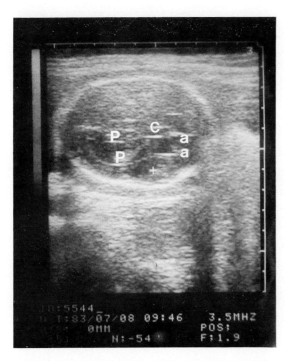

Fig. 11. A transverse section of the fetal head at 23 weeks' gestation. The AHVR and PHVR are arrowed in Figures 9 and 10. C = cavum septi pellucidi, a = dilated anterior horn, P = dilated posterior horn.

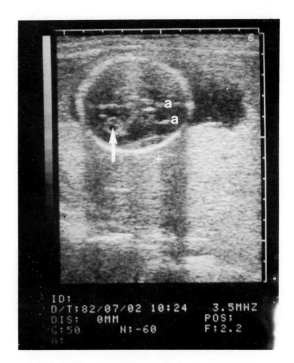

Fig. 12. A transverse section of a fetal head demonstrating a transient cyst of the choroid plexus (*arrow*). a = anterior horn.

NTDs, as the ultrasound diagnosis is the same as for ventriculomegaly associated with spina bifida; however, it is a separate etiologic entity from NTD[24] and shows a different pattern of inheritance. The risk of recurrence of isolated ventriculomegaly is about 3 percent but cases in which the isolated ventriculomegaly is due to aqueduct stenosis show a sex-linked recessive pattern of inheritance and will therefore affect 50 percent of subsequent male infants.

We should introduce a note of caution over scanning patients at risk of sex-linked ventriculomegaly. Although the ventriculomegaly may be apparent at 16 to 18 weeks' gestation it may not appear until later in the pregnancy.[25,26] We, therefore scan such patients every month from 16 to 28 weeks' gestation. In a recent report[27] of ventriculomegaly ultrasonically diagnosed in a fetus of a patient known to be at risk of sex-linked hydrocephalus postmortem did not show aqueduct stenosis, perhaps suggesting that aqueduct stenosis is secondary to the hydrocephalus. This suggests that if termination is carried out on ultrasound evidence and the fetus is male then care should be taken before giving a prognosis because, even if aqueduct stenosis is not present, there may be a sex-linked inheritance pattern.

OTHER CENTRAL NERVOUS SYSTEM ABNORMALITIES

Brain Cysts

Not all intracranial anomalies carry a poor prognosis. We have recently described a transient cyst of the choroid plexus.[28] These lesions are probably developmental and may be seen within the choroid plexus in the body and posterior horn of the lateral cerebral ventricle from 16 weeks' gestation onward (Fig. 12). They are probably always bilateral but reverberation prevents the visualization of the more proximal choroid plexus. In all cases they have disappeared by 26 weeks' gestation and detailed follow-up on the infants has failed to reveal any neurologic abnormality.

Porencephalic cysts, however, have a much gloomier prognosis. They result from resolution of an intracerebral hemorrhage and are most commonly diagnosed postnatally following a grade IV intraventricular hemorrhage. We have diagnosed two such cysts antenatally. One arose spontaneously but the other followed a severe hypoxic insult to the mother. This latter patient was an epileptic who developed status epilepticus during the course of her pregnancy. She required a prolonged period of intermittent positive

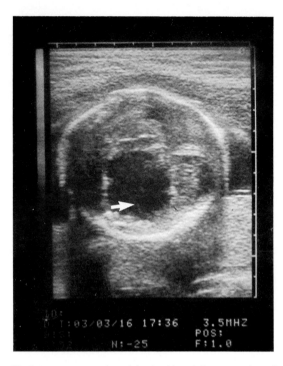

Fig. 13. A transverse section of the fetal head demonstrating a large porencephalic cyst (*arrow*).

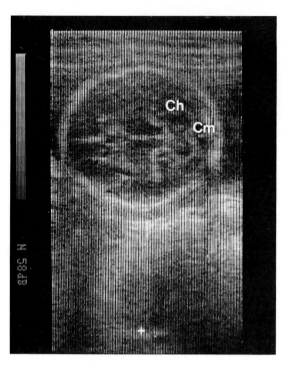

Fig. 14. A suboccipital bregmatic view (sobv) demonstrating a normal cerebellum. ch = cerebella hemisphere, cm = cysterna magna.

pressure ventilation. On recovery her fetus underwent an ultrasound examination to determine its growth pattern and it was noted to have an echo-free space in its brain. We were able to diagnose the porencephalic cyst but the fetus died a few weeks later. A similiar outcome was reported by Awoust et al.[29] in which a porencephalic cyst was diagnosed in a fetus following maternal cardiac and respiratory arrest. These authors were able to record the agonal convulsions of the fetus as it died. The outcome for antenatally diagnosed porencephalic cysts depends upon the size and site. Figure 13 illustrates a porencephalic cyst that appeared to arise spontaneously and for which because of its size the patient underwent a termination of pregnancy. Several intracranial hemorrhages have been detected in utero. Whether the hemorrhage is intraventricular or parenchymal, it results in an echogenic area which over a period of time will either cause hydrocephalus or a porencephalic cyst.[30-32]

Tumors have also been seen in utero. A teratoma[33] and a malignant CNS tumor[34] were recognized because there were numerous abnormal echoes within the brain substance.

Posterior Fossa and Cerebellar Anomalies

Having examined the cerebral ventricles, attention should now naturally turn to the posterior fossa and its contents. The view required to examine the poste-

rior fossa is a suboccipital bregmatic view (Fig. 14). This is obtained by finding the view for the cerebral ventricles and rotating the transducer in a cephalad direction.

Our nomogram of the growth of the cerebellar hemispheres has been published.[23] Essentially the diagnosis of posterior fossa abnormalities is made by comparing the cerebellar hemispheres with each other and by measuring the cysterna magna. The cerebellum may have an absent or hypoplastic vermis in two conditions. The first is the Dandy–Walker malformation in which there is thought to be a relative obstruction to the foramen of Magendie that results in a cyst of the fourth ventricle that destroys the cerebellar vermis. This is a sporadic condition that may be associated with polydactyly and after birth is always associated with excessive enlargement of the head. It is not amenable to surgical decompression although shunting does help. The second condition resulting in absence or hypoplasia of the cerebellar vermis is Joubert syndrome.[35] This is an extremely rare condition in which there is complete or partial agenesis of the cerebellar vermis, resulting in a large fourth ventricle that communicates with the cysterna magna. It is associated with the clinical syndrome of episodic hyperpnea, abnormal eye movements, ataxia, and mental retardation. This syndrome shows an autosomal mode of inheritance and its prenatal diagnosis has only recently been described.[36] It is

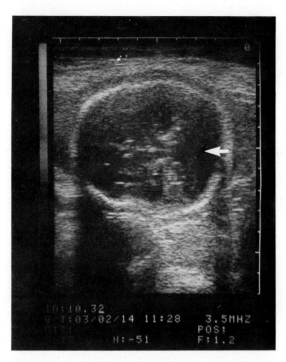

Fig. 15. A suboccipital bregmatic view demonstrating a Dandy–Walker malformation. (See text.)

nosologically different from the Dandy–Walker syndrome but the ultrasound appearances of the two conditions may be remarkably similar. We have succeeded in diagnosing three cases of the Dandy–Walker syndrome (Fig. 15) before 26 weeks' gestation and one case of Joubert syndrome. We made the differentiation upon the family history and not upon the ultrasound appearances.

Another condition with a similar sonographic appearance is an extra-axial posterior fossa cyst. In this syndrome the cerebellum is intact and not hypoplastic. The cerebellum, particularly the echogenic vermis, can be seen between the cyst and the tentorium.[37]

Absence of the cerebellum may occur in trisomies particularly those involving chromosomes 15 or 18. Agenesis may also occur with spina bifida, microcephaly, or hydrocephaly. Unilateral agenesis has been described and may be compatible with a normal existance or may result in spastic diplegia.

Microcephalus

Microcephalus means a small brain enclosed within a small skull. As head growth is determined by brain growth the primary defect in microcephaly lies in the development of the cerebrum.[38] Most authors report microcephalus if the head circumference is equal or less than 3 standard deviations below the mean[39] but if postmortem evidence is available then brain weight

TABLE 8
Causes of Microcephaly

Rubella infection
Cytomegalic virus infection
Toxoplasmosis infection
Severe irradiation
Chronic maternal mercury poisoning
Maternal heroin addiction
Maternal alcoholism
Autosomal recessive condition

should be the criteria. Infants born with microcephalus are always of severely subnormal intellect. As brain growth also affects stature the survivors are often underweight and dwarfed.

Microcephalus may be caused by various factors. Some of the more well-known causes are listed in Table 8. Prenatal diagnosis of this condition is desirable but as there is no structural defect it is not always easy. It may well be that some of the factors causing microcephalus do not operate until late pregnancy and that the diagnosis cannot therefore be made before 26 weeks' gestation. The diagnosis is best made by demonstrating impairment of head growth (biparietal diameter and head circumference) with normal growth of the abdominal circumference and femur. Serial examinations are necessary preferably beginning with a crown–rump length in the first trimester so that gestational age may be accurately established. The subsequent lower growth rate of the head results in a fall in the head circumference to abdominal circumference (H/A) ratio.[40] There is an association with trisomy chromosomal anomalies.

From our referral clinic we have been successful in diagnosing nine patients that were carrying a fetus with microcephaly before 26 weeks' gestation and have not missed any patients. However, as Figure 16 shows, we did not make the diagnosis in one patient until after 24 weeks' gestation. It may well be that in some instances the slowing of the head growth does not occur until after 26 weeks' gestation. We have had no experience of diagnosing microcephaly by comparison of intraorbital distances.[41] (See Chapter 19).

Microcephalus is a diagnosis that may well not be detected on routine scanning at 16 to 18 weeks' gestation. We have missed one from our routine antenatal scanning, which occurred in the pregnancy of a teenage girl.

Rare CNS Abnormalities

Rare CNS abnormalities are listed in Table 7. Iniencephaly is characterized by gross hyperextension of the fetal head with fusion of the occiput to the cervical vertebrae (Fig. 17). Holoprosencephaly is replacement

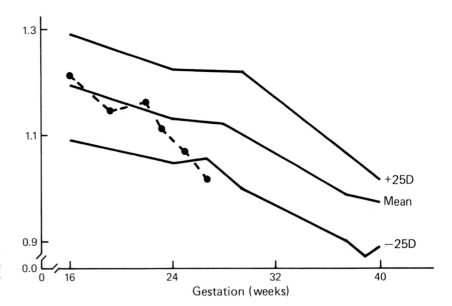

Fig. 16. The head/abdominal circumference ratio chart in a case of microcephaly. Note the diagnosis was not apparent until 24 weeks' after gestation.

of the two lateral cerebral ventricle with a single ventricle in the midline (see Chapter 19.) We have diagnosed such a case in the infant of a diabetic mother. The fetus also had phocomelia. Hydranencephaly is thought to occur when there is occlusion of both carotid arteries early in development. It is easily diagnosed on ultrasound (Fig. 18) in that there is a complete lack of echoes from the contents of the vault as the cerebrum is replaced entirely by fluid and partial or complete absence of the falx.[42] In our case diagnosed before 26 weeks the fetus also had cyclopea and was an example of trisomy 13–15.

Vein of Galen aneurysms are easy to confuse with posterior fossa cysts or porencephalic cysts. These arteriovenous malformations are located in the midline posterior to the quadrageminal cistern. The dilated vein may secondarily compress the aqueduct causing lateral ventricular dilatation. Venous flow within the aneurysm can be detected with Doppler.[43] Theoretically an affected fetus could be salvaged by immediate post-delivery surgery although this has not been achieved in practice.

Abnormalities of the shape of the skull are easily recognized. The dolichocephalic shape of the head with breech presentations is well known to every experienced ultrasonographer. This has to be distinguished from the rare but striking condition of craniostenosis (premature closure of the cranial sutures). We have diagnosed a single case of scaphocephaly (closure of the sagittal suture) because its cephalic index (biparietal diameter × occipital frontal diameter × 100) was only 62 (normal range 70 to 80). The diagnosis was

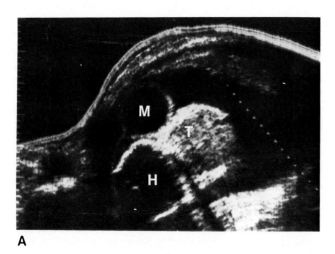

A

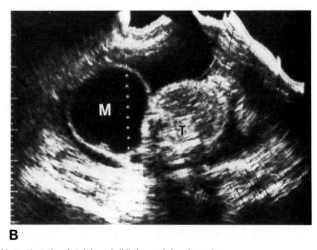

B

Fig. 17. A. Longitudinal view of iniencephalic fetus. Note that the fetal head (H) is unduly close to the trunk (T). A large meningocele (M) is present. **B.** Transverse view. The fetal trunk (T) and the meningocele (M) are seen. (*Courtesy of Roger Sanders, MD.*)

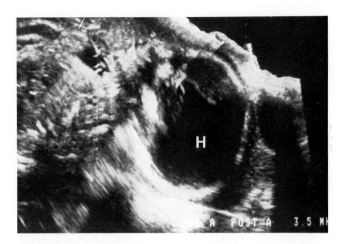

Fig. 18. Hydranencephalus. The skull contains only fluid (H) apart from the brainstem and midbrain. (*Courtesy of Roger Sanders MD.*)

made in the second trimester but as the head circumference grew at a normal rate no action was taken. The child was delivered at term and is now nearly 2 years old. It still has scaphocephaly but is growing normally and has no neurologic abnormalities. Surgery has not been necessary as yet.

We have diagnosed one case of macrocephaly (macrocrania). After discussion of the possible outcome the parents decided to continue with the pregnancy. The biparietal diameter and head circumference were consistently greater than the 90th centile whereas the abdominal circumference and limb measurements grew along the 50th centile. It was born by spontaneous vaginal delivery at term. Its head still is above the 90th centile but at six months of age it has not yet shown any evidence of the remainder of the syndrome of macrocrania that is ataxia and large hands and feet.[44]

In utero infection with toxoplasmosis or cytomegalic inclusion disease can lead to intercranial calcification and ventriculomegaly. A case has been described in which the calcification shadowing caused a confusing ultrasonic appearance.[45]

SUMMARY

We have attempted to demonstrate the place of high resolution ultrasound examination in the diagnosis of structural abnormalities of the central nervous system in the fetus. We hope that we have demonstrated that it is at least as accurate as AFAFP in diagnosing a fetus with a NTD. It has the added advantages, however, in that, as far as we know, it is free from risk (which amniocentesis is not) and that it can predict the type, site, and extent of the lesion accurately. This allows a realistic prognosis to be given to the parents. It will detect many structural abnormalities that

screening with MSAFP will not. It is hoped that the future holds the means to train sufficient sonologists so that every pregnant lady may be offered a high-resolution scan at 16 to 18 weeks' gestation to accurately establish the gestational age, exclude multiple pregnancy and to reassure the mother that her baby is free from structural abnormalities.

REFERENCES

1. Smithells RW, Sheppard S, et al: Possible prevention of neural tube defects by periconceptional vitamin supplements. Lancet i:339, 1980
2. Editorial: Vitamins, neural tube defects and ethics committees. Lancet i:1061, 1980
3. Althouse R, Wald N: Survival and handicap of infants with spina bifida. Arch Dis Child 55:845, 1980
4. Brock DJH: Neural tube defects, in Brock DJH (ed): Early Diagnosis of Fetal Defects. London, Churchill Livingstone, 1982, p 73
5. Smith C: Computer programme to estimate recurrence risks for multifactorial familial disease. Br Med J 1:495, 1972
6. Carter CO, Evans KA: Children of adult survivors with spina bifida cystica. Lancet ii:925, 1973
7. UK collaborative study on AFP in relation to neural tube defects. Lancet i:1323, 1977
8. UK collaborative study on AFP in relation to neural tube defects (second report). Lancet i:651, 1979
9. Report of the Collaborative Study on acetylcholinesterase. Lancet ii:321, 1981
10. An assessment of the hazards of amniocentesis. Report to the MRC by their working party on amniocentesis. Br J Obstet Gynaecol (Suppl 2) 1978
11. NICHD National Register for Amniocentesis Study Group. Midtrimester amniocentesis for prenatal diagnosis. Safety and accuracy. J Am Med Assoc 236:1471, 1976
12. Simpson NE, Dalliare L, et al: Prenatal diagnosis of genetic disease in Canada: Report of the collaborative study. Can Med Assoc 115:739, 1976
13. Campbell S, Johnstone FD, et al: Anencephaly: Early ultrasound diagnosis and active management. Lancet ii:1226, 1972
14. Mannes EJ, Crelin ES, et al: Sonographic demonstration of fetal acrania. Am J Roentgenol 139:181, 1982
15. Campbell S, Pryse Davies J, et al: Ultrasound in the diagnosis of spina bifida. Lancet i:1065, 1975
16. Wald N, Cuckle H, et al: Biparietal diameter measurements in fetuses with spina bifida. Br J Obstet Gynaecol 87:219, 1980
17. Roberts AB, Campbell S: Fetal head measurements in spina bifida. Br J Obstet Gynaecol 87:927, 1980
18. Lorber J: Systematic ventriculographic studies in infants born with meningomyelocoele and encephalocoele: The incidence of development of hydrocephalus. Arch Dis Child 36:381, 1961
19. Campbell S: Diagnosis of fetal abnormalitites by ultrasound, in Milunsky A (ed), Genetic Disorders and the Fetus. New York, Plenum, 1979, p 445

20. Campbell S, Pearce JMF: Ultrasonic visualisation of structural abnormalities of the fetus. Br Med Bull 10: 475, 1983

21. Campbell S, Pearce JMF: Ultrasonic diagnosis of structural fetal anomalies, in Campbell S (ed), Clinics in Obstetrics and Gynaecology (in press)

22. Consensus Report on Fetal Treatment 1982. N Engl J Med 307:1651, 1982

23. Laurence KM: Antenatal detection of nueral tube defects, in Barson AJ (ed), Fetal and Neonatal Pathology. Eastbourne, Praeger 1982, p 76

24. Carter CO: Genetics of common single malformations. Br Med Bull 32:21, 1976

25. Rogers JG, Danks DM: Prenatal diagnosis of sex linked hydrocephaly. Prenat Diag (letter) 3:269, 1983

26. Chervenak FA, Berkowitz RL, et al: The diagnosis of fetal hydrocephalus. Am J Obstet Gynecol 147:703, 1983

27. Egmond-Lindon A, Wladimiroff JW, et al: Prenatal diagnosis of sex-linked hydrocephaly. Prenat Diag 3:245, 1983

28. Chudleigh P, Pearce JMF, et al: Transient cysts of the fetal choroid plexus. Prenat Diag (in press)

29. Awoust J, Paquot J, et al: Convulsions in a human fetus in utero. Presented at the Xth Conference on Fetal Breathing and Movements and Other Fetal Measurement. June 1983, Malmo, Sweden

30. Kim MS, Elyaderani MK: Sonographic diagnosis of cerebroventricular hemorrhage in utero. Radiology 142:479, 1982

31. Lustig-Gillman H, Young BK, et al: Fetal intraventricular hemorrhage: Sonographic diagnosis and clinical implications. J Clin Ultrasound 11:277, 1983

32. Chinn DH, Filly RA: Extensive intracranial hemorrhage in utero. J Ultrasound Med 2:285, 1983

33. Vinters HV, Murphy J, et al: Intracranial teratoma: Antenatal diagnosis at 31 weeks' gestation by ultrasound. Acta Neuropathol 58:233, 1982

34. Shawker TH, Schwartz RM: Ultrasound appearance of a malignant fetal brain tumor. J Clin Ultrasound 11:35, 1983

35. Joubert M, Eisenring JJ, et al: Familial agenesis of the cerebellar vermis. Neurology 19:813, 1969

36. Campbell S, Tzannatos C, et al: The Prenatal Diagnosis of Joubert's syndrome (in press)

37. Dempsey PJ, Koch HJ: In utero diagnosis of the Dandy–Walker syndrome: Differentiation from extra-axial posterior fossa cyst. J Clin Ultrasound 9:403, 1981

38. Warkany J: Congenital Malformations. Chicago: Year Book, 1971, p 767

39. Kurtz AB, Wapner RJ, et al: Ultrasound criteria for in utero diagnosis of microcephaly. J Clin Ultrasound 8:11, 1980

40. Campbell S, Thoms A: Ultrasonic measurement of fetal head to abdomen circumference ratio in the assessment of growth retardation. Br J Obstet Gynaecol 84:165, 1977

41. Mayden K, Tortora M, et al: Orbital diameters: A new parameter for prenatal diagnosis and dating. Am J Obstet Gynecol 144:289, 1982

42. Hidalgo H, Bowie J, et al: In utero sonographic diagnosis of fetal cerebral anomalies. AJR 139:143, 1982

43. Hirsch JH, Cyr D, et al: Ultrasonographic diagnosis of an aneurysm of the vein of Galen in utero by duplex scanning. J Ultrasound Med 2:231, 1983

44. Milunsky A, Cowie VA, et al: Cerebral gigantism in childhood. Paed 40:395, 1967

45. Graham D, Guidi SM, Sanders RC: Sonographic features of in utero periventricular calcification due to cytomegalovirus infection. J Ultrasound Med 1:171, 1982

19 | Ultrasonic Assessment of the Face and Neck

Roger C. Sanders

Since the last edition of this book, much information has become available about the ultrasonic appearances of normal and pathologic structures in the face and neck. Interest in this area has increased since it has become apparent that the intraorbital distance is a relatively easy measurement to perform for which normal standards are now available.[1-3] Measurements have been described for the distance between the inner and outer margins of the orbit[1,2] and between the centers of the orbits[3] (see Appendix 4).

The detailed anatomy of the structures in the region of the face and neck has been elucidated. The orbits are easily recognizable as circular structures with echogenic rims (Fig. 1). With high-quality equipment the globes of the eye can be seen within the orbit and movements of the globe can be observed with real time. Although a number of eye movement patterns have been described,[4] clinical significance has not yet been ascribed to the different movement sequences.

Between the two orbits, a relatively echogenic zone representing the structures in the region of the nose such as the ethmoids and turbinates is visible. The equally echogenic, somewhat triangular, maxilla can be seen immediately inferior to this area. The mandible is visible and munching movements are often seen with real time. The mandible is of similar echogenicity as the maxilla. Subtle echoes from the teeth, lips and tongue can also be identified with the most sensitive systems, and tongue and lip movements and soft tissue defects can be visualized. The teeth are seen as a series of echogenic dots in the maxilla.

Views taken in a more posterior and lateral location will show the fetal ear as a hemispherical structure normally containing two parallel curvilinear ridges (Fig. 2). The typical shape helps in the recognition of the ear and in distinction from pathologic entities. The ear has been mistaken for an encephalocele or neck teratoma.[5]

These organs are visible from early in the second trimester and become more obvious as pregnancy proceeds.

TECHNIQUE

Technique is crucial in observing these relatively subtle structures. After the orbits are located on a standard axial view of the head as for a biparietal diameter, the transducer is placed at right angles in a coronal plane and angled down through the orbits, eventually making the angle sufficiently steep to observe the orbits, maxilla and mandible (Fig. 3). The transducer is rocked backwards and forwards until the ideal plane to show the orbits and, usually separately, the maxilla and mandible is obtained. Measurements are made by finding the orbits on a transverse view and taking a measurement either from the center of the orbit or from the medial or lateral rim to the opposite orbital structure.

A sagittal section through the nose and mouth is also desirable; this can also show the structures in the neck (Fig. 4). Swallowing and chewing movements of the mandible can be observed at frequent intervals with real time; occasionally tongue movements and gulping can be seen (Fig. 5).[6] It has been suggested that such gulping movements may indicate the pres-

258

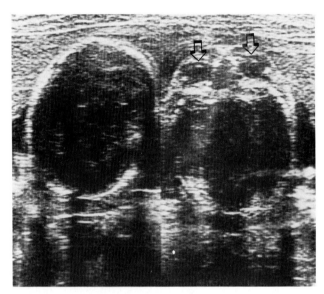

Fig. 1. A transverse view shows the orbits (*arrows*) with the maxilla in between. The rim of the globe of the eye can be seen within the orbits.

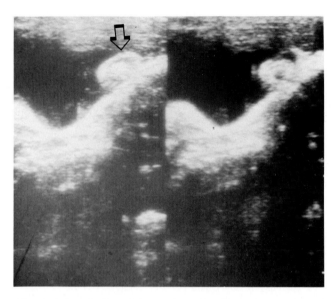

Fig. 2. A lateral view of the neck region shows the ear (*arrow*). Ridges can be seen within it.

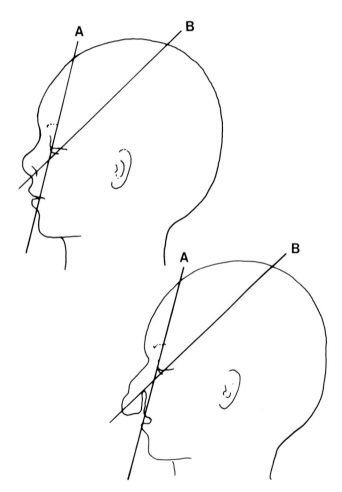

Fig. 3. Diagram showing the technique required to demonstrate a cleft palate. (*Reprinted with permission from Seeds JW, Cefalo RC: Technique of early sonographic diagnosis of bilateral cleft lip and palate. Obstet Gynecol 62:25, 1983.*)

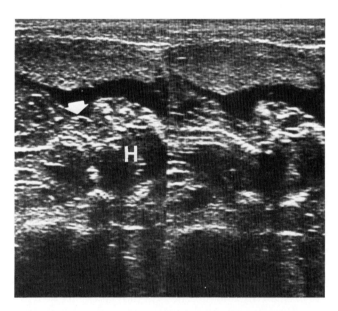

Fig. 4. Longitudinal section showing the fetal head (H), neck and upper chest. The jaw can be seen. The soft tissue of the neck (*arrow*) is the site where esophogeal swallowing movements can be detected with real time.

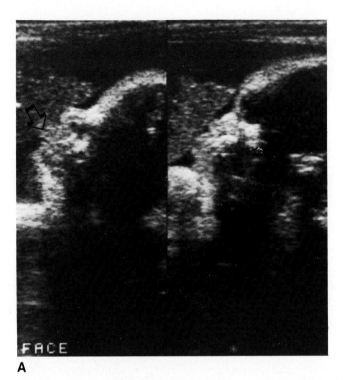
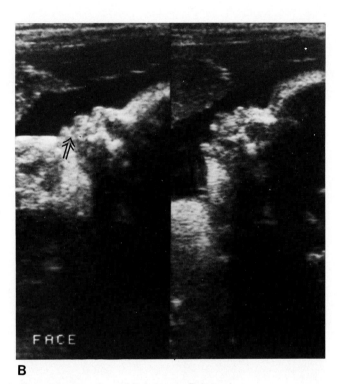

A **B**

Fig. 5. A. Lateral views showing the fetal nose with the lips and tongue (*arrow*) in between. **B.** Lateral views showing the lips and tongue (*arrow*).

ence of tracheoesophogeal atresia; this has yet to be confirmed and they may represent a normal finding.

FACE PROBLEMS

Hypertelorism

An increased interorbital distance is seen in a number of rare syndromes. Only the more common entities are described. An increased interorbital distance is seen with various types of craniosynostosis.[7] We have discovered several types in utero. In Pfeiffer syndrome there is severe coronal craniosynostosis, with hypertelorism and broad spatulated thumbs. The shape of the head is distorted with a brachycephalic appearance. In a very severe variant of Pfeiffer syndrome, the ventricles were markedly dilated and herniated laterally through the cheeks (Fig. 6). Most examples are much milder and usually patients have normal intelligence.

Apert syndrome is a similar condition in which there is craniosynostosis with increased intraorbital distance and webbing of the fingers. Again, the head shape is abnormal with brachycephaly. The hand deformity may be recognizable ultrasonically since the hand is clenched and the fingers are consistently bunched together. Ventriculomegaly may be present and the syndrome is commonly associated with subnormal intelligence. Other types of craniosynostosis

that we can expect to detect by ultrasound include Crouzon syndrome, cephalosyndactyly, acrocephalopolysyndactyly, and oculodentodigital dysplasia. In Crouzon syndrome there is bilateral coronal synostosis, a parrot beak nose, maxillary hypoplasia, choanal atresia and high-arched palate. In oculodentodigital dysplasia there is microphthalmus, a small nose, dental anomalies and syndactyly of fourth and fifth digits. In acrocephalopolysyndactyly there is a digital syndac-

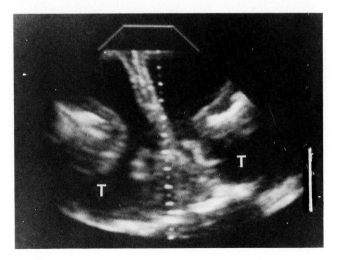

Fig. 6. Transverse view of a fetus with Pfeiffer syndrome showing lateral ventricles with gross hydrocephalus. The temporal horns (T) have herniated into the cheek because of severe craniosynostosis.

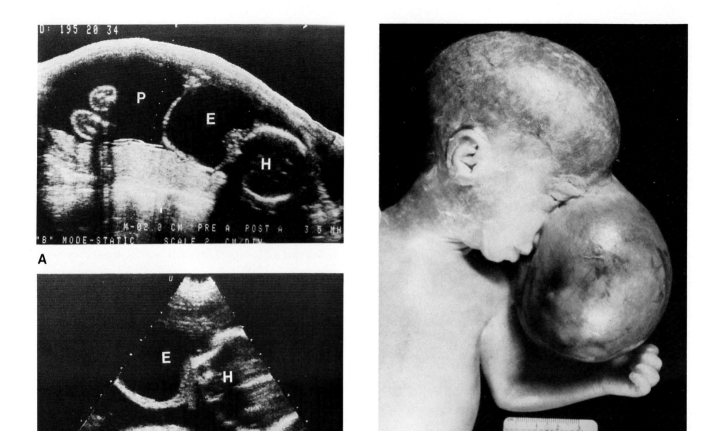

Fig. 7. A. Anterior encephalocele. A large encephalocele (E) can be seen lying anterior to the fetal head (H). There is polyhydramnios (P). **B.** Real time lateral views showed the cystic structure to arise from the anterior aspect of the face above the neck. Facial structures can be seen associated with the encephalocele (E). H = head. **C.** The fetus was aborted. A large anterior encephalocele protrudes between the eyes.

tyly and polydactyly. In craniotelencephalic dysplasia there is hypertelorism, microphthalmus and massive protrusion of the forehead. In all of these syndromes the hypertelorism and the distorted head shape should be recognizable even if the subsidiary anomalies are not.

Anterior Encephalocele. Most encephaloceles are occipital in location (75 percent) but in a minority (about 15 percent), the encephalocele protrudes between the eyes above the nose (Fig. 7). A parietal location is also possible. Anterior encephaloceles cause hypertelorism; they are single cystic dural lined cavities of variable size that may or may not contain brain tissue. Unlike other anomalies in this area this lesion is associated with a skull defect with absence of any bony structure in the nasal region at the site of the encephalocele.

The lesions are usually cystic on ultrasound—a septum may be present along with more echogenic material representing brain tissue on some occasions.[8] The α-fetoprotein level is elevated and polyhydramnios is commonplace. When recognized prior to 22 weeks, continued pregnancy is probably undesirable. The prognosis is poor, although dependent upon the amount of brain tissue contained within the encephalocele.

Hypertelorism has been seen in association with trisomy 8 and 9, triploidy, and XXXX chromosomal anomalies.

Hypotelorism

A decreased intraorbital distance is an indication of a number of anomalies, most associated with central nervous system malformations and some with chromo-

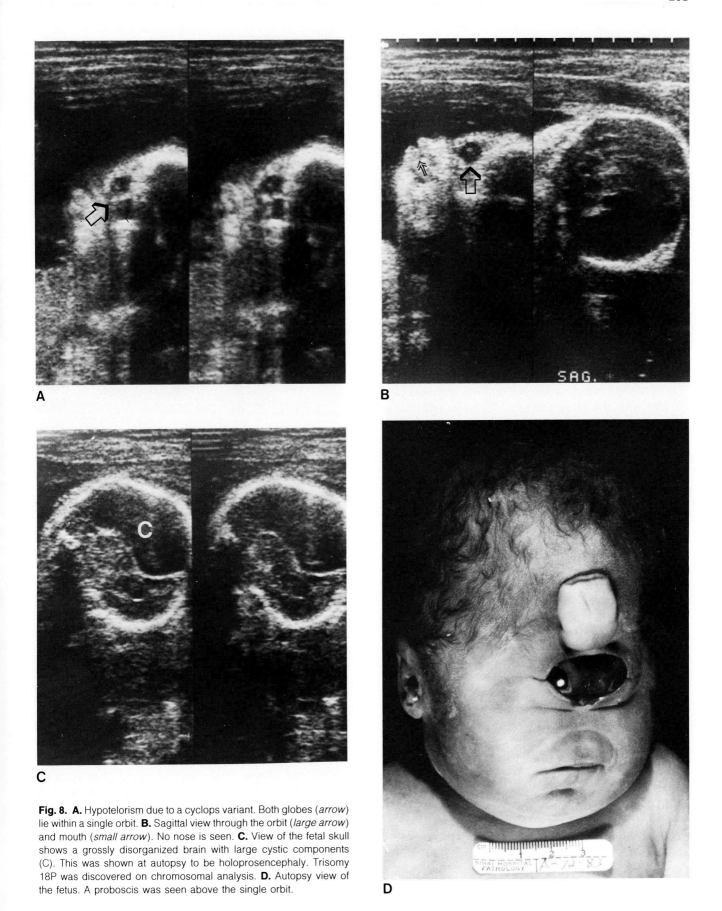

Fig. 8. A. Hypotelorism due to a cyclops variant. Both globes (*arrow*) lie within a single orbit. **B.** Sagittal view through the orbit (*large arrow*) and mouth (*small arrow*). No nose is seen. **C.** View of the fetal skull shows a grossly disorganized brain with large cystic components (C). This was shown at autopsy to be holoprosencephaly. Trisomy 18P was discovered on chromosomal analysis. **D.** Autopsy view of the fetus. A proboscis was seen above the single orbit.

somal anomalies such as trisomy 13 and trisomy 18P. In these syndromes, to a varying degree, the intraorbital structures are hypoplastic or absent.

Five different conditions, all associated with central nervous malformations, have been described. The most severe form is a single orbit—cyclopia. This condition may be associated with a proboscis—a fingerlike protrusion sometimes located above the single eye. There may be one or two eyeglobes present within a single orbit that, indeed, may not be recognizable as an orbit (Fig. 8A–D).[9] Cebocephaly (monkeyhead) is a closely related syndrome in which there is a flat nose in a normal position with hypotelorism, a common optic foramen, an absence of a septum premaxilla, and rudimentary nasal bones and turbinates. Another very similar condition is ethmocephaly, in which there are two orbits extremely close together with no ethmoids or virtual absence of the ethmoidal structures. In all of these syndromes there is an associated intracranial anomaly, which is usually holoprosencephaly—a single fused central ventricle with a disorganized brain. The prosencephalon fails to differentiate into the normal forebrain components. No midline structures are present with the more severe variants, in which case the syndrome is termed alobar holoprosencephaly. Microcephaly is universal and hydramnios is common. Two less severe variants exist in which the degree of hypotelorism is less marked (Fig. 9) and more ethmoidal structures are present, but, again, central nervous system malformations are common. Many of these related conditions are associated with chromosomal anomalies so it is worthwhile looking at the cardiac and skeletal structures that may also be affected by these chromosomal variants. The finding of hypotelorism is usually considered an indication for amniocentesis since there is a strong, though not invariable, association with chromosomal anomalies. Prenatal diagnosis of these syndromes is desirable because the prognosis is hopeless. Neonatal survival ranges from a few days to several months. Intracranial derangement is most often the cause of death.

Phenylketonuria (PKU) is also associated with hypotelorism. It has no other potentially visible sonographic manifestations apart from microcephaly.

Cleft Palate. Cleft palate is commonly seen with trisomy 13, which is a syndrome also associated with hypotelorism and alobar holyprosencephaly. Cleft palate has been recognized on several occasions with ultrasound (Fig. 10).[10] There is a familial incidence of cleft palate, which occurs 4 percent of the time if a sib is affected and 17 percent if both sib and parent are affected. It is more common on the left but may

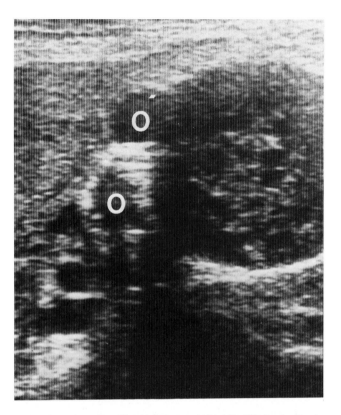

Fig. 9. Hypertelorism with widely separated orbits (O) due to Aperts syndrome with craniosynostosis. The skull shape was brachycephalic.

be bilateral. Maxillary structures are partially or completely absent below the nose. A coronal view angling through the maxilla is crucial in making this diagnosis (Fig. 3). The time gain compensation should be set so that the soft tissues are easily seen. Hypotelorism may be seen in association with cleft palate.

Jaw Problems. Theoretically, it should be possible to recognize micrognathia with ultrasound. It is a component of a number of syndromes associated with chromosomal anomalies. Prominence of the jaw, as in Robert syndrome, has been seen.[11] Certainly with current real-time equipment the jaw is easily visualized; it is only a matter of time before micrognathia is recognized.

Cloverleaf Skull. A prominent forehead area with bossing of the bone has been seen in association with a number of syndromes and is known as the cloverleaf skull. In addition to craniosynostosis,[7] this syndrome has been seen with thanatophoric dwarfism and some of the variants of hypotelorism, such as cyclops, described earlier.

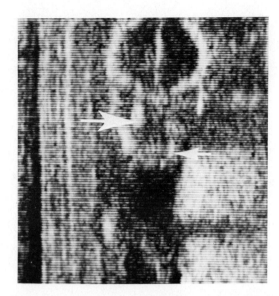

Fig. 10. Cleft palate. The large arrow indicates the absent maxillary ridge. Small arrow identifies the mandibles. (*Reprinted with permission from Seeds JW, Cefalo RC: Techniques of early sonographic diagnosis of bilateral cleft lip and palate. Obstet Gynecol 62:25, 1983.*)

Micrognathia, malar hypoplasia, and hypo- and hypertelorism may occasionally be seen with various types of dwarfism such as camptomelia and achondrogenesis.

NECK PROBLEMS

Cystic Hygroma (Lymphangioma)
Although cystic hygromas occur elsewhere in the body, the neck is by far the commonest site for these lymph-filled cavities which are associated with intradermoid lymphangiactasia 80 percent of the time.[12] These fluid-filled masses arise from the anterior, lateral, or, most commonly, posterior aspect of the fetal neck. A typical cystic hygroma has a wavy membrane around its outer aspect and usually contains one or more septations (Fig. 11).[13-18] The hygroma may be larger than the fetal head. Fetal ascites, polyhydramnios, and an enlarged edematous placenta are commonly present and there may be generalized fetal soft tissue thickening. Other fetal anomalies may be seen in addition such as omphalocele.

An association exists between cystic hygroma and Turner syndrome (Fig. 12).[19] It is thought that the webbed neck seen in Turner syndrome represents a resorbed cystic hygroma.[20] The α-fetoprotein level is often elevated to a very high level in cystic hygroma.[21] Although theoretically surgically resectible, severe de-formities of the face and neck may be unavoidable, as the cystic hygroma can surround the entire head.

Theoretically this condition could be confused with branchial cleft cyst—a smaller cystic structure that arises from the lateral aspect of the neck. Branchial cleft cysts have not yet been reported diagnosed in utero. A nuchal cyst is another cystic structure occurring in an occipital location that can be mistaken for encephalocele or for a posteriorly located cystic hygroma; it is of no pathologic significance.

Fetal Teratoma
Fetal teratoma occur most often in the sacral area but a second site of relatively frequent involvement is in the region of the neck.[22-26] As in other parts of the body, these masses are complex, sometimes containing cystic area or areas of calcification with acoustical shadowing (approximately 40 percent of cases) (Fig. 13). Usually slightly eccentrically located, they may grow to a large size; since they involve the neck areas, they may compromise fetal respiration at birth.[24] Surgical resection is usually possible but segments of the mandible may need to be removed and the operation may be very mutilating. The α-fetoprotein level is sometimes elevated and hydramnios may be present.

Causes of neck masses so far not reported seen by ultrasound include hemangioma, neuroblastoma, and sarcoma.

Goiter
Fetal goiters have been visualized by ultrasound and are ventral in location, symmetric, evenly echogenic structures associated with normal α-fetoprotein. When they are very large, they can cause hyperextension of the fetal neck and problems at delivery.

Normal Variants Confused with Neck Pathology
When there is little amniotic fluid, one might confuse structures outside the fetus with neck or facial problems. Theoretically, a stunted second twin could be mistaken for a neck mass; if the placenta were adjacent to the fetus, it is possible that a subchorionic placental cyst could be confused with an encephalocele or cystic hygroma. The fetal ear has been confused with an encephalocele (Fig. 2).[5] A segment of Wharton jelly was confused with a neck mass.[27]

Much detailed anatomy is involved in the recognition of facial abnormalies. With increasing ultrasonic resolution, further subtle anomalies will be detected in this cosmetically sensitive area.

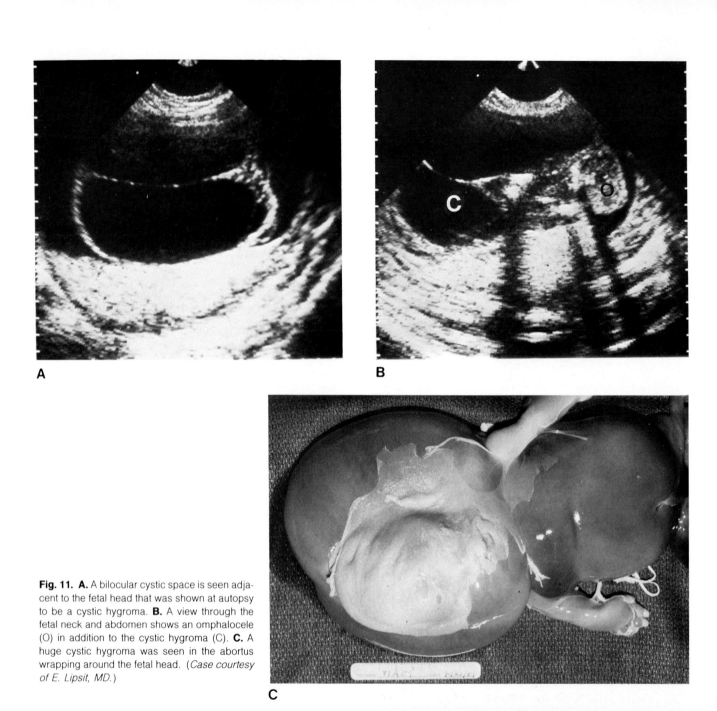

Fig. 11. A. A bilocular cystic space is seen adjacent to the fetal head that was shown at autopsy to be a cystic hygroma. **B.** A view through the fetal neck and abdomen shows an omphalocele (O) in addition to the cystic hygroma (C). **C.** A huge cystic hygroma was seen in the abortus wrapping around the fetal head. (*Case courtesy of E. Lipsit, MD.*)

A

B

C

Fig. 12. Regressing cystic hygroma. An earlier series had shown a large cystic hygroma. This view shows a relatively small cystic structure anterior to the fetal head. Chromosomal analysis showed Turner syndrome. At delivery, only webbing of the neck was found.

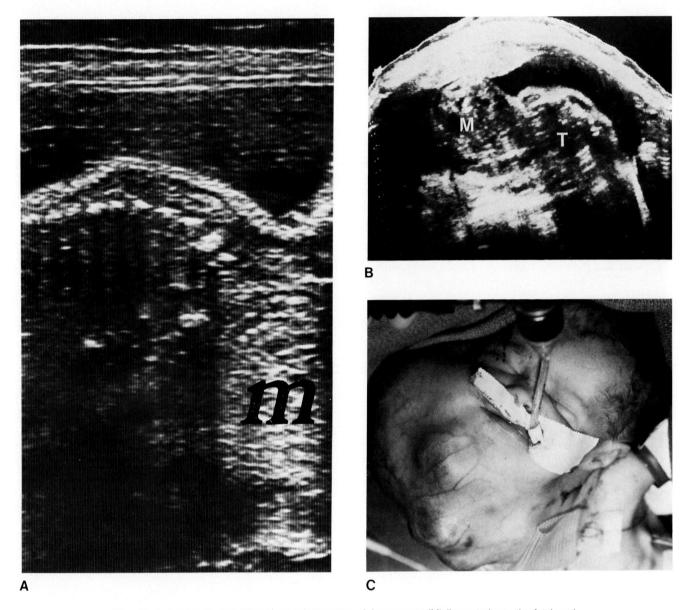

Fig. 13. A. Longitudinal section of a neck teratoma. A large mass (M) lies anterior to the fetal neck above the thorax. **B.** A transverse view through the fetal chest shows the upper thorax (T) with a large mass alongside (M) which represents the teratoma. **C.** Immediately following delivery, the fetus developed respiratory distress. A difficult tracheotomy was performed and the neonate was taken straight to the operating room. The large teratoma was surgically removed. At a 2-year follow-up, there was barely any residual deformity of the jaw.

REFERENCES

1. Mayden KL, Tortora M, Berkowitz R, et al: Orbital diameters: A new parameter for prenatal diagnosis and dating. Am J Obstet Gynecol 144:298, 1982

2. Jeanty P, Dramaix-Wilmet M, Van Gansbeke D, et al: Fetal ocular biometry by ultrasound. Radiology 143:513, 1982

3. Aubry JP, Aubry MC, Briard ML, et al: Mesure prenatale de la distance interorbitaire par echographie appoint dans le depistage des formes mineures d'holoprosencephalie. J Genet Hum 29:395, 1981

4. Levi S, Awoust JT, De Clercq JC: Fetal eye movements (EM) and neurological development. Presented at the World Federation of Ultrasound in Medicine and Biology, 1983

5. Fink IJ, Chinn DH, Callen PW: A potential pitfall in the ultrasonographic diagnosis of fetal encephalocele. J Ultrasound Med 2:313, 1983

6. Bowie JD, Clair MR: Fetal swallowing and regurgitation:

Observation of normal and abnormal activity. Radiology 144:877, 1982

7. Mohr G, Hoffman HJ, Munro IR, et al: Surgical management of unilateral and bilateral coronal craniosynostosis. Neurosurgery 2:83, 1978

8. Nicolini U, Ferrazzi E, Minonzio M, et al: Prenatal diagnosis of cranial masses by ultrasound: Report of five cases. J Clin Ultrasound 11:70, 1983

9. Lev-Gur M, Maklad NF, Patel S: Ultrasonic findings in fetal cyclopia. J Repro Med 28:554, 1983

10. Seeds JW, Cefalo RC: Technique of early sonographic diagnosis of bilateral cleft lip and palate. Obstet Gynecol 62:2S, 1983

11. Hobbins J: Skeletal dysplasia, in Sanders R, James AE (eds), The Principles and Practice of Ultrasound in Obstetrics and Gynecology. New York: Appleton-Century-Crofts, 1980

12. Singh S, Baboo ML, Pathak IC: Cystic lymphangioma in children. Report of 32 cases including lesions at rare sites. Surgery 69:947, 1971

13. Phillips HE, McGahan JP: Intrauterine fetal cystic hygromas: Sonographic detection. AM J Roentgenol 136:799, 1981

14. Frigoletto FD, Birnholz JC, Driscoll SG, et al: Ultrasound diagnosis of cystic hygroma. Am J Obstet Gynecol 136:962, 1980

15. O'Brien WF, Cefalo RC, Bair DG: Ultrasonographic diagnosis of fetal cystic hygroma. Am J Obstet Gynecol 138:464, 1980

16. Shaub M, Wilson R, Collea J: Fetal cystic lymphangioma (cystic hygroma): Prepartum ultrasonic findings. Radiology 121:449, 1976

17. Morgan CL, Haney A, Christakos A, et al: Antenatal detection of fetal structural defects with ultrasound. J Clin Ultrasound 3:287, 1975

18. Young LW, Haimovici H, LaVigne RJ, et al: Radiological case of the month. Am J Dis Child 134:311, 1980

19. Tabor A, Bang J, Philip J: 45,X Karyotype: May the diagnosis be suspected on ultrasonic examination in the second trimester of pregnancy? Prenat Diagnos 1:281, 1981

20. Miller JM, McCarter L, Pai GS, et al: Hygroma cervicis: Antepartum ultrasonic findings. J Repro Med 26:567, 1981

21. Pawlowitzki IH, Wormann B: Elevated amniotic alpha fetoprotein in a fetus with Turner's syndrome due to puncture of a cystic hygroma. Am J Obstet Gynecol 133:584, 1979

22. Patel RB, Gibson JY, D'Cruz CA, et al: Sonographic diagnosis of cervical teratoma in utero. Am J Roentgenol 139:1220, 1982

23. Thurkow AL, Visser GHA, Oosterhuis P, et al: Ultrasound observations of a malignant cervical teratoma of the fetus in a case of polyhydramnios: Case history and review. Eur J Obstet Gynec Reprod Biol 14:375, 1983

24. Kang KW, Hissong SL, Langer A: Prenatal ultrasonic diagnosis of epignathus. J Clin Ultrasound 6:295, 1978

25. Diagnostic oncology case study: Am J Roentgenol 140:507, 1983

26. Schoenfeld A, Edelstein T, Joel-Cohen SJ: Prenatal ultrasonic diagnosis of fetal teratoma of the neck. Br J Radiol 51:742, 1978

27. Corson VL, Sanders RC, Johnson TRB, et al: Mid-trimester fetal ultrasound: Diagnostic dilemmas. Prenat Diagnos 3:47, 1983

20 | Skeletal Dysplasia

John C. Hobbins
Maurice J. Mahoney

INTRODUCTION

In the time elapsed since the second edition of this book, the experience of investigators in prenatal diagnosis has been expanded and ultrasound imagery has improved. However, it will take many more years to describe the full range of expression in individual skeletal dysplasias because of the relative rarity of these conditions. Also, although a few reports have emerged in which some nine different skeletal dysplasias have been diagnosed in utero, our knowledge is incomplete concerning how early in gestation the diagnosis can be made using long bone length in individual conditions.

This chapter first addresses the requisites of an adequate ultrasound examination designed for the patient at risk for fetal skeletal dysplasia. Then a few of the most common (currently catalogued) disorders are discussed.

TECHNIQUES

Measurement of Long Bones

See Appendix 6. The static scanner is not as suitable as a real-time machine in the evaluation of the fetus at risk for skeletal dysplasia simply because the unpredictable fetus rarely is cooperative in curtailing its movement during this often lengthy examination. In our opinion it makes little difference whether or not a linear array or a sector real-time unit is employed.

Measurement of the long bone length should be undertaken very carefully and several measurements of each bone should be accomplished. Since it is theoretically impossible to "overmeasure" the length of a long bone and much more common to underestimate long bone length by tangential cuts through the bone, it is advisable to accept the longest measurement obtained. Also, measurements of a long bone that are in the "east/west" (Fig. 1A) axis are more reliable than when the bone is extending obliquely from the top to the bottom of the screen (Fig. 1B). The speed of sound through the bone is about 4080 m/sec, compared with the normal calibrated velocity of 1540 m/sec in soft tissue. Since ultrasound beams would be at least partially running along the long axis of the bone in an obliquely positioned leg, there is a potential source for error. Fetuses rarely spend prolonged periods of time in the back-down or back-up position, so it is advisable to postpone long bone measurement until the fetus moves onto its side.

Not all of the long bone will be echogenic. For example, when examining abortuses in a waterbath we noticed that ultrasound measurements of long bones were similar to those obtained with a plastic rule at 16 to 18 weeks.[1] The measurements, however, became gradually discordant through 25 weeks, at which time there was a 17 percent difference between ultrasound values and external measurements for the same long bone in the same abortus. It is logical that the reason for the discrepancy is that the cartilagenous ends of the long bone are not echogenic in the late second trimester. Since norms for gestational age are based on in vivo measurements, this phenomenon should not affect one's ability to date the pregnancy

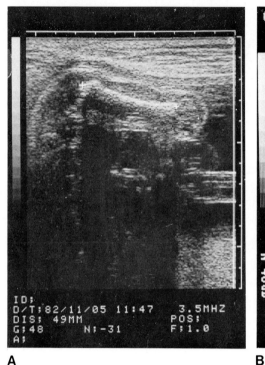 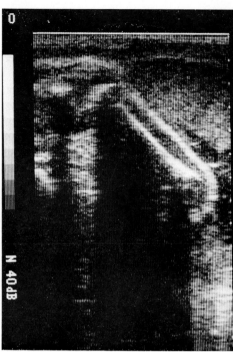

Fig. 1. Typical ultrasonic scans of long bones for length measurements. The measurement is more accurate with the bone in the "east–west" axis (as shown in **A**) than in the oblique or vertical position (as shown in **B**).

A   **B**

or to appreciate abnormal shortening in a fetus at risk for short-limb dysplasia.

There is a suggestion from recent studies that the fetal femur may have less biologic variation than the biparietal diameter (BPD) as pregnancy progresses.[2] This has already led some authors to tout femur length as being superior to the "golden standard" BPD in late gestation. This may not be true because the theoretical advantage of smaller biologic variation is easily outweighed by the greater interobserver error arising from the fact that measurements of femur length are more difficult to make than that of the BPD. For this reason, when a diagnosis of short-limbed dysplasia is entertained based on a limb measurement that is more than 2 standard deviations (SDs) below the mean, it is prudent to reexamine the patient before a definitive diagnosis is made.

Besides determining the length of the long bone, it is important to assess its echogenicity and its ability to cast an acoustic shadow. For example, in osteogenesis imperfecta and in hypophosphatasia the poorly calcified bones may be weakly echogenic and incapable of casting a uniform acoustic shadow (Fig. 2). Also, in achondrogenesis, a recessive condition resulting in markedly shortened limbs, an affected fetus may have a spine that is poorly visualized with ultrasound.

The shape of the bone may provide useful information to the diagnostician. For example, in the normal fetus there is often some bowing of the long bones (camptomelia). In camptomelic dysplasia, however,

this bowing is markedly exaggerated (Fig. 3). In osteogenesis imperfecta the configuration of the bone is distinctive when a fracture is present. We have noticed an overriding fracture in a fetus suffering from the more severe form of the autosomal dominant type of OI (type I). This same finding has also been reported by other investigators.[3]

A careful examination of the long bone should include observation of movement of the fetal extremities. For example, some forms of arthrogryposis are inherited by an autosomal recessive inheritance pattern. Little is known about how early in gestation the limb contractures occur in arthrogryposis, and, as yet, no index cases of successful prenatal diagnosis exist. Nevertheless, in the third trimester one would suspect that the finding of full limb extension in a fetus at risk would mean absence of the condition. However, since no data exist concerning how early in pregnancy limb extension would be compromised in affected fetuses, one could not yet exclude the presence of the condition in the second trimester fetuses by the observation of supple limbs.

Although an attempt should be made to examine all of the bones of fetuses at risk for skeletal dysplasia, there are certain bones or limbs that deserve special attention, depending upon the condition. For example, in some skeletal dysplasias such as achondroplasia, rhizomelic (proximal) shortening is the rule and femur and humerus should be scrutinized. In mesomelic syndromes (medial shortening) such as chondroectodermal dysplasia, the tibia, fibula, radius, and ulna should be carefully evaluated. Often hypoplasia or agenesis of one long bone may be a feature of a more serious fetal condition potentially diagnosable with ultrasound. For example, approximately 20 percent of infants suffering from Fanconi's anemia, an eventually lethal blood disorder with a 25 percent recurrence rate, have hypoplastic radii. Since a hypoplastic radius is extremely rare in the overall population, the demonstration of only one bone on cross section of the lower forearm in a fetus at risk for this disease should confirm the diagnosis. Similarly, the two major features of thrombocytopenia absent radius (TAR) syndrome are implicit in the condition's title. The successful prenatal diagnosis of the condition has already been reported by ultrasound demonstration of absent radii.[4]

The distal extremities are also sites of potentially useful information. It is extremely important to attempt to provide a precise diagnosis for patients suddenly confronted with the news that their second trimester fetus has a skeletal dysplasia, since some conditions are far more serious than others. In dia-

strophic dysplasia, a condition that is not necessarily lethal, affected fetuses will display, among other features, persistently abducted thumbs (hitchhiker thumbs). This feature is potentially demonstrable with ultrasound. Careful examination of the fetal hands is critical to the diagnosis of other severe fetal conditions associated with polydactyly, such as chondroectodermal dysplasia (Ellis–van Creveld syndrome). Clubbing of an extremity may be an isolated finding or noted in association with other anomaly syndromes. For example, Filly identified a club hand in association with a complex limb reduction syndrome.[5]

Occasionally, the sonologist is asked to diagnose a condition only affecting the fetal hands and/or feet. Such a condition is ectrodactyly (split-hand deformity), an autosomal dominant condition affecting one, some, or all of the extremities. Although not a life-threatening condition, it can be extremely disabling. We have successfully excluded this diagnosis in seven fetuses at risk for this condition. In the first case, fetoscopy, an invasive procedure associated with a 5 percent procedure-related fetal loss rate, was used to establish the integrity of the extremities. In the other six cases, however, it was possible to exclude the diagnosis with ultrasound alone. This examination can be very time consuming and tedious but well worth the effort to demonstrate to an extremely anxious couple that their fetus has normal extremities.

Ethical dilemmas abound in the diagnosis of skeletal dysplasias when the condition in question only affects one or more distal extremities. It is not in the design of this chapter to provide discussion of the moral–ethical justification for abortion of a fetus with a defect that is partially correctable with surgery. What one person might consider trivial may be devastating to another, especially if that parent is affected with the condition. It is our opinion that the diagnostician's first responsibility in today's complex society is to provide the most accurate information possible so that parents can be properly counseled concerning the nature of any fetal defect, its natural course and treatment, and the options for management of the pregnancy.

Examination of the Head
In many forms of skeletal dysplasia the head is disproportionately large compared with body size, and in some conditions, such as homozygous achondroplasia or thanatophoric dysplasia, the head may be actually

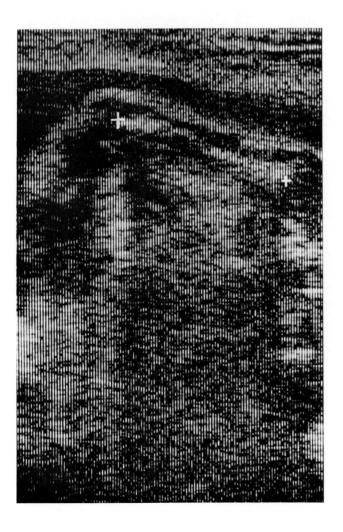

Fig. 2. Humerus at 32 weeks' gestation with decreased acoustic shadowing.

large for gestational age (above the 95th percentile). This should be reflected in ultrasonic measurements of fetal BPD. Since head growth tends to stay within a specific percentile range throughout pregnancy,[6] it is likely that before the 20th to 24th week of gestation BPD measurements would be in a high profile range (75th percentile). Relative disproportion between head and body can be quantitated by measurement of the head-to-abdomen (H/A) circumference ratio. Head circumference measurements should be made at the level of the thalami, and for reasons discussed in other parts of this text, abdominal circumference is measured at the level of the umbilical vein. Campbell[7] has constructed a nomogram for head-to-body ratio that is particularly useful in skeletal dysplasias in which head-to-body disproportion is a feature (Table 1). In some skeletal dysplasias, such as thanatophoric dysplasia, there may be a frank hydrocephaly. In this condition a cloverleaf skull occasionally is present (Fig. 4).[8] A prominent forehead is the rule in heterozygous achondroplasia and thanatophoric dysplasia.

An attempt should be made to visualize the fetal face in different planes when examining a fetus at risk for skeletal dysplasia. It is now possible, for example, to identify cleft lip and palate with ultrasound (see Chapter 19 and Fig. 5).[9,10] Certain skeletal dysplasia syndromes will commonly include a cleft lip and a palate. Among these are Kniest syndrome and Miller syndrome. When a cleft is detected and limbs are shorter than the 5th percentile, these disorders would be part of the differential diagnosis.

In Roberts syndrome facial protuberances are encountered that can be visualized clearly with ultrasound. In the amniotic band syndrome, an acquired condition resulting in limb reduction defects, bizarre craniofacial abnormalities can sometimes be identified.

In severe forms of osteogenesis imperfecta and in congenital hypophosphatasia, the calvarium is poorly mineralized. This phenomenon has been documented by radiographs and ultrasound evaluations at birth. There are two reports in which both conditions were diagnosed in utero by the ultrasonic findings of poorly defined and deformed crania.[11,12] In osteogenesis imperfecta there can be skull fractures that may be ultrasonically definable.

Thorax

The diameter and configuration of the chest may be diagnostic in certain skeletal dysplasias. For example, in asphyxiating thoracic dysplasia the chest is long and narrow. Measurements of thoracic diameter can be compared with data from available nomograms and to measurements of the abdominal perimeter in the same fetus. Also, sagittal scans will reveal the shape

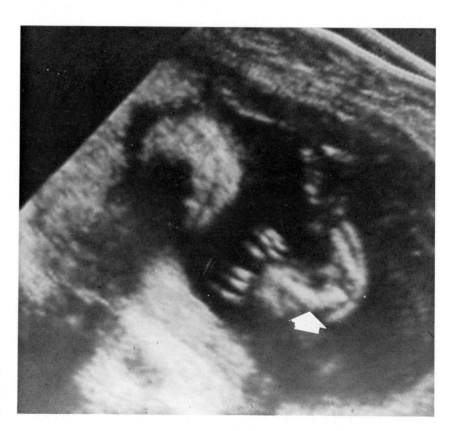

Fig. 3. Twenty-three-week-old fetus with Camptomelic dysplasia demonstrating the severe shortening, thickening and bowing of the humerus and forearm bones (*arrows*). The umbilical cord is seen across the shoulder of the fetus.

of the chest and may permit the identification of a pear-shaped configuration in thanatophoric dysplasia. In osteogenesis imperfecta and hypophosphatasia, the thorax can be somewhat collapsed, especially in late gestation.

In some types of short-limbed dysplasia, such as chondroectodermal dysplasia, cardiac anomalies are common. At present, it is possible with high-resolution real time and M-mode ultrasound to define intracardiac anatomy in the fetus (Fig. 6), making feasible the identification of some cardiac anomalies, such as interventricular septal defects, hypoplastic or single ventricles, and atretic valves.[13] Real-time imaging also permits the observation of the pattern and amplitude of fetal respiratory movements. For example, in thanatophoric dysplasia thoracic excursions may be of small amplitude.

Rib cage and thoracic spine can be visualized with today's ultrasound equipment. With some care it is even possible to count the fetal ribs. Rib fractures, occasionally seen in osteogenesis imperfecta, might well be missed, however. In one recent experience it was impossible to visualize the poorly mineralized spine of a fetus with achondrogenesis.[5]

Fluid accumulations in the pericardial and pleural spaces can easily be appreciated. Since many thanatophoric dysplasia fetuses display varying degrees of

nonimmune hydrops, the finding of a pleural effusion combined with short limbs should lead the investigator to suspect the diagnosis.

Abdomen

Measurement of the abdominal perimeter at the level of the umbilical vein has been extremely useful in assessing fetal weight[14,15] and in evaluating intrauterine growth retardation (IUGR). Since nomograms of abdominal circumference are available,[16,17] the visual impression of abdominal protuberance seen in short-rib polydactyly syndromes and thanatophoric dysplasia can be quantified and compared with normal measurements of abdominal perimeter. Also, since the thorax is small in some forms of skeletal dysplasia, abdominal organs are displaced downward, creating the appear-

TABLE 1
Mean Fetal H/A Circumference Ratios with 5th and 95th Centile Limits Related to Menstrual Age from 13 to 42 Weeks*

Menstrual Age (weeks)	Number of Measure-ments	H/A Circumference Ratio		
		5th Percentile	Mean	95th Percentile
13–14	18	1.14	1.23	1.31
15–16	39	1.05	1.22	1.39
17–18	77	1.07	1.18	1.29
19–20	54	1.09	1.18	1.26
21–22	41	1.06	1.15	1.25
23–24	22	1.05	1.13	1.21
25–26	18	1.04	1.13	1.22
27–28	36	1.05	1.13	1.22
29–30	23	0.99	1.10	1.21
31–32	31	0.96	1.07	1.17
33–34	42	0.96	1.04	1.11
35–36	49	0.93	1.02	1.11
027057 37–38	67	0.92	0.98	1.05
39–40	47	0.87	0.97	1.06
41–42	4	0.93	0.96	1.00

* Values have been combined into 2 weekly groupings to smooth out fluctuations due to small numbers (568 individual measurements).
Reprinted with permission from Campbell S, Thoms A: Ultrasound measurement of the fetal head to abdomen circumference ratio in assessment of growth retardation. Br J Obstet Gynaecol 84:165, 1977.

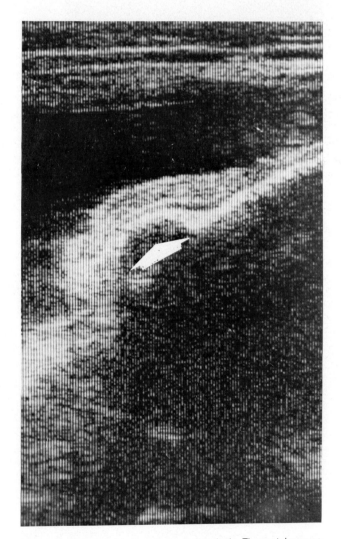

Fig. 4. Cloverleaf skull in thanatophoric dysplasia. The protuberance, marked by the arrow, occurs at the base of the skull and is typical of this malformation.

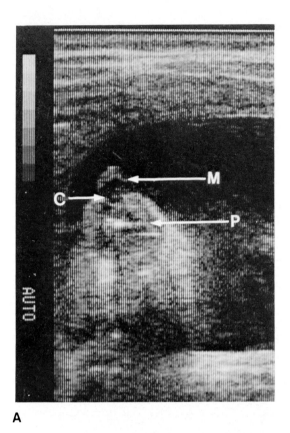

A

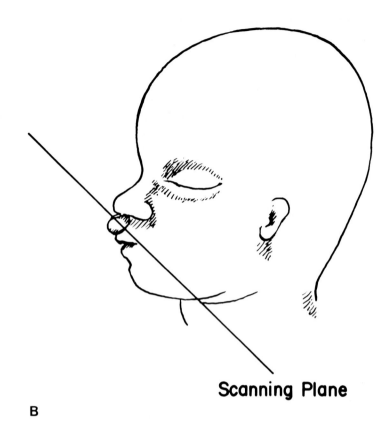

B

Fig. 5. A. Oblique scan through lower part of fetal face showing intact palate, cleft lip, and a mass protruding from lip. **B.** Demonstration of scanning plane.

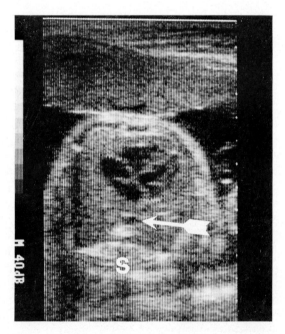

Fig. 6. Four-chamber view of the fetal heart at 26 weeks' gestation. The two ventricles, on the right, are separated by an intact septum and the two atria on the left are connected by the patent foramen ovale. Also note aorta (*long arrow*) and spine (S).

ance of organomegaly. Ascites can be easily appreciated in skeletal dysplasias in which nonimmune hydrops is a feature.

INDIVIDUAL CONDITIONS

Thanatophoric Dysplasia

This condition is one of the more frequently recognized skeletal dysplasias and, as the Greek-derived term suggests, it is uniformly fatal. Most of the reports in the literature of successful diagnoses have been in third trimester patients. Since the findings are so striking and the condition is so serious, it is surprising that more second trimester reports have not emerged. In fact, in one of our cases (Table 2) the fetus was already hydropic by the 22nd week of gestation.

Although recurrences of this condition have been unusual, one author,[18] who reported two instances of thanatophoric dysplasia in one family, was convinced that there was an autosomal recessive variant. Nevertheless, patients can be counseled that recurrence would be unlikely.

Polyhydramnios is the rule in thanatophoric dysplasia. It is also of note that in both of our third trimester patients the L/S ratio was very low (0.4 to 0.6) after 35 weeks.[8] Goodlin also reported the same interesting finding in the third trimester.[18] In only one case was the L/S ratio indicative of pulmonic maturity (>2) after 36 weeks. The polyhydramnios and immature L/S ratio suggest an inability of the fetus to move fluid in and out of its lungs and some compromise of fetal swallowing or absorption. Dye studies performed in one thanatophoric fetus indicated fetal swallowing, but it was impossible to quantify this fetal activity. In one instance, described in the first edition, we observed fetal breathing movements, but they seemed to be of small amplitude. Since the thanatophoric fetus's thorax is narrow, compromised respiratory excursions might be expected. The standard fetal findings in thanatophoric dysplasia are enlarged head (with or without cloverleaf skull), occasional hydrocephalus, hypertelorism, narrow chest, protuberant abdomen, and markedly shortened limbs. In some cases the limbs appear as thick "buds."

Camptomelic Dysplasia

It is not unusual to have some bowing of fetal long bones. However, in one form of short limb dysplasia, camptomelic dysplasia, the abnormally shortened limbs are excessively bowed. The category is actually a "wastebasket" term and undoubtedly includes several different skeletal dysplasias that have not, as yet, been correctly categorized. Because of the condition's heterogenous makeup, a uniform inheritance pattern for the condition would not be expected. Since one of our patients had delivered two offspring with this condition, we suspected an autosomal recessive pattern of inheritance in that family.[17] However, the literature does not support autosomal recessive inheritance for all families. Prominent features include rhizomelic and mesomelic shortening of long bones and generally normally proportioned trunk and head measurements.

Diastrophic Dysplasia

Prenatal diagnosis of diastrophic dysplasia has been published.[19] In this autosomal recessive condition the limbs are exceedingly short (Fig. 7). The head, although appearing large by comparison to other body parts, is generally not above the 50th percentile in BPD. The body seems compressed in configuration. The classical "hitchhiker thumbs" are not uniformly present. This finding, however, is particularly useful in diagnosing the condition if it is observed in a fetus with short limbs. Diastrophic dysplasia is generally not lethal at birth.

TABLE 2
Yale Experience in Detecting Skeletal Dysplasia in Utero

Skeleton and Limbs	Pregnancies Examined At Risk*	Positive Diagnosis in Those At Risk
Achondrogenesis	6	0
Achondroplasia	8	0
Acrocephalosyndactyly (Apert syndrome)	1	0
Adactyly	1	0
Asphyxiating thoracic dysplasia	3	0
Camptomelic dysplasia	6	1
Cartilage-hair hypoplasia (McKusick syndrome)	2	0
Chondroectodermal dysplasia (Ellis–van Creveld syndrome)	2	1
Diastrophic dysplasia	5	1
Ectrodactyly (lobster-claw)	7	0
Fanconi's anemia	1	0
Osteogenesis imperfecta	20	3
Osteopetrosis	7	0
Polydactyly	3	0
Roberts syndrome (renal/skeletal)	4	2
Seckel syndrome (microcephaly, dwarfism)	2	0
Skeletal dysplasia (miscellaneous)	25	1
Spondylo-epiphyseal dysplasia	2	0
Spondylo-thoracic dysplasia (Jarcho–Levin syndrome)	2	0
Thanatophoric dysplasia	9	2
Thrombocytopenia with absent radius syndrome (TAR)	2	1
Total	118	12

* June 1, 1976 to January 28, 1983.

Osteogenesis Imperfecta

This disorder exists in several forms. Subcategories of osteogenesis imperfecta (OI) have recently been described (Table 3),[20] but it is already evident that this classification is not satisfactory and must be regarded as temporary until further genetic and biochemical information is developed. The generally lethal variety in which the infant is seriously affected at birth has been labeled as OI congenita (OI Type II). These infants have poorly mineralized and often collapsed crania. Their sclerae are dark blue. Multiple fractures are noted in the spine, ribs, and long bones. The limbs are symmetrically short and angulated as a result of fracture. If not fractured, they are often bowed. This condition seems to have an autosomal recessive inheritance pattern most of the time.

There are at least three other forms of the disease (OI Tarda) that present less dramatically at birth, including two autosomal dominant forms and one autosomal recessive. The least severe is an autosomal domi-

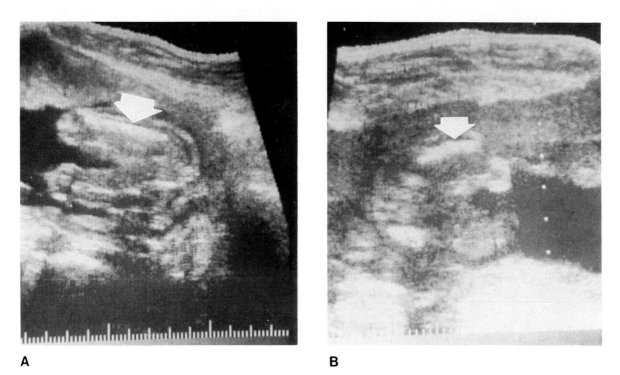

Fig. 7. Ultrasound scan through upper legs (*arrow*) of a normal fetus **(A)** and a fetus with diastrophic dysplasia **(B).**

TABLE 3
Expected Ultrasound Findings in Skeletal Dysplasias

Condition	Inheritance	Head	Chest and Body	Spine	Limbs
1. (a) Achondrogenesis I (Parenti–Fraccaro)	AR*	Thin, poorly mineralized skull	Short chest and body with thin ribs	Low-level echoes from vertebral bodies	Marked symmetrical reduction
(b) Achondrogenesis II (Langer–Saldino)	AR	Increased H:B ratio	Short, barrel-shaped thorax	Low-level echoes from vertebral bodies	Symmetrical reduction, straight
2. Achondroplasia	AD†	Increased HC, BPD, and H:B ratio; bulging forehead			Short limbs, especially femurs and humeruses
3. Asphyxiating thoracic dysplasia	AR		Long, narrow chest with very short ribs		Variable shortening; hexadactyly (occasional)
4. Camptomelic dysplasias	NK‡				
a. long-limbed	NK	Increased HC, BPD, and H:B ratio; micrognathia (profile)	Small, narrow thorax	Perhaps some flattening of spine	Long, thin, and definitely bowed
b. short-limbed normocephalic	NK				Short, broad, angulated
c. short-limbed with craniosynostosis	NK	Increased HC, BPD, and H:B ratio; micrognathia (profile)			Short, broad, angulated
5. Chondroectodermal dysplasia (Ellis–van Creveld syndrome)	AR		Long, narrow chest; congenital heart disease (occasional)		Shortening of both proximal and distal segments; hexadactyly
6. Diastrophic dysplasia	AR				Short with contractures—''hitchhiker'' thumbs
7. Hypophosphatasia	AR	Very thin, with poor mineralization, sometimes collapsed	Thin, poorly visualized ribs	Thin, poorly visualized	Short, thin, ribbon-like; fractures

274

nant variety (Type IV) in which the patient, who does not have blue sclerae, will generally have normal longevity but will be prone to bowing and fracture of long bones and ribs. Radiographic evaluation may not be confirmatory. Of the other two forms, the autosomal recessive, progressively deforming variety (Type III) is generally more severe. The patient will show evidence of Wormian bone formation and will have compromised height and severe limb bowing. Pathologic fractures are common. Type III patients have normal sclerae, which distinguishes them from patients with the remaining autosomal dominant form (Type I), who have similar but less severe features of the disease. Type I patients have blue sclerae.

The fetal areas that deserve ultrasonic scrutiny in patients at risk for OI are the cranium, ribs, spine, and long bones. The skull is poorly mineralized and should appear very thin. Also, as a result of compression, the outline can be irregular. In the lethal form of OI the ribs are often fractured. With ultrasound, the ribs are among the most difficult bones to evaluate thoroughly because on sagittal scan only a small por-

tion of each rib is seen. Transverse scans reveal portions of the rib cage on three sides, but it is virtually impossible to trace each rib around the thorax and, therefore, failure to demonstrate rib fracture does not preclude the diagnosis. The fetal spine can be viewed in its entirety after the 16th week of gestation only if the fetus is in a "back-up" position, and lateral displacement can, thereby, be defined. During pregnancy, the fetus lies on its side approximately 80 percent of the time and one has to evaluate the spine in a series of sagittal scans with a static scanner or with a curved sweep of a real-time transducer. In this position, front-to-back displacement can be noted. Individual spinal segments can best be outlined with carefully spaced transverse scans.

The long bones at birth are thickened and angulated in OI congenita. The shortening should be apparent in the late second trimester. OI can be differentiated from hypophosphatasia by the degree of demineralization of the calvarium (more so with hypophosphatasia) and the thickness of the shortened limbs. In OI congenita the limbs tend to be thickened and broad while

TABLE 3 (Continued)

8. Langer mesomelic dysplasia	AR	Micrognathia			Severe middle segment shortening (forearms, legs)
9. Osteogenesis imperfecta					
a. Type I (blue sclerae)	AD	Normal size			Perhaps mild bowing
b. Type II (blue sclerae, lethal variety)	AR	Thin, often collapsed cranium	Rib fractures	(?) Fractures	Short, broad, and angulated with fractures; femurs especially tend to be broad with marked bowing
c. Type III (normal sclerae)	AR	Thin, but not as marked as Type II	Occasional rib fractures		Fractures possible, broad bones, mild bowing, slightly short
d. Type IV (normal sclerae)	AD	Normal size	Occasional rib fractures		Bowing and occasional fractures
10. Short rib–polydactyly syndromes					
a. Type I (Saldino Noonan)	AR		Narrow thorax, protuberant abdomen	Flat vertebrae	Very short, polydactyly
b. Type II (Majewski)	AR		Narrow thorax, protuberant abdomen		Moderate shortening, polydactyly
11. Spondyloepiphyseal dysplasia congenita (Spranger–Wiedemann)	AD		Short, barrel-shaped chest		Proximal shortening
12. Thanatophoric dysplasia	NK	Increased HC, BPD, and H:B ratio; prominent forehead	Narrow, pear-shaped thorax, protuberant abdomen	Marked flattening of vertebrae	Very short and bowed

* Autosomal recessive.
† Autosomal dominant.
‡ Not known.
Adapted from Sillence DW, Rimoin DL, Lachman R: Neonatal dwarfism. Symposium on Medical Genetics. Ped Clin N Am 25(3):453, 1978

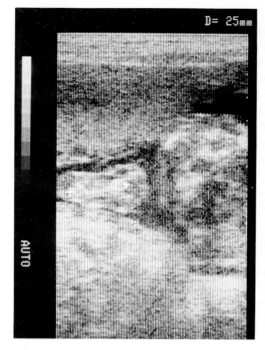
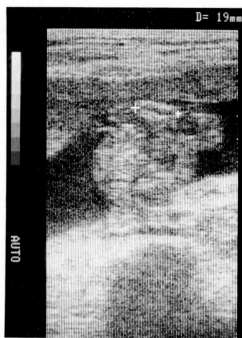

Fig. 8. Marked shortening of **(A)** tibia and fibula and **(B)** femur in 20.4-week fetus at risk of OI Type II.

in hypophosphatasia the long bones are thin and ribbonlike.

Many have felt that OI congenita (Type II) is not truly a primary short-limb dysplasia and that the reduction in limb length is simply a result of fractures in utero or at the time of birth. A literature review at the time of this writing yielded only two cases of OI congenita (Type II) diagnosed in the second trimester.[21,22] In these and in the third trimester cases fractures and abnormal bone configuration accompanied the shortened limb measurements described. We recently, however, identified a fetus with OI congenita (Type II) in the second trimester. Femur measurements were more than 2 SD below the mean for gestation and there was no evidence of fracture (Figs. 8A, 8B). This suggested that the fetus had a defect that exerted a primary effect on bone length.

Previously, we had diagnosed a form of OI tarda (Type I) in the second trimester by demonstration of a femoral fracture at 18 weeks.[1] Recently, we had the opportunity to follow another patient with OI tarda (Type I) prospectively with ultrasound and noticed a difference in the thickness, configuration, and, later, echogenicity of the fetal femurs compared with those of unaffected fetuses.[23] These somewhat subtle changes were manifested in the second trimester in the fetus, who was confirmed at birth to have OI tarda (Type I).

Achondroplasia

This condition has an autosomal dominant inheritance pattern. The heterozygous condition can result when either both parents are heterozygotes or if one parent is a heterozygote. Spontaneous mutations can also arise in normal parents. Homozygous achondroplasia, a 25 percent possibility when both parents have heterozygous disease, is a lethal condition in which there is a significant limb shortening and thoracic narrowing. There is also appreciable head-to-body disproportion. Heterozygous achondroplasia presents as an infant with short limbs, protuberant forehead, and abdomen and chest that are modestly narrowed.

Filly prospectively studied four pregnancies at risk for achondroplasia.[5] Femoral measurements in two heterozygous achondroplastic fetuses did not fall below 99 percent confidence levels until after the second trimester, while homozygous achondroplasia was apparent in one fetus in the early second trimester, at which time bone length was markedly compromised.

Individuals with short-limb dysplasia often marry someone with the same or some other dysplasia. These parents are generally quite sophisticated concerning diagnostic possibilities in skeletal dysplasia. Since it is impossible for sonologists to gain much experience in these rare conditions, these couples can represent a formidable diagnostic challenge.

Acquired Skeletal Defects

There are a few acquired skeletal defects that warrant mention. The association between progestin exposure in the first trimester and limb reduction defects has been overstated. A recent experience suggests that the risk of these defects is very small. Nevertheless, because of an early report suggesting an association,[24] many anxious couples have been offered prenatal diagnosis. It is impossible to assess the cost-effectiveness of scanning all patients exposed to some form of progestin in the first trimester but we suspect the yield, compared with the effort involved, is extremely low.

Amniotic band syndrome occurs when there is a defect in the amnion and a portion of the fetus becomes adherent to the underlying chorion early in gestation. Limb development can be impaired under these restricting circumstances. Affected infants will have a variety of limb, trunk and, occasionally, cranial deformities. Often, one or more limbs will be partially amputated. Sometimes only a distal limb is grotesquely affected. One should suspect the diagnosis when multiple skeletal anomalies are identified that do not seem to fit into any definable pattern.

CONCLUSION

Although the skills required for intrauterine diagnosis of structural anomalies are not commonly available, it is hoped that in the near future tertiary institutions will have the trained personnel required to offer these services on a routine basis. This will greatly augment efforts of the obstetrician, perinatologist, and neonatologist to provide a complete prenatal profile of anomalies in a particular fetus.

ACKNOWLEDGMENT

We wish to thank Ingeborg Venus for her editorial assistance in preparation of this manuscript.

REFERENCES

1. Hobbins JC, Bracken MB, Mahoney KJ: Diagnosis of fetal skeletal dysplasias with ultrasound. Am J Obstet Gynecol 142:306, 1982
2. Yeh MM, Bracero L, Reilly KB, et al: Ultrasonic measurements of the femur length as an index of fetal gestational age. Am J Obstet Gynecol 144:519, 1982
3. Rumack CM, Johnson ML, Zunkel D: Antenatal diagnosis. Clin Diag Ultrasound 8:210, 1981
4. Luthy DA, Hall JG, Graham CB: Prenatal diagnosis of thrombocytopenia with absent radii. Clin Genet 15:495, 1979
5. Filly RA, Golbus MS: Ultrasonography of the normal and pathologic fetal skeleton, in Callen PW (ed), Ultrasonography in Obstetrics and Gynecology. Philadelphia, Saunders, 1983, pp 81–96
6. Sabbagha RE, Hughey M, Depp R: Growth adjusted sonographic age: A simplified method. Obstet Gynecol 51:383, 1978
7. Campbell S, Thoms A: Ultrasound measurement of the fetal head to abdomen circumference ratio in assessment of growth retardation. Br J Obstet Gynaecol 84:165, 1977
8. Chervenak FA, Blakemore KJ, Isaacson G, et al: Antenatal sonographic findings of thanatophoric dysplasia with cloverleaf skull. Am J Obstet Gynecol 146:8, 984–985, 1983
9. Christ JE, Meininger MG: Ultrasound diagnosis of cleft lip and cleft palate before birth. Plastic Reconstr Surg 68:854, 1981
10. Savoldelli G, Schmid W, Schinzel A: Prenatal diagnosis of cleft lip and palate by ultrasound. Prenatal Diag 2:313, 1982
11. Mullivor RA, Mennuti M, Zackai EH, et al: Prenatal diagnosis of hypophosphatasia: Genetic biochemical and clinical studies. Am J Hum Genet 30:271, 1978
12. Woo JSK, Ghosh A, Liang ST, et al: Ultrasonic evaluation of osteogenesis imperfecta congenita in utero. J Clin Ultrasound 11:42, 1983
13. Kleinman CS, Donnerstein RL, Jaffe CC, et al: Fetal echocardiography. A tool for evaluation of in utero cardiac arrythmias and monitoring of in utero therapy: Analysis of 71 patients. Am J Cardiology 51:237, 1983
14. Warsof SL, Gohari P, Berkowitz RL, et al: Estimation of fetal weight by computer-assisted analysis. Am J Obstet Gynecol 128:881, 1977
15. Shepard MJ, Richards VA, Berkowitz RL, et al: An evaluation of two equations for predicting fetal weight by ultrasound. Am J Obstet Gynecol 142:47, 1982
16. Tamura RK, Sabbagha RE: Percentile ranks of sonar fetal abdominal circumference measurements. Am J Obstet Gynecol 138:475, 1980
17. Hobbins JC, Grannum PAT, Berkowitz RL, et al: Ultrasound in the diagnosis of congenital anomalies. Am J Obstet Gynecol 134:331, 1979
18. Goodlin RC, Lowe EW: Unexplained hydramnios associated with a thanatophoric dwarf. Am J Obstet Gynecol 118:873, 1974
19. Mantagos S, Weiss BR, Mahoney MJ, Hobbins JC: Prenatal diagnosis of diastrophic dwarfism. Am J Obstet Gynecol 139:111, 1981
20. Sillence DW, Rimoin DL, Lachman R: Neonatal dwarfism. Symposium on Medical Genetics. Ped Clin N Am 25(3):453, 1978
21. Shapiro JE, Phillips JJ, III, Byers PN, et al: Prenatal diagnosis of lethal perinatal osteogenesis imperfecta (OI Type II). J Pediat 100:127, 1982
22. Elejalde BR, Elejalde MM: Prenatal diagnosis of perinatally lethal osteogenesis imperfecta. Am J Med Genet 14:353, 1983
23. Chervenak FA, Romero RR, Berkowitz RL, et al: Antenatal sonographic findings of osteogenesis imperfecta. Am J Obstet Gynecol 143:228, 1982
24. Nora JJ, Nora AH, Blu J, et al: Exogenous progestogen and estrogen implicated in birth defects. JAMA 240:837, 1978

21 | Diagnostic Ultrasound in Erythroblastosis Fetalis

John T. Queenan
Gregory D. O'Brien

INTRODUCTION

Not so long ago "hydrops" was a term used almost exclusively to describe problems associated with eryth- roblastosis fetalis due to rhesus incompatability. With the success of Rh-immune globulin therapy the conse- quent decreased frequency of erythroblastosis fetalis has resulted in other causes of hydrops of a nonimmu- nologic variety coming to the fore. Nonimmunologic hydrops (NIH) is responsible for 3 percent of fetal mortality. The term "nonimmune hydrops" is now used to describe a group of conditions other than eryth- roblastosis fetalis in which the sonographic features of fluid overload are seen. Sonographic findings that typify hydrops are fetal ascites, pleural effusion, peri- cardial effusion, and skin thickening due to edema. There is almost always polyhydramnios and the pla- centa in most types of nonimmune hydrops is thick- ened and has an abnormal echogenic acoustical texture. The fetal liver and spleen are often enlarged.

The causes of nonimmune hydrops are varied but there is in common an increased venous pressure (Table 1).[1-6] There are other hematologic causes apart from Rh incompatability, such as fetomaternal transfusion, placental chorioangioma with syphoning of the blood that was destined for the fetus to the placenta, twin- to-twin transfusion, and G6 PD deficiency. However, the most common cause of nonimmune hydrops is car- diovascular lesions such as hypoplastic left heart syn- drome or other types of congenital heart disease and functional cardiac problems such as dysrhythymias (e.g., tachycardia) or myocarditis. The nonimmune hy- drops seen with the TORCH group of infections may be due to myocarditis. Obstructive vascular problems may occur outside the heart, as with umbilical vein thrombosis or pulmonary diseases such as cystic ade- nomatoid malformation, lymphangiectasia, pulmonary hypoplasia and diaphragmatic hernia. Some neoplasms such as neuroblastoma and teratoma are thought to cause hydrops either by obstruction or by siphoning off of blood that would otherwise go to the fetal heart.

Chromosomal anomalies such as trisomy 18 or 21 or triploidy can be associated with nonimmune hy- drops. The mechanism by which asphyxiating thoracic dystrophy, achondroplasia, and other forms of dwarf- ism and the cystic hygroma seen with Turner syndrome cause nonimmune hydrops is not entirely clear. The hydrops associated with thanatophopic dwarfism is thought to be related to decreased thoracic compliance. NIH associated with cystic hygroma is thought to be secondary to lymphatic flow disturbances.

Congenital nephrosis causes severe nonimmune hydrops presumably because of edema due to hypoal- bumenia but other renal problems such as hydrone- phrosis and dysplastic kidneys are also associated with nonimmune hydrops. Two maternal causes of non- immune hydrops are known—diabetes mellitus and toxemia.

The causes of nonimmune hydrops are varied but in most instances the condition is fatal. Nevertheless, it is worthwhile trying to establish the diagnosis prior to delivery because a few of the responsible conditions can be treated at birth. The detection of a fetal tumor can be followed by successful surgery. Elective delivery of a twin affected by the twin-to-twin transfusion may be successful. Fetal dysrhythmias often resolve after

TABLE 1
Anomalies Associated with Sonographic Features of Nonimmunological Hydrops

Anatomic Area	Condition	Sonographic Findings
Head	Toxoplasmosis	Intracranial calcification
	Encephalocele	Cystic area arising from head
	Galen aneurysm	Posterior cyst in head
Abdomen	Sacral teratoma	Tumor mass near sacrum or
	Neuroblastoma	kidney
	Duodenal atresia	Double-bubble appearance
	Meconium peritonitis	consider Down syndrome
		Peritoneal calcification
Lungs	Cystic adenomatoid malformation	Cystic spaces in chest
	Diaphragmatic hernia	Stomach and other cystic structures in the chest
Kidneys	Congenital hydronephrosis	Cystic space in kidneys
	Congenital nephrosis	Large kidneys
Heart	Severe congenital heart disease	Chamber enlargement or absence (hypoplastic left heart)
	Myocarditis	Abnormal wall motion
	Dysrhythmias	Rhythm changes
Limbs	Dwarfism	Short limbs
	Osteogenesis imperfecta	Fractures
	Arthrogryposis	Abnormal feet and hands
Twin pregnancy	Twin-to-twin transfusion	Second fetus of small size
Placenta	Chorioangioma	Mass adjacent to or in the placenta
	Syphilis	Thick placenta
Neck	Cystic hygroma	Septated cystic structure generally in the neck region
Cord	Umbilical vein thrombosis	Absent cord pulsation
	Umbilical cord anomalies	Single artery

Adapted from Fleischer AC, Killam AP, et al: Hydrops fetalis. Radiology 141:163, 1981, with permission.

birth and can be treated in utero (see Chapter 15). It is therefore incumbent on the sonographer to perform a comprehensive survey of the fetus. The relevant findings in the different segments of the fetal anatomy which should be sought are shown in Table 1.

In this chapter we shall be concentrating on erythroblastosis fetalis since the other anomalies that cause hydrops are described in various other segments of the text (see Chapters 14–17, 19, and 20).

Erythroblastosis fetalis (EBF) is caused by an incompatibility of erythrocyte antigens between the fetus and the mother. The mother usually becomes isoimmunized by a transplacental hemorrhage or by an incompatible transfusion. Subsequently, maternal antibodies against the fetal antigens cross the placenta and cause a hemolytic anemia in the fetus. If the EBF is mild, there is fetal anemia and neonatal hyperbilirubinemia, which may be managed by phototherapy or exchange transfusion. If the EBF is severe, the hemolysis in the fetus may be so profound that the fetus develops congestive heart failure and dies. When the disease is this severe, hydrops fetalis is generally present.

EBF is unique because the fetal condition is reflected by the bilirubin concentration in amniotic fluid (AF) obtained by amniocentesis. Since serial amniotic fluid bilirubin determinations are often required, diagnostic ultrasound is particularly helpful to facilitate a safe amniocentesis. Ultrasound guidance for this procedure has become a standard of practice.

EBF is also unique because fetal deterioration can be detected by a second modality, ultrasound scanning. Since congestive heart failure occurs secondary to profound fetal hemolysis, certain pathologic changes may be detected by diagnostic ultrasound. Although the earliest indication of worsening fetal condition should be gained from amniotic fluid analysis, anatomic changes in the fetus can be detected by ultrasound scan. This modality is an extremely important aspect of comprehensive care. In some situations, the history and antibody titers may suggest that an amniocentesis is not yet necessary. In such situations sonograms provide an excellent backup. If anatomic changes (polyhydramnios, hyperplacentosis, ascites, or cardiomegaly) occur they can be detected. Once it is established that the fetus has significant EBF, the fetal condition can be monitored sonographically by observations of various pathologic changes. This is especially important once intrauterine transfusions have commenced.

With severe EBF, intrauterine transfusions (IUT) may be necessary. These have become much safer and easier when performed with real-time ultrasound guidance as the main imaging modality rather than fluoroscopy. Not only can radiation to the mother and her fetus be avoided, but real-time ultrasound offers very accurate guidance for performance of an IUT.

Today EBF is being managed predominantly in medical centers where the level of ultrasound scanning expertise for detecting early fetal compromise is high. Diagnostic ultrasound is an essential feature in the management of the fetus with EBF.

DETERMINING GESTATIONAL AGE

Knowing correct gestational age is important in EBF. The timing of the first amniocentesis and the timing of delivery is dependent on gestational age. Accurate gestational age is also important to determine the adequacy of fetal growth during pregnancy.

Most patients with Rh isoimmunization are aware that they have a high-risk pregnancy. Therefore, they usually visit their doctors early in pregnancy, giving them the opportunity to determine gestational age accurately. An accurate menstrual history and an early pelvic exam are an accurate clinical way to determine gestational age. Yet, in the many patients who do not have regular menstrual cycles ultrasound scanning offers the most accurate means of determining gestational age.

The crown–rump length provides a very accurate means of establishing gestational age between 7 and 13 weeks' gestation. If the determination is done carefully, the sonographically derived dates should be accurate within 3 to 4 days. Between 14 and 20 weeks' gestation, the biparietal diameter and fetal femur length provide an accurate means of determining gestational age. Using these modalities together, the clinician can check one against the other to ensure accuracy. If done carefully, accuracy should be within 1 week of gestational age. After 20 weeks the accuracy of ultrasonic dating techniques decreases.

AMNIOCENTESIS

If the Rh-immunized patient has a very low antibody titer, the pregnancy may be monitored by antibody titers alone. Periodic ultrasound scanning can provide back-up monitoring to be sure the fetus is not undergoing unsuspected deterioration.

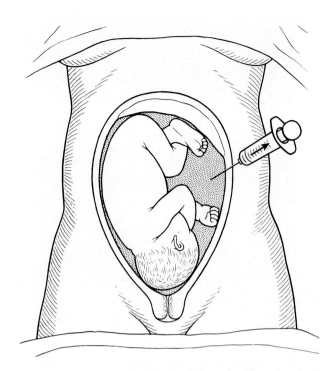

Figure 1. Diagram of method for amniocentesis. (*Reproduced with permission from Queenan JT: Amniocentesis and transamniotic fetal transfusion for Rh disease. Clin Obstet Gynecol 9:491, 1966.*)

If the Rh-immunized patient has an antibody titer that reaches or surpasses the "critical titer," then antibody titers are not a reliable way to follow fetal condition. The critical titer is that level below which the laboratory has not experienced an intrauterine or neonatal death due to EBF. In such situations amniocentesis with AF analysis for bilirubin is the appropriate way to determine fetal condition (Fig. 1).

Ultrasound scanning is an integral part of the amniocentesis procedure. The scan is useful to:

Confirm gestational age

Identify pockets of AF

Avoid placental injury

Avoid fetal injury

Detect twins and congenital malformations.

Pockets of AF are easy to identify with ultrasound scanning. The objective is to identify a pocket of AF that does not require traversing the placenta to obtain AF.

The placenta may be identified easily by ultrasound scanning. If it is posterior, it poses no problem for an amniocentesis. If it is anterior, generally the clinician can find a placenta-free window through which to aspirate AF. If the placenta is anterior and no placenta-free window can be detected, ultrasound scanning can still help to increase the safety of traversing the placenta. The insertion of the umbilical cord

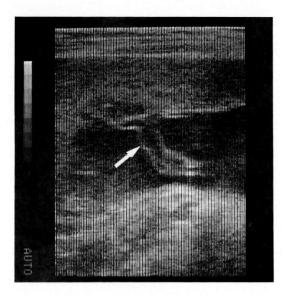

Figure 2. Anterior placenta with cord insertion.

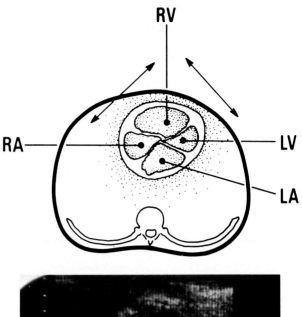

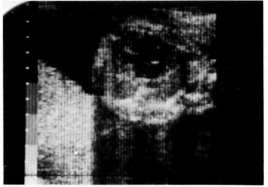

Figure 3. Transthoracic four-chamber sonogram view of the heart and diagram showing method of determining fetal heart size.

on the chorionic plate is identified (Fig. 2). It is dangerous to traverse the placenta at the cord insertion because all of the vessels radiate out from this site. An amniocentesis site over a pocket of AF as far from the cord insertion as possible is selected. Following the amniocentesis, a scan over the site is performed to see if there is any bleeding from the placenta. This would be identified as an echogenic cascade falling through the AF.

Ultrasound scanning permits selection of an amniocentesis site away from vital fetal structures such as the face, neck or thorax. Fetal structures like arms or legs in the amniotic fluid pocket present no problem because usually they will reflexly move away if touched by a needle.

Ultrasound scanning detects multiple pregnancies. In EBF it would be necessary to sample AF from both sacs because one twin could be Rh-negative and the other Rh-positive. If severe congenital malformations like anencephaly are present, it is essential to detect this early to prevent the performance of unindicated procedures.

FETAL CONDITION

In erythroblastosis fetalis, the pathophysiology includes hemolytic anemia, compensatory erythropoiesis with hepatosplenomegaly and congestive heart failure. Many of these pathologic processes cause anatomic changes that can be observed sonographically. These have been well described in the literature.[7-10] Pathologic changes that can be studied on the fetus include

cardiomegaly, hepatosplenomegaly, ascites, umbilical vein dilatation, subcutaneous edema, amniotic fluid volume, and placental thickness.

HEART SIZE

EBF is characterized by a hemolytic anemia in the fetus. When the hemolysis is severe, the fetus is likely to develop congestive heart failure.

A simple method for assessing the fetal heart size is available. A transthoracic four-chamber view of the heart is obtained as illustrated in Figure 3. Measurements are taken by the on-screen calipers of both the long and short axes of this view of the heart. It is preferable to do this without the freeze-frame, as the motion of the cardiac muscle makes it easier to delineate the outer borders of the heart. A simple assessment of heart size or area is made by multiplying the measurements of the long and short axis. A simple graph of the normal heart size was calculated from measure-

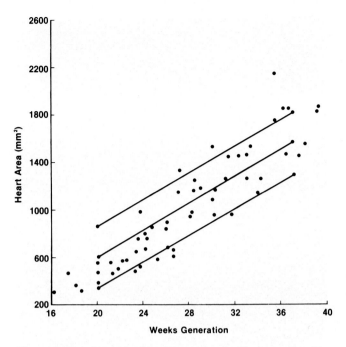

Figure 4. Sample graph of fetal heart size (mm²). (regression line ± SEM).

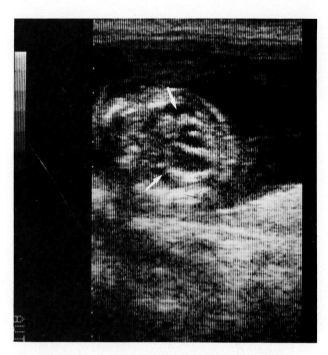

Figure 5. Cardiomegaly with pericardial effusion (*arrows*).

ments on normal fetuses (Fig. 4). Cardiomegaly can be detected in the fetus by using this graph of normal measurements. If cardiomegaly is detected, the heart size may be monitored by serial ultrasound determinations. Figures 5 and 6 show fetal hearts with marked cardiomegaly. Note how distinct all four chambers are. The arrows point to a pronounced pericardial effusion. The heart area measurements greatly exceeded the upper limits of normal for that week of gestation. Figure 7 shows the same fetal heart after an IUT and treatment by digitalizing the mother. There is a marked decrease in heart size and in the size of the pericardial effusion.

ASCITES

Fetal ascites is a definite indication of heart failure in a mother with an elevated Rh titer. The very early diagnosis of fetal ascites may be difficult. Pseudoascites, which may be seen as an artifact on linear array real-time ultrasound scanners, may be confused with ascites; pseudoascites may be recognized because it is not dependent on position (Fig. 8). It is seen in normal pregnancies and therefore has no significance. We like to visualize a section of umbilical vein traversing the falciform ligament in ascitic fluid for a length greater than 3 mm to diagnose ascites. Fetal ascites is present in Figures 9 and 10.

When early ascites is detected it is a definite indication of fetal compromise secondary to heart failure.

Moderate to severe ascites presents very distinctive ultrasound features that would be difficult to overlook.

HEPATOSPLENOMEGALY

Hepatic and splenic enlargement result from the markedly increased erythropoieses in the Rh-affected fetus. This may result in a rapidly increasing abdominal cir-

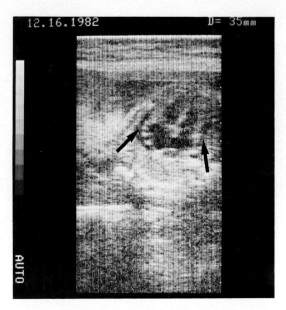

Figure 6. Cardiomegaly with pericardial effusion (*arrows*).

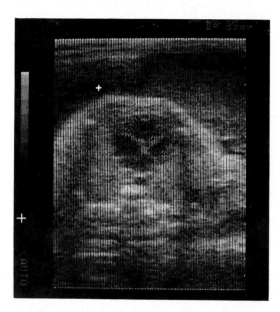

Figure 7. Normal appearing four-chamber view of the heart following fetal therapy.

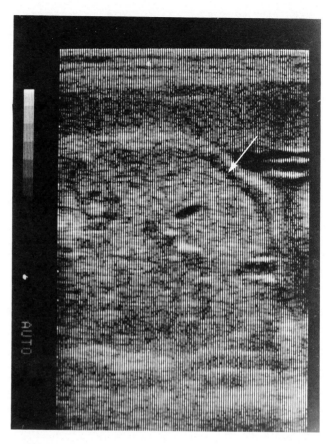

Figure 8. Transverse section of fetal abdomen illustrating pseudoascites (*arrow*).

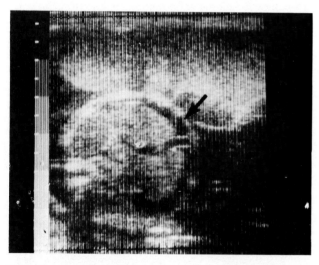

Figure 9. Transverse section of fetal abdomen with "real" ascites (*arrow*).

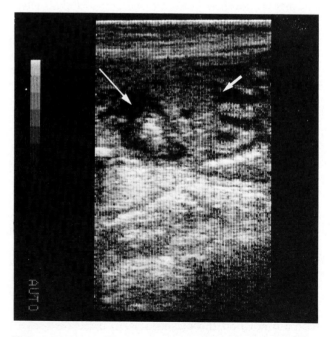

Figure 10. Longitudinal section of hydropic fetus. Long arrow indicates ascites. Short arrow indicates pleural effusion.

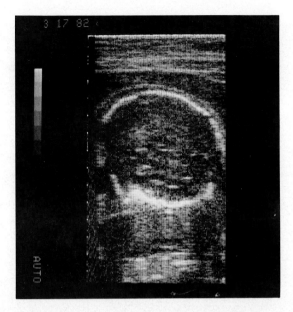

Figure 11. Subcutaneous edema around the fetal scalp.

cumference, which can be followed sonographically. An increase of abdominal girth of greater than 2 cm per week has been described as being significant, although the sensitivity of this technique for detecting hepatosplenomegaly remains to be defined more conclusively.

UMBILICAL VEIN DILATATION

When the fetus develops congestive heart failure, it is reasonable to expect venous distention. Indeed, when there is a combination of venous distention and polyhydramnios, the ultrasound scan can produce a striking picture.

The diameter of the umbilical vein can be measured with electronic calipers. The umbilical vein as it traverses the fetal liver can also be distended with severe EBF. However, due to congestion of the liver and to accelerated erythropoiesis, the ability of the umbilical vein to distend may be compromised. The best area to measure the umbilical vein is in a loop of cord in the AF.

DeVore and associates indicated that increased umbilical vein diameter and the fetal liver size predicted the need for intrauterine transfusions.[9] It was suggested that increased umbilical vein diameters would precede the development of fetal hydrops or increases in amniotic fluid bilirubin. Witter and Graham did not find the umbilical vein diameter to be a useful test in isoimmunized pregnancies.[11] Of the four fetuses with ascites demonstrated on sonogram, three

had sonographic evidence of hydrops. All of these patients had OD at 450 values in Liley zone III. Of these four fetuses with ascites, none had an umbilical vein diameter measured in the liver or in the amniotic fluid that met the criteria of DeVore. Indeed, although the umbilical vessels appear engorged with severe erythroblastosis fetalis, the umbilical vein diameter does not appear to be a reliable indicator of fetal condition.

SUBCUTANEOUS EDEMA

When subcutaneous edema (anasarca) is identified it indicates that the fetus is rapidly deteriorating with hydrops fetalis. Although this finding usually occurs a few days before fetal death, not all fetuses develop this feature before dying in utero. Usually, the initial detectable site is the scalp. Figure 11 illustrates fetal scalp edema. Later the trunk and, finally, the limbs, may be involved.

PLACENTA

With mild EBF, there are no characteristic placental changes detected by ultrasound scanning. With moderate or severe EBF or with hydrops fetalis the placental size may increase. The thickness exceeds 50 mm and the texture may appear homogenous like ground glass (Fig. 12). These findings almost always occur in the presence of the other ultrasound signs of severe EBF.

POLYHYDRAMNIOS

Increased amniotic fluid volume is often associated with hyperplacentosis. There is no strict criteria for an ultrasound diagnosis of polyhydramnios, although, when present in its severest form, there is usually no trouble in making the diagnosis. The fetus can extend its limbs and there is a "bulging" uterine outline. It is usually found with the hydropic fetus, but its appearance in the less severely affected fetus is inconsistent. The presence of polyhydramnios is usually a poor prognostic sign. Oligohydramnios also appears to be a sign of poor prognosis.

MONITORING FETAL CONDITION

Once a fetal abnormality suggesting EBF is detected by ultrasound scanning, this feature may be monitored serially to determine fetal condition. Since the objective

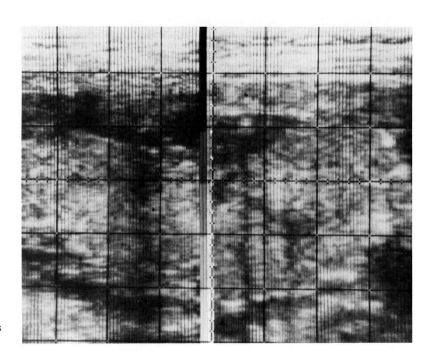

Figure 12. Placenta thickened by erythroblastosis fetalis.

of care is to get as much maturity as possible without letting the fetus die in utero, monitoring fetal heart size or progression of ascites are very valuable predictors of fetal deterioration.

Additionally, fetal movements are very important. The fetus that dies in utero usually becomes very inactive before fetal death. Fetal movement can be determined well by employing a system of counting maternally perceived kicks as with the Cardiff kick count. Alternatively, fetal movement can be quantitated during a scanning session providing an estimate of fetal activity which may not be perceived by the mother.

INTRAUTERINE TRANSFUSIONS

When severe EBF requires that IUTs be used to keep the fetus alive, ultrasound guidance is particularly valuable. First, it avoids the use of x-rays. Second, it facilitates the safe performance of the IUT and third it is vital to monitor the fetus over the next few days to observe the absorption of blood. During the IUT, the real-time transducer may be placed in a sterile bag containing sterile gel so that it may be used during the procedure to guide the proper placement of the needle in the fetal abdomen. For a more complete review of this subject, see Chapter 22 and consult *Modern Management of the Rh Problem.*[12]

Accurate guidance of the needle for the IUT is crucial because of the potential for fetal injury. The marked hepatosplenomegaly requires that the needle be placed in the lower third of the fetal abdomen. The distended fetal bladder can easily be identified and serves as an excellent guide to the area for needle insertion. Proper placement of the needle can be ascertained because injection of air, saline, or blood all cause visible turbulance emanating from the end of the needle.[13] As packed red blood cells are injected the stream of blood can be visualized in the fetal peritoneal cavity. Occasionally one will see a layer of red blood cells in the dependent portion. The appearance of apparent ascites with blood between the fetal liver and abdominal wall can be visualized after 15 to 20 ml have been injected. As the blood is injected the fetal heart is observed by ultrasound so that a bradycardia or arrhythmia can be detected. This may indicate poor tolerance to the procedure. Ascites fluid should be aspirated prior to the procedure.

SUMMARY

Diagnostic ultrasound has become an integral part of managing the isoimmunized pregnancy today. Ultrasound guidance has increased the safety and efficacy of amniocentesis and IUT. Ultrasound scanning gives an accurate means of determining and monitoring fetal condition. Finally, it has allowed the clinician to eliminate x-rays from the management of EBF.

REFERENCES

1. Fleischer AC, Killam AP, et al: Hydrops fetalis: Sonographic evaluation and clinical implications. Radiology 141:163, 1981
2. Perlin BM, Pomerance JJ, et al: Nonimmunologic hydrops fetalis. Obstet Gynecol 57:584, 1981
3. Hutchison AA, Drew JH, et al: Nonimmunologic hydrops fetalis: A review of 61 cases. Obstet Gynecol 59:347, 1982
4. Davis CL: Diagnosis and management of nonimmune hydrops fetalis. J Reprod Med 27:594, 1982
5. Hadlock F, et al: Fetal ascites not associated with Rh incompatibility: Recognition and management with sonography. Am J Roentgenol 134:1225, 1980
6. Garrett W: Gray scale sonography in the diagnosis of hydrops due to fetal lung tumor. J Clin Ultrasound 311:45, 1975
7. Wiener S, Bolognese RJ, et al: Real-time ultrasonography in the diagnosis of erythroblastosis fetalis. Proceedings 25th Annual Meeting of AIUM, 1980
8. Wiener S, Bolognese RJ, et al: Ultrasound in the evaluation and management of the isoimmunized pregnancy. J Clin Ultrasound 9:315, 1981
9. DeVore GP, Mayden K, et al: Dilation of the fetal umbilical vein dilation in rhesus hemolytic anemia: A predictor of severe disease. Am J Obstet Gynecol 141:464, 1981
10. DeVore GR, Donnerstein RL, et al: The diagnostic significance of fetal pericardial effusion using real-time directed M-mode echocardiography. Proceedings 26th Annual Meeting of AIUM, 1981
11. Witter FR, Graham D: The utility of ultrasonically measured umbilical vein diameters in isoimmunized pregnancies. Am J Obstet Gynecol 146:225, 1983
12. Queenan JT: Intrauterine transfusion, in Queenan JT (ed), Modern Management of the Rh Problem, 2nd ed. Hagerstown, MD, Harper and Row, 1977
13. Queenan JT: Erythroblastosis fetalis, in Queenan JT, Hobbins JC (eds), Protocols in High Risk Pregnancy. Oradell, NJ, Medical Economics, 1982

22 | Fetal Therapy

Michael L. Johnson
William Clewell
Dolores Pretorius
Paul Meier
David Manchester

The ultrasonic diagnosis of fetal congenital anomalies has now reached such a sophisticated level that many fetal diseases and malformations can be accurately diagnosed. Detection of fetal disease has dramatic effects on the management of the pregnancy, fetus, and newborn. Harrison has divided fetal diseases into categories based on method of treatment: selective pregnancy termination, delivery at term with planned treatment of the neonate, premature delivery in order to institute treatment, cesarean delivery in order to reduce trauma to the infant, and, finally, fetal treatment.[1] This last category involves the treatment of conditions that cause progressive damage to the fetus, impair further normal development, or threaten fetal life at a stage of pregnancy when premature delivery is not a reasonable option. Though this is a very small segment of the patient population, it has excited immense interest among scientific and lay communities. At times this interest has been out of proportion to the true importance of these developments. Fetal therapy is not a new concept. Long before the first attempts at direct fetal treatment, obstetricians attempted to improve fetal well-being by improving maternal health. In 1963, Liley performed the first intrauterine fetal transfusion for erythroblastosis fetalis.[2] This revolutionized the treatment of this disorder. Intrauterine transfusion remained the only direct treatment for fetal disease until recently and serves as a useful model for more recent attempts at fetal therapy.

PREREQUISITES FOR FETAL THERAPY

Accurate Diagnosis
The most important prerequisite for fetal treatment is an accurate diagnosis. Not only must congenital anomalies be accurately identified, but additional and complicating malformations or diseases must be identified or ruled out. To this end, family histories and consideration of genetic amniocentesis should always be included. Much of what can be learned about a fetus, however, will depend upon the skill and experience on the part of the ultrasonographer and a thorough and complete examination of both the fetus and the mother. This includes visualization and assessment of the fetal brain, heart, pleural cavity, liver, kidneys, bladder, gastrointestinal (GI) tract, skin, spine, and long bones. No organ system should be omitted.

Lesion Responsive to Therapy
Any lesion being considered for in utero treatment must be known to respond to the proposed therapy and, if alleviated, allow more normal fetal development to proceed. The presence of additional diseases or malformations should probably be considered a contraindication to fetal treatment. Additional malformations may render the proposed treatment futile. Applying experimental treatments to the fetus with multiple problems will confuse the interpretation of results and should be avoided if possible. Since premature delivery with neonatal treatment is an acceptable, if not preferable, approach to many of the diseases considered for in utero treatment, it must be carefully considered in every case.

Lesion Is Progressive
It should be demonstrated as well as possible that the lesion is progressive. One cannot justify experimental treatment if the disease appears to be static. Treatment should be attempted only if there is a clear danger of continued and irreversible damage to the fetus.

Capable Medical Team

A multidisciplinary team should be assembled that includes an obstetrician experienced in fetal diagnosis and intrauterine transfusion techniques, an ultrasonographer experienced in the diagnosis of fetal anomalies and percutaneous surgical techniques, a pediatric surgeon experienced in the neonatal management of the disease in question, and a neonatologist who will manage the infant after delivery. The input of experienced dysmorphologists and clinical geneticists is also invaluable. These individuals should all concur in the proposed plan for treatment.

Concurrence of Institutional Review Board

Since interventions involving the fetus are almost all experimental, an institutional review board (IRB) must be consulted and approve any program of fetal treatment. The ethical issues involved in fetal experimentation are complex and careful consideration must be given to fetal, maternal, and professional rights.

Investigative Soundness

Prior to embarking on experimental treatment, provisions must be made for follow-up and evaluation of results. Failure to make such provisions or failure to report results to the medical community constitutes a breach of good research practice and could be construed as unethical.

If these prerequisites are met, the following medical and surgical fetal problems can be considered for in utero therapy.

ERYTHROBLASTOSIS FETALIS

With the development of Rh(D) immune globulin, the number of Rh-sensitized patients has greatly decreased, but erythroblastosis fetalis nevertheless remains an important clinical problem, especially for the major referral centers. Intrauterine transfusion (IUT) was first developed by William Liley in 1963[2] and the technique significantly improved with fluoroscopic guidance. With the advent of high-resolution real-time ultrasound scanners intrauterine transfusion is now even safer and faster and the needles can be placed very accurately in the lower fetal abdomen, avoiding critical organs such as the fetal aorta, liver and spleen.

The technique of ultrasound needle guidance is essentially the same for all fetal therapy. To avoid taking the transducer out of clinical use and avoid any potential damage to the crystals, the transducer itself is not sterilized. The transducer and the cable are placed inside a gas sterilized polyethylene bag. If the bag is contaminated during the procedure, it can be replaced quickly. The face of the transducer is coated with coupling gel prior to insertion into the sterile plastic bag. Using sterilized tape, the bag is securely folded around the transducer such that a single layer of plastic (not a seam) is smoothly applied to the gel-coated face. The outside surface of the plastic bag over the transducer face is then coated with sterile coupling gel. The polyethylene is essentially transparent to ultrasound. As the transducer and cable are covered in sterile plastic, the unit can easily be used in the surgical field for transfusion. The transducer can be placed adjacent to the puncture site during needle placement. Polyethylene trash bags, masking tape, and foil packets of surgical lubricant can all be gas-sterilized together for use in these procedures.

The maternal abdomen is prepped and draped and the mother is mildly sedated but awake. A site on the maternal abdomen is then selected for the introduction of an 18 gauge aortography needle. If possible, the placenta is avoided; a point overlying the anterolateral surface on the lower fetal abdomen is chosen. The fetal bladder is the most useful landmark for identifying the appropriate cephalocaudal level of the fetus for needle entry. If necessary, external version either from breech to vertex or vice versa is carried out to bring the anterolateral surface of the lower fetal abdomen into an appropriate position.

As the transducer is covered with sterile plastic, it can be placed directly adjacent to the point of needle insertion. By carefully keeping the needle and the transducer beam coplanar, the progress of needle insertion can be observed on the ultrasound screen. Contact with the fetal abdomen can be detected both by resistance to advancement of the needle and by indentation of the fetus on the ultrasound screen. The needle is directed toward the fetal bladder or minimally cephalad to it. This keeps the point of penetration within the lower fetal abdomen and well away from the liver and spleen, either of which may be enlarged and vulnerable to laceration. Once the fetus is contacted, the needle is advanced a few more centimeters. Penetration of the fetal abdominal wall is generally easily visualized. The exact depth of needle penetration may be difficult to ascertain by ultrasound scan. The needle occasionally appears longer on the screen than it is because of lateral beam width artifact. It may also appear shorter if it passes out of the plane of the ultrasound beam. Ultrasonic visualization of the needle may be facilitated by sliding the stylet back and forth within the needle lumen. The hollow needle and the needle-stylet assembly have different reflective properties and the moving stylet is easily seen. This gives the operator added confidence in the displayed needle position. The presence of significant fetal ascites aids in the determi-

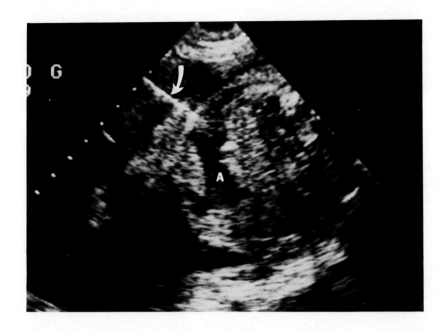

Fig. 1. Real-time ultrasound exam during fetal transfusion demonstrating needle (*curved arrow*) penetrating fetal abdominal wall. Fetal ascites (A) is present.

nation of the depth of penetration into the fetal abdomen. The needle tip can be seen clearly when surrounded by ascitic fluid (Fig. 1).

Once the needle appears to be in the fetal peritoneal cavity, an attempt is made to aspirate any ascites. Occasionally the needle enters the bladder and fetal urine is obtained. This is easily distinguished from ascites by its low protein content and lack of opalescense. If the bladder has been entered, the needle is withdrawn and reinserted slightly cephalad. If ascites is encountered, as much fluid as possible is removed before commencing transfusion. If no fluid is obtained, additional attempts are made to confirm intraperitoneal placement of the needle. A small amount of sterile saline is injected. Intraperitoneal injection should encounter almost no resistance, and it is usually visible on the ultrasound screen because small amounts of air are displaced from the needle. If there is no resistance to the injection, a small amount of air is injected. Bubbles are easily seen on the screen. If they rise to the highest point in the fetal abdomen and remain trapped there, the intraperitoneal placement is almost certain.

Once the peritoneal placement is confirmed, infusion of blood is begun. Fetal heart rate is monitored during the infusion. Specially packed O Rh-negative red blood cells are used, with a hematocrit of 80 to 90 percent. The blood is crossmatched against that of the mother. The cells are infused through the needle in 10-ml increments by syringe. The volume of blood infused is determined according to gestational age by the formula:

$$\text{volume} = (\text{gestational age in weeks} - 20) \times 10. \quad [1]$$

For example, at 28 weeks

$$\text{volume} = (28 - 20) \times 10 = 80 \text{ ml.}$$

The entire volume is given over approximately 30 minutes. If fetal heart rate abnormalities are noted in response to the infusion, it is halted until they have resolved or the procedure is terminated.

Aggressive management of the patient with severe Rh disease has resulted in significant improvement in fetal survival rates.[3-7] Some studies have reported survival rates as high as 100 percent for the nonhydropic fetus and 75 percent in the hydropic fetus.[7] Procedure-related fetal deaths occur in less than 10 percent of cases. Harman et al. demonstrated that one of the most important variables in determining fetal outcome is the experience of the surgical team.[7] Given an experienced team the severely affected fetus below 26 weeks of gestational age and those with hydrops fetalis may now be successfully treated with an appropriate and aggressive approach. It is clear that referral of the severely sensitized patient to a major center with experience and skill in the treatment of this disorder is advisable.

FETAL TACHYCARDIA WITH CONGESTIVE HEART FAILURE

Fetal cardiac arrhythmias are being detected with increasing frequency due to the proliferation of real-time equipment and the increase in electronic fetal monitoring. Persistent fetal tachycardia can result in congestive heart failure and hydrops fetalis. In any fetus with ascites, pleural effusions, or skin edema, a careful examination of the fetal heart is imperative. As fetal tachycardia may be intermittent, measurement of the fetal heart rate and rhythm a number of times is advisable. In addition, a careful anatomic analysis of the fetal heart is necessary. Although the fetus with arrhythmia usually has normal cardiac anatomy, arrhythmias have been associated with various anatomic defects, including intracardiac tumors. We have detected five fetuses with supraventricular tachycardia, four of whom had fetal hydrops. All had evidence on fetal echocardiogram of ventricular failure. They all had a heart rate over 240 beats per minute. Four had no anatomic abnormalities. The fifth had an intracardiac tumor, presumed to be a rhabdomyoma. The mothers were digitalized and the fetal heart rate returned to normal in three of the cases. In the fourth, additional therapy with propranol and verapamil was tried after an initial failure of digitalis to correct the rate. When these drugs also failed, the woman was treated with sustained high doses (0.75 mg/day) digoxin. After 1 week the fetal heart rate converted and the hydrops resolved. In the fifth case, with the intracardiac tumor, the rate converted with digitalis but maternal toxemia of pregnancy necessitated delivery before there was time to see resolution of the hydrops.

High-dose maternal digoxin therapy has been almost universally successful in converting fetal supraventricular tachycardia. Since maternal clearance of the drug is increased in pregnancy, higher doses are needed to achieve and maintain therapeutic blood concentrations. Caution must be exercised in the treatment, however, as these doses can produce toxicity in the mother. Since free (non–protein bound) drug crosses the placenta and equilibrates with the free drug concentration in the mother, it may take several days after the mother has reached therapeutic blood concentration for the fetus to equilibrate. Intravenous administration of digoxin to mother can deliver drug to the fetus more rapidly by producing bolus effects, but, again, care must be taken to avoid maternal toxicity.

URINARY TRACT OBSTRUCTION

As with many fetal anatomic problems, obstructive uropathy is a spectrum of disorders. As in children, obstruction can occur at a variety of levels in the fetal urinary tract. Unilateral ureteropelvic junction (UPJ) obstruction is one of the most common lesions. Depending on its severity, this lesion leads to variable degrees of unilateral hydronephrosis. If the obstruction is severe and early in gestation, it may lead to unilateral

cystic renal dysplasia. Obstruction may occur less commonly at almost any other point in the urinary tract, including the ureterovesicle junction and the urethra. Ureteral obstruction is generally unilateral and, thus at worst, results in unilateral renal damage. Rarely, it may be bilateral. Urethral obstruction, as produced by posterior urethral valves, results in bilateral dilatation of the urinary tract and, if severe, may result in bilateral renal dysplasia. This can be fatal to the newborn infant. Fetal renal failure from any cause results in profound oligohydramnios and this is associated with pulmonary hypoplasia. Severely affected infants generally die of pulmonary insufficiency before their renal disease becomes a significant factor in their survival.

In cases of bilateral urinary tract obstruction due to urethral valves or bilateral UPJ obstruction, there is danger of progressive renal damage and neonatal death. Because the primary problem in these disorders is obstruction, it seems reasonable that diversion of urine around the obstruction should prevent further damage. Since urethral obstruction is more common than bilateral UPJ obstruction, the most common site of diversion should be from the bladder to the amniotic cavity. Although bilateral ureterostomies was reported in one case, cystostomy has been and will remain the more common and generally preferable operation.[10-15] Diversion of fetal urine around urethral obstruction has been accomplished by ultrasound-guided placement of shunts leading from the bladder to the amnion. In this procedure a needle is inserted into the fetal bladder and then a shunt is inserted either over or through the needle into the bladder. The shunt is then displaced from the needle as the needle is withdrawn so that the distal end is left in the amnion. This operation has been carried out in a number of centers in this country and in Europe. The procedure appears to be quite feasible and many successful shunt placements have been reported. Successful outcome, as measured by neonatal survival, however, has been much less rewarding owing largely to associated pulmonary hypoplasia. Survival rates reported to date have ranged from 30 percent in fetuses treated at less than 20 weeks of gestation, to 20 percent in fetuses treated after 20 weeks of gestational age. The survival rate does not appear to be affected by the presence or absence of oligohydramnios or hydronephrosis.

Patient selection in obstructive uropathies is very difficult. The fetus with severe obstruction early in gestation may be doomed to cystic renal dysplasia and death. Rarely are these patients good candidates for fetal intervention. Many fetuses with moderate obstruction but who still maintain urinary output will probably survive without prenatal treatment. Between these two extremes is a group of individuals with moderate to severe obstruction and progressive renal damage who might be helped by intervention. The difficulty is to distinguish this group from each of the other groups. Clearly, gestational age is an important criteria. Beyond 32 weeks of gestation, expectant management of premature delivery may be preferable to fetal treatment. At more immature gestational age candidates for treatment must be distinguished from the fetuses with irreversible renal damage and the fetuses with nonprogressive disease. Decreasing amniotic fluid volume or oligohydramnios may distinguish the candidate from the fetus with nonprogressive disease. The extent of irreversible renal damage is more difficult to detect. A two-stage experimental approach to this situation has therefore been proposed. First, fetal urinary tract catheterization with external drainage is performed in order to assess fetal urine production. Although precise normal values are not known for all gestational ages, the absence of urine flow implies a poor prognosis and no further intervention may be considered. If significant urine production is present, then in utero urinary tract diversion should be attempted.

Clearly, treatment of fetal urinary tract obstruction by means other than premature delivery is experimental. Patient selection criteria are not well established. Risks and benefits of treatment are not fully known, and the long-term prognosis for treated and surviving infants is unknown. Because we lack precise selection criteria many treated fetuses may die of their disease and its consequences despite intervention. It is also clear, however, that some treated survivors might have survived without in utero treatment.

Fetal Hydrocephalus

Obstructive hydrocephalus is dilatation of the cerebral ventricular system associated with an increase in cerebral spinal fluid pressure and has an incidence of 0.5 to 1.8 per thousand births.[16] The causes of congenital hydrocephalus are multiple.[17,18] The majority of cases presenting at birth have no clear-cut etiology and are probably due to a combination of genetic and environmental influences (multifactorial inheritance). A minority of cases are inherited as X linked (2 percent) traits or are due to autosomal recessive disorders. Fetal infection (cytomegalo virus, toxoplasmosis or rubella) may also cause hydrocephalus. The distribution of causes of hydrocephalus presenting in the fetus, however, is unknown. With the advent of high-resolution real-time ultrasound it is now possible to confidently diagnose fetal hydrocephalus prior to 18 menstrual weeks.[19-21] Extreme care must be exercised, however, as a number of false positive diagnoses have been made. No therapy should be instituted without a second opinion by an experienced ultrasonographer.

Given multiple possible etiologies, it is vitally important that every effort be made to determine the specific etiology in individual cases. Appropriate investigations include careful ultrasound examination, karyotype, viral cultures and serology as well as a careful genetic family history. It is important to note, however, that many cases of congenital hydrocephalus will occur without relevant antecedent family or pregnancy history.

The cerebral spinal fluid (CSF) hypertension in congenital hydrocephalus can be caused by a number of specific mechanical problems in the brain. Complete or partial obstruction of the cerebral aqueduct is probably the most common. Communicating hydrocephalus, in which there is obstruction to absorption of cerebral spinal fluid by the subarachnoid granulations, can also cause congenital hydrocephalus. Dandy–Walker malformation and Arnold–Chiari myelodysplasia cause internal hydrocephalus due to obstruction at the level of the fourth ventricle. Fetal hydrocephalus secondary to intraventricular hemorrhage has been seen.[22,23]

The prognosis for congenital hydrocephalus is quite variable and depends upon the etiology as well as the time of onset and severity of the process. The management of the pregnancy complicated by fetal hydrocephalus is made more difficult by our incomplete knowledge of its natural history. In some cases the process is relentlessly progressive throughout gestation and results in a grossly distorted fetal head and profound brain damage. In other cases hydrocephalus appears to arrest spontaneously or is only slowly progressive; occasionally it appears to resolve completely.

In recent years a number of attempts have been made to treat hydrocephalus in utero.[24,25] The goal of these procedures has been to relieve CSF hypertension temporarily while awaiting fetal maturity with the hope of arresting progressive brain damage.

The percutaneous placement of a ventricular amniotic shunt for the relief of fetal hydrocephalus was first reported in 1982.[26] This entailed the insertion of a needle through the maternal abdominal wall and uterus into the dilated fetal lateral ventricle under ultrasound guidance. A silastic shunt containing a one-way valve was inserted through the needle and left to extend from the ventricle to the amniotic space (Fig. 2). At the time of shunt placement in our first case, 23 weeks of gestation, the LVW/HW ratio was 0.87. Following shunt placement this ratio declined to 0.50 and the cortical mantle became correspondingly thicker. After shunt placement the ventricles were asymmetric with the shunt ventricle (right) consistently smaller than the left. Between 32 and 34 weeks the shunt appeared to stop functioning. The LVH/HW ratio increased and the fetal biparietal diameter was found to be 10 cm. Following delivery by cesarean section it was found that the shunt was obstructed by an ingrowth of tissue from the ventricular end.

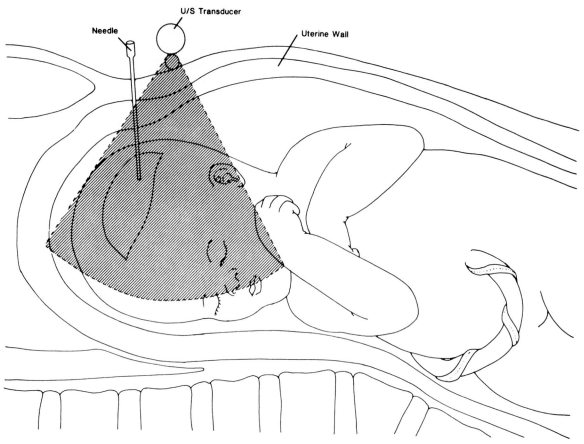

Fig. 2. Schematic diagram depicting needle placement in fetal head under ultrasound guidance. The needle should be within the plane of the ultrasound at all times.

The infant had a ventricloperitoneal shunt placed on the first day of life and was discharged at 28 days of age. This infant had a family history consistent with x-linked aquaductal stenosis. At birth he had flexion contractures of both hands and duplication of the distal phalanx of the left thumb. At 2 years of age he has profound psychomotor retardation.

Four additional fetuses have been treated at the University of Colorado School of Medicine with similar procedures. None of these have had significant family histories or other apparent etiologies for the hydrocephalus. In two infants the shunts became displaced from the fetal head several days to weeks after placement. In both cases the ventricles rapidly enlarged again and a second shunt was placed. In these two infants the LVW/HW ratio returned to almost normal following in utero shunting. Both were delivered at 32 weeks of gestation by cesarean section following spontaneous rupture of membranes. Both had ventricloperitoneal shunts in the neonatal period. The third fetus had spontaneous rupture of membranes the day after in utero shunt placement. He was delivered by cesarean section 3 weeks later at 28 weeks of gestation.

He had a ventricloperitoneal shunt and was doing well at discharge from the nursery.

A fifth fetus was found to have no pressure gradient from his lateral ventricle to the amnion at the time of operation. Although his ventricles were clearly enlarged, the lack of significant pressure elevation suggested that drainage would be of no value and a shunt was not placed. The pregnancy was subsequently terminated. Pathologic examination of the fetal brain showed no evidence of aquaductal stenosis. There was also no histologic evidence of elevated intraventricular pressure. In a subsequent case in which elective pregnancy termination occurred without attempted fetal treatment, definite aquaductal obstruction was found as well as ventriculomegaly, but there was no histologic evidence of elevated ventricular pressure. These cases indicate that one must interpret with caution the histologic evidence for hydrocephalus.

The postnatal development of these infants with in utero shunts has ranged from the severe retardation seen in the first case to essentially normal development in the second. Given the uncertainties as to the course of fetal hydrocephalus and its multiple etiologies, such variation is not surprising. To date over 24 fetuses have been treated with similar operations in several centers. No significant maternal morbidity has been reported. There has been one procedure-related fetal death and three deaths due to associated congenital anomalies. Although detailed developmental data are not yet available on the surviving infants, approximately 48 percent are considered normal neurologically, 10 percent mildly abnormal, and 42 percent severely retarded, at a mean follow-up age of approximately 9 months.

The limited experience with experimental in utero treatment of hydrocephalus precludes any conclusions as to its efficacy at this time. It also raises several difficult questions regarding moral and ethical issues and allocation of human resources that are beyond the scope of this chapter.[27] Several generalizations can be made, however. Treatment with ventricular amniotic shunts can decrease ventricular size and prevent further progression of the disease. On the other hand, duration of benefit has been limited by shunt dislodgement and obstruction. As these are both mechanical or technical problems, it seems likely that they can eventually be overcome. In cases of progressive ventriculomegaly due to increased intracranial pressure, fetal shunting can restore normal anatomy (as seen on ultrasound and computerized tomography) and result in an infant with a normal size head and normal size ventricles. Some of these infants will have completely normal neurologic and developmental exams at discharge from the nursery and 1 year of age. As encouraging as these findings are, it is also clear that some infants will be significantly retarded, even with apparently successful treatment. The developmental prognosis probably depends as much on the etiology of the hydrocephalus as it does on the severity or stage of pregnancy when the shunting is performed.

In selecting patients for fetal shunt placement several criteria must be met. First, other serious anomalies should be excluded as thoroughly as possible. This requires a very meticulous ultrasound examination, utilizing the most sophisticated equipment and interpretation. Amniocentesis for karotype and α-fetoprotein should be performed. Second, the procedure should probably not be performed beyond 32 weeks of gestation because neonatal survival is quite good in modern nurseries at that stage. Third, consultation involving obstetricians, ultrasonologists, pediatricians, geneticists, pediatric neurosurgeons, and psychosocial services must be obtained. Lastly, and most importantly, the family must be completely informed of the risks, benefits, and experimental nature of the procedure before being asked to consent to it.

Fetal shunting for hydrocephalus is and will remain for some time to come an experimental procedure.

Criteria for patient selection, operative technique, and equipment continue to evolve. It will be several years before meaningful follow-up data are available to assess the benefit of this procedure. Extraordinary caution in patient selection and follow-up is mandatory during this experimental period.

REFERENCES

1. Harrison MR, Golbus MS, Filly RA: Management of the fetus with a correctable congenital defect. JAMA 246:774, 1981
2. Liley AW: Intrauterine transfusion of foetus in haemolytic disease. Br Med J 2:1107, 1963
3. Acker D, Frigoletto FE, Birnholz JC, et al: Ultrasound-facilitated intrauterine transfusions. Am J Obstet Gynecol 138:1200, 1980
4. Berkowitz RI, Hobbins JC: Intrauterine transfusion utilizing ultrasound. Obstet Gynecol 57:33, 1981
5. Clewell WH, Dunne MG, Johnson ML, et al: Fetal transfusion with real-time ultrasound guidance. Obstet Gynecol 57:516, 1981
6. Larkin RM, Knochel JQ, Lee TG: Intrauterine transfusions: New techniques and results. Clin Obstet Gynecol 25:303, 1982
7. Harman CR, Manning FA, Bowman JR, et al: Severe RH disease-poor outcome is not inevitable. Am J Obstet Gynecol 145:823, 1983
8. Harrigan JT, Kangos JJ, Sikka A, et al: Successful treatment of fetal congestive heart failure secondary to tachycardia. N Engl J Med 304:1527, 1981
9. Wiggins JW, Clewell W, Johnson ML, et al: Successful diagnosis and therapy of arrhythmias, congestive heart failure in the fetus. Submitted for publication.
10. Harrison MR, Filly RA, Parer JT, et al: Management of the fetus with a urinary tract malfunction. JAMA 246:635, 1981
11. Harrison MR, Golbus MS, Filly RA, et al: Fetal surgery for congenital hydronephrosis. N Engl J Med 306:591, 1982
12. Golbus MS, Harrison MR, Filly RA, et al: In utero treatment of urinary tract obstruction. Am J Obstet Gynecol 142:383, 1982
13. Blane CE, Koff SA, Bowerman RA, et al: Nonobstructive fetal hydronephrosis: Sonographic recognition and therapeutic implication. Radiol 147:95, 1983
14. Manning FA, Harman CR, Lange IR, et al: Antepartum chronic fetal vesicoamniotic shunts for obstructive uropathy: A report of two cases. Am J Obstet Gynecol 145:819, 1983
15. Kramer SA: Current status of fetal intervention for congenital hydronephrosis. J Urol 130:641, 1983
16. Robertson RD, Sarti DA, Brown WH, et al: Congenital hydrocephalus in two pregnancies following the birth of a child with neural tube defect: Etiology and management. J Med Genet 18:105, 1981
17. Bay C, Kerzin L, Hall B: Recurrence risk in hydrocephalus. Birth Defects: Original Article Series 15(5C):95, 1979

18. Habib Z: Genetics and genetic counseling in neonatal hydrocephalus. Obstet Gynecol Surv 36:529, 1981

19. Johnson ML, Dunne MG, Mack LA, et al: Evaluation of fetal intracranial anatomy by static and real-time ultrasound. J Clin Ultrasound 8:311, 1980

20. Hadlock FP, Deter RL, Park SK: Real-time sonography: Ventricular and vascular anatomy of the fetal brain in utero. Am J Roentgenol 136:133, 1981

21. Denkhaus H, Winsberg F: Ultrasonic measurement of the fetal ventricular system. Radiology 131:781, 1979

22. Kim MS, Elyaderani MK: Sonographic diagnosis of cerebroventricular hemorrhage in utero. Radiology 142:479, 1982

23. McGahan JP, Haessloin HC, Meyer M, et al: Sonographic recognition of in utero interventricular hemorrhage. Am J Roentgenol 142:171, 1984

24. Machejda M, Hodgen JD: In utero diagnosis and treatment of non-human primate fetal skeletal anomalies. I. Hydrocephalus. JAMA 246:1093, 1981

25. Birnholz JC, Frigoletto FD: Antenatal treatment of hydrocephalus. N Engl J Med 304:1021, 1981

26. Clewell WH, Johnson ML, Meier PR, et al: A surgical approach to the treatment of fetal hydrocephalus. N Engl J Med 306:1320, 1982

27. Elias S, Annas G: Perspectives on fetal surgery. Am J Obstet Gynecol 145:807, 1983

23 | Ultrasonography and Diabetes Mellitus in Pregnancy

E. Albert Reece
John C. Hobbins

INTRODUCTION

Pregnancy may coexist with almost every known acute and chronic disease. Diabetes mellitus, by virtue of its frequency and its metabolic derangements, is one of the most significant medical complications of pregnancy. The gestational process requires an optimal endocrine milieu; therefore, the concurrence of diabetes and pregnancy raises concerns about normal fetal growth and development.

Prior to the availability of insulin, diabetes mellitus was usually incompatible with survival to reproductive age or fertility, and a term gestation in a diabetic gravida was rarely achieved. Today, as a result of insulin usage, diabetes is one of the most frequently encountered problem associated with pregnancy. Improvements in the overall perinatal care given especially to the diabetic patient have significantly decreased the perinatal morbidity and mortality among this group.[1,2]

The effects of diabetes mellitus in pregnancy may be manifested in many ways, some of which are associated with fetal and neonatal illnesses and death. This chapter will address primarily those effects that can readily be evaluated by ultrasonography, including:

1. The estimation of gestational age.
2. Fetal congenital anomalies.
   a. Skeletal and central nervous system malformations.
   b. Cardiac abnormalities.
   c. Renal anomalies.
   d. Gastrointestinal malformations.
   e. Other anomalies.
3. Polyhydramnios either on an idiopathic basis or associated with congenital anomalies.
4. Intrauterine growth retardation.
5. Fetal macrosomia.
6. Assessment of fetal well-being.
7. The placenta.

ESTIMATION OF GESTATIONAL AGE

The need for accurate estimation of gestational age is self-evident, especially in the diabetic patient in whom growth abnormalities may occur and in whom the progress of pregnancy postdates is usually not allowed. The clinical estimation of gestational age is somewhat unsatisfactory in most cases since it has been reported that 20 to 40 percent of pregnant women fail to recall the exact date of the last normal menstrual period (LNMP).[3] Physical examination using fundal height also is undesirable for accuracy of gestational age estimation in the diabetic pregnancy. Studies relating fundal height assessment to gestational age have been shown to have an accuracy of no more than ±6 weeks at the 90 percent confidence level.[3]

Ultrasonography in the first trimester allows for the estimation of gestational age using crown–rump length with a range of 4.7 days at the 95% confidence level. Between 12 to 26 weeks the BPD measurement provides reliable estimates. Beyond 30 weeks there is progressive increase in variations, and the establishment of accurate gestational age is less satisfactory. The femur length measurement correlates with gestational age particularly during 14 to 22 weeks, with a range of 6.7 days at the 95 percent confidence level.[3-5]

In diabetics, since some fetal areas are affected more than others, more study will be required before it will be ascertained which fetal parameter will be best in dating pregnancies. Perhaps a combination of measurements will be most efficient, but as of yet, it is not known how to "weigh" each parameter since an average may not be appropriate. A study is in progress in our laboratory to answer this question.

CONGENITAL ANOMALIES

An association between diabetes mellitus and fetal congenital anomalies has been suspected since the nineteenth century. As early as 1885, it was reported that congenital malformation occurred in two infants of diabetic mothers (IDM).[6,7] Despite improved management of the diabetic pregnancy, the incidence of fetal congenital anomalies still remains a major cause of illness and death among IDMs. Congenital abnormalities have now replaced respiratory distress syndrome as the leading cause of death in some centers caring for diabetic pregnancies.[6-8] These anomalies are reported to be responsible for approximately 40 percent of all perinatal deaths.[9,10] The frequency of congenital anomalies among diabetic offspring is estimated at 3 to 6 percent of all infants at birth, representing a two- to threefold increase in children of diabetic mothers.[11-14] Kucera[15] has reported a 4.8 percent incidence, while Naeve[16] found greater than a twofold difference. An increased incidence and severity of malformations have been reported in infants of diabetic mothers with varying degrees of vasculopathy. A frequency of occurrence among such diabetic offspring was estimated to be 4.4 percent in White's classes A, B, and C, 9.7 percent in class d, and 16.7 percent in class f, with an overall incidence of 6.4 percent in all diabetic offspring as compared with 2 percent in the general population.[8,11,12,14]

The current view regarding the pathogenesis of congenital malformations in IDMs is that organogenesis is disrupted by the hyperglycemia of diabetes. In animal models the teratogenic effect of maternal glucose has been demonstrated by the experimental production of hyperglycemia during organogenesis.[17-20] In humans, there is suggestive evidence of a similar pathogenesis. Glycosylated hemoglobin (HbA$_{1C}$) is a normal minor hemoglobin distinguished from hemoglobin A by the nonenzymatic addition of a glucose moiety to the amino terminal valine of the beta chain. This glycosylation occurs throughout the life span of a red blood cell (RBC), being influenced by the average glucose concentration to which the RBC has been exposed.

The measured HbA$_{1C}$, expressed as a percentage of total hemoglobin, provides an integrated, retrospective index of glucose control over the 4 to 6 weeks preceding its determination.[21-23] It has been reported that there is a significantly higher incidence of major congenital anomalies in the offspring of diabetic women with elevated first trimester HbA$_{1C}$ values. Of the major congenital anomalies observed, 5.1 percent were associated with HbA$_{1C}$ determinations between 7.0 and 8.5 percent, and 22.4 percent of these malformations were associated with a HbA$_{1C}$ level equal to or greater than 8.6 percent.[13] This finding is quite consistent with the work of Mills et al.,[7] who, using a developmental morphologic dating system of each organ primarily involved in diabetic congenital anomalies, showed that such malformations usually occurred prior to the seventh week of gestation.[7,17,24-26] Pederson and others have demonstrated that improved diabetic control may reduce the incidence of congenital malformations in IDMs.[10,14,20,23,26] There also is preliminary information showing that IDMs having congenital anomalies may show a "growth lag" in the first trimester of pregnancy as compared with their counterparts who are free of malformations.[24-26] This finding deserves further investigation, because if these data can be corroborated by large prospective studies, then early growth curtailment by itself may be an indicator of fetal anomalies. It should be noted, however, that in spite of this large body of information suggesting an increased frequency of fetal congenital anomalies among diabetic offspring, there are authors, notably Farquhar,[27] who have failed to demonstrate an increased rate of congenital malformations among such infants. Despite Farquhar's finding, a review of the literature has revealed a particular cluster of anomalies that are most commonly present in infants of diabetic mothers (see Table 1).[15,27-29]

Improved high-resolution gray scale ultrasound equipment has made it possible to delineate fetal anatomy, and consequently the in utero detection of fetal congenital anomalies. Such diagnoses can usually be made early enough in the second trimester, thus allowing patients the option of pregnancy termination.

Skeletal and Central Nervous System Malformations

The caudal regression syndrome or phocomelic diabetic embryopathy is very rare, although it is the most typical and commonly associated lesion with maternal diabetes. The anomaly occurs in about 0.2 to 0.5 percent of infants of diabetic pregnancies. The rate of occurrence represents approximately a 200-fold increase over the rate seen in the general population.[7,8] This lesion probably results from a defect in the mid-posterior axis mesoderm of the embryo before the fourth

TABLE 1
Congenital Anomalies in Infants of Diabetic Mothers

I. Skeletal and central nervous system
  A. Caudal regression syndrome
  B. Neural tube defects excluding anencephaly
  C. Anencephaly with or without herniation of neural element
  D. Microcephaly
II. Cardiac
  A. Transposition of the great vessels with or without ventricular septal defect.
  B. Ventricular septal defects
  C. Coarctation of the aorta with or without ventricular septal defect or patent ductus arteriosus
  D. Atrial septal defects
  E. Cardiomegaly
III. Renal anomalies
  A. Hydronephrosis
  B. Renal agenesis
  C. Ureteral duplication
IV. Gastrointestinal
  A. Duodenal atresia
  B. Anorectal atresia
  C. Small left colon syndrome
V. Other
  A. Single umbilical artery

week of gestation, resulting in absence or hypoplasia of caudal structures.[12,30] Although experimental studies have demonstrated similar skeletal malformations by the use of high doses of insulin in embryonic chicks and mammals, other studies have implicated hypoglycemia in the genesis of fetal malformations.[11] It is unclear whether fetal malformations in the insulin-treated animal models resulted from the high insulin dosage or the metabolic effects of insulin. Several other studies in animals have shown that insulin administration that maintains euglycemia has reduced the incidence of fetal malformations.[17,19,29-31]

Hyperinsulinism has been demonstrated in human fetuses induced by excessive glucose transport from mother to fetus. The embryo, however, is unable to mount a hyperinsulinemic response in the very early gestation (during organogenesis) and thus is theoretically protected from the potential teratogenic effects of fetal insulin. Knowledge of the exact pathogenesis of malformations in IDMs is limited; however, it is apparent that a well-controlled glycemic state is associated with a lower incidence of fetal malformations.[20,29]

Neural Tube Defects. Maternal serum α-fetoprotein (MSAFP) screening programs include only about 2 to 3 percent of pregnancies requiring sonographic evaluation to exclude neural tube defects (NTD).[32] The diabetic pregnancy is at high risk for neural tube anomalies, with a reported incidence of 19.5 per 1000 in the

diabetic gestation, as compared with 1 to 2 per 1000 in the general population.[33]

Baker[17] created an experimental model of diabetes in rats using streptozotocin infusion during the period of organogenesis. The incidence of neural tube (lumbosacral) defects in the saline-treated group was significantly higher than the insulin-treated group ($p < 0.005$). Diabetes occurring after the period of organogenesis did not affect the incidence of NTD. These data suggest that the high incidence of neural tube anomalies seen in IDMs may be associated with hyperglycemia, resulting from poorly controlled diabetes during the period of organ differentiation.[17]

It should be emphasized that approximately 90 percent of children born with NTD are delivered by women without a previously affected child; therefore, routine MSAFP in the diabetic gestation is warranted. Caution should, however, be exercised in the interpretation of MSAFP determinations in the diabetic pregnancy since there have been reports of lower MSAFP values per gestational age in this group of patients.[32,33] First trimester growth lag in IDMs has been one of the proposed explanations for the lower MSAFP values noted in diabetic pregnancies. A high percentage of false positive results (about 95 percent) is associated with this test. For example, for every 1000 patients screened with MSAFP, approximately 50 to 75 patients will have two elevations of more than 2.5 multiples above the median. Only 20 of these will require amniocentesis, since the remaining patients will be found on ultrasound evaluation to have erroneous dating, intrauterine demise, or multiple gestations. Of the 20 patients requiring amniocentesis, only 1 to 2 will have an amniotic fluid elevation of more than 5 SD above the mean for the gestation.[34] NTD can usually be diagnosed by ultrasonography following elevated α-fetoprotein values (maternal serum and amniotic fluid).

The diagnosis of spinal defects is often difficult, especially when the lesions are small, and thus requires meticulous attention to the subtle sonographic findings in that area. In the longitudinal scan, if the fetus is lying with the vertebral column anteriorly ("back-up" position), two lines will be seen representing the posterior elements and the vertebral body (Fig. 1). If the fetus is lying transversely ("back-transverse" position), three lines will be visualized. These lines represent the vertebral body in the middle and the posterial elements on either side (Fig. 2). As the transducer is moved from the normal area towards the defect, the middle line disappears and the lateral lines diverge (Fig. 3). This divergence may not be seen in smaller lumbar defects; however, on transverse or sagittal sections confirmation of defects usually can be made (see Fig. 4). The "back-down" position is unsatisfactory in the evalua-

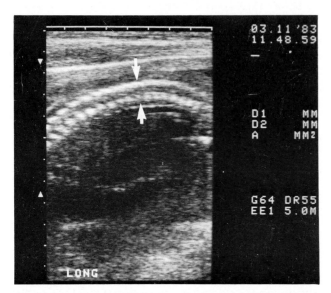

Fig. 1. Sagittal scan of the fetal vertebral column, with the fetus in the "back-up" position. Two lines are visualized (*arrows*) representing the posterior elements and the vertebral body.

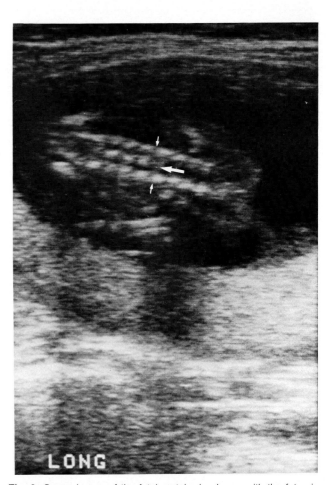

Fig. 2. Coronal scan of the fetal vertebral column, with the fetus in the "back-transverse" position. Note the three lines visualized depicting the vertebral body in the middle and the posterior elements on either side (*arrows*).

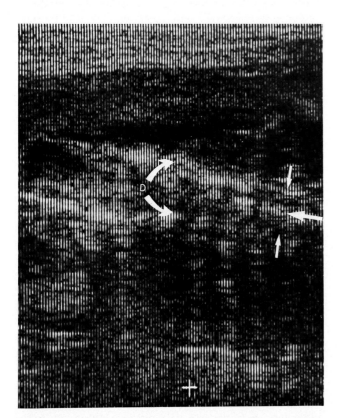

Fig. 3. Coronal scan of the fetal vertebral column. The fetus is lying in the "back-transverse," and three lines are visualized (*straight arrows*). A divergence of the lateral lines can be seen and loss of middle line at the site of the defect (*curved arrows*, D = defect).

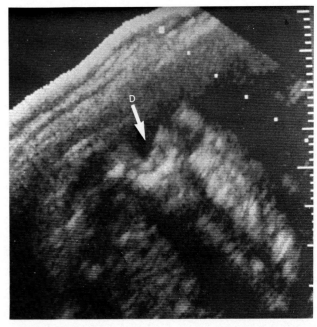

Fig. 4. Transverse scan of an open neural tube defect (D = defect).

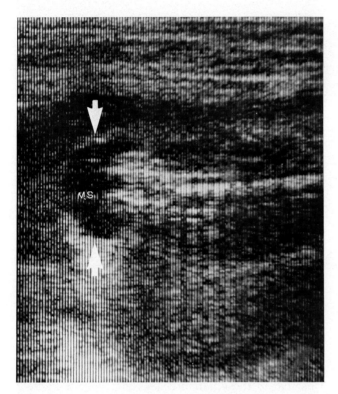

Fig. 5. Transverse scan of neural tube defect depicting a saccular herniation (*arrows*) arising from the open neural lesion (MS = meningeal sac).

tion of neural tube defects. The sacral spine, on occasion, cannot be completely evaluated because of poorly defined landmarks in that area.[35,36] Herniations including meningoceles or myeloceles present ultrasonically as saccular protrusions from the fetal spine (Fig. 5).[5,37,38]

Anencephaly. This is the most common anomaly affecting the central nervous system, with an increased incidence of 0.57 percent in the diabetic pregnancy. This represents a threefold increase over that expected in the normal population (0.19 percent). The recurrence risk is 4 percent following a single affected fetus, but 10 percent after two successively affected fetuses.[3,8,39]

Anencephaly results from a failure of the neural tube to close completely at the cranial pole during fusion of the neural folds to form the forebrain. This occurs between the second and third week of development. The cerebral hemispheres (telencephalon) are usually absent while the brainstem and portions of the midbrain are usually present. Absence of the cranial vault is a constant finding, although portions of cranial bones may be present. Common varieties of NTD include rachischisis, spina bifida, meningocele, and myelomeningocele, occurring in approximately 50 percent of anencephalics.[3]

The diagnosis of anencephaly is usually made in patients referred for gestational age estimation; in patients with elevated α-fetoprotein, or by the presence of hydramnios, occurring in about 40 to 50 percent of cases. The sonographic diagnosis can be made by the fifteenth week of gestation because of the presence of poorly formed cranial bones (Figs. 6,7).[35] It should be noted, however, in early pregnancy that occasionally the fetal head enters the pelvis and sometimes gives a mistaken impression of anencephaly. The experienced sonographer will have little difficulty in differentiating this normal variant.[37,38]

Other conditions that may be confused with anencephaly include severe microcephaly, or amniotic band syndrome involving the head, where portions of the cranial vault are absent. The distinction between anencephaly and the other conditions can be made by the symmetrical absence of the calvarium seen in anencephaly.[3]

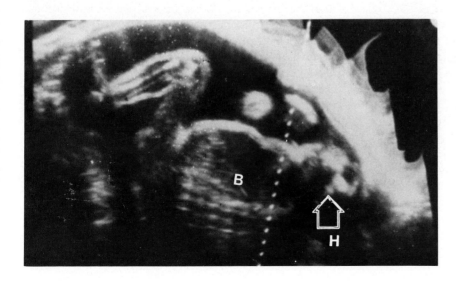

Fig. 6. An anencephalic fetus. Poorly visualized cranial bones (*arrow*) are diagnostic of this condition (B = body).

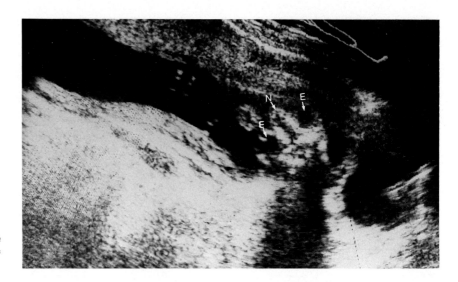

Fig. 7. Anencephalic. Facial structures can be seen (*arrows*), but calvarium is absent (N = nose, E = eye).

Microcephaly. Microcephaly is an uncommon condition, with an estimated incidence of 1 in 6200 to 8500 births. In a retrospective study of the diabetic offspring, Naeve[16] has reported an increased rate of occurrence. This condition may occur as an inherited autosomal recessive trait associated with parental consanguinity or the Meckel–Gruber syndrome (polydactyly, encephalocele, polycystic kidneys, and microcephaly), chromosomal abnormalities, or environmental damage. In the diabetic pregnancy, the exact cause of the retarded fetal head growth is unclear.

Microcephaly is defined as an abnormally small head for gestational age. The sonographic diagnosis can be established by an occipitofrontal or biparietal diameter of the fetal head reduced to 3 SD or more below the mean.[3] This diagnosis can be further supported by an abnormal cephalic index determination (BPD/occipitofrontal diameter > 80 percent), suggesting a rounded head, a head circumference predictive of a much earlier gestational age,[40] or head-to-body ratio below the fifth percentile.[41]

The finding of a normal BPD in a patient at high risk for microcephaly virtually excludes the disorder in the late gestation. The differentiation between symmetrical intrauterine growth retardation (IUGR) and microcephaly may be difficult. A recent report by O'Brien and Queenan[42] has utilized the femur length in the diagnosis of IUGR. The differentiation of symmetrical IUGR from microcephaly was not specifically addressed in this study; nevertheless, this biometric parameter may serve as a useful adjunct to current methods of diagnosing IUGR, and the possible exclusion of microcephaly.

Cardiac Anomalies

The incidence of congenital heart disease (CHD) is much greater in infants of diabetic mothers (IDM) than in infants of nondiabetic mothers and is probably the most common fetal anomaly in the diabetic pregnancy. Rowland, Hubbell, and Nadas,[43] in a series of 470 IDMs, reported an incidence of CHD approximating 4 percent in these patients. This incidence is fivefold that seen in the general population (8 per 1000). Pedersen, Tygstrup, and Pedersen,[14] however, in a series of 853 IDM found a 1.7 percent incidence of CHD. In the diabetic pregnancy the risk of congenital heart disease is 1:39, as compared with 1:20 for infants whose parents have cardiac lesions.[44]

The major cardiac anomalies include transposition of the great vessels, ventricular septal defect and coarctation of the aorta (Table 1). The overwhelming majority of cardiac malformation are transpositions of the great vessels. The significance of this excess number of great vessel lesions among IDMs is unclear.[8,44]

Pedersen, Tygstrup, and Pedersen[14] demonstrated a direct relationship between the rate of CHD in IDMs and the increasing degree of vascular complications. Neave,[16] in a prospective study of 2592 IDMs, correlated the malformation rate with severity and duration of maternal diabetes. Other authors have associated age at onset of diabetes with the incidence of congenital malformations.[12,45,46]

Fetal echocardiography has facilitated the identification of fetuses with various types of cardiac malformations, particularly septal defects, coarctation, transposition, and cardiomegaly (Figs. 8–10).[36,47–49] Cardiac septal hypertrophy, which occurs frequently in IDMs, may also be detected by this modality (Fig. 11). In addition to delineating normal and abnormal cardiac anatomy, fetal echocardiography quantitates ventricular function and measures various cardiac dimensions.[49–53] Cardiac volume can be measured by

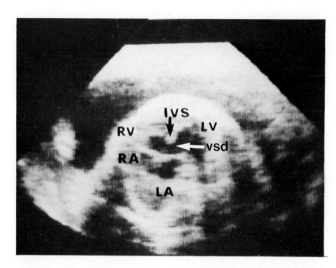

Fig. 8. Ventricular septal defect (vsd) diagnosed in utero. (RV = right ventricle, RA = right atrium, LA = left atrium, LV = left ventricle. (*Courtesy of C. Kleinman.*)

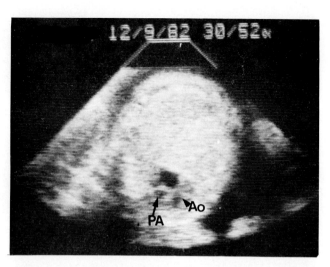

Fig. 9. Short-axis (transverse view of the heart of a fetus at 30 weeks' gestation). Normal anatomy at the level of the great arterial origins results in a circular aortic cross section with a curvilinear right ventricular outflow tract ("circle and sausage" view). In this fetus the two great arterial origins are circular in this view. This fetus was subsequently diagnosed to have transposition of the great arteries. While this fetus was not the fetus of a diabetic mother, this study does demonstrate the feasibility of visualizing this cardiac abnormality using fetal echocardiography. (Ao = aorta; PA = pulmonary artery). (*Courtesy of C. Kleinman.*)

obtaining dimensions of the heart in the longitudinal (*a*) and transverse (*b*) views and using the formula of an ellipsoid: $a \times b^2 \times 0.5233$. Nomograms are available for comparison across gestational ages (Tables 2,3).

A distinctive pattern of severe asymmetrical hypertrophy of the interventricular septum has been described in symptomatic neonates.[54] This finding became known as hypertrophic cardiomyopathy, Kleinman and Hobbins[55] have also noted this finding in utero. They observed in a poorly controlled diabetic marked hypertrophy (>3 mm) of the interventricular septum (IVS). Four weeks later, following improvement in the glycemic control, the IVS returned to normal size (<3 mm). A study was subsequently conducted on the left ventricular free wall and the interventricular septal dimensions of well-controlled

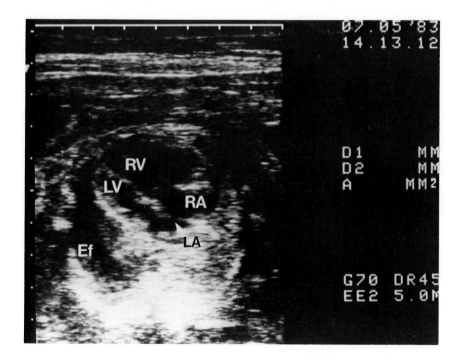

Fig. 10. Four-chamber view of the heart of a fetus at 32 weeks' gestation. There is relative cardiomegaly with disproportionate enlargement of the right ventricular cavity (RV). The normal ratio of RV to left ventricular (LV) dimension is 1.0 to 1.2. In this case the RV/LV ratio is greater than 2.0. There is a moderately large pleural effusion (Ef). (RA = right atrium; LA = left atrium). (*Courtesy of C. Kleinman.*)

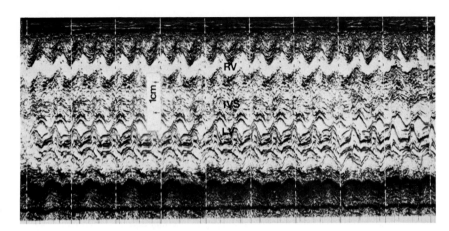

Fig. 11. Thickened interventricular septum (IVS) (RV = right ventricle, LV = left ventricle). (*Courtesy of C. Kleinman.*)

diabetics in comparison with the normal population. There was no statistically significant difference in the size of the IVS and left ventricular free wall between these groups (Table 4).[55] This phenomenon of cardiac hypertrophy has been attributed to poor glycemic con-

TABLE 2
The Cardiac Diameters

Week	Transverse				Longitudinal		
	5th	50th	95th		5th	50th	95th
12	4	5	6	||	5	6	7
13	5	6	7	||	6	7	9
14	6	7	8	||	8	9	10
15	7	8	10	----	9	10	12
16	8	10	11	||	10	12	14
17	9	11	13	||	12	14	16
18	10	12	15	||	13	15	18
19	11	14	16	||	14	17	20
20	13	15	18	||	16	19	22
21	14	17	20	||	18	21	24
22	15	18	21	||	19	23	26
23	16	20	23	||	21	24	28
24	18	21	25	||	22	26	30
25	19	23	27	----	24	28	32
26	20	24	28	||	25	30	34
27	22	26	30	||	27	32	36
28	23	27	32	||	28	33	38
29	24	29	34	||	30	35	40
30	25	30	35	||	31	37	42
31	26	32	37	||	32	38	44
32	28	33	38	||	33	40	46
33	29	34	40	||	34	41	47
34	30	35	41	||	35	42	49
35	30	37	43	----	36	43	50
36	31	38	44	||	37	44	51
37	32	39	45	||	37	45	52
38	33	39	46	||	38	46	53
39	33	40	47	||	38	46	54
40	33	41	48	||	38	46	55
	mm	mm	mm		mm	mm	mm

Reprinted with permission from Jeanty P, Romero R: Ultrasonography in Obstetrics. New York, McGraw-Hill, 1984.

trol and the effects of hyperinsulinism. Cardiomegaly is noted to be present in approximately 50 percent of IDMs without associated congenital heart disease. The weight of these infant's heart at postmortem examination may exceed 2 SD above the mean. Based on these findings, some authors have suggested excess glycogen deposition as a possible etiologic factor in diabetic cardiomegaly. In fact, Hurwitz and Irving,[56] using Best's carmine stain, have demonstrated increased glycogen in the myocardium. This finding has been confirmed.[57]

It is of interest that cardiac hypertrophy observed in some IDMs is not demonstrable in macrosomic infants of nondiabetic mothers. Despite the clinical and histologic similarities, the hypertrophic cardiomyopathy of IDMs differs from other forms of obstructive cardiomyopathy. The diabetic form is both transient and nonfamilial, and resolves without the need for positive inotropic agents.[49,58] Disproportionate septal hypertrophy (DSH), defined as a ratio of interventricular septum to left ventricular posterior wall >1:3, is the rule, although it may be an occasional nonspecific finding in normal infants who are asymptomatic at birth. The presence of DSH on echocardiogram in an IDM is highly suggestive of hypertrophic cardiomyopathy and further evaluation is indicated.[49,59] Echocardiographic measurement of the thickness of interventricular septum has been proposed as a possible indicator of maternal diabetic control. At the present time, however, more data are needed for support of such a proposal. Neonates of diabetic mothers, however, have been evaluated by cardiac septal measurements. Those neonates with severe heart failure had a more prominent hypertrophy of the interventricular septum.[54,60]

Fetal lambs subjected to hypoxia-related ductus arteriosus constriction had excess smooth muscle in the pulmonary vasculature. Cardiac hypertrophy was postulated to be a compensatory phenomenon, designed to maintain cardiac output in the face of hypoxic

TABLE 3
The Cardiac Volume

Age	Percentile		
	5th	50th	95th
10	.011	.021	.038
11	.018	.033	.059
12	.038	.067	.119
13	.072	.127	.224
14	.128	.225	.395
15	.213	.374	.655
16	.336	.588	1.031
17	.504	.883	1.546
18	.726	1.271	2.224
19	1.008	1.764	3.086
20	1.356	2.373	4.150
21	1.776	3.106	5.433
22	2.273	3.975	6.951
23	2.851	4.987	8.722
24	3.519	6.155	10.765
25	4.282	7.490	13.103
26	5.150	9.008	15.758
27	6.130	10.723	18.757
28	7.232	12.649	22.123
29	8.458	14.795	25.877
30	9.812	17.163	30.023
31	11.284	19.743	34.545
32	12.857	22.505	39.392
33	14.498	25.388	44.459
34	16.155	28.301	49.579
35	17.750	31.107	54.512
36	19.180	33.626	58.952
37	20.308	35.642	62.554
38	20.966	36.913	64.989
39	20.903	37.156	66.046
40	19.478	35.580	64.993
	cm³	cm³	cm³

Reprinted with permission from Jeanty P, Romero R: Ultrasonography in Obstetrics. New York, McGraw-Hill, 1984.

changes in the pulmonary circulation. Although this may be a somewhat logical way to explain cardiac hypertrophy, there are no data to support this hypothesis in IDMs.[13]

Echocardiography may be used as an adjunctive tool in the clinical evaluation of cardiac anatomy and function of diabetic pregnancies at or beyond 20 weeks'

gestation. The information obtained can be essential in the management of these patients. For example, if some cardiac anomalies such as hypoplastic ventricle are identified early, the option of pregnancy termination may be chosen by the parent. If diagnosis occurs later in the pregnancy, this information will be useful for counseling purposes and in enabling the pediatric and/or surgical team to make appropriate preparations. Fetal arrhythmias may also be elucidated by this modality, as well as the evaluation of any cardiac compromise secondary to inadequate cardiac function. The delineation of the type of arrhythmia allows for institution of the most appropriate therapy.

Although the causative factors have not been clearly identified, nevertheless the associated increased incidence of CHD in the diabetic pregnancy is clear. The antenatal control of diabetes offers a possible preventive role to the development of cardiac and other diabetes associated fetal congenital anomalies. Echocardiograpy can provide useful information regarding cardiac anatomy and function, thus influencing significantly the clinical management of the diabetic gestation at risk for cardiac disease.

Renal Anomalies

An increased rate of occurrence of urological anomalies among diabetic offsprings was noted by Kucera.[15] Some of these malformations include ureteral duplication, renal agenesis, and hydronephrosis.[12,15]

The measurement of the abdominal circumference (AC) at the level of the umbilical vein is a good index of fetal mass and fetal abdominal girth. A transverse scan at a slightly lower level will reveal the kidneys as circular structures on either side of the vertebral column (Fig. 12).[35,61] A nomogram has been established (Table 5) to compare the mean kidney circumference with the abdominal circumference (KC/AC ratio). This nomogram originally designed for use in polycystic kidney disease is also useful in renal diseases resulting in hydronephrosis, a common anomaly in the diabetic offspring. Serial sonographic evaluations, however, will be necessary to confirm such a diagnosis (Fig. 13).[3,35,36,62]

TABLE 4
Comparison of Left Ventricular Free Wall and Interventricular Septum Between Well-Controlled Diabetics and Normals

Gestational Age	Left Ventricular Free Wall		Interventricular Septum	
	Diabetic	Nondiabetic	Diabetic	Nondiabetic
19–26	2.6 ± 0.9 mm	2.9 ± 1.2 mm	2.9 ± 0.4 mm	3.1 ± 2.2 mm
26–35	2.8 ± 0.6 mm	2.9 ± 0.8 mm	2.9 ± 0.7 mm	3.1 ± 1.0 mm
35–40	3.4 ± 1.1 mm	3.2 ± 0.9 mm	3.9 ± 1.3 mm	3.6 ± 1.2 mm
	$p = NS$		$p = NS$	

Courtesy of Talner et al. Reproduced with permission.

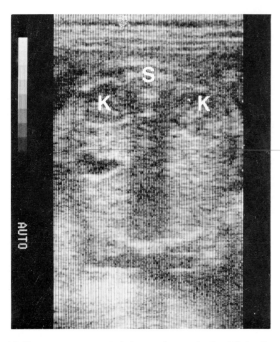

Fig. 12. Transverse scan of abdomen demonstrating bilaterally normal appearing kidneys (S = spine, K = kidney).

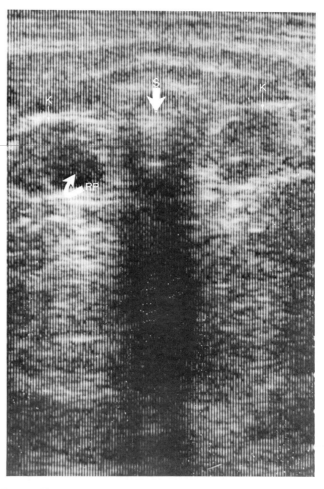

Fig. 13. Transverse scan of the abdomen at the level of the kidneys demonstrating the vertebral column and bilaterally hydronephrotic kidneys with dilated renal pelvices (K = kidney, S = spine, RP = renal pelvis).

The fetal bladder can be identified as early as 18 weeks. Identification of the fetal bladder at any time in the gestation precludes the diagnosis of nonfunctioning kidney or renal agenesis. The absence of the fetal bladder may mean recent voiding or inadequate renal function. Recent voiding is a less likely possibility, since a residual urine volume is usually maintained following voiding. A diagnostic test may be employed using a single intravenous injection of furosemide. If there is satisfactory functioning of the urinary system, the fetal bladder will be visualized by ultrasound within half an hour of the maternal diuretic infusion. The persistent inability to visualize this organ is strongly suggestive evidence of inadequate renal function, and further evaluation for renal disease would be indicated.[3,35]

Renal agenesis is one of the most common causes of inadequate renal function in a diabetic gestation. The sonographic findings highly suggestive of this disease include absent or poor renal shadows, no demonstrable bladder, as well as oligohydramnios (Fig. 14).

Imaging the adrenal glands may occasionally give a mistaken impression of kidneys; however, with experience and the use of improved resolution real-time equipment, the sonographer should have little difficulty in distinguishing these two organs and, thus, making the diagnosis of renal agenesis (Fig. 15). A paucity of fluid in the area of the fetal limbs will be noted, revealing a sonographic pattern of crowding

(Fig. 16).[12,35] Neonates with this condition either are stillborn or die of pulmonary hypoplasia shortly after birth. Associated anomalies are common, including Potters facies, duodenal atresia, and Meckel's diverticulum.[28]

Gastrointestinal Malformations

The most common gastrointestinal disorders associated with diabetes, in order of occurrence, are (1) imperforate anus, (2) small bowel atresia, and (3) small left colon syndrome.

The diagnosis of imperforate anus and small left colon syndrome is generally made in the neonate. A presumptive diagnosis of these conditions may be made in the presence of dilated loops of bowel and/or associated skeletal and cardiac defects (Fig. 17).[63,64]

Duodenal atresia may occur singly or in combination with other congenital anomalies, particularly of

TABLE 5
Kidney Biometry

Week	Volume Percentile			Length Percentile			Width Percentile			Thickness Percentile		
	5th	50th	95th	5th	50th	95th	5th	50th	95th	5th	50th	95th
20	—	2	5.6	21	28	36	10	14	18	11	15	19
21	—	3	6	22	29	36	10	14	18	11	15	19
22	—	3	6.4	22	30	37	10	14	18	12	16	20
23	—	3	6.8	23	30	37	11	15	19	12	16	20
24	—	4	7.2	24	31	38	11	15	19	13	17	21
25	0.6	4	7.6	24	31	39	11	15	19	13	17	21
26	1	4	7.9	25	32	39	12	16	20	14	18	22
27	1.4	5	8.3	26	33	40	12	16	20	14	18	22
28	1.8	5	8.7	26	33	40	12	16	20	14	18	22
29	2.1	6	9.1	27	34	41	13	17	21	15	19	23
30	2.5	6	9.5	27	34	42	13	17	21	15	19	23
31	2.9	6	9.9	28	35	42	13	17	21	16	20	24
32	3.3	7	10.3	29	36	43	14	18	22	16	20	24
33	3.6	7	10.7	29	36	43	14	18	22	17	21	25
34	4	8	11.1	30	37	44	14	18	22	17	21	25
35	4.4	8	11.5	30	38	45	15	19	23	17	21	25
36	4.8	8	11.9	31	38	45	15	19	23	18	22	26
37	5.2	9	12.3	32	39	46	15	19	23	18	22	26
38	5.5	9	12.6	32	39	47	16	20	24	19	23	27
39	5.9	9	13	33	40	47	16	20	24	19	23	27
40	6.3	10	13.4	33	41	48	16	20	24	19	23	27
	cm³	cm³	cm³	mm	mm	mm	mm	mm	mm	mm	mm	mm

The Computed Kidney Perimeter to Abdomen Perimeter Ratio

$$\frac{(\text{kidney width} + \text{kidney thickness})}{(\text{anteroposterior abdominal diameter} + \text{transverse abdominal diameter})} = 23\%$$

+/− 5% for the 5th and 95th percentile, the normal range is between 19% or 28%

The Measured Kidney Perimeter to Abdomen Perimeter Ratio

	Gestational Age (in Weeks)					
	< 17	17–20	21–25	26–30	31–35	36–40
ratio =	28%	30%	30%	29%	28%	27%
5th–95th	24–32%	24–36%	26–34%	24–33%	22–34%	19–35%

Reprinted with permission from Jeanty P, Romero R: Ultrasonography in Obstetrics. New York, McGraw-Hill, 1984.

the gastrointestinal, cardiovascular and, occasionally, of the skeletal system. This lesion can be identified quite readily by its characteristic sonographic findings including polyhydramnios and the so-called double bubble sign. This sign represents distension of the stomach and duodenum secondary to the distal obstruction. Other gastrointestinal lesions are less specific for diabetes (Fig. 18).[65,66]

Other Anomalies

A single umbilical artery occurs in about 6.4 percent of IDMs, representing a fivefold increase over the control population. Froehlich and Fujikura[61] examined the collaborative study data collected between 1959 to 1963 and reported an incidence of associated malfor-

mations in 28.6 percent of infants in whom a single umbilial artery was encountered. These malformations include inguinal hernia (3.95 percent), polydactyly (3.44 percent), vertebral anomalies (2.95 percent), talipes or clubfoot (2.95 percent), multiple anomalies of the heart and great vessels (2.95 percent), hypoplasia of the lung (2.47 percent), and malformation of the skin. Velamentous insertion of the umbilical cord was found in 5.9 percent of cases. The umbilical cord vessels are easily identifiable by ultrasonography on transverse section (Figs. 19,20).[61] In the diabetic gestation the detection of a single umbilical artery on ultrasound should lead to further sonographic evaluations of the skeletal and cardiovascular systems to exclude the presence of malformations.

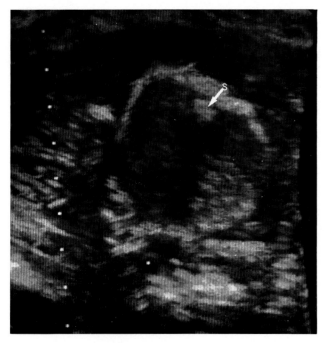

Fig. 14. Transverse scan of the abdomen illustrating the absence of kidneys in a patient with renal agenesis (S = spine).

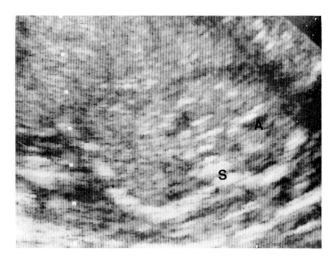

Fig. 15. Transverse scan of the abdomen depicting vertebral column, absent kidneys and enlarged adrenal glands masquerading as a kidney (S = spine, A = adrenal).

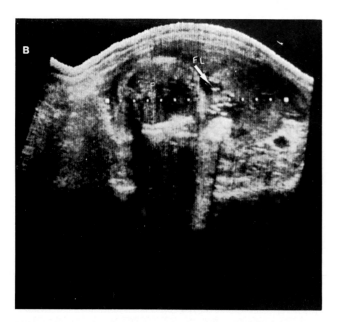

Fig. 16. Severe oligohydramnios. Fetal structures with minimal surrounding fluid noted (FL = fluid, F = fetus).

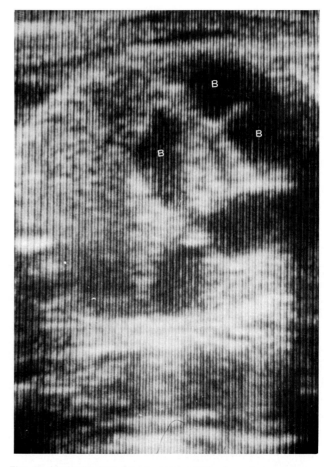

Fig. 17. Markedly dilated loops of bowel (B = bowel).

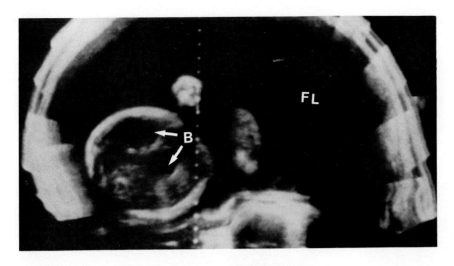

Fig. 18. Severe polyhydramnios and duodenal atresia. The dilated duodenum and stomach appear ultrasonically as two echolucent areas (B) referred to as the "double bubble sign.") (FL = fluid).

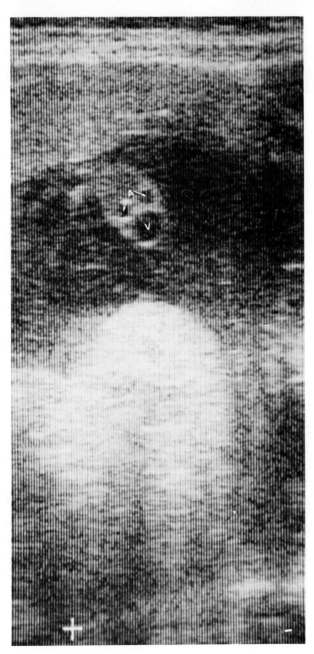

Fig. 19. Transverse scan of a normal umbilical cord with three vessels: two arteries (A), one vein (V).

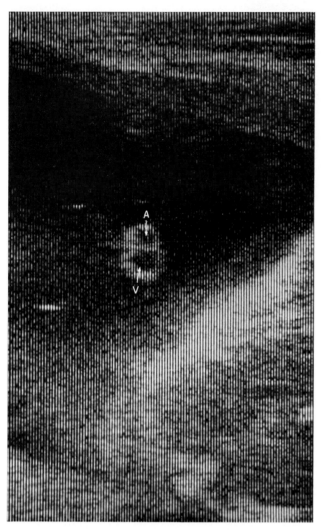

Fig. 20. Transverse scan of the umbilical cord with two vessels: one artery and vein (A = artery, V = vein).

POLYHYDRAMNIOS

Polyhydramnios is the excessive accumulation of amniotic fluid occurring in about 0.7 to 1.5 percent of all pregnancies.[67] The volume of amniotic fluid increases linearly until the 38th week of gestation when a mean volume of 1000 cm³ is present. Subsequently, the amniotic fluid volume decreases to about 250 cm³ at 43 weeks' gestation.[35]

Eighty percent of cases of hydramnios are idiopathic, or associated with the diabetic state which accounts for the larger proportion. The remaining 20 percent of cases are associated with major fetal abnormalities.[67-70] Hobbins et al.[35] reported an incidence of 2.8 percent, with fetal congenital anomalies associated with 18 percent of the cases.

The etiologic basis for polyhydramnios is not always clear. In diabetes mellitus, the proposed mechanisms for hydramnios are (1) increase in amniotic fluid osmolality due to increased glucose, (2) fetal polyuria resulting from fetal hyperglycemia, or (3) decreased fetal swallowing. Experimental work has not provided strong support for any of these hypotheses.[67,71]

Although gastrointestinal abnormalities are frequently associated with polyhydramnios, central nervous system (CNS) anomalies are the most common fetal malformations associated with hydramnios, and constitute about 45 percent of the total. Anencephaly accounts for approximately 80 percent of these CNS anomalies.[67,72]

The sonographic evaluation of a gestation complicated by hydramnios reveals excessive amniotic fluid with displacement of the fetus toward the posterior aspect of the uterine cavity (Fig. 21). Fetal extremities appear to be separated by vast spaces of amniotic fluid. Calculation of the total intrauterine volume (TIUV) permits a semiquantitative determination of hydramnios. TIUV measurements outside the 95 percent confidence limit for a given gestational age confirm an enlarged intrauterine volume. Follow-up evaluations may also utilize serial TIUV determinations (Fig. 22, Table 6).[12] The diagnosis of polyhydramnios is usually only made in the third trimester, since amniotic fluid volumes are generally normal in the first and second trimesters in those cases where polyhydramnios is noted in the third trimester.[62,67,73]

Following a diagnosis of polyhydramnios, scrutiny of fetal morphology and the placenta is essential. A biochemical evaluation for diabetes mellitus is also indicated, since diabetes is one of the conditions most frequently associated with an increased amniotic fluid volume.

INTRAUTERINE GROWTH RETARDATION

Intrauterine growth retardation is discussed in detail in Chapter 11.

Infants are considered growth retarded when their birth weight falls at or below the tenth percentile for a given gestational age. Other less stringently used criteria include the presence of tissue wasting or fetal malnutrition.[74-77]

IUGR is associated with conditions that predispose to uteroplacental vascular insufficiency, namely juvenile onset diabetes mellitus, hypertension, preeclampsia, renal disease, heavy smoking, anemia, maternal malnutrition, and cardiac disease.[78]

Diabetic pregnancies, when associated with vascu-

311

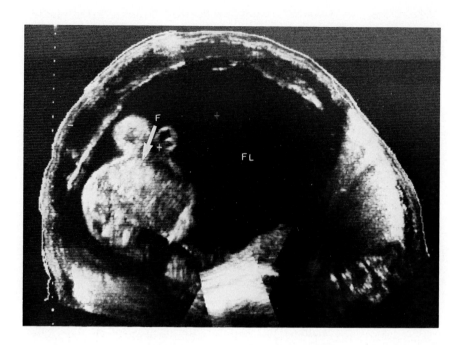

Fig. 21. Severe polyhydramnios (FL = fluid, F = fetus). (*Reprinted with permission from Hobbins JC, Winsberg F, Berkowitz RL: Ultrasonography in Obstetrics and Gynecology. Baltimore, Williams and Wilkins, 1983.*)

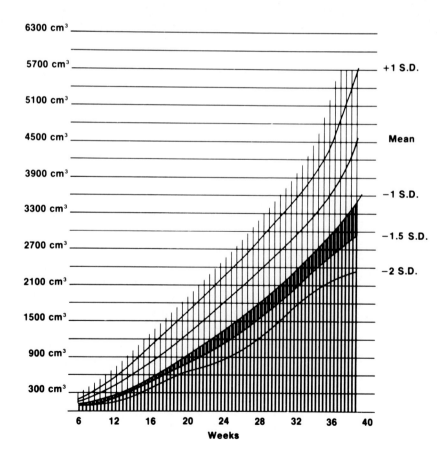

Fig. 22. Total intrauterine volume. (*Reprinted with permission from Gohari P, Berkowitz RL, Hobbins JC: Prediction of intrauterine growth retardation by determination of total intrauterine volume. Am J Obstet Gynecol 127:255,1977.*)

TABLE 6
Intrauterine Volume

Week	−2 SD	−1.5 SD	−1 SD	Mean	+1 SD	SD
6	89	104	120	152	184	32
7	88	112	137	188	239	51
8	87	120	155	224	293	69
9	86	128	172	260	348	88
10	106	148	192	280	368	88
11	126	168	212	300	388	88
12	139	206	276	416	556	140
13	152	244	340	532	724	192
14	262	334	409	558	708	150
15	372	424	477	584	691	107
16	483	514	546	610	674	64
17	594	605	615	636	657	21
18	664	698	734	804	875	71
19	734	792	852	972	1092	120
20	763	876	993	1228	1462	235
21	792	960	1134	1483	1832	349
22	825	992	1166	1513	1860	347
23	859	1025	1197	1542	1887	345
24	934	1104	1282	1636	1991	355
25	1009	1184	1366	1730	2094	364
26	961	1200	1448	1945	2441	497
27	914	1216	1530	2159	2788	629
28	943	1263	1596	2263	2929	667
29	972	1310	1662	2366	3070	704
30	1357	1640	1935	2525	3115	590
31	1742	1970	2208	2684	3160	476
32	1871	2101	2341	2820	3300	480
33	2000	2232	2473	2956	3439	483
34	2263	2464	2674	3094	3513	420
35	2526	2697	2875	3231	3587	356
36	2329	2628	2940	3563	4186	623
37	2132	2559	3004	3894	4784	890
38	2269	2752	3255	4262	5268	1007
39	2405	2945	3506	4629	5752	1123
	← IUGR →	← Grey Zone →	← Normal →			

Reprinted with permission from Jeanty P, Romero R: Ultrasonography in Obstetrics. New York, McGraw-Hill, 1984.

lopathy (White's classes D,F,H,R, and T), may result in retarded fetal growth. The exact pathogenesis of this growth delay is unclear. Since vascular disease in diabetes undoubtedly affects the placenta, some have assumed that placental vascular insufficiency with resulting decrease in transfer of nutrients is responsible for IUGR. Nevertheless, other factors may also be partially responsible. For example, insulin is a growth hormone, involved in the stimulation of insulin-sensitive tissues. The interplay between hormone and target tissue may contribute to alterations in fetal growth.[79] Insulin receptors have been demonstrated in various tissues, including adipose tissue, liver, fibroblasts, and red blood cells. The magnitude of response by a target tissue to insulin is dependent on the concentration of plasma insulin and the tissue sensitivity to insulin. Resistance to insulin may occur at different levels, evidenced by impaired response of the target organs and decreased receptor binding capacity, which has been observed in the hepatic animal cell plasma membrane, cardiac and skeletal muscle, and adipose tissue.

There are experimental models in which the fetal pancreas has been removed or destroyed using chemical agents, resulting in retarded fetal growth, poor adipose tissue formation, and failure of muscle mass development.[13] Recent data indicate that monocytes of newborn infants have increased number of insulin receptors and increased receptor affinity, suggesting that there might be an integral relationship between insulin and fetal growth and development.[13] The information that is currently available has led to the etiologic hypothesis of Hill regarding retarded fetal growth in the diabetic pregnancy. Under conditions in which fetal insulin is absent, or in which end organ sensitivity is altered, marked intrauterine growth retardation may occur.[79] IUGR seems to be a late gestation phenomenon, since most of these infants achieve a weight comparable to that of a 29- to 32-week fetus and appear to gain little additional weight beyond this gestational age.[79]

The intrauterine detection of retarded fetal growth by clinical means is possible in approximately 30 percent of affected pregnancies.[76] Ultrasonography, therefore, offers an objective, reliable, and more effective means of identifying retarded intrauterine fetal growth.

Biparietal Diameter (BPD) Determinations

Calculated estimates of weekly increments for the size of the BPD are available[41]; hence, when comparing the observed increase in BPD with the expected rate of growth one should be able to identify growth-retarded fetuses when the head is affected in the growth curtailment. However, the BPD alone is often an unsatisfactory means of assessing IUGR because the fetus suffering from placental compromise will often "spare" its head in the early stages of IUGR. This determination, utilized singly, fails to identify about 20 to 50 percent of affected cases.[41,76,80] Serial measurements of the BPD when used adjunctively with other measurements can be quite useful.

Total Intrauterine Volume (TIUV)

This method presumes that IUGR is manifested by total diminution of fetal and placental size as well as amniotic fluid volume. The TIUV is calculated by measuring the longitudinal (L), transverse (T), and anteroposterior (AP) dimensions of the uterus and using the condensed formula for an ellipse: $V = 0.5233 \times L \times T \times AP$.[81] The problem, however, in using this method of evaluation singly, is that the symmetrically growth-retarded fetus and the small normal fetus may fall into an indeterminate zone (gray zone) (Fig. 22, Table 5). Additional measurements are therefore necessary to discriminate between these two groups. The severely growth-retarded fetus, however, will almost always be screened in by this method. This technique has been largely supplanted by other methods, which depend on real-time equipment rather than a contact scanner needed to perform a TIUV.

Sonographic Estimated Fetal Weight (SEFW)

This method utilizes determinations of the BPD and the abdominal circumference (AC) obtained at the level of the umbilical vein. The calculation of SEFW has been described elsewhere.[82-85] Comparing the weight obtained on the patient under study with a nomogram of SEFW for gestational age, the diagnosis of IUGR can be made readily and a weight deficit can be quantified.

Other Methods for IUGR Detection

Several other methods mentioned in another chapter have been proposed for the diagnosis of IUGR including the trunk circumference at the level of the portal branch of the ductus venosus, head-to-body ratio, hourly fetal urine production rate (HFUPR), and semiquantitative estimation of amniotic fluid volume.[76]

Ultrasonography utilized in the diabetic pregnancy is an essential adjunctive tool in the antenatal assessment of fetal growth. Following the identification of retarded intrauterine growth, antepartum fetal testing and serial ultrasonograms will become essential for follow-up evaluation and timing of clinical intervention.

FETAL MACROSOMIA

The infant of the diabetic mother (IDM) is classically described as plump, plethoric, and cushingnoid. Their resemblance is sometimes more striking to other IDMs than to their siblings.[13]

Macrosomia is defined as a fetal weight in excess of 4000 g or a birth weight above the 90th percentile per gestational age.[49,86,87] Fetuses weighing more than 4000 g account for 10 percent of all deliveries, while infants whose birth weights are 4500 g or more account for approximately 1 percent of deliveries.[73]

The macrosomic IDM is at high risk for multiple

complications, including stillbirths and intrapartum trauma. The perinatal mortality in macrosomic infants is twice that for appropriate-for-gestational age infants. Maternal and perinatal morbidity and mortality increase in direct relation to increasing birth weight of the large infant.[87,88] Houchang et al.,[89] in a retrospective study, reported that during the intrapartum period the incidence of labor augmentation by oxytocin, shoulder dystocia, and cesarean section deliveries were significantly greater in the presence of fetal macrosomia. Macrosomic fetuses, however, did not experience greater fetal distress than the appropriate-for-gestational weight term-size fetuses. Infants experiencing birth injuries, including shoulder dystocias, are known to have serious immediate and long-term morbidity. Benedetti and Gabbe[90] found shoulder dystocia in the macrosomic infant to be enhanced in the presence of prolonged second stage of labor and midpelvic delivery. These data underscore the importance of the antenatal detection of fetal growth acceleration and the need for expectant intrapartum management.

The etiology of hypersomatism or macrosomia is thought to be secondary to fetal hyperinsulinemia resulting from maternal hyperglycemia. The fetal pancreas is stimulated by elevated blood glucose to increase production and to release insulin. Pedersen has proposed that the concomitant presence of excessive substrate and insulin enhance fetal glycogen synthesis, lipogenesis, and protein synthesis. There are experimental data supporting insulin as a growth hormone. The administration of insulin to fetal rats and lambs has resulted in increased size of the newborn and deposition of fat in adipose tissue.[13,14,23,54,91-93] Experimental diabetes in rhesus monkeys noted findings consistent with some of the clinical observations made in humans.[13] There was no change in brain weight, while visceral organs and adipose tissue were significantly enlarged. In vitro experiments have demonstrated selective tissue responses to insulin administration in which insulin-sensitive tissues exhibited increased lipid and triglyceride synthesis.[13] Increase in fetal levels of deoxyribonucleic acid (DNA) and proteins have been demonstrated in animal models indicating cellular hyperplasia and hypertrophy in some organs and body areas.[93]

Fetal macrosomia is characterized by a disparity in the growth rates of various tissues, depending on their insulin sensitivity. Increased weight of the insulin sensitive tissues including liver, pancreas, heart, lungs, adrenals (see Fig. 23) has been demonstrated in IDMs.[13,94] The brain (an insulin insensitive tissue) is reported by some to weigh less in IDMs than in nondiabetic controls.[95-97] This finding is probably reflected

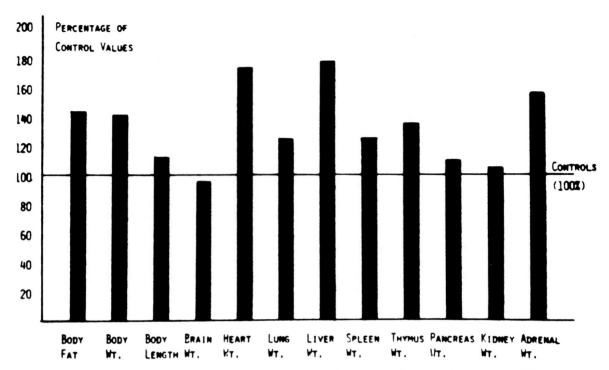

Fig. 23. Tissue sensitivity to insulin of infants of diabetic mother and of controls as measured by their weights. (*Reprinted with permission from Merkatz IR, Adams PAJ: The Diabetic Pregnancy. A Perinatal Perspective. New York, Grune and Stratton, 1979.*)

clinically in the sonographic biparietal diameter (BPD) measurement that has been reported by Aantaa and Forss[98] to be smaller than controls, especially during the 20th through 32nd week of pregnancy. This difference in BPD determination is statistically significant.[98] Other authors, notably Murata and Martin,[68] have found the BPD of IDMs to be similar to that of controls.

Although fetal hyperinsulinemia seems to be strongly implicated in the genesis of fetal macrosomia, accurate determination of fetal blood insulin levels is difficult. Insulin-treated diabetics form antibodies that cross the placenta and interfere with the measurements of fetal insulin levels. Hyperinsulinemia has been documented in the umbilical cord blood and the neonate, however. Increased amniotic fluid insulin levels have also been reported. It should be recalled, however, that amniotic fluid insulin is of fetal origin, since maternal insulin does not traverse the placenta. The appearance of amniotic fluid insulin correlates with pancreatic β-cell activity, and significant hypertrophy and hyperplasia of the pancreatic islet cells have been demonstrated in IDMs in response to maternal hyperglycemia.[13,71,99]

Ultrasonography offers the possibility of identifying in utero macrosomia, thus providing essential information which will affect the clinical management of these patients.

The Biparietal Diameter (BPD)

The BPD determination has been the subject of much investigation and conflicting findings.

Murata and Martin[68] have reported no difference in the BPD between IDMs and nondiabetic controls during the 13th through the 37th week of gestation. Measurements after the 37th week, however, were slightly larger than those in the nondiabetic group. These findings were the same in White's classes A, B, C, and D. Opposite findings were reported by Aantaa and Forss,[98] where the BPD in diabetic fetuses was statistically significantly smaller than controls during the 20th through 32nd week of pregnancy. There was no difference in BPD during the 36th through 40th week of gestation. Most authors do agree that the BPD is not significantly larger in the infant of the diabetic mother as compared with nondiabetic controls. Sonographic measurements of the fetal BPD is therefore of little value in the detection of evolving fetal macrosomnia.[99]

The growth rate, however, seems to be consistent with that found in controls. In normal pregnancy, the fetal BPD increases after the 32nd week by an average of 1.6 to 1.8 mm/week. This increase is less rapid as term approaches. The infant of the diabetic mother shows no significant deviation in growth rate in the BPD determination.[100]

Abdominal Size Determination

Many of the intraabdominal organs are insulin sensitive, and thus accelerated growth would be expected in the presence of fetal hyperinsulinemia. The sonographic fetal abdominal transverse diameter (FATD) has been shown to be useful in the antepartum diagnosis of fetal macrosomia. In approximately 50 percent of IDMs, the abdominal circumference determined at the level of the ductus venosus exceeded 2 SD above the mean for diabetics between 28 and 32 weeks' gestation, suggesting a diagnosis of accelerated fetal growth.[99] The neonatal evidence of fetal macrosomia corroborated the sonographic findings. Campbell and Thoms[41] have constructed a nomogram of head-to-abdominal circumference ratio with mean, 5th, and 95th percentile levels ranging from the 13th to the 42nd week of gestation, which may be useful in assessing head-to-body proportions. At Yale, all diabetic patients receive serial sonographic evaluations including an estimated fetal weight and head-to-body ratio assessment. We have found that the abdominal circumference determination is more reproducible than chest measurement and the information derived may be interpreted across gestational ages for evidence of evolving fetal macrosomia. Grandjean et al[96] utilized this FATD measurement as an indicator for the detection of gestational diabetes. They found that the FATD, when greater than the 95th percentile, was a more sensitive indicator in the detection of gestational diabetes than was a past history of diabetes in the family, obesity, prior macrosomia, hydramnios, glucosuria, or prior stillbirths. It should be noted, however, that an increase in the abdominotransverse diameter may occur in the presence of normal birth weight and biparietal diameter per gestational age.

Chest Size Determination

The chest size is also affected by the effects of diabetes. Most of the intrathoracic organs are insulin sensitive and increased growth of these organs has been demonstrated in IDMs, both in pathologic specimens and by ultrasonography. Wladimiroff, Bloemsma, and Wallenburg[88] obtained a chest size measurement by a cross-sectional dimension immediately caudad to the fetal heart pulsation. Using this single determination, they reported a detection rate of fetal macrosomia of 80 percent in relation to the 90th percentile of the mean weight for gestation, and 47 percent in relation to the 95th percentile of normal. Houchang et al.[89] have utilized a chest circumference measurement in a ratio to head size in identifying macrosomic infants at high risk for traumatic delivery. Neonates experiencing shoulder dystocia had significantly greater shoulder-to-head ratio (4.8 ± 2.1 compared with a control of 3.3 ± 1.3), and chest-to-head disproportion (1.6 ± 2.2 compared with a control of 0.2 ± 1.8) than those macrosomic neonates delivered without shoulder dystocia. Elliot et al.,[86] in an attempt to predict diabetic macrosomia using ultrasonography, calculated a diabetic macrosomic index (chest circumference minus BPD). From this study 87 percent of the infants weighing greater than 4000 g had a macrosomic index of ≥1.4. Of these infants, 27 percent experienced shoulder dystocia.

Although the antenatal sonographic measurement of chest-to-head size ratio may be useful in selecting patients at risk for obstructed or traumatic deliveries, it should be noted that sonographic determination of chest sizes may be difficult due to lack of precise landmarks and irregular outline.

Sonographic Estimated Fetal Weight (SEFW)

Several formulas are now available for the calculation of intrauterine fetal weight following the sonographic determination of appropriate dimensions.[82-85]

The BPD measurement alone is an inexact predictor of fetal weight. Cephalometry in conjunction with other fetal biometric parameters result in an improved estimation of in utero fetal weight. Thompson and Makowski,[101] using the BPD and cross-sectional views of the fetal thorax, estimated birth weight within ±660 g (2 SD); Lunt and Chard[74] measured the BPD and cross-sectional area of the fetal thorax at the level of the heart, constructing a skull thoracic area multiple index (STAM). The range of error in 95 percent of the population was ± 430 g (2 SD); Warsof et al.[85] obtained BPD, AC, total intrauterine volume (TIUV), and estimated fetal weight by computer analysis and reported that birth weight was most precisely predicted using abdominal circumference and BPD together, with a standard deviation of 106 g/kg of fetal weight.

Campbell and Wilkin[102] obtained fetal AC at the level of the umbilical vein and using a second-degree polynomial regression formula, were able to predict birth weights, with confidence limits dependent on the size of measurement.

With the availability of the SEFW, objective assessment of fetal weight may be made and the appropriate route of delivery chosen, thus obviating some of the morbidity and even mortality that may be associated with the macrosomic infant. Sack,[103] in a review of the complications associated with macrosomic infants delivered vaginally and weighing 10 or more pounds, reported 10.3 percent postpartum hemorrhage, 10.0 percent shoulder dystocia, 7.2 percent perinatal mortality, 11.4 percent neurologic complication, and 4.5 percent infant death.

Following the diagnosis of fetal macrosomia, attention should be given to anthropometric proportions. If disproportion exists between abdomen and head, or thorax and head, consideration should be given to the potential for obstructed labor and/or traumatic delivery. Head-to-body disproportion can also be assessed from measurements of abdominal circumference and head circumference.[41] Houchang et al.[89] reported a 1.6 chest–head circumference difference and a 4.8 shoulder–head circumference difference as constituting anthropometric disproportion and thus indicated the possibility of shoulder dystocia during labor. They recommended cesarean section delivery in the presence of anthropometric disproportion in macrosomic infants.

Ultrasonography, therefore, not only can identify fetal macrosomia but can also provide other information essential to the clinical management of the pregnancy and to the route of delivery utilized.

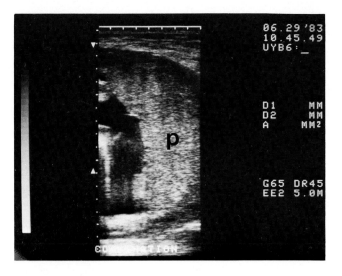

Fig. 24. Grade 0 placenta (P = placenta).

ASSESSMENT OF FETAL WELL-BEING

Recent attention has been directed toward intrauterine fetal breathing movements (FBM), recorded by real-time ultrasound, as an indicator of fetal health.[14]

Normal fetuses spend about 30 percent of their time breathing, with peaks in breathing activity occurring postprandial and between 4:00 and 7:00 AM. Apneic periods may last as long as 120 minutes. Breath-to-breath intervals were generally 0.5 to 1.0 seconds in the 30-week fetus compared with an interval of 1.0 and 1.5 seconds in the 38- to 39-week fetus.[5] Fetal tachypnea has been a diagnosis generally made by qualitative assessment. Nevertheless, the rare observation of rapid FBM has been observed almost exclusively in poorly controlled diabetics.[104-106] Real-time ultrasound has become a popular tool for observing typical diaphragmatic movements made during fetal breathing. During inspiration the chest wall moves inward by about 2 to 5 mm, and the abdominal wall moves outward by 3 to 8 mm, producing paradoxical excursions of the anterior thoracoabdominal wall.[5]

THE PLACENTA

The sonographic descriptions of placental morphology and maturation have been described by Grannum and Hobbins[60] and a grading system has been introduced based on these findings. There is a predominance of Grade I placentas in the third trimester diabetic classes A and B, while in diabetics with end organ disease there is a higher rate of Grade III placentas than is found in a normal population. At present, these obser-

vations are anecdotal and must be quantified by data from large studies. It is of interest, that it is rare for a Grade 0 placenta (the least mature type) to be seen after 30 weeks gestation in a normal pregnancy. This finding, however, is not unusual in a diabetic. In fact, the finding of a Grade 0 placenta (Fig. 24) after 30 weeks in an otherwise normal pregnancy should alert the physician to suspect glucose intolerance. Since the placenta is a fetal organ and may mature in parallel with intrafetal organs, such as the lung (which tends to mature more slowly in the diabetic), it is not surprising that less mature appearing placentas are seen in diabetics (Fig. 25).

Placental thickness is also affected by diabetes. In the nonvascular form of the disease (White's classes A, B, and C), there is increased placental thickness. For example, a placental thickness of 4 cm or greater is often seen in patients with the nonvascular form of the disease. In diabetics with vasculopathy (White's classes D,F,R,H, and T) the converse is true, i.e., placental thickness is often less than 3 cm.[60] The clinical significance of these alterations in placental morphology is not entirely clear but may be related to the fetal biochemical and morphologic development.

RECOMMENDATIONS FOR THE ADJUNCTIVE USE OF ULTRASOUND IN THE MANAGEMENT OF DIABETIC PREGNANCIES

1. Excellent blood glucose control is the obvious goal in the management of all diabetic pregnancies.

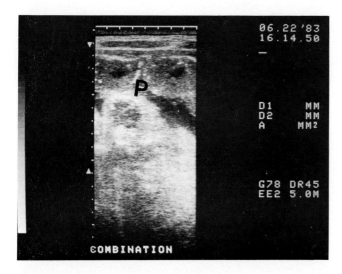

Fig. 25. Grade III placenta (P = placenta).

2. First trimester glycosylated hemoglobin (HbA$_{1c}$) determinations, since if this value is elevated the risk of fetal congenital anomalies is increased.
3. First trimester ultrasound examination for gestational age estimation in order that subsequent evaluations for growth abnormalities become more precise.
4. α-Fetoprotein (AFP) at 14 to 16 weeks, recognizing that the diabetic pregnancy is at high risk for neural tube defects (NTD). Sonographic evaluation for NTD may become necessary if AFP level is elevated.
5. Fetal echocardiography at 18 to 22 weeks for the assessment of cardiac anatomy and function.
6. Ultrasonogram profile at 18 to 22 weeks. At this examination there is careful scrutiny of the entire fetal anatomy for evaluation of gross fetal congenital anomalies.
7. Follow-up sonographic examinations every 4 to 6 weeks, particularly for fetal growth and estimated fetal weight. Attention should also be given to fetal breathing movements, amniotic fluid volume, and placental status. Fetuses identified as either macrosomic or growth retarded may benefit from more frequent examinations toward term.
8. At term, especially in the absence of vasculopathy (Classes A, B, and C) a SEFW and head-to-body ratio should be obtained prior to delivery. In the presence of fetal macrosomia (>4000 g) and anthropometric disproportion, consideration should be given to a cesarean section delivery.
9. Assessment of the total intrauterine volume may be useful in the patient in whom hydramnios is suspected.

SUMMARY

Pregnancies complicated by diabetes occur in as much as 2 to 3 percent of the obstetric population. Although remarkable improvements have been made in the prognosis of these patients, the perinatal mortality in the diabetic pregnancy still remains approximately 2 to 3 times higher than in the nondiabetic population. Major congenital malformations seem to be the principal contributor to the perinatal death rate. Abnormal fetal growth is also associated with increased perinatal morbidity and mortality.

Ultrasonography offers the potential for the detection of congenital anomalies, assessment of fetal weight and well-being as well as the evaluation of the placental status and amniotic fluid volume. Using sonography as an adjunctive form of fetal surveillance allows for the improved clinical management of pregnancies complicated by diabetes.

ACKNOWLEDGMENT

We wish to thank Ingeborg Venus, M.S. for her editorial assistance.

REFERENCES

1. Bolognese RJ, Schwarz RH: Perinatal Medicine: Management of the High Risk Fetus and Neonate. Baltimore, Williams and Wilkins, 1977, pp 470–474
2. Pildes RS: Infants of diabetic mothers. N Eng J Med 289:902, 1973
3. Callen PW: Ultrasonography in Obstetrics and Gynecology. Philadelphia, Saunders, 1983, pp 21–37
4. Depp R: How ultrasound is utilized by the perinatologist. Clin Obstet Gynecol 20:315, 1977
5. Hobbins JC, Winsberg F, Berkowitz RL: Ultrasonography in Obstetrics and Gynecology, 3rd ed. Baltimore, Williams and Wilkins, 1983, pp 203–206
6. Mills JL: Malformations in infants of diabetic mothers. Teratology 25:385, 1982
7. Mills JL, Baker L, Goldman AS: Malformations in infants of diabetic mothers occur before the seventh gestational week. Implications for treatment. Diabetes 28:292, 1979
8. Soler NG, Walsh CH, Malins JM: Congenital malformations in infants of diabetic mothers. J Med 178:303, 1976
9. Karlsson K, Kjellmer I: The outcome of diabetic pregnancies in relation to the mother's blood sugar level. Am J Obstet Gynecol 112:213, 1972
10. Pedersen J, Molsted-Pedersen L, Andersen B: Assessors of fetal perinatal mortality in diabetic pregnancy. Anal-

ysis of 1,332 pregnancies in the Copenhagen series, 1946–1972. Diabetes 23:302, 1974

11. Gabbe SG: Congenital malformations in infants of diabetic mothers. Obstet Gynecol Survey 32:125, 1977

12. Gabbe SG, Cohen AW: Diabetes mellitus in pregnancy; in Bolognese RJ, Schwarz R, Schneider J (eds), Perinatal Medicine: Management of the High Risk Fetus and Neonate. Baltimore, Williams and Wilkins, 1982

13. Merkatz IR, Adam PAJ: The Diabetic Pregnancy. A Perinatal Perspective. New York, Grune & Stratton, 1979

14. Pedersen IM, Tygstrup I, Pedersen J: Congenital malformations in newborn infants of diabetic women. Correlation with maternal diabetic vascular complications. Lancet 1:1124, 1964

15. Kucera J: Rate and type of congenital anomalies among offspring of diabetic women. J Rep Med 7:61, 1971

16. Neave C: Congenital malformations in offspring of diabetics. Ph.D. thesis, Harvard University, Boston, 1967

17. Baker L, Egler JM, Klein SH, et al.: Meticulous control of diabetes during organogenesis prevents congenital lumbosacral defects in rats. Diabetes 30:955, 1981

18. Beard RW, Lowy C: Commentary. The British Survey of Diabetic Pregnancies. Br J Obstet Gynaecol 89:783, 1982

19. Horii K, Watanabe G, Ingalls TH: Experimental diabetes in pregnant mice. Prevention of congenital malformations in offspring by insulin. Diabetes 15:194, 1966

20. Editorial: Abnormal infants of diabetic mothers. Lancet 1:633, 1980

21. Miller E, Hare JW, Cloherty JP, et al: Elevated maternal hemoglobin Alc in early pregnancy and major congenital anomalies in infants of diabetic mothers. N Engl J Med 304:1331, 1981

22. Watkins PJ: Congenital malformations and blood glucose control in diabetic pregnancy. Br Med J 284:1357, 1982

23. Ylinen K, Raivio K, Teramo K: Hemoglobin Alc predicts the perinatal outcome in insulin-dependent diabetic pregnancies. Br J Obstet Gynaecol 88:961, 1981

24. Pedersen JF, Molsted-Pedersen L: Early growth delay predisposes the fetus in diabetic pregnancy to congenital malformation. Lancet 1:739, 1982

25. Pedersen JF, Molsted-Pedersen L: Early fetal growth delay detected by ultrasound marks increased risk of congenital malformation in diabetic pregnancy. Br Med J 283:269, 1981

26. Pedersen JF, Molsted-Pedersen L: Early growth retardation in diabetic pregnancy. Br Med J 1:18, 1979

27. Farquhar JW: The child of the diabetic woman. Arch Dis Childhood 34:76, 1959

28. Rubin A, Murphy DP: Studies in human reproduction. III. The frequency of congenital malformations in the offspring of nondiabetic and diabetic individuals. J Pediatr 53:579, 1958

29. Oakley NW, Beard RW, Turner RC: Effect of sustained maternal hyperglycemia on the fetus in normal and diabetic pregnancies. Br Med J 1:466, 1972

30. Bruyere HJ, Viseskul C, Optiz JM, et al.: A fetus with upper limb amelia, "Caudal Regression" and Dandy–Walker defect with an insulin-dependent diabetic mother. Eur J Pediar 134:139, 1980

31. Mintz DH, Chez RA, Hutchinson DL: Subhuman primate pregnancy complicated by streptozotocin-induced diabetes mellitus. J Clin Invest 51:837, 1972

32. Wald NJ: Maternal serum alpha-fetoprotein measurement in antenatal screening for anencephaly and spina bifida in early pregnancy. Report of U.K. Collaborative study on alpha-fetoprotein in relation to neural tube defects. Lancet 1:1323, 1977

33. Milunsky A: Prenatal diagnosis of neural tube defects. The importance of serum alpha-fetoprotein screening in diabetic pregnant women. Am J Obstet Gynecol 142:1030, 1982

34. Burrow GN, Ferris TF: Medical complications during pregnancy. Philadelphia, Saunders, 1982, pp 121–122

35. Hobbins JC, Grannum PAT, Berkowitz RL, et al: Ultrasound in the diagnosis of congenital anomalies. Am J Obstet Gynecol 134:331, 1979

36. Jeanty P, Romero R: Ultrasonography in Obstetrics. New York, McGraw Hill, 1984

37. Campbell S: Early prenatal diagnosis of neural tube defects by ultrasound. Clin Obstet Gynecol 20:35, 1977

38. Campbell S, Prysedy J, Coltart TM, et al.: Ultrasound in the diagnosis of spina bifida. Lancet 1:1065, 1975

39. Cunningham ME, Walls WJ: Ultrasound in the evaluation of anencephaly. Radiol 118:165, 1976

40. Hadlock FP, Deter RL, Harrist RB, et al: Fetal head circumference: Relation to menstrual age. Am J Roentgenol 138:649, 1982

41. Campbell S, Thoms A: Ultrasound measurement of the fetal head to abdomen circumference ratio in the assessment of growth retardation. Br J Obstet Gynaecol 84:165, 1977

42. O'Brien GD, Queenan JT: Ultrasound fetal femur length in relation to intrauterine growth retardation. II. Am J Obstet Gynecol 144:35, 1982

43. Rowland TW, Hubbell JP, Nadas AS: Congenital heart disease in infants of diabetic mothers. J Pediatr 83:815, 1973

44. Mitchell SC, Sellman AH, Westphal MC, et al: Etiologic correlates in a study of congenital heart disease in 56,109 births. Am J Cardiol 28:653, 1971

45. Comess LJ, Bennet PH, Man MB, et al: Congenital anomalies and diabetes in the Pima Indians of Arizona. Diabetes 18:471, 1969

46. Koller O: Diabetes and pregnancy. Acta Obstet Gynecol Scand 32:80, 1953

47. Kleinman CS: Fetal echocardiography, in Sanders RC (ed), Ultrasound Annual. New York, Raven, 1982, p 321

48. Lange LW, Sahn DJ, Allen HD, et al: Qualitative real-time cross-sectional echocardiographic imaging of the human fetus during the second half of pregnancy. Circulation 62:799, 1980

49. Way GL, Wolfe RR, Eshaghpour E, et al: The natural history of hypertrophic cardiomyopathy in infants of diabetic mothers. J Pediatr 95:1020, 1979

50. Allan LD, Tynan MJ, Campbell S, et al: Echocardiographic and anatomical correlates in the fetus. Br Heart J 44:444, 1980

51. Allan LD, Tynan M, Campbell S, et al: Identification of congenital cardiac malformations by echocardiography in midtrimester fetus. Br Heart J 46:358, 1981

52. Crawford CS: Antenatal diagnosis of fetal cardiac abnormalities. Annals of Clinical and Laboratory Science 12:99, 1982

53. Sahn DJ, Lange LW, Allen HD, et al: Quantitative real-time cross-sectional echocardiography in the developing normal human fetus and newborn. Circulation 62:588, 1980

54. Vohr BR, Lipsitt LP, Oh W: Somatic growth of children of diabetic mothers with reference to birth size. J Pediatr 97:196, 1980

55. Kleinman C, Hobbins JC: Cardiomegaly and septal hypertrophy in the infant of diabetic mothers. Unpublished data.

56. Hurwitz D, Irving IC: Diabetes and pregnancy. Am J Med Sci 194:85, 1937

57. Miller HC: The effect of diabetic and prediabetic pregnancies on the fetus and newborn infant. J Pediatrics 29:455, 1946

58. Gutgesell HP, Speer M, Rosenberg HS: Further characterization of the hypertrophic cardiomyopathy of infants of diabetic mothers. Am J Cardiology 41:406, 1978

59. Halliday HL: Hypertrophic cardiomyopathy in infants of poorly controlled diabetic mothers. Arch Dis Childhood 56:258, 1981

60. Grannum PA, Hobbins JC: The placenta. Symposium. Radiol Clin N Am 20:353, 1982

61. Froehlich LA, Fujikura T: Significance of a single umbilical artery. Am J Obstet Gynecol 94:274, 1966

62. Hobbins JC: Use of ultrasound in complicated pregnancies. Clin Perinatol 7:397, 1980

63. Davis WS, Campbell JB: Neonatal small left colon syndrome. Am J Dis Child 129:1024, 1975

64. Duhamel B: From the mermaid to anal imperforation: The syndrome of caudal regression. Archives Dis Childhood 36:152, 1961

65. Atwell JD, Klidjian AM: Vertebral anomalies and duodenal atresia. J Pediatric Surg 17:237, 1982

66. Lees RF, Alford BA, Norman A, et al: Sonographic appearance of duodenal atresia in utero. Am J Roentgenol 131:701, 1978

67. Alexander ES, Spitz HB, Clark RA: Sonography of polyhydramnios. Am J Roentgenol 138:343, 1982

68. Murata Y, Martin CB: Growth of the biparietal diameter of the fetal head in diabetic pregnancy. Am J Obstet Gynecol 115:252, 1973

69. Santos-Ramos R, Duenhoelter JH: Diagnosis of congenital fetal abnormalities by sonography. Obstet Gynecol 45:279, 1975

70. Wladimiroff JW, Barentsen R, Wallenburg HCS, et al: Fetal urine production in a case of diabetes associated with polyhydramnios. Obstet Gynecol 46:100, 1975

71. Susa JB, McCormick KL, Widness JA, et al: Chronic hyperinsulinemia in the fetal rhesus monkey. Effects on fetal growth and composition. Diabetes 28:1058, 1979

72. Jacoby HE, Charles D: Clinical conditions associated with hydramnios. Am J Obstet Gynecol 94:910, 1966

73. Houchang D, Modanlou HD, Dorchester WL, et al: Macrosomia—Maternal, fetal, and neonatal implications. Obstet Gynecol 55:420, 1980

74. Lunt RM, Chard T: A new method for estimation of fetal weight in late pregnancy by ultrasonic scanning. Br J Obstet Gynaecol 83:1, 1976

75. McCallum WD: Fetal cardiac anatomy and vascular dynamics. Clin Obstet Gynecol 24:837, 1981

76. Sabbagha RE: Intrauterine growth retardation, in Sabbagha RE (ed), Diagnostic Ultrasound. Hagerstown, MD, Harper & Row, 1980

77. Tamura RK, Sabbagha RE: Assessment of fetal weight, in Sabbagha RE (ed), Diagnostic Ultrasound. Hagerstown, MD, Harper & Row, 1980, pp 93–102

78. Sanders RC: The role of ultrasound in the evaluation of intrauterine growth retardation, in Sanders RC (ed), The Principles and Practice of Ultrasonography in Obstetrics and Gynecology, 2nd ed. New York, Appleton-Century-Croft, 1980

79. Hill DE: Effect of insulin on fetal growth. Semin Perinatol 2:319, 1978

80. Sabbagha RE, Barton BA, Barton FB: Sonar biparietal diameter. Am J Obstet Gynecol 126:485, 1976

81. Gohari P, Berkowitz RL, Hobbins JC: Prediction of intrauterine growth retardation by determination of total intrauterine volume. Am J Obstet Gynecol 127:255, 1977

82. Compogrande M, Todros T, Brizolara M: Prediction of birth weight by ultrasound measurements of the fetus. Br J Obstet Gynaecol 84:175, 1977

83. Deter RL, Hadlock FP, Harrist RB, et al: Evaluation of three methods for obtaining fetal weight estimates using dynamic image ultrasound. J Clin Ultrasound 9:421, 1981

84. Shepard MJ, Richards VA, Berkowitz RL, et al: An evaluation of two equations for predicting fetal weight by ultrasound. Am J Obstet Gynecol 142:47, 1982

85. Warsof SL, Gohari P, Berkowitz RL, et al: The estimation of fetal weight by computer-assisted analysis. Am J Obstet Gynecol 128:881, 1977

86. Elliott JP, Garite TJ, Freeman RK, et al: Ultrasonic prediction of fetal macrosomia in diabetic patients. Obstet Gynecol 60:159, 1982

87. Golditch IM, Kirkman K: The large fetus. Management and outcome. Obstet Gynecol 52:26, 1978

88. Wladimiroff JW, Bloemsma CA, Wallenburg HCS: Ultrasonic diagnosis of the large-for-dates infant. Ostet Gynecol 52:285, 1978

89. Houchang D, Modanlou HD, Komatsu G, et al: Large-for-gestational-age neonates: Anthropometric reasons for shoulder dystocia. Obstet Gynecol 60:417, 1982

90. Benedetti TJ, Gabbe SG: Shoulder dystocia. A complication of fetal macrosomia and prolonged second stage of labor with midpelvic delivery. Obstet Gynecol 52:526, 1978

91. Kim YS, Young K: A new animal model for fetal macrosomia in diabetic pregnancy. Exp Molec Pathol 35:388, 1981

92. Kim YS, Yoon YJ, Jatoi I, et al: Fetal macrosomia in diabetic multiparous animals. Diabetologgia 20:213, 1981

93. Kim YS, Yoon YJ, Jatoi I, et al: Fetal macrosomia in experimental maternal diabetes. Am J Obstet Gynecol 139:27, 1981

94. Naeye RL: Infants of diabetic mothers: A quantitative morphologic study. Pediatrics 35:980, 1965

95. Driscoll SG: The pathology of pregnancy complicated by diabetes mellitus. Med Clin N Am 49:1053, 1965

96. Grandjean H, Saramon MF, De Mouzo J, et al: Detection of gestational diabetes by means of ultrasonic diagnosis of excessive fetal growth. Am J Obstet Gynecol 138:790, 1980

97. Murray SR: Hydramnios. A study of 846 cases. Am J Obstet Gynecol 88:65, 1964

98. Aantaa K, Forss M: Growth of the fetal biparietal diameter in different types of pregnancies. Radiology 137:167, 1980

99. Ogata ES, Sabbagha R, Metzger BE, et al: Serial ultrasonography to assess evolving fetal macrosomia. JAMA 243:2405, 1980

100. Jouppila P, Ylostalo P, Pystynen P: Fetal head growth measured by ultrasound in the last few weeks of pregnancy in normal, toxemic and diabetic women. Acta Obstet Scand 49:367, 1970

101. Thompson HE, Makowski EL: Estimation of birth weight and gestational age. Obstet Gynecol 37:44, 1971

102. Campbell S, Wilkin D: Ultrasonic measurement of fetal abdomen circumference in the estimation of fetal weight. Br J Obstet Gynaecol 82:689, 1975

103. Sack RA: The large infant. A study of maternal, obstetric, fetal and newborn characteristics; including a long-term pediatric follow-up. Am J Obstet Gynecol 104:195, 1969

104. Boddy K, Dawes GS: Fetal breathing. Br Med Bull 31:3, 1975

105. Manning FA, Heaman M, Boyce D, et al: Intrauterine fetal tachypnea. Obstet Gynecol 58:399, 1981

106. Romero R, Chervenak FA, Berkowitz RL, et al: Intrauterine fetal tachypnea. Am J Obstet Gynecol 144:356, 1982

24 | The Sonographic Evaluation of Multiple Gestation Pregnancy

Clifford S. Levi
Edward A. Lyons

INTRODUCTION

Although multiple gestation pregnancies account for approximately 1 percent of all births,[1-3] the perinatal mortality among twins in North America is approximately 13 to 14 percent, which is 5 to 10 times the perinatal mortality rate for singleton pregnancies.[4-6] Ultrasound plays an important role in the detection of multiple gestation pregnancy, and the evaluation of each fetus throughout gestation to assess fetal well-being.

Embryologically, twins may arise from the fertilization of two separate ova by two separate spermatazoa (dizygotic twins) or from the division of a single fertilized ovum (monozygotic twins). Dizygotic twins (zygote refers to a fertilized egg) are more common, occurring with a frequency of approximately 1 in 80 to 90 births. The frequency of dizygotic twinning is variable and is influenced by maternal age and parity as well as hereditary influences and racial background. The use of pharmacologic agents, including gonadotropins and clomiphene, to stimulate ovulation is also associated with an increased incidence of dizygotic twins. Monozygotic twins occur with a frequency of approximately 1 in 250 births. The overall perinatal mortality of monozygotic twins is 2.5 times greater than the perinatal mortality of dizygotic twins.[5]

Higher numbers of fetuses may arise from multiple zygotes or a division of a single zygote or a combination of both processes. The ratio of multiple gestation pregnancies to twin pregnancies increases with the use of gonadotropins or clomiphene (Fig. 1).[7]

CLINICAL FEATURES

The history and physical examination may be helpful in raising the physician's index of suspicion of a twin pregnancy; however, up to 50 percent of twin gestations have gone to term undiagnosed. A strong maternal family history of dizygotic twins is associated with an increased incidence of dizygotic twinning. Even higher orders of multifetal pregnancies should be suspected when the pregnancy has resulted from the pharmacologic stimulation of ovulation.

In the second trimester, physical examination usually reveals a uterus that is "large for dates," i.e., uterine size is greater than would be normally be expected at that menstrual age. In addition to a multiple gestation pregnancy, the differential diagnosis of the large for dates uterus includes a normal gestation with an inaccurate menstrual history, fibroids, polyhydramnios, hydatidiform mole, or, in diabetic mothers, fetal macrosomia.[7] An adnexal mass or elevation of the uterus by distended bladder may mimic a large for dates uterus. The most common outcome, about 65 percent in our experience, of sonographic evaluation referred because of a large for dates uterus is an entirely normal uterus, fetus, placenta, and amniotic fluid volume.

In the second and third trimester, the diagnosis of twins may be made by palpation of more than one fetal head or auscultation of two fetal hearts. This becomes difficult in the fat patient, in the presence of polyhydramnios, or with a large anterior placenta.

By physical examination it is often difficult to

make the diagnosis of twins early in gestation. In various reports, the rate of twin pregnancies going to term undiagnosed has ranged from as low as 5 percent to as high as 50 percent. In one center the routine use of ultrasound in obstetrics was associated with a reduction of the mean gestational age of twin detection from 35 to 20 weeks.[8]

Attempts have been made to identify a hormonal assay that can be used to differentiate a singleton fetus from a multiple gestation pregnancy. Maternal serum levels of human chorionic gonadotropin (hCG) and human placental lactogen (hPL) are related to the placental mass and are statistically higher in multiple gestation pregnancy than in singleton pregnancies.[9-11] A maternal serum hPL level that is greater than 1 SD above the mean in the second or third trimester suggests the presence of a twin pregnancy[10]; however, if the pregnancy is complicated by fetoplacental dysfunction the hPL level may not be elevated, and the diagnosis of twins may be missed. Knight et al.[11] demonstrated a twin detection rate of only 45.9 percent when the 90th percentile of the hPL level for singletons was used as a cutoff point.

In a study by Thiery et al.[9] maternal serum hCG levels were elevated significantly in five of nine twin pregnancies in the first trimester and in 72 percent of 39 twin pregnancies in the second and third trimester.

Knight et al.[11] demonstrated a twin detection rate of 78.3 percent of 37 twin pregnancies using the 90th percentile of maternal serum α-fetoprotein (AFP) in singletons as a cutoff point.

The combined use of hPL and AFP assays in the study by Knight et al.[11] raised the twin detection rate to only 80 percent. Thiery et al.[9] demonstrated a twin detection rate of 95 percent when either or both of the maternal serum levels of hPL or hCG were elevated greater than 1 SD above the mean for singleton pregnancies. They felt that the hormonal levels were too inconsistent throughout pregnancy to be useful as a screening test, but elevated levels of either hCG or hPL should alert the obstetrician to the possibility of a twin pregnancy.

Maternal serum AFP levels are currently used as a screening test for fetal neural tube defects (NTD). Twin pregnancies act as false positives in these NTD screening programs. The mean AFP level for twins is approximately 2.5 multiples of the mean calculated for normal singleton pregnancies (MOM).[12] In a twin pregnancy when the serum AFP level is greater than 5 MOM the outcome is significantly worse than those with levels less than 5 MOM. In a study by Ghosh et al.[12] over 50 percent of those twin pregnancies with a serum AFP level greater than 5 MOM ended in abor-

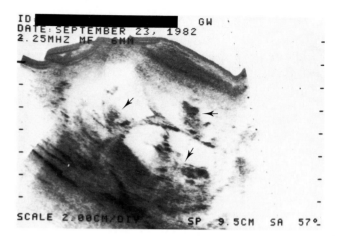

Fig. 1. Triplets at 13 weeks in a 29-year-old female with polycystic ovaries. Ovulation was induced with clomiphene citrate. Arrows point to the three fetuses. Fetal heart and fetal movement was demonstrated in each.

tion, still birth, fetus papryaceous, or were associated with either concordant or discordant neural tube defects.[13]

COMPLICATIONS

The most frequent cause of perinatal mortality in multiple gestation pregnancy is premature delivery associated with low birth weight (less than 2500 g). Often intrauterine growth retardation is a contributing factor, especially in monovular twins.

In a recent large American study, Naeye and coworkers[5] demonstrated that 60 percent of perinatal deaths in twins were due to amniotic fluid infections, 11 percent were due to premature rupture of the membranes, 8 percent were due to monovular twin transfusion syndrome, 8 percent were due to large placental infarcts, and 7 percent were due to congenital anomalies. Congenital anomalies in twins are twice as frequent as in singleton fetuses.

Other maternal complications that occur more commonly in twins include hypertension, maternal anemia, postpartum hemorrhage, abruptio placentae, placenta previa, vasa previa, polyhydramnios, and complications arising in labor such as dystocia and complications related to position and lie.[7]

SONOGRAPHIC EVALUATION OF MULTIGESTATIONAL PREGNANCY

As with all sonographic examinations a careful and complete examination is essential. Many feel that a complete study should include evaluation with an ar-

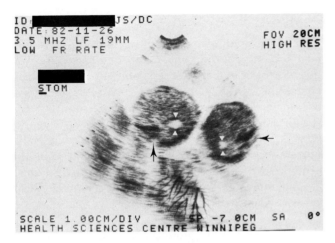

Fig. 2. Real-time scan in a transverse plane through both fetal abdomens in twins at 24.5 weeks. Stomach and spine are well demonstrated in both fetuses. White arrowheads, stomach; black arrow, spine.

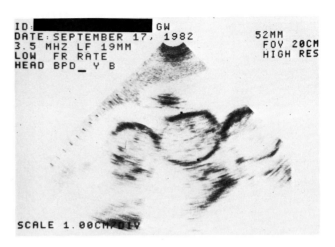

Fig. 3. Real-time scan through all three fetal heads in triplets at 21 weeks' menstrual age.

ticulated arm static scanner and a real-time scanner, either a linear array or sector type. The static study should include a predetermined matrix of parasagittal (longitudinal) and transverse sections of the entire uterus. These can be 1 or 2 cm apart, depending on the size of the uterus. This is important in that it allows adequate documentation of the intrauterine contents. In the late second and third trimesters with overlying fetal parts, it may be very difficult to identify the second fetus. Unless meticulous care is taken, it is not uncommon to miss a third or even fourth fetus. It is very important clinically to identify the triplet or quadruplet gestations, as the rate of prematurity and other obstetric complications rises significantly.

The real-time study is crucial, as well, to evaluate each fetus individually. The combination of both a static and real-time study should maximize the information retrieved. Each fetus must be examined completely and measurements including biparietal diameter, abdominal diameter, and femoral lengths should be obtained for each individual fetus.

In the breech fetus the biparietal diameter is not as consistent or reliable as in the cephalic presentation. The use of femoral lengths to date, or at least confirm dating, has gained wide acceptance recently.

In order to verify the presence of a multifetal gestation and ensure accuracy of the number of fetuses present a part of each fetus that can be easily identified as belonging to that fetus should be included on a single scan (e.g., two fetal heads, fetal abdomens, or thoraces) (Figs. 2,3). On occasion in the flexed fetus one can record the head and abdomen as two apparently unconnected separate structures, leading to a misinterpretation at a later time.

OVULATION INDUCTION ON MULTIFETAL PREGNANCY

Ultrasound is a reliable indicator of follicle maturation in ovulation induction with human menopausal gonadotropin (hMG) or clomiphene citrate.[14-18] (See Chapter 37.) In spontaneous follicle growth (those individuals who are not receiving exogenous stimulation) rapid growth of a dominant, usually single, follicle occurs during the 4 to 5 days prior to ovulation and reaches a size of 20 to 25 mm. In contrast, the nondominant follicles grow slowly, to reach a maximum size of 12 to 14 mm. In the gonadotropin stimulated ovary, more than one follicle may exhibit rapid growth prior to ovulation.[14]

In ovulation induction a course of hMG or clomiphene citrate is given to stimulate follicular growth. Serial (often daily) ultrasound examinations are used to assess follicular growth. When the maturing follicle reaches approximately 20 mm in diameter, hCG is administered to "trigger" ovulation.

Some investigators suggest that when three or more dominant follicles are present in the stimulated ovary, the incidence of a multifetal pregnancy is much higher and the "triggering dose" of hCG should be withheld and ovulation induction should be attempted again in the next cycle.[19]

EARLY TWINS

In the mid 1970s several reports were published describing the high incidence of concomitant blighted ova and normal intrauterine gestation. This seemed

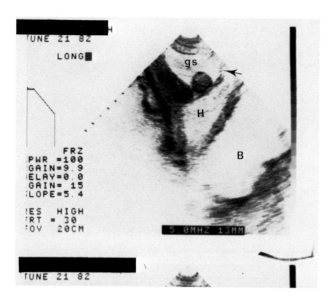

Fig. 4. Implantation bleed in a singleton pregnancy at 12 weeks' menstrual age mimicking a second gestational sac. No fetal echoes are present in the pseudosac. gs, gestational sac; H, implantation bleed or pseudosac; B, bladder; arrow, chorionic membrane.

to be followed by abortion of the blighted ovum, with no effect on the normal gestational sac. This did not seem to be a reasonable hypothesis, as the incidence of twinning would have had to be over 75 percent of all pregnancies. We advanced the hypothesis that the second sac actually represented a normal finding; an implantation bleed with blood filling the endometrial cavity not yet filled with the enlarging gestational sac. One should be able to see the second space or sac in most early gestations (5 to 8 weeks). The pseudosac never contains a fetus but may contain some solid material due to echogenic blood clot (Figs. 4–7).

MEMBRANES AND PLACENTAE

In the sonographic evaluation of the multiple gestation pregnancy the location and number of placentae and the presence of membranes separating the fetuses must be identified. In dizygotic twins, each fetus will have its own separate chorionic and amniotic sacs (Fig. 8). At approximately 5 to 7 weeks' menstrual age dizygotic twins may be seen sonographically as two completely separate sacs (Fig. 9). Later the chorionic and amniotic membranes of each sac in apposition will fuse and, on sonographic examination, only one membrane will be seen separating the two fetuses. Two placentae or one fused placenta will be present (Figs. 10–12).

The exact type of monozygotic twinning and the relationship of membranes and placentae that will arise depends on the stage of gestational development of the zygote at the time of division. At 2 days, between the two-cell, or blastomere, stage and the sixteen-cell (morula) stage, division will result in two separate chorionic and two separate amniotic sacs or dichorionic diamniotic twins (Fig. 8).

Sonographically a diamniotic dichorionic gestation from a single fertilized ovum (monozygotic) is indistinguishable from a gestation due to two fertilized ova (dizygotic twins). As with the dizygotic twin the presence of two separate placenta or one fused placenta depends on their proximity of implantation (Figs. 10,11).

If division of the zygote occurs during the blastocyst stage after the inner cell mass forms (about day 4 through 8 fetal life), the chorion will have already developed. Division of the inner cell mass will give rise to two fetuses developing in separate amniotic sacs but within a single chorionic sac, i.e., monochorionic

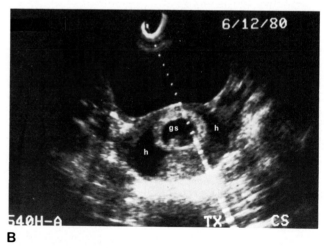

Fig. 5. A. Gestational sac with fetal pole at 7.5 weeks' menstrual age. **B.** Gestational sac and fetal pole in the same patient at 10 weeks' menstrual age. A pseudosac (h) has developed in the interval between the two examinations clearly demonstrating that it is an implantation bleed rather than a second gestational sac. gs, gestational sac; h, implantation bleed. (*Courtesy of CRB Merritt, MD, Ochsner Clinic, New Orleans.*)

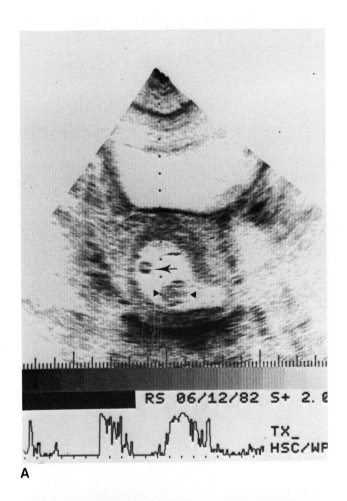

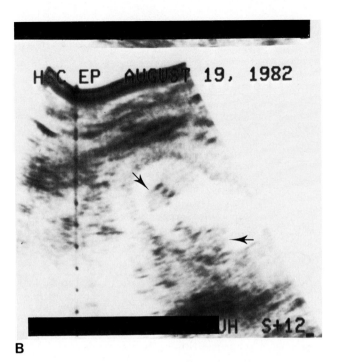

Fig. 6. A. Singleton fetus at 9.5 weeks' menstrual age. The arrowheads indicate the fetal abdomen. The arrow points to the secondary yolk sac which is a normal finding and should not be misinterpreted as a small second fetus. The membrane within the gestational sac is the amniotic membrane. **B.** Twins at 9.5 weeks. The arrows point to both fetuses. Fetal heart and fetal movement could be demonstrated in both fetuses.

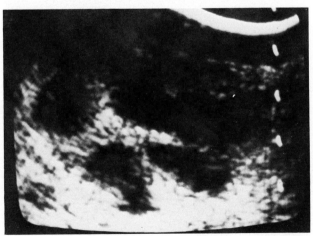

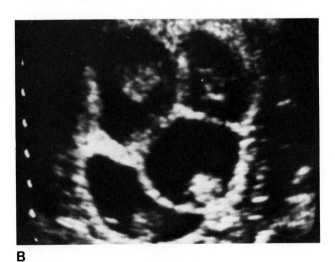

Fig. 7. A. Four gestational sacs at 9 weeks' menstrual age following hMG stimulation. **B.** A fetus is demonstrated within each gestational sac indicating quadruplets. Fetal heart and fetal movement could be identified in each fetus. (*Courtesy of M. Gillieson, M.D., Ottawa General Hospital. Reprinted from Lyons EA, Levi CS: Ultrasound in the first trimester of pregnancy. RCNA 20(2), June 1982. With permission from W. B. Saunders.*)

326

MONOZYGOTIC TWINS   MEMBRANES AND PLACENTAE   DIZYGOTIC TWINS

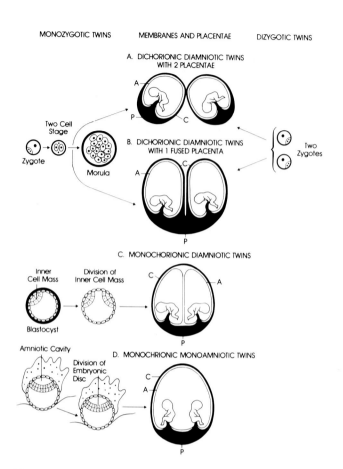

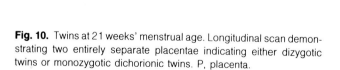

Fig. 8. Dichorionic diamniotic twins with two placentae or one fused placenta may be formed either by two separate zygotes or by the division of a single zygote between the two-cell stage and the morula stage. Monochorionic diamniotic twins are formed by division of the inner cell mass during the blastocyst stage. Monochorionic monoamniotic twins are formed by division of the embryonic disc during the blastocyst stage after the formation of the amniotic cavity. A, amniotic membrane; C, chorionic membrane; P, placenta.

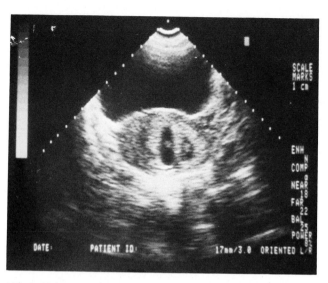

Fig. 9. Twins at 8 weeks' showing two separate sacs separated by chorion. (*Courtesy Mrs. Gail Wiebe, Health Sciences Centre, Winnipeg, Canada.*)

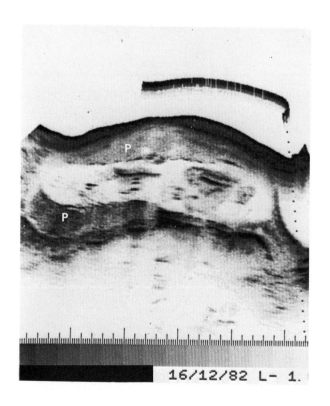

Fig. 10. Twins at 21 weeks' menstrual age. Longitudinal scan demonstrating two entirely separate placentae indicating either dizygotic twins or monozygotic dichorionic twins. P, placenta.

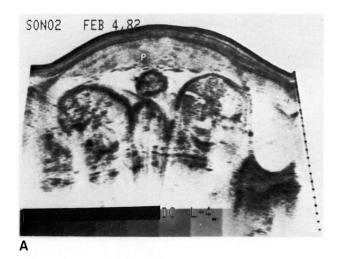
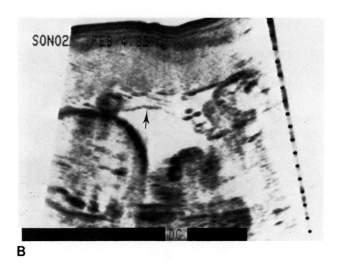

Fig. 11. A. Twins at 34 weeks' menstrual age. Longitudinal scan demonstrating a single anterior placenta in a twin pregnancy. P, placenta. **B.** The arrow points to a membrane separating the two fetuses.

diamniotic, monozygotic twins (Fig. 8). These twins will share a common placenta because of the common chorionic sac. Occasionally large arteriovenous anastomoses are present within the common placenta, with resultant monovular twin transfusion syndrome (vide infra). Monochorionic diamniotic monozygotic twins are the most common form of monozygotic twinning (Fig. 11).

Once the amniotic cavity has formed, by approximately 8 days' fetal life, division of the embryonic disc will result in a monochorionic monoamniotic twinning. Both fetuses will lie within a common amniotic and chorionic sac and no membrane will be demonstrable sonographically separating them. The importance of this finding cannot be overstated because of the extremely high fetal mortality rate. This most commonly is secondary to intertwining of the umbilical cords with obstruction of blood flow to one or both of the fetuses. In order to exclude the presence of monoamniotic twinning a careful attempt in all cases should be made to demonstrate and document a membrane between the fetuses. (Figs. 13,14.) Monochorionic monoamniotic twins represent approximately 4 percent of monozygotic twins.

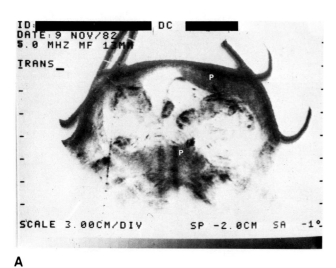
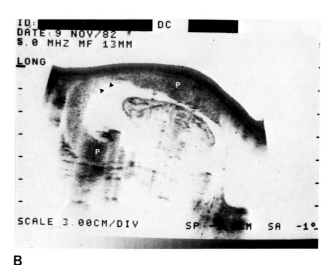

Fig. 12. A. Twins at 24 weeks' menstrual age. Transverse scan through the maternal abdomen in a twin pregnancy demonstrating placental tissue posteriorly as well as anterolaterally to the left. **B.** A longitudinal scan 3 cm to the left of the midline, however, demonstrates continuity of the placental tissue (*arrowheads*) that appeared to be separate on the transverse scan. P, placenta.

If incomplete division occurs after the formation of the embryonic disc conjoined twins may result. Whenever twins are present and a membrane has not been demonstrated separating the fetuses the possibility of conjoined twins must be considered. The index of suspicion should increase if the fetuses face each other; the absence of this finding does not rule out conjoined twins, however. When both of these twins are nearly completely formed the joined areas are usually the thorax anteriorly. When the duplication is less complete the attachment is often lateral (Fig. 15).

GROWTH RATES

Until approximately 26 to 28 weeks the biparietal diameters and growth rate of twins are similar to that of healthy singleton fetuses and the same growth rate curves apply. Early in the third trimester some investigators have noted a gradual slowing of the growth in twins as compared to singletons.[20-22] As a result both twins will "fall off" the singleton growth curve. Crane et al. found no significant difference in the growth of concordant twins and appropriate gestational age singletons in the third trimester.[3] Controversy still exists concerning growth rates of twins in the third trimester and subsequent studies should cast some light on this subject. It has been shown, however, that the birth weights of twins born after 30 weeks' gestation are less than those of singletons of the same gestational age[23] and the accelerated postnatal growth

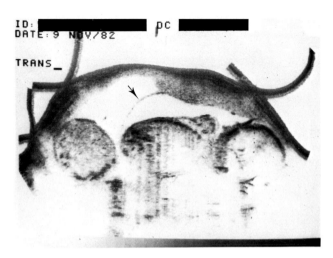

Fig. 13. Twins at 24 weeks' menstrual age. Transverse scan through the maternal abdomen in a twin pregnancy clearly demonstrating a membrane (*arrow*) separating the two fetuses.

that ensues suggests some degree of in utero malnutrition.[24]

A difference of 5 mm or greater in biparietal diameter (BPD) between twins suggests discordant growth. Discordant growth is defined as a weight difference in twins at birth of greater than 25 percent. A biparietal diameter of less than or equal to 4 mm is usually not associated with discordant growth. Discordant growth is present in 20 to 30 percent of fetuses with a difference in BPD of 5 mm or greater. When the difference in BPD is 7 mm or greater the incidence of fetal death

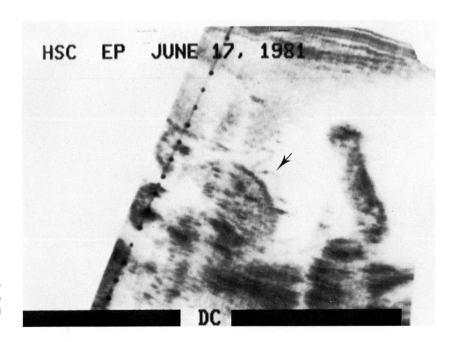

Fig. 14. Twins at 24.5 weeks' menstrual age. The two fetuses are separated by a membrane (*arrow*): however, visualization of the membrane was difficult and could only be demonstrated with very careful scanning.

increases significantly (Fig. 16).[23] It is important to note that discordancy does not occur in all twins with an intrapair difference in BPD, and other signs of growth retardation must be present before the diagnosis can be made. Molding of the fetal skull may account for the difference in BPD but the most common cause is probably measurement error. The BPD is known to be poorly correlated with birth weight. Serial examination and evaluation of growth is vital.

The finding of discordant growth appears to be caused by two distinct clinical syndromes: (1) monovular twin transfusion syndrome and (2) IUGR of one fetus while the other fetus develops normally.

As the name suggests, monovular twin transfusion occurs only in monozygotic twins and is seen almost invariably in those cases with one placenta or one fused placenta. Approximately 15 to 20 percent of monozygotic twins will have some degree of twin-to-twin transfusion caused by large subchorionic vascular communications. Blood is shunted to the recipient fetus, which becomes volume overloaded while the donor fetus becomes anemic and hypovolemic. This usually results in a growth-retarded donor and a hydropic recipient. An important differential feature between monovular twin transfusion syndrome and simple IUGR in one fetus is that the former occurs in the second trimester and the latter does not begin until the third trimester.[25]

In the overperfused twin in monovular twin transfusion syndrome polyhydramnios and hydrops may ensue, whereas the underperfused twin may have oligohydramnios (Fig. 17). Premature labor is common and these pregnancies usually do not reach the third trimester. The perinatal mortality rate is high. Occasionally the hydropic fetus may die and become macerated (fetus papyraceous), with the underperfused twin surviving. With the resultant correction of the intertwin shunting the surviving underperfused twin may exhibit increased growth and be relatively normal at birth.

Discordant growth diagnosed in the third trimester is associated with a better prognosis and may be the result of IUGR in one fetus. The cause of discordant growth may be due to asymmetric fetal nutrition and placental insufficiency in the smaller growth-retarded fetus. The larger fetus is usually normal and does not have evidence of hydrops or polyhydramnios and will have a normal biophysical profile.

HETEROTOPIC PREGNANCY

Heterotopic pregnancy is coexistent intrauterine and ectopic pregnancy. Heterotopic pregnancy is very rare and occurs with a frequency of approximately 1 in

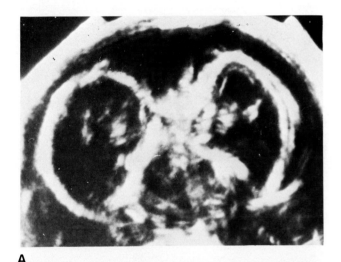

A

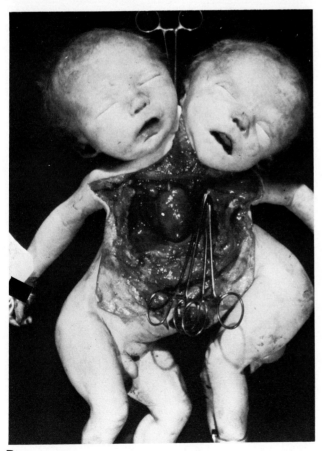

B

Fig. 15. A. Two fetal heads are present immediately adjacent to one another with both fetuses facing posteriorly. Serial scan planes through the fetus revealed a single thorax diagnostic of conjoined twins. **B.** The conjoined twins at postmortem.

30,000 pregnancies. Because the early diagnosis of ectopic pregnancy depends on a nongravid uterus and a positive pregnancy test the diagnosis of heterotopic pregnancy is very difficult. The diagnosis will be clear-cut sonographically only when a gestational sac with a fetus can be demonstrated in the adnexa in combination with an intrauterine gestational sac and fetus.

UTERINE CONGENITAL ANOMALIES

An exceedingly rare occurrence is a twin gestation associated with a bicornuate uterus in which each uterine horn contains a single gestation. It is more common to see a singleton gestation in one horn and to confuse the decidual reaction in the nongravid horn for a second gestational sac.

HYDATIDIFORM MOLE ASSOCIATED WITH PREGNANCY

Hydatidiform moles have been classified into two distinct groups: (1) the complete or classical mole; and (2) the partial mole with an associated fetus (alive or dead) and a triploid karyotype.[26-28] (See Chapter 29.)

Complete hydatidiform moles may rarely be associated with a normal fetus, usually as a result of a dizygotic twin pregnancy in which one of the pair of twins has developed into a mole.[27,29-31] Metastatic disease has never been demonstrated to arise from a partial mole[26]; however, a complete mole associated with a live fetus has the same malignant potential and local invasiveness as any other complete mole.[27,30] The complete mole associated with a normal fetus may be seen sonographically as a discrete mass of molar tissue separate from the placenta. Molar tissue adjacent to the placenta may represent either a partial mole or a complete mole.

Sauerbrei et al. point out that the role of ultrasound is to raise the suspicion of a hydatidiform mole, but the diagnosis should be confirmed by hCG levels because a missed abortion or a partially necrotic leiomyoma may result in a similar appearance.[31]

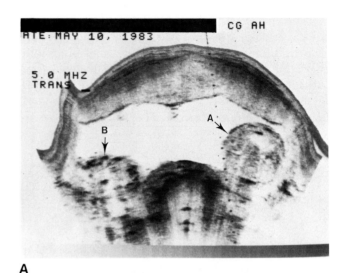

A

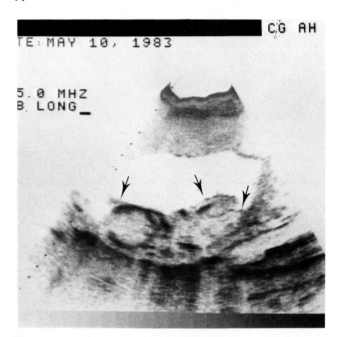

B

Fig. 16. A. Transverse scan through the maternal abdomen of a 23-year-old female with twins at 24 weeks' menstrual age. No evidence of fetal cardiac pulsation or fetal movement could be demonstrated in the twin to the maternal right (twin B). Twin A is a normal appearing fetus with associated polyhydramnios. **B.** Longitudinal scan through twin B demonstrating a small compressed fetus and oligohydramnios consistent with fetus papyraceous. The arrows point to the membrane separating the two gestational sacs. **C.** Longitudinal scans through twin A.

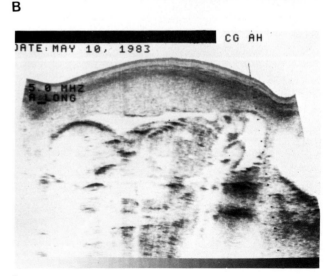

C

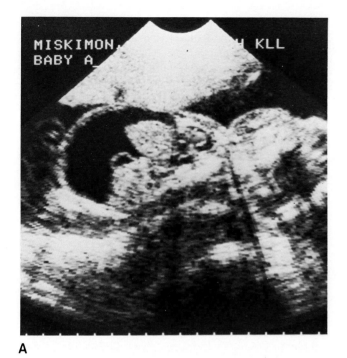
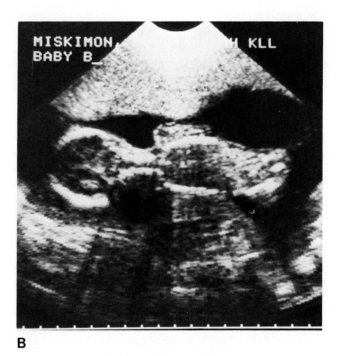

A   **B**

Fig. 17. Twin-to-twin transfusion syndrome. **A.** Fetus shows evidence of severe fetal ascites (A) and skin thickening (*arrow*). This fetus subsequently died. **B.** Fetus is small and does not show fetal ascites. Fetus B survived.

MISCELLANEOUS

Fetal anomalies may occur in one or more fetuses in a multiple gestation pregnancy. To rule out genetic abnormalities, amniocentesis is necessary, with careful sampling of both sacs. Real-time monitoring of the needle aspiration will aide in successful sampling, but, in addition, a nontoxic dye such as methylene blue can be used to color the first sac after sampling. The second sac should of course have clear fluid.

Fetus papyraceous is the result of one of the twin gestations dying while the other continues to grow normally (Fig. 17). Often with the death of one fetus hydramnios occurs, leading to premature labor and delivery, with the resultant death of the second fetus. If one fetus dies and the pregnancy continues the dead fetus may be partially reabsorbed and flattened by the enlarging surviving twin. The end result is a paper-thin second sac and fetus that may even be overlooked at delivery.

SUMMARY

For optimal obstetrical management it is important that the presence of a multifetal pregnancy be diagnosed as early as possible. Careful sonographic technique and evaluation should result in virtually a 100 percent yield in the diagnosis of multifetal pregnancy. The future considerations include invasive procedures and fetal surgery in utero by ultrasonic guidance.

REFERENCES

1. Neilson JP: Detection of the small-for-dates twin fetus by ultrasound. Br J Obstet Gynaecol 88:27, 1981
2. O'Connor MC, Arias E, Royston JP, et al: The merits of special antenatal care for twin pregnancies. Br J Obstet Gynaecol 88:222, 1981
3. Crane JP, Tomich PG, Kopta M: Ultrasonic growth patterns in normal and discordant twins. Obstet Gynecol 55:678, 1980
4. Hawrylyshyn PA, Barkin M, Bernstein A, et al: Twin pregnancies—A continuing perinatal challenge. Obstet Gynecol 59:463, 1982
5. Naeye RL, Tafari H, Judge D, et al: Twins: Causes of perinatal death in 12 United States cities and one African city. Am J Obstet Gynecol 131:267, 1978
6. Powers WF: Twin pregnancy complications and treatment. Obstet Gynecol 42:795, 1973
7. Pritchard JA, Macdonald PC: Multifetal pregnancy, in Hellman LM, Pritchard JA (eds), Williams Obstetrics, 16th ed. New York, Appleton-Century-Crofts, 1980
8. Persson PH, Grennert L, Gennser G, et al: On improved outcome of twin pregnancies. Acat Obstet Gynecol Scand 58:3, 1979

9. Thiery M, Dhout M, VandeKersckhove D: Serum hCG and hPL in twin pregnancies. Acta Obstet Gynecol Scand 56:495, 1976

10. Gennser G, Grennert L, Kullander S, et al: Human placental lactogen in screening for multiple pregnancies. Lancet 1:274, 1975

11. Knight GJ, Kloza EM, Smith DE, et al: Efficiency of human placental lactogen and alpha-fetoprotein measurement in twin pregnancy detection. Am J Obstet Gynecol 141:585, 1981

12. Ghosh A, Woo JSK, Rawlinson HA, et al: Prognostic significance of raised serum alpha-fetoprotein levels in twin pregnancies. Br J Obstet Gynecol 89:817, 1982

13. Finlay D, Dillon A, Heslip M: Ultrasound screening in a twin pregnancy with high serum alpha-fetoprotein. J Clin Ultrasound 9:514, 1981

14. Fink RS, Bowes LP, Mackintosh CE, et al: The value of ultrasound for monitoring ovarian responses to gonadotrophin stimulant therapy. Br J Obstet Gynaecol 89:856, 1982

15. Funduk-Kurjak B, Kurjak A: Ultrasound monitoring of follicular maturation and ovulation in normal menstrual cycle and in ovulation induction. Acta Obstet Gynecol Scand 61:329, 1982

16. Bryce RL, Shuter B, Sinosich MJ, et al: The value of ultrasound, gonadotropin, and estradiol measurements for precise ovulation prediction. Fertil Steril 37:42, 1982

17. Seibel MM, McArdle CR, Thompson IE, et al: The role of ultrasound in ovulation induction: A critical appraisal. Fertil Steril 36:573, 1981

18. Hackeloer BJ, Fleming R, Robinson HP, et al: Correlation of ultrasonic and endocrinologic assessment of human follicular development. Am J Obstet Gynecol 135:122, 1979

19. Gottesfeld K: Personal communication, 1983

20. Divers WA, Hemsell DL: The use of ultrasound in multiple gestations. Obstet Gynecol 53:500, 1979

21. Leveno KJ, Santos-Ramos R, Duenhoelter JH, et al: Sonar cephalometry in twins: A table of biparietal diameters for normal twin fetuses and a comparison with singletons. Am J Obstet Gynecol 135:727, 1979

22. Houlton MCC: Divergent biparietal diameter growth rates in twin pregnancies. Obstet Gynecol 49:542, 1977

23. Leveno KJ, Santos-Ramos R, Duenhoelter JH, et al: Sonar cephalometry in twin pregnancy: Discordancy of the biparietal diameter after 28 weeks' gestation. Am J Obstet Gynecol 138:615, 1980

24. Haney AF, Crenshaw MC Jr, Dempsey PJ: Significance of biparietal diameter differences between twins. Obstet Gynecol 51:609, 1978

25. Wittmann BK, Baldwin VJ, Nichol B: Antenatal diagnosis of twin transfusion syndrome by ultrasound. Obstet Gynecol 58:123, 1981

26. Szulman AE, Surti U: The clinicopathologic profile of the partial hydatidiform mole. Obstet Gynecol 59:597, 1982

27. Callen PW: Ultrasonography in evaluation of gestational trophoblastic disease, in Callen PW (ed), Ultrasonography in Obstetrics and Gynecology. Philadelphia, Saunders, 1983

28. Szulman AE, Philippe E, Boue JG, et al: Human triploidy: Association with partial hydatidiform moles and nonmolar conceptuses. Hum Pathol 12:1016, 1981

29. Fisher RA, Sheppard DM, Lawler SD: Twin pregnancy with complete hydatidiform mole (46,XX) and fetus (46,XY): Genetic origin proved by analysis of chromosome polymorphisms. Br Med J 284:1218, 1982

30. Block MF, Merrill JA: Hydatidiform mole with coexistent fetus. Obstet Gynecol 60:129, 1982

31. Sauerbrei EE, Salem S, Fayle B: Coexistent hydatidiform mole and live fetus in the second trimester. An ultrasound study. Radiology 135:415, 1980

25 | Sonography of the Placenta

Beverly A. Spirt
Lawrence P. Gordon
Eugene H. Kagan

INTRODUCTION

The recent improvements in ultrasound imaging systems have enabled the sonographer to examine the placenta in much greater detail than was previously possible. With bistable equipment, one could easily identify the placenta by its typical "speckled" appearance and the strong line of echoes emanating from the chorionic plate. Placental localization was determined with 95 percent accuracy,[1] and this was of prime importance to exclude placenta previa and to locate the placenta prior to amniocentesis. With the advent of gray scale, the accuracy of placental localization approaches 100 percent, and it has now become possible to examine both the internal structure of the placenta and the retroplacental area. This chapter describes the sonographic appearance of the normal placenta as well as some physiologic and pathologic variations.

THE NORMAL APPEARANCE OF THE PLACENTA

The placenta is first identified by sonography at approximately 8 weeks' menstrual age. At this time a thickening of a portion of the gestational sac, representing the decidua basalis and chorion frondosum, is visible (Figs. 1A, B). By 10 to 12 weeks, the sac is elongated, and the diffuse granular texture of the placenta is clearly apparent (Fig. 2). This texture is produced by echoes emanating from the villous tree, which is bathed in maternal blood. The placenta retains this general sonographic texture throughout pregnancy, with some variation to be discussed below.

At the end of the 12th week, the amnion and chorion fuse, forming an avascular membrane surrounding the amniotic cavity. A portion of this membrane, along with the underlying fetal vessels and trophoblast, forms the fetal surface of the placenta known as the "chorionic plate." The chorionic plate provides a strong acoustic interface with the adjacent amniotic fluid, resulting in a distinct line of echoes (Fig. 3).

The basal plate does not have a specific echo pattern and cannot be identified sonographically unless it becomes calcified near term. However, the echo pattern of the placenta is readily distinguishable from that of the retroplacental myometrium (and decidua basalis), which appears relatively sonolucent when compared to the placenta (Fig. 2). The myometrium can be visualized throughout pregnancy although it progressively thins towards term. That portion of the myometrium which is contrasted with amniotic fluid may appear relatively echogenic and should not be confused with placental tissue (Fig. 2).

During the third month of gestation placental septa develop. These are composed of decidua and trophoblast and extend from the basal plate towards the fetal surface. They divide the maternal surface into 15 to 20 lobes, which are not known to have any physiologic significance.[2] Unfortunately in the ultrasound literature these lobes have incorrectly been called cotyledons. The term cotyledon refers only to the functional unit of the placenta as determined by the branching pattern of the villous tree and includes the

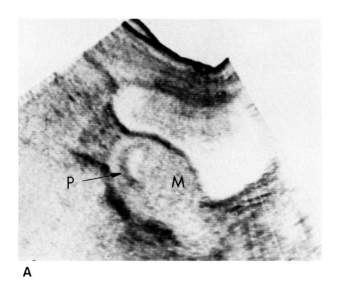
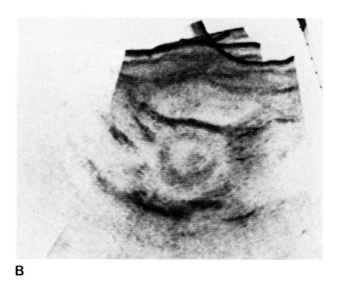

A   B

Fig. 1. Longitudinal **(A)** and transverse **(B)** scans of the uterus at 8 weeks' gestational age show the gestational sac, early placenta (P), and thickened myometrium (M).

primary stem villus with its derivatives.[2] See Chapter 4. Each cotyledon is further subdivided into a variable number of lobules. Because of the confusion, it has been suggested that the term cotyledon not be used when referring to the primate placenta.[2]

At the end of the fourth month, the placenta has attained its final thickness and shape[2]; however, circumferential enlargement continues into the third trimester.

Maternal blood flows to the placenta via the spiral arterioles that terminate at the base of the placenta, supplying blood to the intervillous space. Blood drains from the placenta through endometrial veins, which are present all along the base of the placenta[3-6] as well as in the septa. These veins are often visible sonographically, particularly if the placenta is posterior in location (Fig. 4). This appears to be related to gravity: the veins associated with a posterior placenta are more dependent, and are therefore more likely to be distended when the patient is supine.[7,8]

In order to examine the placenta most effectively, one must use a transducer with optimal frequency and focal length. So-called echo-spared areas in the mature placenta, which have been described by several au-

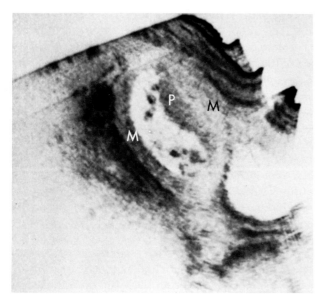

Fig. 2. Longitudinal sonogram at 12 weeks' gestational age clearly shows the placenta (P), which is anteriorly located. The retroplacental myometrium (M) appears relatively sonolucent, while the myometrium on the posterior wall appears more echogenic.

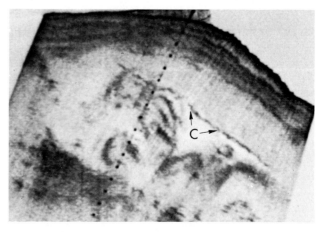

Fig. 3. A clearly defined chorionic plate (C) is seen on this third-trimester longitudinal sonogram.

thors,[9-11] are probably a result of inappropriate transducer selection and gain settings (Fig. 5). There is no corresponding lesion in the placenta.

Placental Calcification

Placental calcium deposition is a normal physiologic process that occurs throughout pregnancy.[2] Macroscopic plaques appear in the third trimester, most commonly after 33 weeks.[13,14] The calcium is primarily deposited in the basal plate and septa, but it is also found in the villi and in the perivillous and subchorionic spaces. Plaques of calcium are readily detected by sonography as very strong intraplacental echoes that do not produce significant acoustic shadows[7] (Fig. 6). Septal calcifications result in the circular configuration seen in heavily calcified placentas (Fig. 7). This has been incorrectly described as a cotyledonous pattern,[12] but it in fact reflects the lobes as defined by the maternal septa.

The incidence of placental calcification increases exponentially with increasing gestational age, beginning at about 29 weeks (Fig. 8).[13] More than 50 percent of placentas show some degree of calcification after 33 weeks. There is no increased calcification in postmature placentas.[15,16] Placental calcification has also been correlated with primigravidity,[13,14] season of the year,[17] and maternal serum calcium levels.[18,19]

Correlations have been reported between the degree of placental calcification and fetal lung maturity in the obstetric literature.[12] Placentas have been graded on a 0 to III basis depending on the presence of echogenic "commalike" densities[14] which actually represent calcium[12] (Fig. 7). It has been suggested that a grade III placenta is a reliable sign of fetal lung maturity, thus obviating the need for amniocentesis. However, multiple cases have been reported in which fetuses with heavily calcified grade III placentas had immature lungs, as indicated by low lecithin-to-sphingomyelin ratios.[20-22] We believe that the relationship postulated between placental calcification and fetal lung maturity is in fact spurious. Both of these variables are known to increase with increasing gestational age, but it does not follow that they increase with respect to each other.[22a]

VARIATIONS IN SHAPE

Permanent

Usually the placenta consists of one main mass. However, in 0.14 to 3 percent of placentas, succenturiate (accessory) lobes are present.[2,23,24] These consist of separate masses of chorionic villi connected to the main

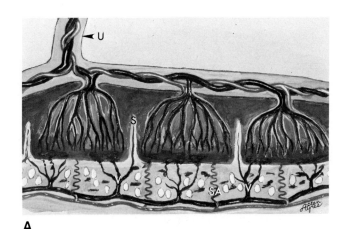

A

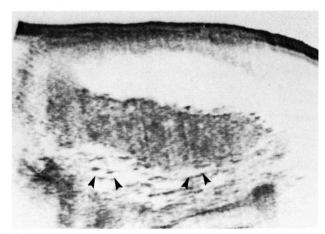

B

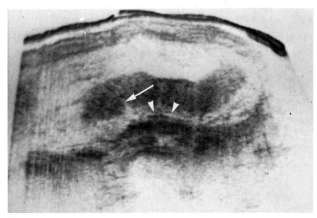

C

Fig. 4. A. Diagram of placental circulation. U, umbilical cord; SA, spiral arterioles; V, draining veins; S, septum. (*Reprinted with permission from Spirt BA, Kagan EH: Sonography of the placenta. Semin. Ultrasound 1:293, 1980, Grune & Stratton, Inc.*) **B** and **C.** Sonograms demonstrating the venous drainage of the placenta (*arrowheads*), including a septal vein (*arrow*).

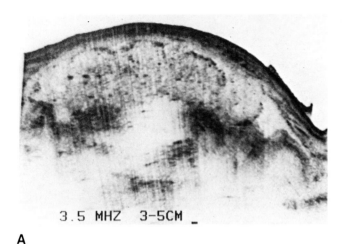

A

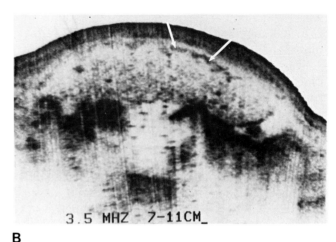

B

Fig. 5. Longitudinal scan at 39.5 weeks obtained with **(A)** 3.5 mHz, short internal focus (3 to 5 cm) transducer and **(B)** 3.5 mHz, long internal focus (7 to 11 cm) transducer. Note the spurious areas of relative sonolucency beneath the calcification in the basal plate (*arrows*) in **B.** (*Reprinted with permission from Spirt BA, Kagan EH: Sonography of the placenta. Semin Ultrasound 1:293, 1980, Grune & Stratton, Inc.*)

placenta by vessels within the membrane. A succenturiate lobe may also be continuous with the placenta via a bridge of chorionic tissue. Succenturiate lobes may be demonstrated by sonography[25] (Fig. 9). It is important to diagnose a succenturiate lobe antenatally because of the following complications: it may be retained in utero, resulting in postpartum hemorrhage; it may overlie the internal cervical os; or the vessels that connect it to the main mass of the placenta may traverse the internal os (vasa previa) and rupture during labor, causing fetal blood loss.

A placenta in which the fetal membranes do not extend to the edge of the placenta, so that the chorionic plate is smaller than the basal plate, is called placenta extrachorialis. The attachment of the fetal membranes to the chorionic plate forms a ring that may be flat (circummarginate) or folded (circumvallate) (Fig. 10). The former has no clinical significance whereas the latter is associated with a higher incidence of premature labor, threatened abortion, perinatal mortality, and marginal hemorrhage.[2,26,27] To our knowledge, neither of these has been diagnosed sonographically.

Other variations of placental shape that are of clinical significance include the annular or ring-shaped placenta, and placenta membranacea, in which chorionic villi cover most or all of the surface of the gestational sac. These are both associated with ante- and postpartum hemorrhage. They have not been documented sonographically.

Temporary

The appearance of the placenta and myometrium may vary with different degrees of bladder filling.[7,28] This

effect occurs most commonly in the second trimester. It may be necessary to repeat the examination following voiding to exclude the presence of a placenta previa (Fig. 11).

Transient myometrial thickening results from normal uterine contractions (Braxton–Hicks) that occur in the second trimester and are imperceptible to the mother. Either time-lapse echography[29] or real-time scanning may be used to demonstrate the appearance and disappearance of a local thickening of the placenta and/or myometrium. It is often possible to follow a contraction as it moves along the uterus (Fig. 12), causing localized thickening of placenta and myometrium that changes with respect to time.

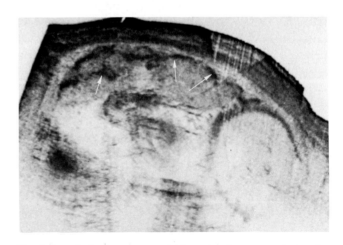

Fig. 6. Longitudinal sonogram at 37 weeks shows an anterior placenta with typical pattern of calcification (*arrows*).

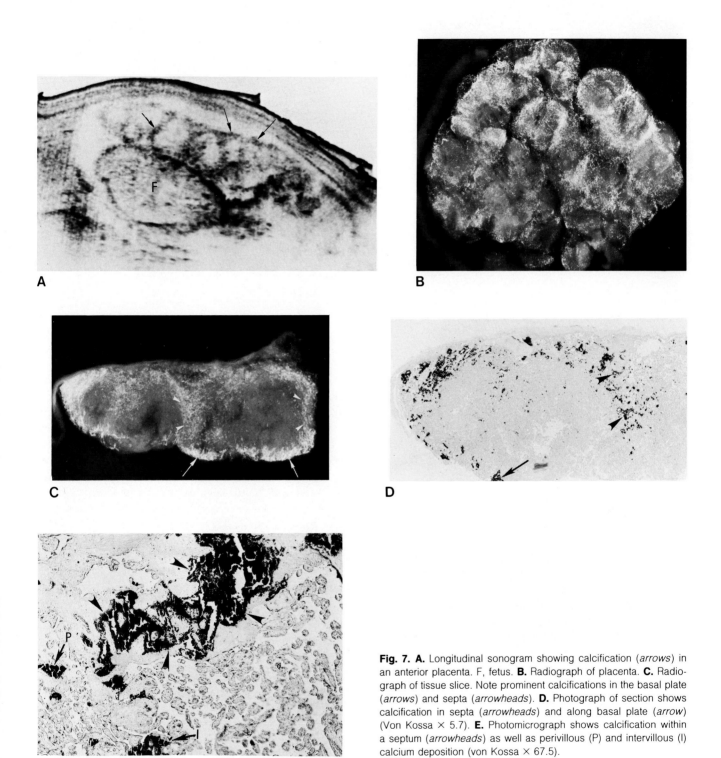

Fig. 7. A. Longitudinal sonogram showing calcification (*arrows*) in an anterior placenta. F, fetus. **B.** Radiograph of placenta. **C.** Radiograph of tissue slice. Note prominent calcifications in the basal plate (*arrows*) and septa (*arrowheads*). **D.** Photograph of section shows calcification in septa (*arrowheads*) and along basal plate (*arrow*) (Von Kossa × 5.7). **E.** Photomicrograph shows calcification within a septum (*arrowheads*) as well as perivillous (P) and intervillous (I) calcium deposition (von Kossa × 67.5).

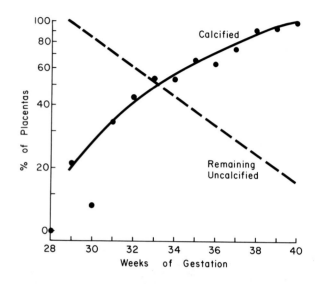

Fig. 8. Placental calcification vs. gestational age. (*Reprinted with permission from Spirt BA, Cohen WN, Weinstein HM: The incidence of placental calcification in normal pregnancies. Radiology 142:707, 1982.*)

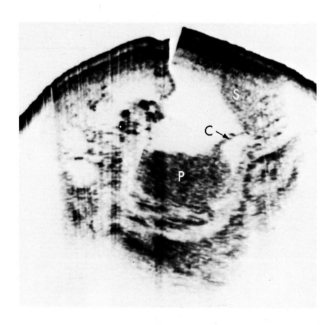

A

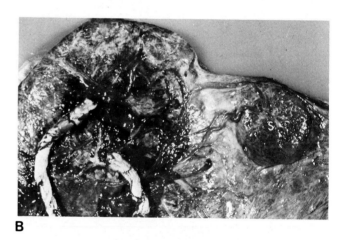

B

Fig. 9. A. Transverse sonogram at 28 weeks demonstrates posterior placenta (P) with left succenturiate lobe (S). C = elevated membranes over a sonolucent space representing a submembranous hematoma, confirmed at delivery. **B.** Gross examination of the placenta shows a succenturiate lobe (S). (*Reprinted with permission from Spirt BA et al: Antepartum diagnosis of a succenturiate lobe. Sonographic and pathologic correlation. J Clin Ultrasound 9:139, 1981.*)

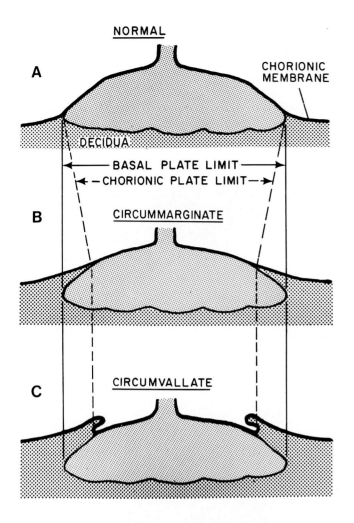

NORMAL

A

CHORIONIC
MEMBRANE

DECIDUA

←——— BASAL PLATE LIMIT ———→
←—CHORIONIC PLATE LIMIT—→

B   CIRCUMMARGINATE

C   CIRCUMVALLATE

Fig. 10. Cross-sectional diagram comparing extrachorial placentas with the normal placenta. **A.** Normal placenta, showing the transition of membranous to villous chorion at the placental edge. **B.** Circummarginate placenta in which the transition of membranous to villous chorion occurs at a distance from the placental edge. **C.** Circumvallate placenta, similar to **B** except for a fold in the chorionic membrane. (*Reprinted with permission from Spirt BA, Kagan EH: Sonography of the placenta. Semin Ultrasound 1:293, 1980, Grune & Stratton, Inc.*)

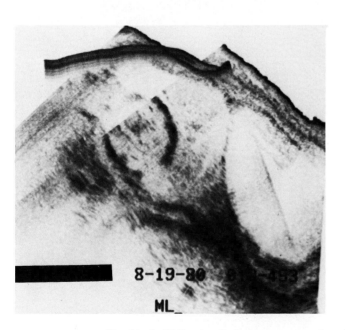
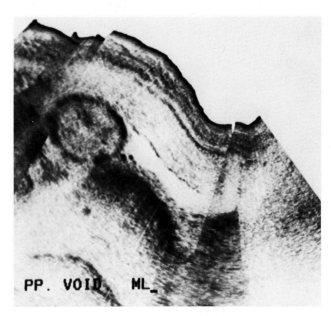

Fig. 11. A. Midline longitudinal scan suggestive of placenta previa. The overdistended bladder is compressing the anterior portion of the lower uterine segment against the posterior wall. **B.** Midline longitudinal scan following voiding shows the placenta away from the cervix. (*Reprinted with permission from Spirt BA, Gordon LP, Kagan EH: The placenta: Sonographic-pathologic correlations. Semin Roentgenol 17:219, 1982, Grune & Stratton, Inc.*)

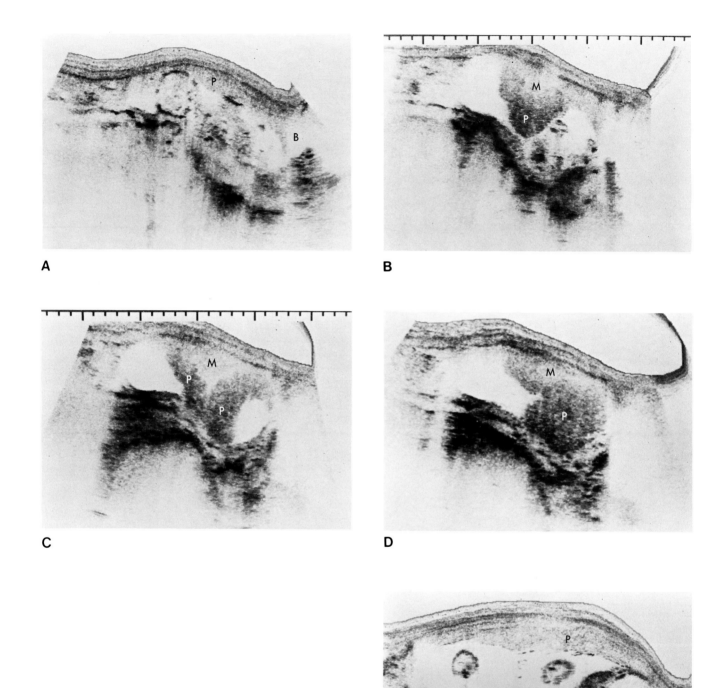

Fig. 12. A. Longitudinal sonogram at 17 weeks' gestational age shows fetus in breech position and anterior placenta. B, bladder. **B.** Approximately 20 minutes later a thickening of placenta (P) and myometrium (M) is seen. **C.** Ten minutes later, the contraction is more pronounced. **D.** Fifteen minutes later, following voiding, the placenta appears to be primarily in the inferior region of the uterus. **E.** Follow-up study at 30 weeks shows anterior placenta.

TABLE 1
Macroscopic Lesions of the Placenta

	Incidence (full term un-complicated pregnancies, in percent)	Etiology	Microscopic Description	Clinical Significance
Intervillous thrombosis	36	Bleeding from fetal vessels	Laminated fibrin and fetal (nucleated) red cells surrounded by villi	Fetal-maternal hemorrhage (e.g., Rh sensitization)
Massive perivillous fibrin deposition	22	Pooling and stasis of blood in intervillous space	Fibrosed villi entrapped in fibrin	Apparently none
Septal cyst	19	Obstruction of septal venous drainage by edematous villi	Small cyst (5 to 10 mm) within septum containing acellular fluid	Apparently none
Infarct	25	Thrombosis of maternal vessel or retroplacental hemorrhage	"Ghost villi"	Dependent upon extent and associated condition
Subchorionic fibrin deposition	20	Pooling and stasis of blood in subchorionic space	Laminated subchorionic fibrin without villi: secondary cyst formation may occur	Apparently none
Massive subchorial thrombus (Breus's mole)	Undetermined (rare)	Massive pooling and stasis due to extensive venous obstruction	Fresh thrombus with no villi	Abortion or premature onset of labor
Hydatidiform change		1. Complete mole	Trophoblastic hyperplasia of all villi	Predisposes to choriocarcinoma
		2. Triploidy; partial mole	Trophoblastic hyperplasia of some villi	Associated with symptoms of preeclampsia
Chorioangioma	1	Vascular malformation	Multiple capillaries in a loose stroma	Usually none, dependent upon size
Teratoma	Rare	?	Tissue elements of three embryonic germ layers	None
Metastatic lesions	Rare	Melanoma, Ca breast, Ca bronchus most frequent		

MACROSCOPIC LESIONS OF THE PLACENTA

Table 1 lists the known macroscopic lesions of the placenta (Fig. 13). Of these, subchorionic fibrin deposition, intervillous thrombosis, perivillous fibrin deposition, hydatidiform change, and chorioangioma have been diagnosed sonographically.

Subchorionic Fibrin Deposition

Subchorionic sonolucent areas may be demonstrated in approximately 10 to 15 percent of obstetric sonograms. These correspond to areas of subchorionic fibrin deposition in the term placenta[30] and are apparently clinically insignificant[2,31] (Figs. 14–16). Subchorionic fibrin refers to laminated collection of fibrin between the chorionic plate and placental villi. It is a result of pooling and stasis of maternal blood in the intervillous space beneath the chorion,[2] which leads to thrombosis and secondary fibrin deposition. Cystic degeneration of the fibrin sometimes occurs.

A rare pathologic entity that might produce a subchorionic sonolucent lesion is massive subchorial thrombosis (Breus's mole). This entity often leads to premature delivery, and a large, fresh subchorionic hematoma is found on gross examination. The pathogenesis is thought to be extensive venous obstruction leading to massive pooling and stasis.[2] This process is considered by Fox to be unrelated to the mechanism that produces subchorionic fibrin deposition.

Intervillous Thrombosis

Intervillous thromboses are intraplacental areas of hemorrhage with variable gross appearance depending upon the age of the lesion. Fresh lesions are dark red, but with aging change to brown, yellow, and finally

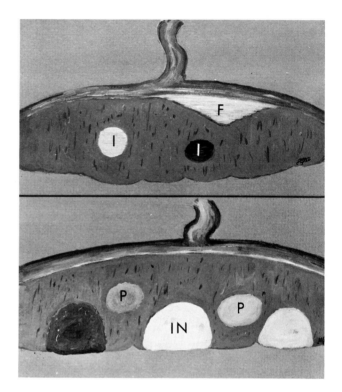

Fig. 13. Common macroscopic lesions of the placenta. Subchorionic fibrin deposition (F) appears as laminated yellow-white plaques, sometimes associated with fresh clot and secondary cyst formation. Intervillous thrombosis (I) appears as round to oval lesions varying from red to laminated white, depending on age. Perivillous fibrin deposition (P) is seen as nonlaminated plaques varying from brown to white depending on age. True infarcts (IN) appear as dark red to white nonlaminated lesions adjacent to the basal plate.

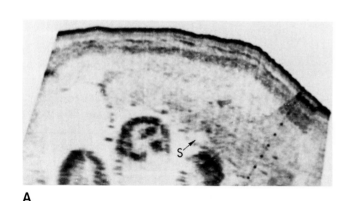

A

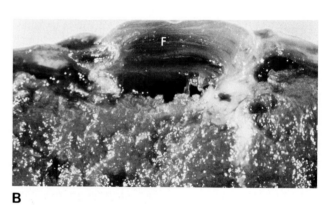

B

Fig. 14. A. Routine sonogram at 38 weeks shows subchorionic sonolucent space (S). **B.** Cross section of the gross lesion shows organizing thrombus with laminated fibrin deposition (F).

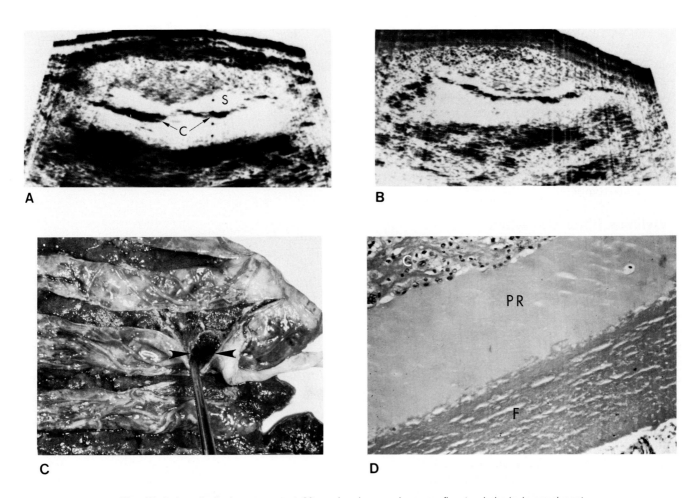

Fig. 15. A. Longitudinal sonogram at 29 weeks shows a large confluent subchorionic sonolucent space (S). C, thickened chorionic plate. **B.** At 34 weeks, this subchorionic sonolucent space appears smaller. **C.** The chorionic membrane contains areas of thickening and opacity. Multiple subchorionic cysts are present (*arrowheads*) **D.** The cyst wall is composed of fibrin (F), which is undergoing cystic degeneration. Proteinaceous material (PR) is present within the cystic space (H and E × 320). C, chorion. (*Reprinted with permission from Spirt BA, Kagan EH, Rozanski RM: Sonolucent areas in the placenta: Sonographic and pathologic correlation. Am J Roentgenol 131:961, 1978.*)

white. Usually there are visible laminations that microscopically are seen to be composed of layers of fibrin. Both fetal and maternal red blood cells are present suggesting that a leakage of fetal cells from a villous tear stimulates maternal coagulation.[32] Intervillous thromboses occur in 3 to 50 percent of term placentas from uncomplicated pregnancies.[2]

Intervillous thromboses appear sonographically as sonolucent intraplacental lesions that vary in size from a few millimeters to several centimeters[33,34] (Fig. 17). They may extend to the subchorionic space or the basal plate, and may be detected by ultrasound as early as 19 weeks.[34] The incidence of intervillous thrombosis is increased in cases of Rh isoimmunization.[33,35,36] It has been suggested that the presence of intervillous thrombosis in Rh negative mothers might result in isoimmunization.[33]

Perivillous Fibrin Deposition

Perivillous fibrin deposition results from pooling and stasis of blood in the intervillous space. The lesions are seen as nonlaminated plaques, varying in color from brown to white depending on age. Sonographically, they appear as intraplacental sonolucent lesions (Fig. 18).

Infarcts

Placental infarcts result from coagulation necrosis of villi and occur most commonly at the base of the placenta, varying in size from a few millimeters to many centimeters. Although small infarcts are found in 25 percent of placentas of uncomplicated pregnancies, they occur with increased frequency in pregnancies complicated by preeclampsia and essential hypertension. Small infarcts have no clinical significance, since up to 30 percent of the villi may be lost without affecting placental function.[2]

We have as yet been unable to document placental infarcts sonographically. We suspect that this may be due to the composition of infarcts; i.e., villi, even "ghost villi" that are present in infarcts, are not echolucent. The sonolucent lesions that we have documented have been composed of either fibrin (see above) or fluid (e.g., hydatidiform change, see below).

Hydatidiform Change

Multiple diffuse intraplacental sonolucent lesions are abnormal and usually represent hydatidiform

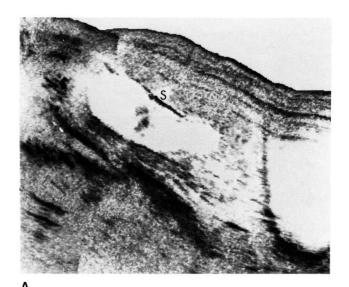

A

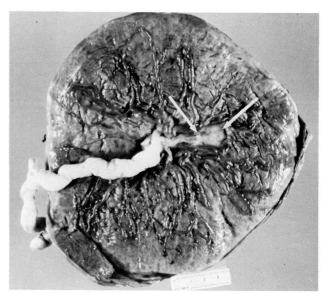

B

Fig. 16. Longitudinal sonograms at **(A)** 13.5 weeks and **(B)** 20.3 weeks demonstrate subchorionic sonolucent space (S). Gross examination **(C)** of the placenta shows corresponding gray-white lesion (*arrows*).

C

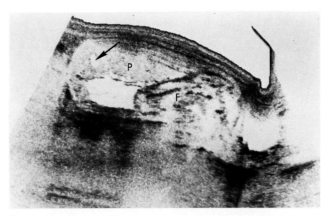

A

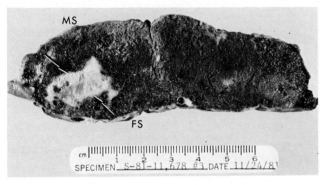

B

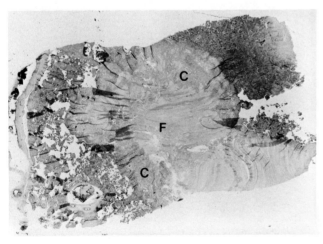

C

Fig. 17. **A.** Longitudinal sonogram at 29.5 weeks demonstrates sono-lucent intraplacental lesion (*arrow*) in superior aspect of the placenta (P). F, fetus. **B.** Gross specimen cut at right angles through lesion in Figure 17A shows that the lesion (*arrows*) is composed of lami-nated fibrin. MS, maternal surface; FS, fetal surface. **C.** Microscopic section shows laminated bands of fibrin (F), (C) represents coagula-tion necrosis of surrounding villi. (*Reprinted with permission from Spirt BA, Gordon LP, Kagan EH: Intervillous thrombosis: Sonographic and pathologic correlation. Radiology 147:197, 1983.*)

change.[29,37] Hydatidiform change may be separated into two groups. See Chapter 29. First is the complete or classical mole (Fig. 19) where there is hydatidiform swelling of all villi, a diploid karyotype, and absence of an embryo. (A viable fetus may coexist with a true mole in the case of a twin pregnancy with one twin surviving.) Second is the partial mole showing areas of molar change alternating with normal villi (Fig. 20). A fetus may be present and is often triploid (69 chromosomes) (Fig. 21). Microscopically, both show tro-phoblastic hyperplasia, although it is usually less prominent in the partial mole, which has other distinc-tive microscopic features.[38-40]

Clinically, partial moles may present with early onset of preeclampsia in the second trimester. Careful pathologic study, including cytogenetic analysis and monitoring of chorionic gonadotropin levels, is war-ranted in such cases. A few cases of partial moles that progressed to trophoblastic disease requiring chemo-therapy have been reported.[41,42]

Primary Neoplasm (*Chorioangioma*)

There are two primary nontrophoblastic tumors of the placenta: the relatively common chorioangioma and the rare teratoma. The chorioangioma is a vascular mal-formation seen in approximately 1 percent of carefully studied placentas.[2] Small tumors occur within the pla-centa while large tumors may protrude from the fetal surface. The microscopic appearance is that of prolifer-ating capillaries present in a loose fibrous stroma.

Sonographically, large chorioangiomas appear as well circumscribed intraplacental mass lesions with a complex echo pattern[43] (Fig. 22). Large lesions are asso-ciated with fetal hydrops, cardiomegaly and congestive heart failure, low birth weight, premature labor, or fetal demise,[44-46] while small lesions usually have no associated problems.

THE PLACENTA IN MATERNAL AND FETAL DISORDERS

The most constant placental abnormality in cases of Rh incompatibility, diabetes, anemia, and preeclampsia is variation in size. A method for determining the vol-ume of the placenta by sonographic examination has been described[47]; however, visual assessment is usually sufficient to judge whether a placenta is too large or too small.

The placenta may be markedly enlarged in cases of hemolytic disease of the newborn. This appears to be secondary both to villous edema and to hyperplasia of the villous tree.[2] The amount of villous edema may vary in different areas of the same placenta. Sono-

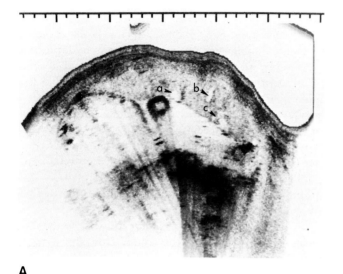

A

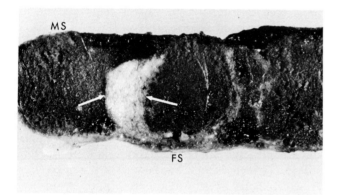

B

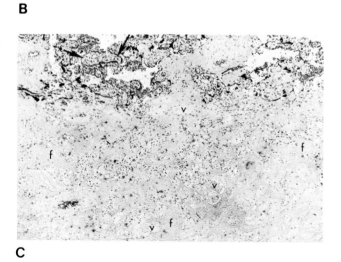

C

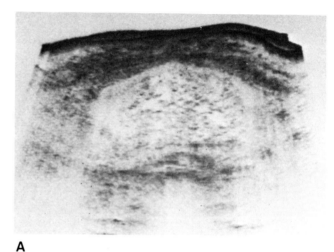

A

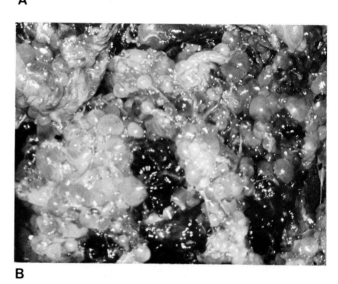

B

Fig. 18. A. Transverse sonogram at 31 weeks shows three intraplacental sonolucent lesions (a, b, c). **B.** This placenta contained multiple areas of perivillous fibrin deposition. Gross specimen at right angles to lesion ''a'' in **A** shows an irregular, nonlaminated collection of perivillous fibrin (*arrows*). FS, fetal surface, MS, maternal surface. **C.** Fibrin (f) separates the villi (v) and obliterates the intervillous space. Normal villi surrounded by maternal red cells are present at the periphery (*arrows*). (H and E × 55)

Fig. 19. A. Sonogram of hydatidiform mole showing vesicular echo pattern. **B.** Gross specimen shows multiple grape-like cysts. (*Courtesy of Dr. David Jones, Department of Pathology, SUNY Upstate Medical Center, Syracuse, New York.*) (*Reprinted with permission from Spirt BA, Kagan EH, Rozanski RM: Sonolucent areas in the placenta: Sonographic and pathologic correlation. Am J Roentgenol 131:961, 1978.*)

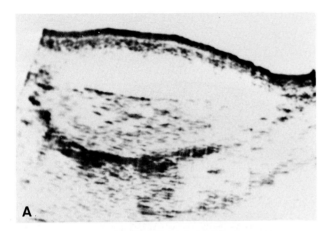
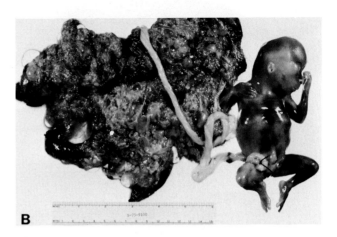

Fig. 20. A. Longitudinal sonogram of a preeclamptic patient at 17 weeks shows multiple intraplacental sonolucent areas. Fetal movement was present. **B.** The patient's condition worsened and a hysterotomy was performed. The placenta contained areas of cystic (hydatidiform) change alternating with normal placental tissue. Chromosomes were not obtained. (*Reprinted with permission from Spirt BA, Kagan EH, Rozanski RM: Sonolucent areas in the placenta: Sonographic and pathologic correlation. Am J Roentgenol 131:961, 1978.*)

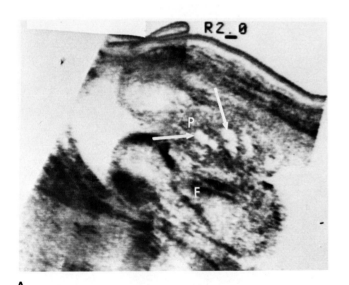
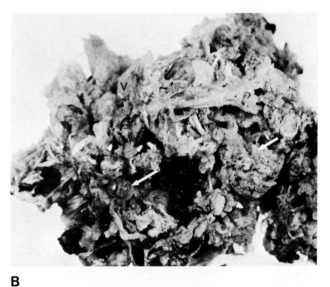

Fig. 21. A. Longitudinal sonogram at 20 weeks shows multiple sonolucent lesions (*arrows*) in the placenta (P). F, fetus. A hysterotomy was performed because of severe maternal hypertension and a triploid female infant with multiple anomalies was delivered. (*Courtesy of Dr. Edward Bell, Crouse-Irving Memorial Hospital, Syracuse, New York*). **B.** Gross photograph of placenta shows areas of normal villi (V) coexisting with areas of hydatidiform change (*arrows*). (*Reprinted with permission from Spirt BA, Gordon LP, Kagan EH: The placenta: Sonographic-pathologic correlations. Semin Roentgenol 17:219, 1982, Grune & Stratton, Inc.*)

348

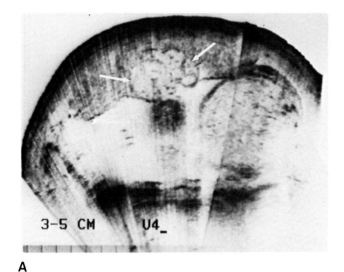

A

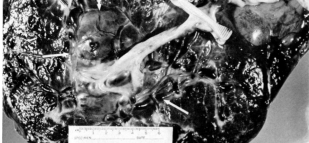

B

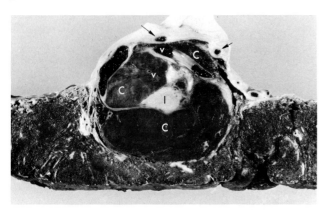

C

Fig. 22. A. Transverse sonogram at 24 weeks shows large solid subchorionic mass (*arrows*). **B.** At delivery, a large subchorionic chorioangioma was found beneath the cord insertion (*arrows*). **C.** Cross section of the tumor shows vessels (v) of varying size within the lesion. C, chorioangioma; I, infarct. Vessels from cord (*arrows*) course over subchorionic margin. (*Reprinted with permission from Spirt BA et al: Antenatal diagnosis of chorionangioma of the placenta. Am J Roentgenol 135:1273, 1980.*)

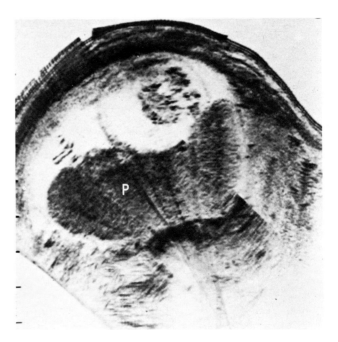

A

B

Fig. 23. A. Materno–fetal Rh incompatibility. Transverse scan at 28 weeks shows grossly enlarged placenta. Marked fetal ascites is present. (*Courtesy of Dr. Edward Bell, Crouse-Irving Memorial Hospital, Syracuse, New York*). **B.** Microscopically, villi are cellular with persistence of cytotrophoblasts (*arrows*). Only mild edema is present (H and E × 100).

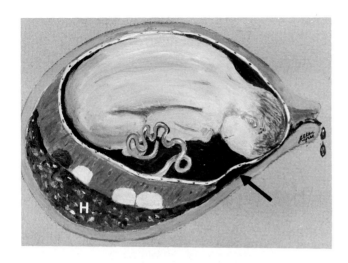

Fig. 24. Artist's drawing of a retroplacental hematoma (H) with submembranous dissection (*arrow*) and external bleeding. Placental infarcts are present.

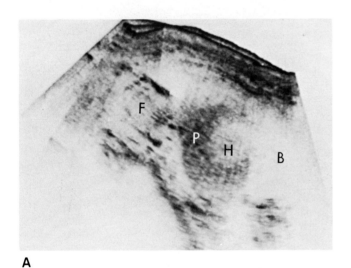

A

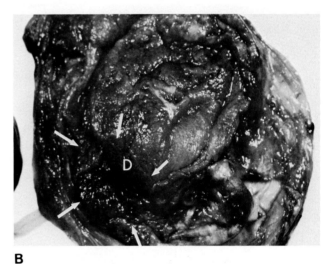

B

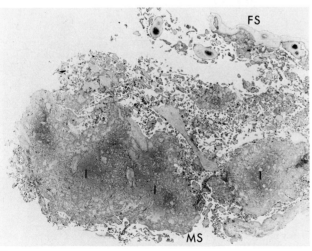

C

Fig. 25. A. Midline longitudinal scan at 18 weeks shows a 3.5 cm retroplacental mass (H). P, placenta; B, bladder; F, fetus. **B.** A hysterotomy was performed due to severe disseminated intravascular coagulation. An area of hemorrhage was found covering the lateral portion of the basal plate and extending to the placental margin and over the chorionic membrane (*arrows*). A depression in the placenta (D) was present at the site of the hematoma. **C.** Microscopic section through area (D) above shows infarcts (I) based on the maternal surface (MS) at the site of the hematoma. FS, fetal surface. (*Reprinted with permission from Spirt BA, Kagan EH, Aubry RH: Clinically silent retroplacental hematoma: Sonographic and pathologic correlation. J Clin Ultrasound 9:208, 1981.*)

graphic examination shows a large placenta (Fig. 23) with an echo pattern that is similar to that of normal placentas. Septal cysts are frequent, due to mechanical obstruction of septal venous drainage by the villous edema.[2] These have not been diagnosed sonographically. The incidence of intervillous thrombosis is increased in Rh incompatibility.

Placentas of diabetic mothers are often unduly large due to villous edema.[2] Septal cysts are more frequent in these placentas as well. Placentas of mothers who are severely anemic also tend to be large but histologically normal.[2]

Placentas from preeclamptic mothers tend to be slightly smaller than the norm.[2] There is a high incidence of placental infarction in such patients, ranging

from 33 percent of mild cases to 60 percent of severely affected patients. In half of the latter group, placental infarcts involving more than 5 percent of the placental tissue are present. This has not as yet been well documented sonographically.

There is an increased incidence of retroplacental hematomas in preeclampsia patients,[2] which undoubtedly accounts in part for the increased incidence of infarction in these patients.

Placentitis, or infection of the placenta, occurs in two ways. Hematogenous spread secondary to maternal sepsis results in inflammation of the basal plate and chorionic villi. Ascending infections, on the other hand, occur as infectious agents enter from the birth canal. This results in inflammation of the amniotic sac

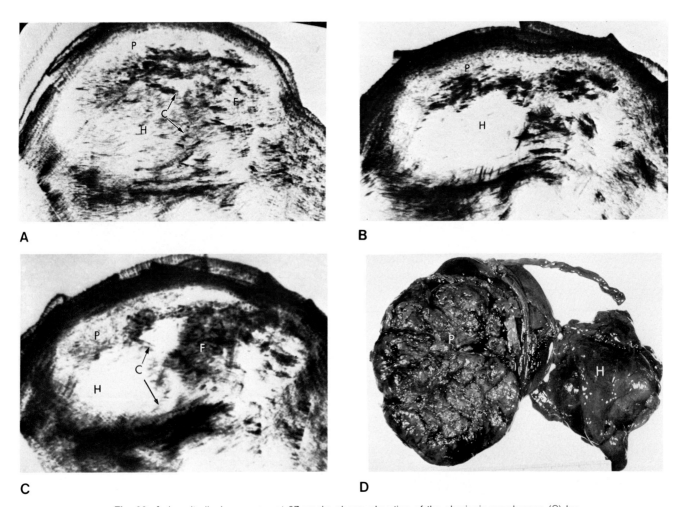

Fig. 26. A. Longitudinal sonogram at 27 weeks shows elevation of the chorionic membranes (C) by a large echogenic hematoma (H). P, placenta; F, fetus. The patient had presented in shock with bright red vaginal bleeding at 27 weeks. **B.** At 29 weeks the hematoma appears echo-free. **C.** Subsequent sonogram at 31 weeks shows a decrease in size of the hematoma. (*Courtesy of Dr. Edward Bell, Crouse-Irving Memorial Hospital, Syracuse, New York*). **D.** A firm contracted hematoma (H) was delivered separate from the placenta (P), but covered with membranes. (*Reprinted with permission from Spirt BA, Kagan EH, Rozonski RM: Abruptio placenta: Sonographic and pathologic correlations. Am J Roentgenol 133:877, 1979.*)

and fetal membrane. The ascending route is more common and typically follows prolonged rupture of membranes. In either case, the placentas usually appear normal on gross examination. Macroscopic lesions have occasionally been observed with *Listeria monocytogenes*[48] and *Proteus mirabilis*[49] infection.

RETROPLACENTAL HEMORRHAGE

Bleeding from placenta previa usually occurs near or at term, while retroplacental or marginal hemorrhage may occur as early as the first trimester. Retroplacental hemorrhage may manifest itself in three ways: (1) external bleeding without formation of a significant in-trauterine hematoma, (2) formation of a retroplacental or marginal hematoma with or without external bleeding, and (3) formation of a submembranous clot at a distance from the placenta with or without external bleeding[47,50] (Fig. 24). Sonographic examination in cases of antepartum bleeding is often negative probably because most of the bleeding is external.

A significant retroplacental or marginal hematoma will appear as a sonolucent or complex mass on sonography[47,50] (Fig. 25,26). A hematoma that collects beneath the placental membranes at a distance from the placenta will appear sonographically as a sonolucent or mixed collection beneath the elevated membranes[47] (Fig. 27,28).

The size of the hematoma may be followed by

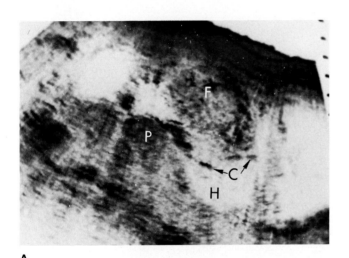

A

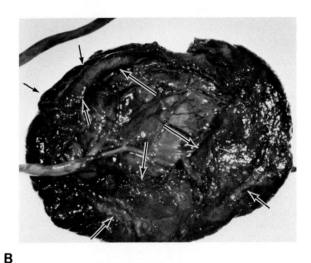

B

C

Fig. 27. A. Longitudinal sonogram at 16 weeks shows elevation of the chorionic membranes (C) adjacent to the placenta. The sonolucent collection (H) represents a hematoma. This patient had experienced painless vaginal bleeding beginning at 12 weeks. **B.** Gross examination shows a circumvallate placenta with a thick rim of organized blood clot (*arrows*) at the transition zone and extending over a large part of the chorionic membrane. **C.** Cross section shows a circumvallate configuration with a fold of chorionic membrane on fetal surface (*arrow*), and attached fibrin and blood clot (H). (*Reprinted with permission from Spirt BA, Kagan EH: Sonography of the placenta. Semin Ultrasound 1:293, 1980, Grune & Stratton, Inc.*)

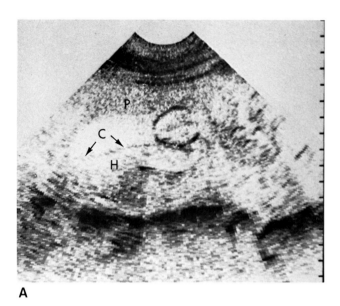

A

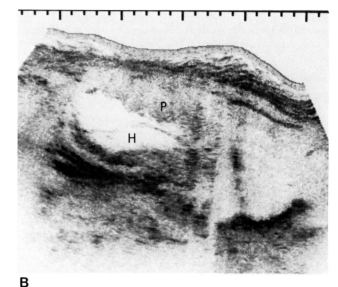

B

C

Fig. 28. A. Oblique sector scan at 13.5 weeks shows elevation of the chorionic membranes (C) over an echogenic collection (H) representing a hematoma. This hematoma is on the opposite side of the uterus from the placenta (P). The patient had experienced painless vaginal bleeding beginning at 13 weeks. (*Courtesy of Dr. Edward Bell, Crouse-Irving Memorial Hospital, Syracuse, New York*). **B.** Longitudinal and **C.** transverse scans at 16.4 weeks shows the hematoma (H) has become sonolucent. P = placenta, F = fetus. The hematoma appeared smaller on follow-up examination. Gross examination of the placenta showed a thickened tan area involving the membranes opposite the placenta which microscopically represented fibrin.

serial ultrasound examinations. Follow-up study may indicate that the lesion has disappeared, but careful examination of the placenta following delivery will show a thin layer of organized hematoma along the membranes.

Retroplacental hemorrhage has an incidence of about 4.5 percent.[2,50] The incidence of marginal hemorrhage, which may be associated with circumvallate placenta and low-lying placenta, is 1.9 percent. Marginal hemorrhage in cases of low implantation of the placenta is thought to be due to traction of the myometrial fibers during obliteration of the lower uterine segment, which causes separation of the spongy and compact layers of decidua, leading to hemorrhage.[51]

The clinical significance of retroplacental hemorrhage is dependent upon the size and extent of the lesion. Disseminated intravascular coagulation may oc-

cur in cases of retroplacental hemorrhage as a result of tissue injury.

In summary, improved anatomic resolution with gray scale instrumentation and real-time imaging has made it possible to accurately delineate internal changes within the placenta. Correlation of these observations with pathologic and clinical circumstances provides greater insight into the normal and abnormal development of this short-lived organ.

REFERENCES

1. Gottesfeld KR, Thompson HE, Holmes JH, et al: Ultrasonic placentography. A new method for placental localization. Am J Obstet Gynecol 96:538, 1966
2. Fox H: Pathology of the placenta, in Bennington JL (ed),

Major Problems in Pathology. Philadelphia, Saunders, 1978

3. Crawford JM: Vascular anatomy of the human placenta. Am J Obstet Gynecol 84:1543, 1962

4. Ramsey EM, Corner GW, Donner MW: Serial and cineradioangiographic visualization of maternal circulation in the primate (hemochorial) placenta. Am J Obstet Gynecol 86:213, 1963

5. Wigglesworth JF: Vascular anatomy of the human placenta and its significance for placental pathology. J Obstet Gynecol Br 76:979, 1969

6. Ramsey EM: Circulation in the maternal placenta of the Rhesus monkey and man with observations on the marginal lakes. Am J Anat 98:159, 1956

7. Spirt BA, Kagan EH, Rozanski R: Sonographic anatomy of the normal placenta. J Clin Ultrasound 7:204, 1979

8. Smith DF, Foley DW: Real-time ultrasound and pulsed doppler evaluation of the retroplacental clear area. J Clin Ultrasound 10:215, 1982

9. Haney AS, Trought WS: The sonolucent placenta in high-risk obstetrics. Obstet Gynecol 55:38, 1980

10. Winsberg F: Echographic changes with placental aging. J Clin Ultrasound 1:52, 1973

11. Fisher CC, Garrett W, Kossoff G: Placental aging monitored by gray scale echography. Am J Obstet Gynecol 124:483, 1976

12 Grannum PAT, Berkowitz RL, Hobbins JC: The ultrasonic changes in the maturing placenta and their relation to fetal pulmonic maturity. Am J Obstet Gynecol 133:915, 1979

13. Spirt BA, Cohen WN, Weinstein HM: The incidence of placental calcification in normal pregnancies. Radiology 142:707, 1982

14. Tindall VR, Scott JS: Placental calcification. A study of 3,025 singleton and multiple pregnancies. J Obstet Gynecol Br 72:356, 1965

15. Wentworth P: Macroscopic placental calcification and its clinical significance. J Obstet Gynecol Br 72:215, 1965

16. Jeacock MK: Calcium content of the human placenta. Am J Obstet Gynecol 87:34, 1963

17. Fujikura D: Placental calcification and seasonal difference. Am J Obstet Gynecol 87:46, 1963

18. Mull JW, Bill AH: Variations in serum calcium and phosphorus during pregnancy. Am J Obstet Gynecol 27:510, 1934

19. Paupe, J, Colin J, Politis E, et al: Variations physiologiques de la calcémie chez la mère au moment de l'accouchement dans le cordon et chez le nouveau-né. Biol Neonat 3:357, 1961

20. Quinlan WR, Cruz AC: Ultrasonic placental grading and fetal pulmonary maturity. Am J Obstet Gynecol 142:110, 1982

21. Kollitz J, Dattel BJ, Key TC, et al: Acute respiratory distress syndrome in an infant with grade III placental changes. J Ultrasound Med 1:205, 1982

22. Harman CR, Manning FA, Stearns E, et al: The correlation of ultrasonic placental grading and fetal pulmonary maturation in five hundred sixty-three pregnancies. Am J Obstet Gynecol 143:941, 1982

22a. Spirt BA, Gordon LP: The placenta as an indicator of fetal maturity—fact and fancy. Semin Ultrasound (in press), 1984

23. Earn AA: Placental anomalies. Can Med Assoc J 65:118, 1951

24. Torpin R, Hart BF: Placenta bilobata. Am J Obstet Gynecol 42:38, 1941

25. Spirt BA, Kagan EH, Gordon LP, et al: Antepartum diagnosis of a succenturiate lobe. Sonographic and pathologic correlation. J Clin Ultrasound 9:139, 1981

26. Scott JS: Placenta extrachorialis (placenta marginata and placenta circumvallate): A factor in antepartum hemorrhage. J Obstet Gynecol Br 67:904, 1960

27. Naftolin F, Khudr G, Benirschke K, et al: The syndrome of chronic abruptio placentae, hydrorrhea, and circumvallate placentae. Am J Obstet Gynecol 116:347, 1973

28. Zemlyn S: The effect of the urinary bladder in obstetrical sonography. Radiology 128:169, 1978

29. Buttery B, Davison G: The dynamic uterus revealed by time-lapse echography. J Clin Ultrasound 6:19, 1978

30. Spirt BA, Kagan EH, Rozanski RM: Sonolucent areas in the placenta: Sonographic and pathologic correlation. Am J Roentgenol 131:961, 1978

31. Benirschke K, Driscoll SG: The Pathology of the Human Placenta. New York, Springer, 1967

32. Kaplan C, Blanc W, Elias J: Identification of erythrocytes in intervillous thrombi: A study using immunoperoxidase identification of hemoglobins. Hum Pathol 13:554, 1982

33. Hoogland HJ, de Haan J, Vooys GP: Ultrasonographic diagnosis of intervillous thrombosis related to Rh isoimmunization. Gynecol Obstet Invest 10:237, 1979

34. Spirt BA, Gordon LP, Kagan EH: Intervillous thrombosis: Sonographic and pathologic correlation. Radiology 147:197, 1983

35. Javert CT, Reiss C: The origin and significance of macroscopic intervillous coagulation hematomas (red infarcts) of the human placenta. Surg Gynecol Obstet 94:257, 1952

36. Devi B, Jennison RF, Langley FA: Significance of placental pathology in transplacental hemorrhage. J Clin Path 21:322, 1968

37. Naumoff P, Szulman AE, Weinstein B, et al: Ultrasonography of partial hydatidiform mole. Radiology 140:467, 1981

38. Szulman AE, Surti U: The syndromes of hydatidiform mole. I. Cytogenetic and morphologic correlations. Am J Obstet Gynecol 131:665, 1978

39. Szulman AR, Surti U: The syndromes of hydatidiform mole. II. Morphologic evolution of the complete and partial mole. Am J Obstet Gynecol 132:20, 1978

40. Szulman AE, Philippe E, Boue JG, et al: Human triploidy: Association with partial hydatidiform moles and nonmolar conceptuses. Hum Pathol 12:1016, 1981

41. Szulman AE, Wong LC, Hsu C: Residual trophoblastic disease in association with partial hydatidiform mole. Obstet Gynecol 57:392, 1981

42. Berkowitz RS, Goldstein DP, Marean AR, et al: Proliferative sequelae after evacuation of partial hydatidiform mole (Letter.) Lancet 2:804, 1979

43. Spirt BA, Gordon LP, Cohen WN, et al: Antenatal diagnosis of chorioangioma of the placenta. Am J Roentgenol 135:1273, 1980
44. Battaglia MC, Woolever CA: Fetal and neonatal complications associated with recurrent chorioangiomas. Pediatrics 41:62, 1967
45. Wallenburg HCS: Chorioangioma of the placenta. Obstet Gynecol Surg 26:411, 1971
46. Leonidas JC, Beatty EC, Hall RT: Chorioangioma of the placenta. Radiology 123:703, 1975
47. Spirt BA, Kagan EH, Rozanski RM: Abruptio placenta: Sonographic and pathologic correlation. Am J Roentgenol 133:877, 1979
48. Steele PE, Jacobs DS: Listeria monocytogenes macroabscesses of placenta. Obstet Gynecol 53:124, 1979
49. Ravid R, Toaff R: Solitary abscess of the placenta in a pregnancy treated by cerclage. Int Surg 61:553, 1976
50. Spirt BA, Kagan EH, Aubry RH: Clinically silent retroplacental hematoma: Sonographic and pathologic correlation. J Clin Ultrasound 9:203, 1981
51. Wilkin P: The placenta, umbilical cord, and amniotic sac, in Gompel S, Silverberg SG (eds), Pathology of Gynecology and Obstetrics, 2nd ed. Philadelphia, Lippincott, 1977

26 | Ultrasound Evaluation of Obstetric Problems Relating to the Lower Uterine Segment and Cervix

Faye C. Laing

INTRODUCTION

Ultrasound plays a major role in helping obstetricians evaluate the pregnant uterus. To date its primary focus has been on the fetus and its development. With the advent of real-time scanning, observers have been able to closely monitor the development of the fetus and chronicle physiologic activities such as breathing, swallowing, and other important intrauterine movements.

Paradoxically, the organ that houses the fetus during the approximate 9 months from conception to birth has received relatively little critical attention, and knowledge of the uterus remains scant. This relative lack of knowledge is somewhat surprising considering the fact that ultrasonographers perform many more uterine than fetal examinations. It is almost as if the uterus and the dramatic changes it undergoes during pregnancy are taken for granted or forgotten once the fetus becomes prominent.

Nonetheless, the uterus and cervix each play important roles during pregnancy and parturition. Because of its ability to view these regions and the changes they undergo during pregnancy, ultrasound functions as an extension of the physical examination in determining if abnormalities such as placenta previa or incompetent cervix are present. Although fetal and maternal morbidity and mortality have decreased because of ultrasonic diagnosis of conditions affecting the lower uterine segment and cervix, their precise pathophysiology remains to be determined.

This chapter reviews the role of ultrasound in evaluating the lower uterine segment and cervical regions. It emphasizes normal anatomy and abnormal conditions such as placenta previa and incompetent cervix. Hopefully, future applications of ultrasound will help to solve some of the mysteries surrounding these conditions.

ANATOMIC CHANGES DURING PREGNANCY

The nongravid uterus consists of two parts: a thick-walled, muscular portion with a triangular configuration known as the body or corpus; and a primarily fibrous portion with a cylindrical shape known as the neck or cervix. At the junction between the body and cervix uteri is a circumferential band of tissue known as the isthmus. Although anatomically considered part of the uterine body, the isthmus functions in a distinctive manner.

The size relationship of the uterine body and cervix is age dependent. In a young child the cervix is twice the length of the uterine body, whereas in a nulliparous woman the cervix is approximately one-third to one-half the length of the body.[1]

During pregnancy the uterus changes dramatically in size, shape, and weight (Fig. 1). In its nongravid state it is approximately 7½ cm long, pear-shaped and weighs about 40 g. Near term it is greater than 20 cm long, oval or rounded and weighs approximately 1000 g.[2] With pregnancy its most striking anatomic change is hypertrophy of smooth muscle fibers within the corpus. The isthmus also changes markedly as it develops into the lower uterine segment. In a nongravid state the isthmus measures approximately 1 cm in

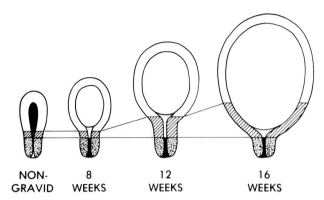

NON-GRAVID   8 WEEKS   12 WEEKS   16 WEEKS

Fig. 1. In the nongravid state and early in pregnancy, the uterine isthmus (parallel lines) is a 1-cm wastelike constriction between the uterine body and cervix (*stippled*). It elongates during the third month of pregnancy and unfolds into the lower uterine segment by about 16 weeks. The cervix does not lengthen during pregnancy but widens and develops a viscus mucus plug (*solid black*) within the endocervical canal.

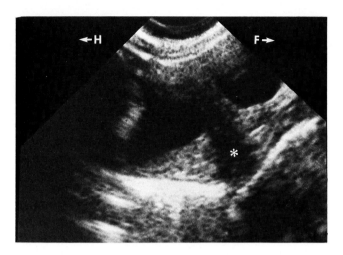

Fig. 2. An insufficiently distended maternal urinary bladder causes the sound beam to reflect from the bladder–uterine interface away from the ultrasound transducer. This results in lack of sound penetration and a relative acoustic shadow (*) in the vicinity of the lower uterine segment and cervix.

length and can be identified as a slight waistlike constriction between the uterine body and cervix. Histologically it differs from the upper portion of the uterine body by being lined with a somewhat atrophic endometrium.[3] During the third month of pregnancy the isthmus elongates. As pregnancy continues its musculature unfolds and develops into the lower uterine segment to accommodate the products of conception. Compared to the body, this portion of the uterus has a thinner muscular wall, a less well-developed decidua, and loosely attached fetal membrane.[3] At term the lower uterine segment comprises approximately one-fourth of the uterus and is 7 to 10 cm in length.[3,4] During parturition it plays a passive role with its muscular fibers relaxing and elongating. This is in contradistinction to the actively contracting muscular fibers of the upper portion of the uterine body.[5]

The uterine cervix also undergoes important changes with pregnancy. Although it does not elongate appreciably, remaining approximately 2½ to 3 cm in length, it thickens primarily as a result of marked proliferation of the endocervical mucosa. At term the mucosa is approximately 3 to 6 mm in depth and occupies about one-half of the entire bulk of the cervix.[3,4] In addition the cervical connective tissue stroma becomes edematous and undergoes hypertrophy and hyperplasia.[4] The cervical mucous is also significantly modified by the formation of a viscous mucous plug that fills the cervical canal.[3,4]

ULTRASOUND EVALUATION OF THE LOWER UTERINE SEGMENT AND CERVIX

In a nonpregnant uterus, neither the isthmus nor cervix is well defined by ultrasound. A slight posterior inden-

tation at the expected level of the isthmus may occasionally be present on ultrasound studies, although this may be due to a focal impression from an adjacent vertebral body.

A uterine landmark that can be readily identified is the central cavity echo, depicted as a highly specular reflection within the central portion of the uterus. Echoes emanating from the vaginal mucosal folds are also easily seen as highly specular echoes coursing in an oblique posterior cranial to anterior caudal direction. Despite the visibility of these two anatomic landmarks, the intervening normal cervix cannot be clearly seen. This is perhaps due to a paucity of endocervical canal mucous and lack of sufficient acoustic contrast between the uterine body and cervix. Although the uterine corpus is primarily muscular tissue and the uterine cervix is primarily fibrous connective tissue, their echo textures are indistinguishable.

During pregnancy the cervix becomes readily visible, although the isthmus and lower uterine segments remain difficult, if not impossible, to define. The ability to evaluate these areas correctly is critically dependent upon the degree of bladder filling. If the bladder is empty or insufficiently distended, the uterine corpus often becomes markedly anteverted. In this position the caudal aspect of the anterior uterine wall lies either oblique or parallel to the ultrasound beam. Sound reflecting off this tissue plane courses *away* from the ultrasound transducer, thereby producing a poor image of the lower aspect of the uterus (Fig. 2). Overdistention of the urinary bladder compresses the anterior and posterior uterine walls and results in a number of problems, not the least of which is false elongation

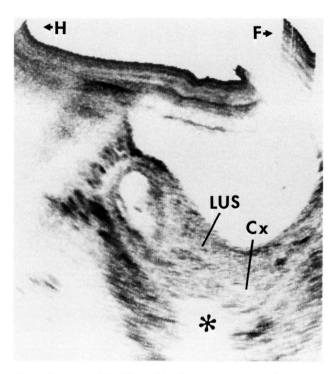

Fig. 3. Cul-de-sac fluid (*) provides the necessary acoustic contrast for visualizing the elongated lower uterine segment (LUS) in this gravid uterus. Until the LUS unfolds, between the 12th and 16th week, the products of conception remain in the upper portion of the uterine body. The echo texture of the cervix (Cx) cannot be distinguished from the LUS.

of the cervix.[6] It can also lead to a false positive diagnosis of placenta previa or a false negative diagnosis of incompetent cervix, two entities that are subsequently discussed. Unfortunately, a precise formula for proper bladder distention is not available. One recommendation is to consider appropriate filling to exist when the uterine wall is convex toward the bladder.[7] If there is a question about the appearance of the lower uterus or cervix, it is frequently necessary to perform sequential scans with various degrees of bladder filling. Most often the patient is requested to void partially, after which the scan is repeated.

When the isthmus elongates between the 8th and 12th weeks of pregnancy, the products of conception remain in the upper portion of the uterine body (Fig. 3).[4] Because of identical echo textures, ultrasound cannot distinguish the elongated isthmus from the cervix. By 16 weeks the uterine cavity elongates because of unfolding of the lower uterine segment. The fetus now occupies all of the available intrauterine space.[4] Ultrasonographically, the lower uterine segment blends imperceptibly with the upper portion of the corpus and cannot be identified as a separate structure. The walls of the lower uterine segment gradually approach one another, ultimately joining with an acute angulation

at the level of the internal cervical os. The endocervical canal, which can be clearly identified as a highly specular echo, is continuous with the internal os (Fig. 4). Its echogenic character is most likely due to viscous mucus which fills the canal during pregnancy. In addition, a rim of relatively sonolucent tissue is frequently noted circumferentially surrounding the echogenic canal. This is probably due to the endocervical mucosa whose thickness doubles during pregnancy. The external cervical os is not routinely visualized because of insufficient acoustic contrast between the external os and vagina. In cases where fluid has been introduced into the vagina, however, it can be readily identified.

CONDITIONS AFFECTING THE LOWER UTERINE SEGMENT

Placenta Previa
The most significant pathologic condition affecting the lower uterine segment is placenta previa. Although considered a fairly uncommon occurrence, observed clinically in 1 out of 200 deliveries (0.5%),[8] sonographers see a higher incidence of this entity because 93 percent of women with placenta previa experience significant vaginal bleeding. From a sonographer's point of view approximately 7 to 11 percent of women with second and third trimester vaginal bleeding will have placenta previa.[9,10]

Although the specific cause for placenta previa is not understood, most authorities agree that the ovum implants abnormally low in this condition.[8,11,12] A common theme in the development of placenta previa is defective decidual vascularization.[13] A known association exists, for example, between lower uterine incision scars for cesarean section or myomectomy and the location of subsequent placental implantations.[8] Placenta previa is also more common in older women and in multiparas, possibly because endometrial scarring occurs with increasing age or repeated pregnancies.[13] The scarring is felt to cause inadequate placental blood supply, for which the placenta compensates by becoming thinner and occupying a greater surface of the uterus.[8,13] A consequence of greater placental attachment is an increased probability for encroachment upon the internal os.

The clinical course and outcome of placenta previa depends to some extent upon the position of the placenta relative to the cervical os. The term central or total previa implies that the implantation completely covers the internal os. This is the severest form of previa, occurring in approximately one-third of cases.[12] In a partial previa the internal os is partially covered by the placenta, while in a low-lying previa the placental edge lies low enough to be palpated by an examining finger introduced through the cervix but does not extend over the os.[13]

The clinical hallmark of placenta previa is painless vaginal bleeding, which usually occurs in the third trimester but can occur as early as 20 weeks.[8] The bleeding, which consists of maternal blood originating from the intravillous space, develops when there is separation of the placental margin from underlying tissues. The site of placental implantation is most often disturbed in the third trimester because of accompanying alterations within the lower uterine segment, and because of cervical effacement and dilatation. The earlier in pregnancy the lower uterine segment begins to form, and the lower the previa, the earlier the first episode of bleeding.[8]

Since ultrasound placentography was first described by Gottesfeld in 1966,[14] many papers have been published attesting to its great accuracy for placental localization and diagnosing placenta previa. In the past decade ultrasound has become the procedure of choice for evaluating patients with possible placenta previa, replacing all previous diagnostic modalities. Although ultrasonographic localization of the placenta and establishment of its position relative to the internal os initially appeared to be a relatively straightforward examination, it soon became apparent that in 5 to 7 percent of cases, false positive diagnoses were made.[9,15,16] Two major and unrelated causes are believed to be responsible for these diagnostic errors.

The first, and probably most important cause, relates to placental "migration," first described by King in 1973.[17] Although the precise mechanism for placental "migration" is not fully understood, most authorities ascribe this phenomenon to differential growth rates between the uterus and placenta.[7,18,19] At 16 weeks' gestation the placenta occupies approximately one-half of the internal uterine surface.[17] Because the placenta grows more slowly than the uterus, at term it occupies only one-quarter to one-third of the uterine surface (Fig. 5).[17] Several studies have shown that in 63 to 91 percent of patients diagnosed as placenta previa during the second trimester, "normal implantation" will be present at term.[15,16,18,19] This is most likely due

Fig. 4. A. The highly echogenic portion of the cervix (—▶), is due to the presence of a viscus mucus plug within the endocervical canal. B. A parasagittal scan to one side of the endocervical canal reveals a relative sonolucency (▶◀) which is most likely due to thickened endocervical mucosa. This appearance should not be mistaken for premature cervical dilatation. C. A transverse scan over the cervix confirms the central echogenic mucus plug (—▶) surrounded on either side by relatively sonolucent tissue (▶). The peripheral portion of the cervix is primarily fibrous connective tissue, whose echo texture is indistinguishable from the muscular lower uterine segment.

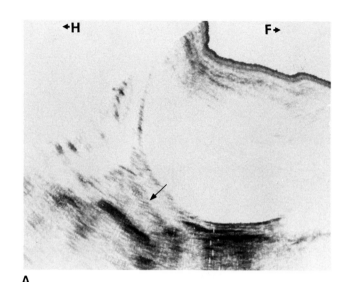

A

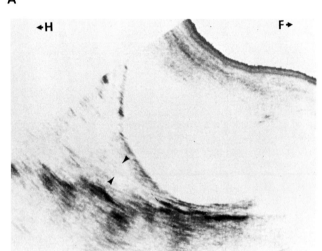

B

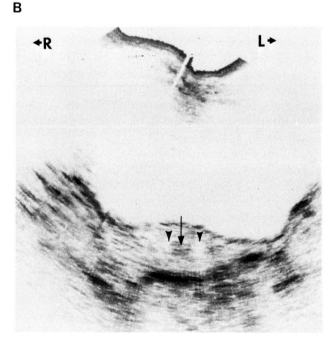

C

to the relatively greater growth and elongation of the lower uterine segment compared to the growth of the attached placenta. The net effect is that with time the initially diagnosed low-lying or placenta previa is carried away from the lower uterine segment toward the

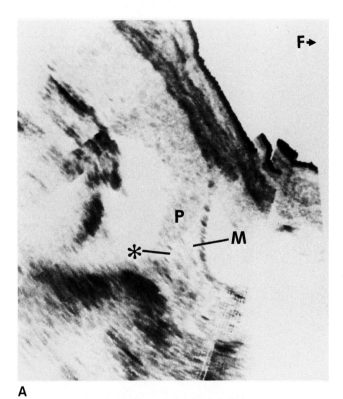

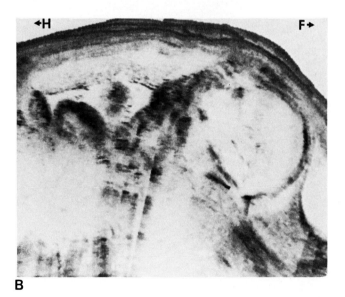

Fig. 5. A. This patient presented at 28 weeks' gestation with painless vaginal bleeding. The sonogram reveals a partial anterior placenta previa (P) as well as a small amount of blood in the proximal endocervical canal (*). The myometrial (M) texture is readily distinguished from that of the placenta. **B.** At term, an anterior placenta is present without previa. The patient underwent an uncomplicated vaginal delivery.

uterine fundus. The reverse phenomenon, i.e., placental migration toward the cervical os, has not been observed.

Recently, ultrasonographers have attempted to predict in which cases placental "migration" will occur. An interesting study by Gillieson, Winer-Mural, and Muram[7] has shown that placentas located on the anterior wall are much more likely to convert to a normal position than those on the posterior wall. Additionally it was found that conversion did not occur with placentas attached to both the anterior and posterior uterine walls. Although these findings are based upon observation of relatively few patients, they are interesting and merit further investigation.

The second cause for misdiagnosing a normal implantation as a placenta previa relates to technical problems associated with an overfilled urinary bladder.[9,18,20,21] Apposition of the lower anterior and posterior uterine walls occurs because of the weight and pressure of the filled bladder. In cases of placental attachment to a portion of the lower uterine segment, bladder-induced compression can result in an image that appears as if placental tissue fills the entire lower uterine segment, or even crosses the internal os (Fig. 6). The obvious solution to this problem is to rescan these patients after partial voiding.

A focal uterine contraction in the region of the lower uterine segment is a much more unusual cause for falsely diagnosing placenta previa. Careful attention to technical factors usually permits the experienced sonographer to recognize subtle textural differences between placental and myometrial tissues (Fig. 7). In addition, correct placental localization can often be made by identifying a relatively clear subplacental zone caused by adjacent vascular channels coursing through the decidual basalis.[22]

Although a false positive diagnosis of placenta previa is worrisome to the patient, her family, and the obstetrician, it does not ultimately harm either the mother or her baby. The same cannot be said if the diagnosis of placenta previa is missed. Although a false negative sonographic diagnosis of placenta previa is uncommon, occurring in less than 2 percent of cases,[9,23,24] its sequelae can be profound with regard to fetal and maternal morbidity and mortality. A false negative diagnosis is most likely to occur when the fetal head prevents visualization of a posterior placenta previa.[10] In 98 percent of patients with cephalic presentations, posterior or low-lying placentas and their relationship to the internal cervical os can be ascertained by scanning the mother in a Trendelenberg position and applying gentle upward traction on the fetal head.[25]

Two other situations exist that can cause confusion and potential failure to recognize and diagnose

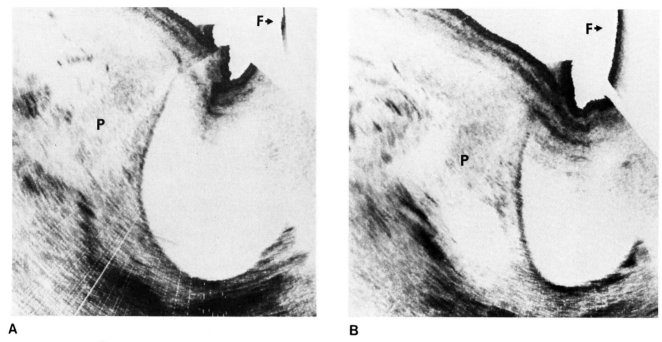

Fig. 6. A. An overly distended urinary bladder caused this anterior placenta (P) to appear as if it covered the internal cervical os. **B.** A repeat scan following partial bladder emptying shows a normally implanted anterior placenta.

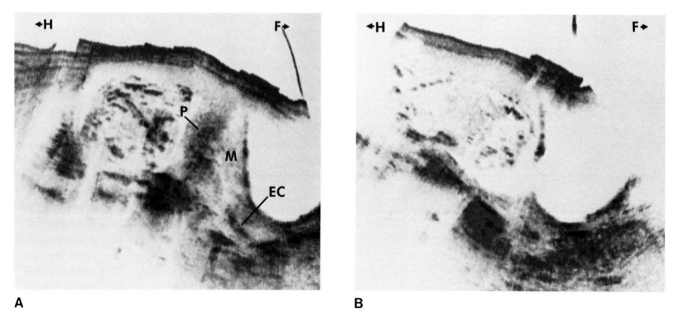

Fig. 7. A. A transient focal uterine contraction (M) of the lower uterine segment can cause rotational changes and lead to a false positive diagnosis of placenta previa. Note the textural change between the thickened myometrium (M) and placenta (P). The endocervical canal (EC) is well seen. **B.** A repeat scan obtained 15 minutes later shows a normally implanted anterior placenta. The myometrium has thinned and is inapparent on this scan.

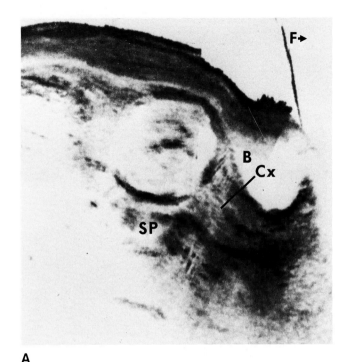

A

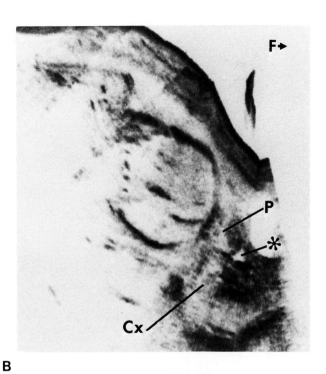

B

Fig. 8. A. This longitudinal scan shows the fetal head closely applied to the maternal urinary bladder (B) and sacral promontory (SP). The placenta is not visible on this scan. Cx = cervix. **B.** An oblique parasagittal scan in the same patient shows a marginal anterior placenta previa (P). The small sonolucent area (*) is due to blood interposed between the placenta and cervix (Cx). *(Reprinted with permission from Laing FC: Placenta praevia: Avoiding false-negative diagnoses. J Clin Ultrasound 9:109, 1981.)*

placenta previa.[26] Although most placentas are located on the anterior, posterior, or fundic portions of the uterus, occasionally attachment will be to the lateral wall in the vicinity of the lower uterine segment. Most sonographers diagnose placenta previa only when placental tissue is interposed between the presenting part and maternal bladder, or if the distance between the presenting part and sacral promontory is 1½ cm or greater.[27] In women with lateral placenta previa, conventional scans will show close apposition of the fetal head to the maternal bladder and sacrum (Fig. 8). This appearance does *not* guarantee absence of a placenta previa. Before excluding a previa, it is necessary to examine the lower uterine segment and cervical areas with multiple angled and oblique views. This can be most expeditiously performed with high-resolution real-time equipment.

A second potential problem in diagnosing placenta previa can occur in patients with blood in the region of the internal cervical os. The blood can sometimes be mistaken for amniotic fluid and can result in a misdiagnosis of "normal" (Fig. 9). This problem can be overcome by careful scanning that will reveal that the fluid in question is interposed between placental tissue

and the cervical os. This extremely important clue, which is commonly present in women who have significant bleeding at the time of the ultrasound examination, should not be overlooked.

Placenta Accreta, Increta, and Percreta

Placenta accreta, increta, and percreta, although rare, appear to have become more common. Their incidence is usually reported as 1 per 7000 deliveries,[28] but recently it has been clinically diagnosed in approximately 1 per 2500 deliveries.[29] This condition occurs when defective decidual formation causes abnormal attachment of the placenta to the uterine wall. In placenta accreta the chorionic villi are in direct contact with the uterine muscle, while in placenta increta and percreta, the villi invade or penetrate through the uterine wall, respectively. Similar to placenta previa, this condition tends to occur in areas of uterine scarring. It is therefore not surprising that it has been reported in association with placenta previa in nearly two-thirds of cases, and in patients who have had prior cesarean sections in approximately one-fourth of cases.[29]

Ultrasound has recently played a role in evaluating this extremely serious condition, which if not properly

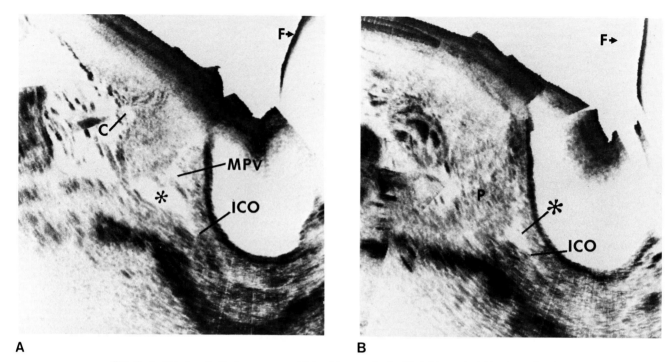

Fig. 9. A. This longitudinal scan was obtained in a patient with brisk vaginal bleeding. The large sonolucent collection (*) abutting the internal cervical os (ICO) could be confused with amniotic fluid. A small subchorionic cyst (C) and marginal placental vein (MPV) are also evident. **B.** A repeat scan with slight change in transducer angulation clarifies that the sonolucent material is clearly interposed between the placenta (P) and internal cervical os (ICO). (*Reprinted with permission from Laing FC. Placenta praevia: Avoiding false-negative diagnoses. J Clin Ultrasound 9:109, 1981.*)

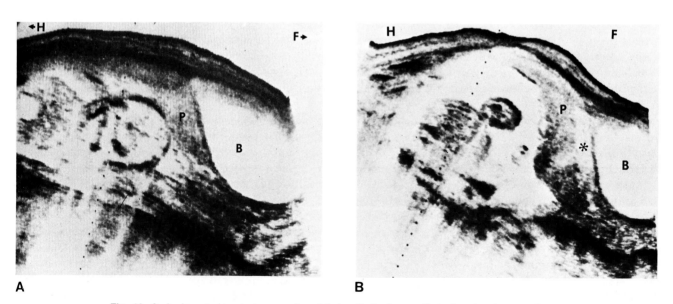

Fig. 10. A. A placenta increta is present on this longitudinal scan. Note that the placenta (P) abuts the uterine wall–bladder (B) interface. **B.** Normally, as in this patient with an anterior placenta previa, a subplacental sonolucent space (*) can be readily identified. This is due to vascular channels coursing through the decidua basalis. (*Reprinted with permission from Tabsh KMA, Brinkman CR III, King W: Ultrasound diagnosis of placenta increta. J Clin Ultrasound 10:288, 1982.*)

diagnosed and treated, can rapidly lead to maternal exsanguination (Fig. 10).[30] Because the decidua is defective in these women, the normally visualized subplacental sonolucent space will be absent. Although ultrasonographic assessment may be impossible in patients with posterior placentas, many affected women will have anterior placentas because of placental attachment in the vicinity of prior cesarean scars. The placental–subplacental complex should therefore be carefully scrutinized in any patient with an anterior placenta previa or prior uterine incision.

CONDITIONS AFFECTING THE CERVIX

During pregnancy, the cervix undergoes appreciable widening. Its length remains similar to that measured in the nongravid state, namely 2.5 to 3 cm.[4] One ultrasonographic study that attempted to measure the cervix found that during pregnancy its length averaged 3.7 cm with a range of 1.9 to 6 cm.[6] Because technical difficulties often preclude identification of precise anatomic landmarks, and because an overfilled urinary bladder falsely elongates cervical measurements, it was felt that the numbers obtained were somewhat exaggerated. Although ultrasonographic evaluation of the cervix should attempt to approximate length, from a diagnostic and clinical viewpoint, it is more important to evaluate the appearance of the endocervical canal. In a normal pregnancy the mucous plug fills the nondilated endocervical canal and is readily visualized as a highly echogenic line. At term and during labor, the cervix thins and dilates to accommodate fetal passage.

Three clinical situations have been described in which the cervix dilates prior to term. These include premature labor, inevitable abortion, and incompetent cervix.[31] Because ultrasound is the only available method for directly visualizing the region of the internal os and endocervical canal, it can play a major role in aiding obstetric management for these conditions. The ultrasound findings for each of these conditions may be similar or identical. The clinical presentation and history are most useful for distinguishing one entity from another.

Premature labor consists of the spontaneous onset of palpable, regularly occurring uterine contractions between the 20th and 37th weeks of pregnancy.[32] The clinical diagnosis can be difficult. Waiting until labor is obviously counterproductive, since therapeutic success is equated with the time it is started. Physical examination shows varying degrees of cervical effacement and/or dilatation, depending upon the course of labor. The decision of whether or not an attempt should be made to arrest premature labor must be an

individual one in each case. Ultrasound demonstration of a close endocervical canal is a favorable sign that may influence the obstetrician to attempt to delay labor in order to allow continued fetal growth and development. If, on the other hand, the ultrasound examination reveals marked cervical dilatation with prolapse of the amniotic sac, therapy is of little value and spontaneous delivery soon occurs.[33]

Although women with an incompetent cervix may also have cervical dilatation, this group differs from women in premature labor or those experiencing inevitable abortion because in this condition, which typically occurs in the second trimester, cervical dilatation is painless, bloodless, and tends to recur with each successive pregnancy.[34] The causes of incompetent cervix are obscure and are probably multiple. A common theme appears to be cervical trauma; for example, women who have undergone dilatation and curettage, or cauterization, appear to be at increased risk.[34] Anatomic factors may also contribute to the development of cervical incompetence; there appears to be excessive smooth muscle with an altered collagen-to-muscle ratio within the cervices of these women.[35] An interesting but poorly understood association exists between incompetent cervix and women who have been exposed to diethylstilbesterol in utero. Five of nine patients with this history developed evidence of cervical incompetence, and, in addition, had cervical hypoplasia. Finally, hormonal influences upon the sphincteric ring, which is felt to exist at the junction of the lower uterine segment and internal os, may also play a role in incompetent cervix.[4] This sphincter is normally tightly contracted during pregnancy but is relatively relaxed under the influence of estrogen.

There are several indications for ultrasound examination of women who carry the diagnosis of incompetent cervix. Because the best time to treat this condition is between the 14th and 18th week of pregnancy,[36] i.e., before significant cervical dilatation occurs, it is important to assess the fetus for possible anomalies, or to ascertain that a molar pregnancy is not present. A second indication is for diagnosis or confirmation of this condition. The ultrasonographic hallmark of cervical incompetence is visualization of fetal parts and/or amniotic fluid within a dilated endocervical canal (Fig. 11). Attention must be paid to technical aspects of the study because an overdistended maternal bladder compressing the anterior and posterior cervical walls can give the false impression of a closed cervix (Fig. 12).[31,37] In suspicious cases, our laboratory examines this area using real-time equipment with the patient standing. In the erect position, gravitational pressure from uterine contents can force amniotic fluid into the proximal endocervical canal such that a mild,

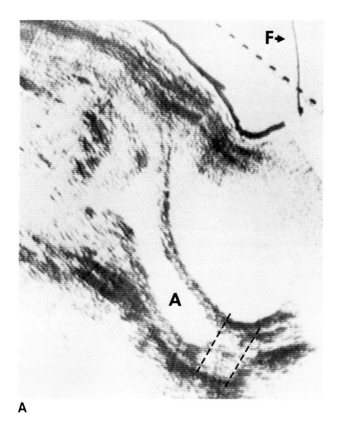

A

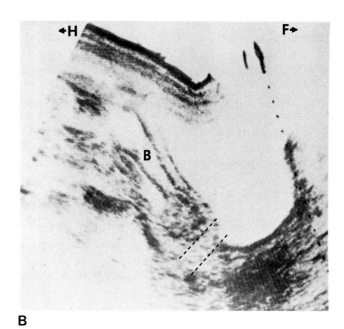

B

Fig. 11. Dilatation of the endocervical canal should be diagnosed when either amniotic fluid (A) or a fetal part (B) is present in the endocervical canal. The visible portion of the cervix (*between dotted lines*) is approximately 1 to 2 cm in these cases. Space between markers is 1 cm.

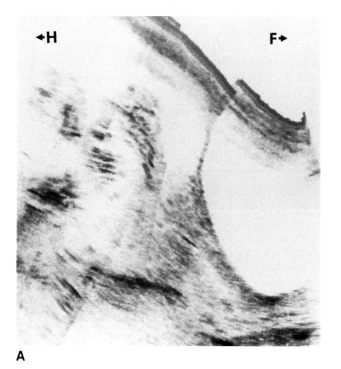

A

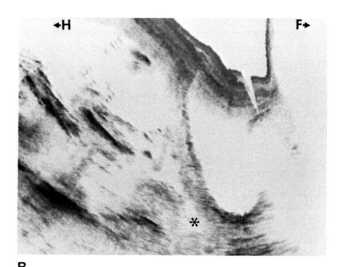

B

Fig. 12. A. An overly distended urinary bladder can cause apposition of the anterior and posterior uterine walls and give the false impression of a closed cervix. **B.** A repeat scan after partial voiding reveals an incompetent cervix with amniotic fluid (*) within the dilated endocervical canal. Note the similarity of this scan with Figure 4B.

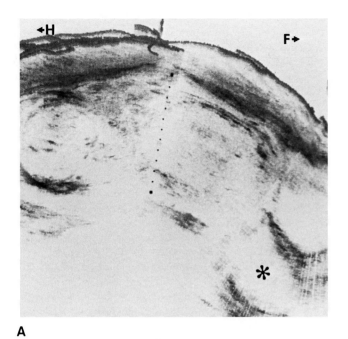
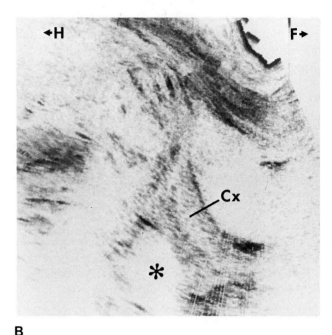

A

B

Fig. 13. A. This midline pelvic sonolucency (*) is compatible with a large amount of fluid in the endocervical canal. **B.** A scan slightly off midline reveals that the cystic mass (*) is posterior to a normal-appearing cervix (CX = cervix canal). The cervix is frequently not positioned in the midline.

albeit significant, amount of cervical dilatation can be visualized at the earliest possible time. Occasionally, the normal lucent endocervical mucosa or paracervical fluid collections can mimic a fluid-filled endocervical canal on ultrasound images (Figs. 4,13). Real-time examination can prevent mistakes of this type by readily establishing precise anatomic relationships.

The final indication for performing an ultrasound study in women with cervical incompetence is to evaluate patients following placement of a cervical cerclage (Fig. 14). Both the 5-mm-wide Mersiline tape suture employed in the Shirodkar procedure and the No. 2 nylon suture used in the McDonald procedure can be visualized as hyperechoic linear structures with variable posterior acoustic shadowing.[38] Ultrasound can be used to locate the position of the suture material relative to the external os and to evaluate for possible protrusion of membranes beyond the sutures before it is clinically evident. As ultrasound forges into the area of interventional techniques, perhaps it will soon be used to guide suture placement during the application of the cerclage.

CONCLUSION

Although the precise etiologies for placenta previa and premature cervical dilatation remain to be determined,

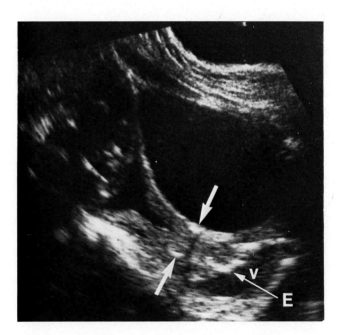

Fig. 14. A longitudinal scan in a patient who had a cerclage because of an incompetent cervix reveals high amplitude echoes with variable shadowing (—▶) due to the suture material. The distance from the sutures to the external cervical os (E) can be readily measured after introducing water into the vagina (V). (*Reprinted with permission from Parulekar SG, Kiwi R: Ultrasound evaluation of sutures following cervical cerclage for incompetent cervical uteri. J Ultrasound Med 1:223, 1982.*)

ultrasound is a major tool in diagnosing these important conditions. Prior to the advent of ultrasound, most patients with painless third trimester vaginal bleeding were treated expectantly, i.e., they were put to bed and were given appropriate fluid replacement. They were all considered to have a placenta previa until a definitive double setup vaginal examination was performed, usually at 36 to 37 weeks.[8] Ultimately, only one-third of this group was diagnosed as placenta previa.[11] The economic and emotional strain on the patient, her family, as well as the obstetrician, was not inconsiderable. Fortunately, ultrasound can now be used to reassure the majority of these women that placenta previa is absent.

Evaluation of the endocervical canal by ultrasound can similarly reassure many patients and physicians by ascertaining that it appears normal. In patients in whom ultrasound diagnoses or confirms premature dilatation, an appropriate course of action can be undertaken at the earliest possible time.

REFERENCES

1. Taslitz N: Anatomy of the female reproductive system, in Iffy L, Kaminetzky HA (eds), Principles and Practice of Obstetrics and Perinatology, 1st ed. New York, Wiley, 1981, pp 43–64
2. Harrison RG: The urogenital system, in Romanes GF (ed), Cunningham's Textbook of Anatomy, 10th ed. London, Oxford University Press, 1964, p 514
3. Percival R: Normal pregnancy, in Holland and Brews' Manual of Obstetrics, 14th ed. Edinburgh, Churchill Livingstone, 1980, pp 66–67
4. Greenhill JP, Friedman EA: Effects of pregnancy on the maternal organism, in Biological Principles and Modern Practice of Obstetrics, 1st ed. Philadelphia, Saunders, 1974, pp 105–109
5. Percival R: Normal labour, in Holland and Brews' Manual of Obstetrics, 14th ed. Edinburgh, Churchill Livingstone, 1980, pp 317–319
6. Zemlyn S: The length of the uterine cervix and its significance. J Clin Ultrasound 9:267, 1981
7. Gillieson MS, Winer-Mural HT, Muram D: Low-lying placenta. Radiology 144:577, 1982
8. Goplerud CP: Bleeding in late pregnancy, in Danforth DN (ed), Obstetrics and Gynecology, 3rd ed. Hagerstown, Maryland, Harper and Row, 1977, pp 378–384
9. Bowie JD, Rochester D, Cadkin AV, et al: Accuracy of placental localization by ultrasound. Radiology 128:177, 1978
10. Scheer K: Ultrasonic diagnosis of placenta previa. Obstet Gynecol 42:707, 1973
11. Greenhill JP, Friedman EA: Placenta previa, in Biological Principles and Modern Practice of Obstetrics, 1st ed. Philadelphia, Saunders, 1974, pp 415–425
12. Kelly JV, Iffy L: Placenta previa, in Iffy L, Kaminetzky HA (eds), Principles and Practice of Obstetrics and Perinatology, 1st ed. New York, Wiley, 1981, pp 1105–1120
13. Hellman LM, Pritchard JA: Placenta previa and abruptio placentae, in Hellman LM, Pritchard JA, (eds), Williams' Obstetrics, 14th ed. New York, Appleton-Century-Crofts, 1971, pp 609–638
14. Gottesfeld KR, Thompson HE, Holmes JH, et al: Ultrasonic placentography—A new method for placental localization. Am J Obstet Gynecol 96:538, 1966
15. Rizos N, Doran TA, Miskin M, et al: Natural history of placenta previa ascertained by diagnostic ultrasound. Am J Obstet Gynecol 133:287, 1979
16. Wexler P, Gottesfeld KR: Early diagnosis of placenta previa. Obstet Gynecol 54:231, 1979
17. King DL: Placental migration demonstrated by ultrasonography. Radiology 109:167, 1973
18. Goldberg BB: The identification of placenta praevia. Radiology 128:255, 1978
19. Mittelstaedt CA, Partain CL, Boyce IL Jr, et al: Placenta praevia: Significance in the second trimester. Radiology 131:465, 1979
20. Williamson D, Bjorgen J, Baier B, et al: Ultrasonic diagnosis of placenta previa: Value of a postvoid scan. J Clin Ultrasound 6:58, 1978
21. Zemlyn S: The effect of the urinary bladder in obstetrical sonography. Radiology 128:169, 1978
22. Callen PW, Filly RA: The placental–subplacental complex: A specific indicator of placental position on ultrasound. J Clin Ultrasound 8:21, 1980
23. Reed MF: Ultrasonic placentography. Br J Radiology 46:255, 1973
24. Dunster GD, Davies ER, Ross FGM, et al: Placental localization: A comparison of isotopic and ultrasonic placentography. Br J Radiology 49:940, 1976
25. Jeffrey RB, Laing FC: Sonography of the low-lying placenta: Value of Trendelenburg and traction scans. Am J Roentgenol 137:547, 1981
26. Laing FC: Placenta previa: Avoiding false-negative diagnoses. J Clin Ultrasound 9:109, 1981
27. Grannum PA, Hobbins JC: The placenta. Radiol Clin N Am 20:353, 1982
28. Breen JL, Neubecker R, Gregori CA, et al: Placenta accreta, increta, and percreta. Obstet Gynecol 49:43, 1977
29. Reed JA, Cotton DB, Miller FC: Placenta accreta: Changing clinical aspects and outcome. Obstet Gynecol 56:31, 1980
30. Tabsh KMA, Brinkman CR III, King W: Ultrasound diagnosis of placenta increta. J Clin Ultrasound 10:288, 1982
31. Sarti DA, Sample WF, Hobel CJ, et al: Ultrasonic visualization of a dilated cervix during pregnancy. Radiology 130:417, 1979
32. Abdul-Karim RW, Beydoun SN: Premature labor, in Iffy L, Kaminetzky HA (eds), Principles and Practice of Obstetrics and Perinatology, 1st ed. New York, Wiley, 1981, pp 1457–1469
33. McGahan JP, Pillips HE, Bowen MS: Prolapse of the amniotic sac ("Hourglass membranes"). Radiology 140:463, 1981

34. Hellman LM, Pritchard JA: Abortion and premature labor, in Hellman LM, Pritchard JA, (eds), Williams' Obstetrics, 14th ed. New York, Appleton-Century-Crofts, 1971, pp 493–534
35. Buckingham JC, Buethe RA Jr, Danforth DN: Collagen–muscle ratio in clinically normal and clinically incompetent cervices. Am J Obstet Gynecol 91:232, 1965
36. Charles D: Cervical incompetence, in Iffy L, Kaminetzky HA (eds), Principles and Practice of Obstetrics and Perinatology, 1st ed. New York, Wiley, 1981, pp 597–602
37. Bernstine RL, Lee SH, Crawford WL, et al: Sonographic evaluation of the incompetent cervix. J Clin Ultrasound 9:417, 1981
38. Parulekar SG, Kiwi R: Ultrasound evaluation of sutures following cervical cerclage for incompetent cervix uteri. J Ultrasound Med 1:223, 1982

27 | Sonography of the Umbilical Cord

David Graham
Joan Campbell
Karen L. Litchfield

FORMATION OF THE UMBILICAL CORD

The umbilical cord is formed in the early weeks of embryogenesis from a fusion between the body stalk (which contains the umbilical arteries, umbilical veins, and allantois) and the yolk stalk (which contains the omphalomesenteric stalk and remnant of the original yolk sac attachment). During this process, the two umbilical veins fuse to form a single vessel and the omphalomesenteric vessels are obliterated. The result is an umbilical cord, covered by amnion and containing a single umbilical vein, and two umbilical arteries supported in Wharton jelly, a gelatinous substance that consists mainly of collagen in addition to elastin and muscle. Although the walls of the umbilical vessels have a large proportion of muscle, they lack collagen and elastin and so are able to change configuration with changes in osmotic pressure in the amniotic fluid.

STRUCTURE AND FUNCTION OF THE UMBILICAL CORD

The umbilical cord is quite variable in length, and normally contains two umbilical arteries and a single larger umbilical vein surrounded by a clear gelatinous Wharton jelly. A layer of amnion covers the umbilical cord except near the fetal insertion where an epithelial covering is substituted. The arteries wind around the umbilical vein in a spiral fashion, and, since the vessels are longer than the cord itself, there are a number of foldings and tortuosities producing protrusions or false knots on the cord surface. The umbilical vein provides

oxygenated blood to the fetus, and, on reaching the fetal abdominal wall passes through the liver posteriorly and cephalad to terminate at the portal sinus (the main left portal vein). Deoxygenated blood from the fetal aorta passes to the hypogastric arteries, which wind superiorly and medially to enter the cord as the umbilical arteries.

The Wharton jelly that surrounds the vessels apparently has a protective function protecting the vessels from undue torsion and compression.[1]

Although the site of cord insertion is usually central into the placenta eccentric cord insertion may occur in 48 to 75 percent of placentas[2,3] and in 5 to 6 percent of cases marginal or velamentous insertion of the cord may occur.[4]

SONOGRAPHIC ANATOMY OF THE NORMAL CORD

The umbilical stalk and the yolk sac may be occasionally seen in the late first trimester, adjacent to the anterior abdominal wall of the fetus (Fig. 1). In the second and third trimesters the cord is much more readily visualized, especially where there is excess amniotic fluid. In longitudinal section, a portion of the cord will be seen as a series of parallel lines (Fig. 2), while in transverse section, the arteries and umbilical vein may be seen as three separately circular luciencies.

Pulsations, occurring at the same rate as fetal heart rate may be seen with real time. More commonly several portions of cord are visualized, giving a "stack of coins" appearance.

Where there is oligohydramnios, the cord may be difficult or impossible to visualize sonographically, even in late pregnancy.

By scanning near the center of the placenta, the insertion site of the cord may be demonstrated as a V- or U-shaped sonolucent area adjacent to the choronic plate (Fig. 3). At the insertion of the cord into the anterior abdominal wall of the fetus the origins of the umbilical vein and hypogastric arteries may be visualized (Fig. 4).

ABNORMALITIES OF CORD LENGTH

Although the average cord length is 55 cm, a normal range of cord length of 30 to 120 cm may be seen.[5] Extremes of cord length may occur from apparently no cord (achordia)[6] to lengths up to 300 cm.[5] Excessively long cords may predispose to vascular occlusion by thrombi and by true knots and also to cord prolapse during labor. Rarely, excessively short umbilical cords may be responsible for abruptio placentae, uterine inversion, or intrafunicular hemorrhage.[5] Although abnormalities of cord length may predispose to a number of these pathologic entities, it is impossible to determine umbilical cord length prior to delivery with current sonographic techniques.

ABNORMALITIES OF CORD POSITION

Normally loops of umbilical cord lie anterior to the fetal abdominal wall and adjacent to the limbs. In a number of instances, however, there may be loopings of the cord around the fetal neck or limbs or, alternatively, loops of cord may lie between the fetal presenting part and the lower uterine segment (funic presentation). The most important umbilical cord malpositions include prolapses, knots and neck, body and shoulder loopings. Kamina and deTourris,[7] in a series of 1750 deliveries, found 4 prolapses, 232 neck loopings, 45 shoulder loopings, and 13 cord knots. Walker and Pye found an incidence of nuchal cord of 17% at delivery.[8] This is not clinically diagnosable until delivery but has been recognized prenatally with ultrasound by demonstration of a loop of cord passing around the fetal neck (Fig. 5).[7,9,11] Although in singletons coiling of the cord around the neck is an uncommon cause of fetal death, in monoamniotic twins a significant portion of the high perinatal mortality rate is attributed to umbilical cord problems.[5]

Occasionally loops of the cord may be seen lying between the fetal presenting part and the lower seg-

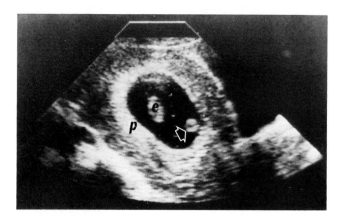

Figure 1. Yolk sac. Longitudinal section through a first trimester gestational sac showing the embryo (e) and the yolk sac (*arrow*), and developing placenta (p).

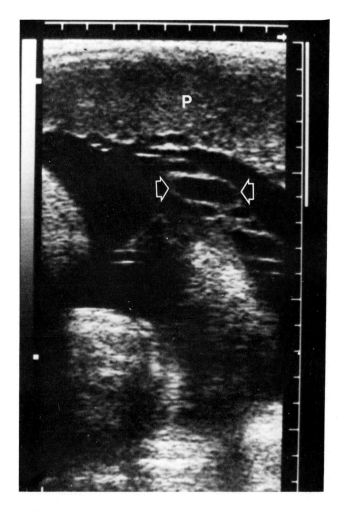

Figure 2. Longitudinal, and normal cord. Section of normal cord near placental insertion showing the parallel line (*open arrows*) representing the walls of the umbilical vein and smaller umbilical arteries. Placenta (P).

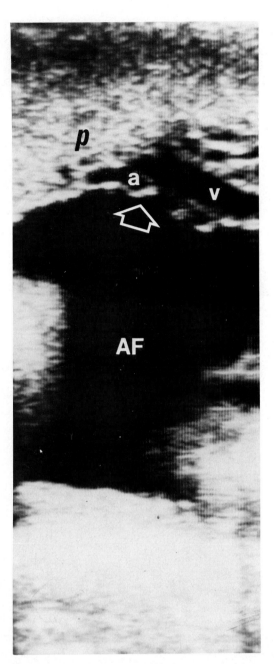

Figure 3. Insertion of cord into placenta. In this third trimester placenta the insertion of the cord vessels into the placenta is clearly visualized (*arrow*). Placenta (p), umbilical vein (v), umbilical artery (a), amniotic fluid (AF).

ment. It is important to recognize this since such a position predisposes to cord prolapse and possible fetal death at the time of rupture of the membranes. Funic presentation is more common with malpresentations such as breech or transverse lie.

Knotting of the cord, which usually occurs secondary to excessive fetal motion, occurs in approxi-mately 1.1 percent of deliveries and has an asso-ciated perinatal loss of 6.1 percent. True knot of the cord has not as yet been reported as being diagnosed prenatally.

SINGLE UMBILICAL ARTERY (SUA)

Although the normal umbilical cord contains two um-bilical arteries, a single umbilical artery may be seen in approximately 1 percent of all singleton births, 5 percent of twins, and 2.5 percent of abortuses.[12] Ber-nischke and Brown first described a relationship be-tween SUA and fetal malformations showing an in-creased incidence of genitourinary tract anomalies.[12] The incidence of SUA has been found to be increased in pregnancies subsequently ending in abortion, tri-somy D or E, the offspring of diabetic mothers, and in black patients.[13,14]

Although there is a fourfold increase in perinatal mortality associated with SUA,[15] some of these deaths may be secondary to the major congenital malforma-tions associated with SUA while others remain unex-plained. In following infants with SUA, Froehlich and Fujikura[16] found a high mortality (14 percent), but in those who survived infancy, serious anomalies were no more common than in a control group, whereas Bryan and Kohler,[17] following 98 infants, found that previously unrecognized malformations become appar-ent in 10.

Prenatal sonographic diagnosis of SUA in two fe-tuses at 34 and at 36 weeks has been reported by Jassani and Brennan.[13] The first infant subsequently died in utero and the second showed evidence of mild left hydronephrosis.

Umbilical Cord Masses

Masses of the umbilical cord, which are quite uncom-mon, have diverse etiologies. Such masses, or apparent masses, may be caused by:

1. False knots
2. True knots
3. Hematoma
4. Allantoic duct cyst
5. Neoplasms
6. Umbilical hernia
7. Omphalocele or gastroschisis

False knots, which clinically have no importance, essentially represent a varix of the umbilical vessels and are recognized grossly by a protrusion from the cord. Sonographically, they may be recognized by ir-regular protrusions from the cord.

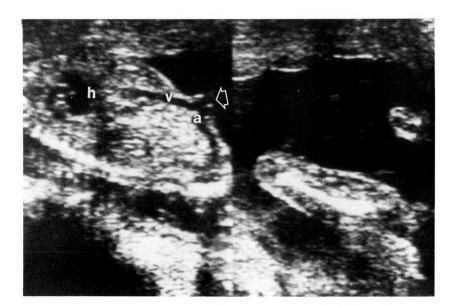

Figure 4. Insertion of cord into fetus. Sagittal section of a midtrimester fetus showing insertion of the cord (*arrow*) into the anterior abdominal wall. Division into the umbilical vein (v) and hypogastic artery is shown. Heart (h).

True knots are thought to be caused by excessive fetal movement and may, if they become tight, lead to vascular occlusion with fetal death in utero. They have not been described sonographically in utero and their diagnosis would most likely be serendipitous.

Umbilical cord hematoma is a rare occurrence in late pregnancy and labor[18-20] and has been reported by Dippel,[20] in a comprehensive review, to have an incidence of 1 in 5505 deliveries. Such hematomas most commonly occur from rupture of the wall of the umbilical vein and may occur secondary to mechanical trauma between fetal and maternal tissues, traction on a short cord or on loops of cord around the fetus or a rare congenital weakness in a vessel wall.[18] Umbilical cord hematoma is associated with a very high perinatal loss—in Dippel's series 47 percent of the infants were stillborn. One mechanism of FDIU may be compression of umbilical vessels by the increased pressure of blood filling the Wharton jelly in the substance of the cord.[18]

Prenatal diagnosis of umbilical cord hematoma has been reported by Ruvinsky and Wiley[19] in a patient referred at 32 weeks of gestation with FDIU. The ultrasound examination showed a 6 × 8 cm sonolucent, septated intrauterine mass adjacent to the fetal abdomen.

Allantoic duct cysts may occur along the course of the cord and may be either true cysts or false cysts.[5] True cysts are usually quite small and represent remnants of the umbilical vesicle or of the allantois whereas false cysts result from liquefaction of Wharton jelly and may reach considerable size. Such allantoic cysts even when large usually do not jeopardize fetal circulation. Sachs[21] has reported the prenatal diagnosis

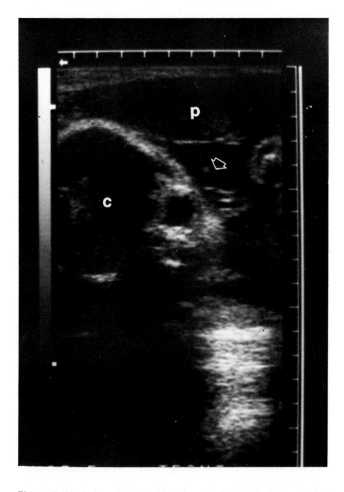

Figure 5. Nuchal cord. In this third trimester fetus with demonstrated variable decelerations on a non-stress test there is sonographic evidence of a loop of cord (*arrow*) wrapped around the fetal neck. Fetal cranium (c), placenta (p).

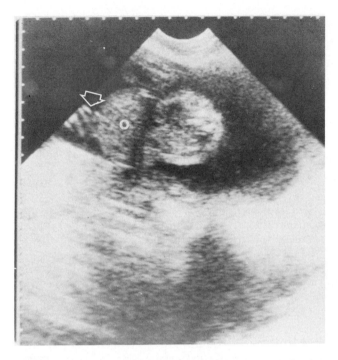

Figure 6. Omphalocele. Transverse section of the fetal trunk showing a large omphalocele (o). The umbilical cord (*arrow*) is implanted at the apex of the omphalocele.

of a 5-cm cystic mass within the umbilical cord, several centimeters from the abdominal wall, at 21 weeks of gestation. Visualization of vessels in the lateral wall of the mass and an intact anterior abdominal wall allowed exclusion of other pathologies.

Neoplasms of the umbilical cord, which are quite rare, are usually angiomyxomas, myxosarcomas, dermoids, and teratomas, of which the most common is the angiomyxoma.[22] These more commonly occur in a location near the placental margin. Hemangioma of the cord has been reported as a cause of increased amniotic fluid α-fetoprotein.[23]

Umbilical hernia, which is one of the most commonly encountered abnormalities in early infancy,[24] is especially common in black and low-birth-weight infants.[25-27] Umbilical hernias are usually not significant clinically and close spontaneously in the first 3 years of life. Umbilical hernia has been reported as being more common in trisomy 21, congenital hypothyroidism, mucopolysaccharidoses, and Beckwith syndrome.[24]

Sonographically, umbilical hernia may be recognized as a protrusion from the anterior abdominal wall, with a normal insertion of the umbilical vessels.

Omphalocele and gastroschisis represent abnormalities of closure of the anterior abdominal wall. With omphalocele there is a midline umbilical defect with pro-

trusion of abdominal structures such as bowel and liver into the base of the umbilical cord (Fig. 6), producing a sonographic appearance of a mass adjacent to the anterior abdominal wall, covered with a membrane and into the apex of which the umbilical cord appears to insert. There is a high incidence of other anomalies, e.g., intestinal, cardiac, and renal anomalies.

With gastroschisis a paraumbilical abdominal wall defect results in protrusion of bowel and other intraabdominal contents into the amniotic fluid. The cord inserts normally and the gastroschisis will therefore appear as a complex mass adjacent to the base of the cord.

UMBILICAL VEIN DIAMETER AS A PREDICTOR OF FETAL DISEASE

Measurement of the diameter of the umbilical vein both in the amniotic fluid and as it passes through the liver has been proposed by Mayden[28] and by DeVore[29] as a predictor of the severity of Rhesus or other isoimmunization. The umbilical vein diameter in the amniotic fluid was found consistently to be the larger of the two measurements. It was suggested that the umbilical vein might dilate within the liver and in the amniotic fluid in response to severe Rh disease and that this dilatation might precede any rise in the ΔOD 450. In a subsequent communication it appeared that the measurement was only of predictive value when increased and that normal values might be obtained in severely affected infants. Witter and Graham,[30] in a study of severely affected infants found that, although in no instance was the umbilical vein diameter outside the normal range quoted by DeVore, in several normal patients idiopathic enlargement of umbilical vein diameter was obtained.

REFERENCES

1. Browne FJ: Abnormalities of the umbilical cord which may cause fetal death. J Obstet Gynaec Br Emp 32:17, 1925
2. Kohorn EI, Walker RMS, et al: Placental localization. Am J Obstet Gynecol 103:868, 1969
3. Purola E: The length and insertion of the umbilical cord. Ann Chir Gynecol 57:621, 1968
4. Fox H: Pathology of the placenta. Philadelphia, Saunders, 1978, pp 426–457
5. Pritchard JA, Macdonald PC: Williams Obstetrics, 16th ed. New York, Appleton-Century-Crofts, 1980
6. Browne FJ: On the abnormalities of the umbilical cord which may cause antenatal death. J Obstet Gynaecol Br Emp 32:17, 1925

7. Kamina P, DeTourris H: The diagnosis of umbilical cord complications with the help of ultrasonic tomography. Electromedica 2:77, 50, 1977

8. Walker CW, Pye BG: The length of the human umbilical cord: A statistical report. Brit Med J 1:546, 1960

9. Spellacy WN, Gravem H, et al: The umbilical cord complications of true knots, nuchal coils and cords around the body. Am J Obstet Gynecol 94:1136, 1966

10. Vintzileos AM, Nochimson DJ, et al: Ultrasonic diagnosis of funic presentation. J Clin Ultrasound 11:510, 1983

11. Jouppila P, Kirkinen P: Ultrasonic diagnosis of nuchal encirclement by the umbilical cord: A case and methodological report. J Clin Ultrasound 10:59, 1982

12. Bernischke K, Driscoll SG: The Pathology of the Human Placenta. New York, Springer, 1967

13. Jassani MN, Brennan JN, et al: Prenatal diagnosis of single umbilical artery by ultrasound. J Clin Ultrasound 8:447, 1980

14. Peckham CH, Yerushalmy J: Aplasia of one umbilical artery: Incidence by race and certain obstetric factors. Obstet Gynecol 26:359, 1965

15. Froehlich LA, Fujikura T: Significance of a single umbilical artery. Am J Obstet Gynecol 94:274, 1966

16. Froehlich L, Fujikura T: Follow-up of infants with single umbilical artery. Pediatrics 52:6, 1973

17. Bryan EM, Kohler HG: The missing umbilical artery. II. Pediatric follow-up. Arch Dis Child 50:714, 1975

18. Roberts-Thomson ME: The hazards of umbilical cord haematoma. Med J Aust 1:648, 1973

19. Ruvinsky ED, Wiley TL, et al: In utero diagnosis of umbilical cord hematoma by ultrasonography. Am J Obstet Gynecol 140:833, 1981

20. Dippel AL: Hematomas of the umbilical cord. Surg Gynecol Obstet 70:51, 1940

21. Sachs L, Fourcroy JL, et al: Prenatal detection of umbilical cord Allantoic cyst. Radiol 145:445, 1982

22. Novak ER, Woodruff JD: Novaks Gynecologic and Obstetric Pathology. Philadelphia, Saunders, 1967

23. Barnson AJ, Donnai P, et. al: Hemangioma of the cord: Further cause of raised maternal serum and liquor alpha-fetoprotein. B Med J 281:1251, 1980

24. Bell MJ: Umbilical and other abdominal wall hernias, in Holder TM and Ashcroft KW (eds), Pediatric Surgery. Philadelphia, W.B. Saunders, 1980

25. Crump EP: Umbilical hernia: I. Occurrence of the infantile type in negro infants and children. J Pediatr 40:214, 1952

26. Evans A: The comparative incidence of umbilical hernias in colored and white infants. J Natl Med Assoc 33:158, 1941

27. Jackson DJ, Moglen LH: Umbilical hernia: A retrospective study. Calif Med 113:8, 1970

28. Mayden K: The umbilical vein diameter in Rhesus isoimmunization. Med Ultrasound 4:119, 1980

29. DeVore GR, Mayden K, et al: Dilatation of the fetal umbilical vein in rhesus hemolytic anemia: A predictor of severe disease. Am J Obstet Gynecol 141:464, 1981

30. Witter FR, Graham D: The utility of ultrasonically measured umbilical vein diameters in isoimmunized pregnancies. Am J Obstet Gynecol 146:225, 1983

28 | Amniocentesis: Current Concepts and Techniques

Lawrence D. Platt
Lynden M. Hill
Greggory R. DeVore

Amniocentesis was first suggested more than 90 years ago by Schatz.[1] However, it was not until 1919 that Hinkel described a patient with polyhydramnios in whom transabdominal amniocentesis was used to relieve an overdistended uterus.[1] During the next 30 years, interest in amniocentesis was sporadic because the diagnostic usefulness of obtaining amniotic fluid was limited. At that time, amniotic fluid was believed to be a stagnant pool protecting the fetus but having no properties of clinical value.

Studies within the last decade, however, have emphasized a complex interrelationship between mother and fetus in the formation and rapid turnover of amniotic fluid which has resulted in a number of clinical applications. In the early 1950s, Beevis[2] reported his work on the amniotic fluid of Rh-sensitized women. In the 1960s, Mandelbaum utilized bilirubin content in the amniotic fluid as a means to assess fetal maturity.[3] In 1971, Gluck and Kulavich[4] developed the lecithin–sphinglemyelin ratio to measure pulmonary maturity from a sample of amniotic fluid. Since then it has become the standard test against which other predictors of fetal maturity (shake test, felma or microviscometry, Foam Stabilization Index, and ultrasound) must be compared. After the development of amniotic fluid cell culture techniques, amniocentesis was extended to the second trimester in order to detect fetal chromosomal and biochemical abnormalities.

The use of amniocentesis has increased exponentially since 1970. In the next few years, with the increasing use of maternal serum α-fetoprotein (AFP) screening for neural tube defects, this rise will certainly continue when amniocentesis is performed for evalua-

tion of amniotic fluid AFP. Although amniocentesis had been performed for a number of years prior to the wide scale availability of ultrasound, the advantages of sonography in conjunction with this procedure are now apparent to the obstetrician.[5-7]

SECOND TRIMESTER AMNIOCENTESIS

Amniocentesis may be performed as early as the 14th week from the last menstrual period. However, both the volume of amniotic fluid and the percent of viable cells present within the fluid are limited.[6] As a result, we believe the ideal gestational age for genetic amniocentesis to be 16 to 18 weeks of menstrual age.

The average time needed for determination of fetal karyotype during the past few years has changed. For example, at Los Angeles County/USC Medical Center, the average time was about 13 to 14 days 1 year ago. More recently, this has shortened considerably. At the Genetics Institute, a regional laboratory, the average time for specimen preparation is currently 8.7 days. At the Mayo Clinic, it is 16 ($\pm$ 3) days when samples are obtained on the premises. Amniotic fluid sent via the mail from surrounding areas is 20 ($\pm$ 6) days. The Mayo Clinic experience seems to emphasize the advantage of transporting the patient, rather than the amniotic fluid sample, to the institute performing the cell culture. However, this has not been the case at the Genetics Institute in Alhambra, California.

It is obvious that no set plan of management for these patients can be followed in all medical centers. There are some centers in which a preliminary examination and counseling session are performed around the 12th week from the LMP. At this time, an ultrasound examination will determine fetal viability and confirm the patient's dates. Based upon this examination, a date for the amniocentesis is given. Other institutions, including our own, have found it useful to perform the counseling session and the ultrasound examination at around the 17th week of gestation. In this fashion, the patient is spared extra waiting and requires only one appointment for both of these procedures. In spite of the fact that the vast majority of women referred to our program request amniocentesis for maternal age, either a geneticist or genetic associate counsels every patient. Each patient is afforded a full genetic evaluation and a pedigree is obtained. It is not unusual to obtain other information that demonstrates the need for a more detailed examination or a possible need for further tests such as fetoscopy or biochemical testing of the amniotic fluid.

During the past few years, results obtained with ultrasound prior to second trimester amniocentesis have been conflicting. Although some studies report a marked reduction in the failure rate, incidence of multiple needle insertions and proportion of bloody taps,[8] others do not.[9] There appears to be a variety of explanations for these observations, including the interval between the ultrasound and amniocentesis, the person performing the ultrasound, the person performing the amniocentesis, and whether or not ultrasound-guided amniocentesis was used. At our respective institutions, both the ultrasound and amniocentesis are performed by the same individual. Thus, we feel that this additional hand/eye coordination reduces the risk of the procedure, the incidence of bloody taps and multiple punctures.[7,10,11]

At the time of the amniocentesis, fetal viability, placental localization, and the quantity of amniotic fluid are evaluated. Obvious congenital malformations may be detected and the presence or absence of twins determined. We have utilized linear-array real-time ultrasound exclusively for the past 6 years and have found this to be a major advantage in determining the site for amniocentesis and in actually carrying out the procedure.

Criteria for a safe amniocentesis site include (1) the absence of fetal trunk or vertex, (2) avoidance of the placenta, (3) an adequate pocket of amniotic fluid, and (4) as close to the midline abdominal position for the needle insertion as possible. Previously,[7] we described a technique for identification of an amniocentesis site with real-time ultrasound. In that technique, the real-time transducer identified an ideal site away from the fetus and where the largest pocket of fluid was found. The site was marked with the backside

of a needle, the abdomen was then wiped dry, and the skin prepped. The needle, was placed to the depth determined by the ultrasound examination. Following the amniocentesis, the fetus was revisualized with ultrasound to confirm fetal viability.

Recently, however, we have demonstrated[12] that the use of a direct ultrasound guidance technique is superior to the above described method. Using this approach, ultrasound is used to identify the ideal tap site away from the fetus and placenta with the largest pocket of amniotic fluid. With the transducer still directed at that site, the skin is prepped with an iodine solution, the transducer doubly draped, and, under real-time guidance, the needle inserted into the amniotic cavity, with the tip of the needle being clearly identified on the monitor screen. We have chosen to utilize local anesthetic because this allows for the controlled placement of the needle. Real-time-directed amniocentesis has been used successfully in over 2000 amniocenteses with a marked reduction in the number of multiple punctures, and almost entirely eliminated bloody or failed taps. In the authors' personal experience (LDP, GRD) there have been no failed amniocenteses during the past 2 years with this technique. Additional advantages of the ultrasound-guided technique allow for fetal manipulation when fetal parts continue to be in the way of the proposed site of amniocentesis.

Often, there seems to be insufficient amounts of fluid at 16 to 17 weeks and the patient is asked to return in 1 week, at which time we have found this procedure to be much simpler. Additionally, an anterior placenta may be present in up to 40 percent of the cases. Hence, the criteria outlined for a safe tap may not be adequately fulfilled. The patient should be advised when the placenta must be traversed in order to obtain a specimen of amniotic fluid since this risk of the procedure appears to be increased.[13] Far lateral taps are restricted because of the presence of the uterine vessels. Occasionally, we have found that either emptying or filling the bladder seems to add to the rotation of the uterus and a clear site appears to become present. It has not been our policy to expect the patient to come to our office with a full bladder. We simply ask her not to void prior to the visit. In this fashion, we can fill or empty the bladder depending upon the need. Although the technique of bladder filling appears to be helpful in those cases in which a site clear of the placenta cannot be determined, it is clear that without direct ultrasound guidance, some difficulty was encountered when patients were asked to void following the site location. It is, therefore, compulsory to either scan the patient again to determine the site location, or leave the bladder full. Naturally,

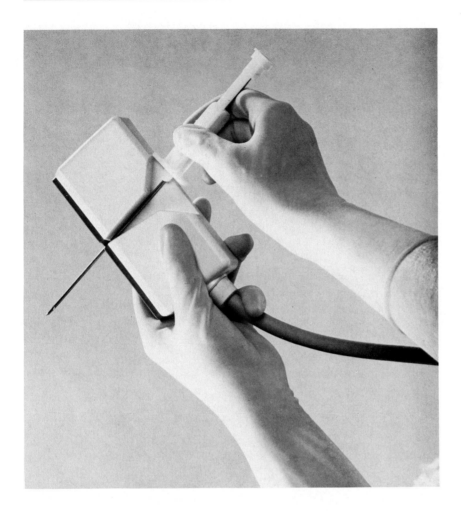

Fig. 1. A linear array transducer with a through transducer needle guide.

the concern that the site be selected away from the bladder is real. Lower quadrant or suprapubic taps, when not preceded by bladder emptying, can lead to inadvertent bladder aspiration.

Some authors recommend the use of needle-guiding transducers. A variety of transducers have been developed for that technique (Fig. 1). The earliest included transducers for static B-scan, which had a mid-bore site and the needle could be easily followed on either the A-scan or static B-scan. Several manufacturers have developed needle guides for linear-array transducers, but these proved to be either bulky or not worthwhile as they require sterilization after each procedure. In our own laboratory, it is not unusual to perform up to 15 procedures a day and this would either require many transducers or a significant delay between procedures. To overcome this, several manufacturers have created side-pods, but not all of the obstacles were overcome. Several of the sector transducers have disposable guides with a glove technique (Fig. 2), and these have proved to be useful for some investigators. Our technique appears to be most useful, as it can be utilized without the additional need of

transducers or guides. A glove or sterile surgical drape, coupled with sterile ultrasound gel, which is readily available (Fig. 3), can be utilized to further ensure the sterility of the procedure.

ANESTHESIA

There does not appear to be a uniform recommendation upon the use of local anesthetic. It has been our personal preference to use local anesthesia, as it not only offers definite pain relief but seems to add an additional psychologic component to many patients who recognize that the physician is attempting to do all in his/her power to eliminate discomfort secondary to the procedure. We recommend that a small needle be used to create a skin wheel and then inject down to the peritoneum, but not to the level of the uterus, where myometrial contractions can be rapidly stimulated with the use of a local anesthetic. By continually talking to the patient during the procedure, additional psychologic support can be offered. It is our belief that, with local anesthetic, readjustment of the needle can be done

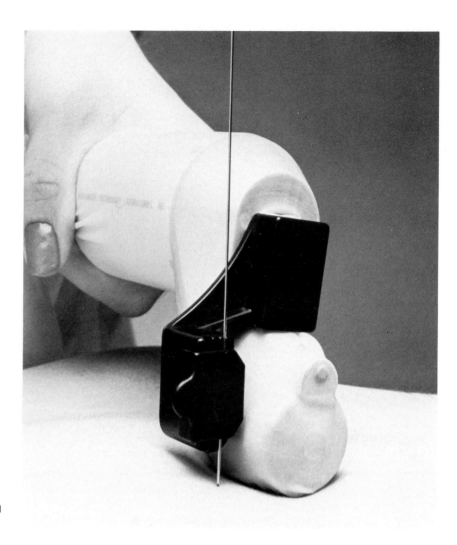

Fig. 2. A sector transducer with laterally placed needle guide.

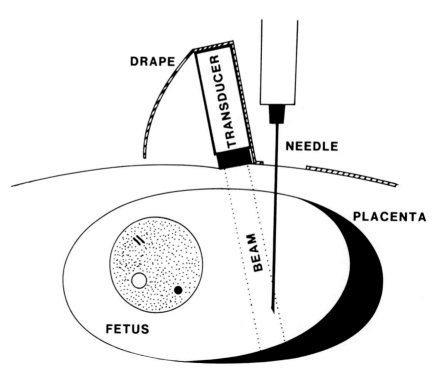

Fig. 3. Schematic of the transducer placed with its relationship to the needle.

with a greater degree of ease should the need arise. The use of local anesthetic also allows for a more controlled needle placement under ultrasound guidance.

NEEDLE SELECTION AND PLACEMENT

All of our amniocentesis procedures are carried out with disposal 20 gauge, 9-cm length needles. Other centers have chosen a smaller needle, a 22 gauge, for this technique. Occasionally, large, obese patients may require a longer needle. This can be determined prior to the performance of the amniocentesis by measuring the depth of insertion identified on the ultrasound oscilliscope. Occasionally, the membranes may be pushed ahead and a "membrane tenting" may be produced.[12] This yields a dry tap unless the needle is withdrawn slightly and advanced in a rapid fashion. Once the needle is inserted into the amniotic cavity, the stylette is withdrawn and several droplets of the fluid allowed to run from the hub of the needle in order to reduce contamination from maternal cells. Some investigators have recommended that 3 ml of fluid first be obtained and discarded because of potential contamination. This has not proven necessary in our own experience of more than 3000 amniocenteses, where we simply discard one to two drops. Although this may have previously been a problem, [14-16] the growth of maternal cells has been nonexistent in our laboratory.

Although the Los Angeles County laboratory has successfully cultured cells from as little as 6 to 7 ml and the Mayo Clinic as little as 3 ml of amniotic fluid, we routinely try to obtain 20 to 25 ml in a single syringe. To prevent needle tracks from occurring, some authors advocate the replacement of the stylette into the needle prior to withdrawing the needle.

In order to avoid the possibility of bacterial contamination, some laboratories recommend that the specimen be transported immediately to the laboratory within the syringe that was used for the procedure. We have not found this necessary, have routinely placed the fluid into plastic disposable tubes, and are not aware of any problems with bacterial contamination.

PATIENT RESPONSE

The patient will occasionally feel intermittent cramping or experience high leakage of fluid following a second trimester amniocentesis, which should gradually resolve within 48 hours. Patients have often experienced pain in the groin area on the side in which the needle is being inserted. Other patients have experienced a pressure or pain sensation in the vaginal vault during the procedure. This referred pain appears to be dependent upon the site of insertion.

Amnionitis following amniocentesis can be severe and can lead to a necessary interruption of pregnancy. All signs that suggest this process must be carefully evaluated. Each Rh-negative unsensitized woman whose husband is Rh-positive or whose blood type is unknown receives Rh immune globulin.[17] We have found at least a threefold increase in sensitization following genetic amniocentesis if this is not done.

At one time, twins were considered a contraindication to second trimester amniocentesis.[11] However, amniocentesis can be safely performed in multiple gestation. In most cases, a membrane can be recognized between the fetuses in the second trimester (Fig. 4). Thus, two separate sites for amniocentesis may be selected. The procedure for twins is as follows: A site for the first amniocentesis is determined. Following successful removal of fluid, one-half ml of indigo carmine dye is instilled into the amniotic cavity and the uterus is moved about. The patient may be asked to stand up and move about in order to disburse the dye within the amniotic sac. The patient is then rescanned, and a second site distant from the first on the opposite side of the membrane is selected. Once again under ultrasound guidance, the second sac is tapped. Clear fluid from the second sac indicates successful puncture. If the dye is identified, this represents a puncture of the first sac. Methylene blue should not be utilized, as this has been demonstrated to lead to hemolysis of red cells in the fetus or newborn.

Over the past 3 years, we have evaluated 20 sets of twins in our practice. Because of the increased chance of discordance and the difficulty in selecting what the patient would do if one fetus was abnormal, four families declined amniocentesis. Amniocentesis was successfully carried out in all instances where it was attempted and no fetal morbidity or mortality occurred in this group. The importance of performing twin amniocentesis in the second trimester has been demonstrated in several studies.[18,19] Discordance for chromosomal abnormalities or biochemical disorders has been recognized. Selective termination of one of two twins has been performed in the Scandinavian countries, in the United Kingdom, as well as in North America. Although this process raises many ethical and moral issues, the decision, at present, must remain with the physician and patient.

ALTERNATIVES TO SECOND TRIMESTER AMNIOCENTESIS

Current studies are under way at many medical centers to evaluate the role of transcervical chorionic villi

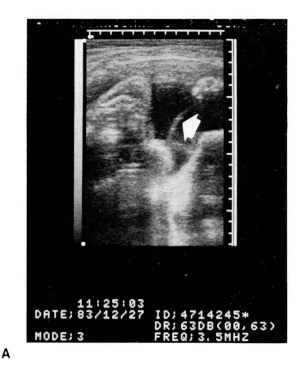

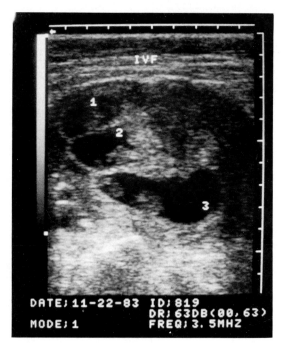

A   **B**

Fig. 4. A. Demonstrates twin membrane (*arrow*). **B.** Real-time image of a triplet pregnancy with membranes seen.

biopsy. This technique involves obtaining tissue in the first trimester of pregnancy for chromosomal and biochemical analysis. The technique holds promise as the method of choice for prenatal diagnosis.

Several methods have been described. The blind approach attempts to aspirate trophoblastic tissue via catheter without the benefit of either fetoscope or ultrasound guidance. Not surprisingly, this method produces less than 50 percent positive samples. Another method involves the use of fiberoptic fetoscope to identify the ideal site for aspiration. Finally, a technique has recently been employed that utilizes real-time ultrasound to guide the catheter to the ideal site (Fig. 5). Preliminary studies demonstrate the method to be highly effective in obtaining an adequate sample.[20]

THIRD TRIMESTER AMNIOCENTESIS

Prior to the wide-scale utilization of ultrasound, only three sites were recommended for third trimester amniocentesis: (1) suprapubic; (2) in the area of the fetal small parts; and (3) nuchal. Each had its own advantages and disadvantages. If a suprapubic site is selected, occasionally the presenting part cannot be elevated or the placenta may be unknowingly penetrated. Characteristically, the fetal back is along one side of the uterus and the placenta along the other. Thus, if the placenta is anterior, amniocentesis in the area of the small parts may, likewise, result in placental laceration and subsequent hemorrhage. The pocket of fluid about the nuchal area is small. Occasionally, an assistant can pull the vertex toward the midline, thus preventing a tap from occurring too far laterally. If the umbilical cord is around the fetal neck, it will be immobilized and, hence, more likely to be penetrated than if it were free floating.[21]

Ultrasound has given the obstetrician the ability to select the safest site after evaluating fetal and cord position, placental localization, and the presence of a sufficient pocket of amniotic fluid. In Figure 6, the site of cord implantation may be readily appreciated, whereas Figure 7 illustrates a large vessel traversing the placenta close to the cord insertion. Hence, a site away from this area will reduce the risk of vessel laceration and hemorrhage should transplacental amniocentesis be necessary. When this does occur, the smallest needle required to perform amniocentesis should be utilized (22 gauge). The technique is the same as described above for second trimester amniocentesis. If the placenta is located posteriorly (Fig. 8), amniocentesis is usually performed without difficulty. When a placenta does not cover the full anterior wall of the uterus, a safe area is rapidly identified. Lateral pockets of amniotic fluid may be approached directly (Fig. 9) or from a more medial position, thus avoiding the uterine vessels.

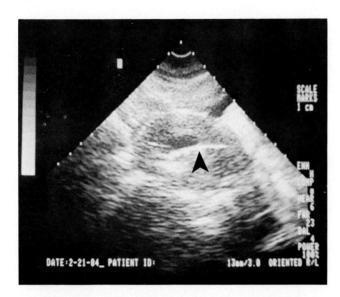

Fig. 5. Catheter tip seen in the area of the chorionic villi (*arrowhead*).

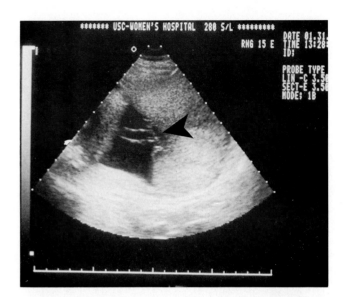

Fig. 6. Scan of the placenta with cord insertion easily seen (*arrowhead*).

OTHER INDICATIONS

Two new indications for second trimester amniocentesis have become apparent; premature labor and premature rupture of the membranes. In both of these, not only are fetal maturity studies evaluated, but so too is the presence of bacteria and white cells in the amniotic fluid. In both situations, the use of amniocentesis has been shown to be helpful in identifying those patients in whom fetal lung maturation is present and in whom the etiology of premature rupture of membranes or premature labor can be determined. It has been recognized that infection has been related to both of these problems. Upon obtaining amniotic fluid with careful ultrasound guidance, the amniotic fluid is evaluated for bacteria and white cells by performing a Gram stain. If identified, these pregnancies are usually interrupted. Conversely, in the absence of any abnormal Gram stain and negative culture, these pregnancies have been shown to be safely prolonged, with improved fetal outcome.

Finally, sonography may also provide information necessary to prevent useless attempts at amniocentesis. Figure 10 is a transverse scan of a severely growth retarded fetus at term. The fetal body is closely aligned against the placenta and uterine side walls. There appears to be no safe amniotic fluid site available for sampling. This case can be managed clinically without an almost certainly futile and dangerous attempt at amniocentesis. It must be emphasized that small pockets of fluid also lead to increased risk of injury. One recent case of a severely growth retarded infant with a very small fluid pocket in the nuchal area led to a

laceration of the eyelid (Fig. 11). Table 1 outlines some of the complications that have been reported with second and third trimester amniocentesis.

SAFETY AND COMPLICATIONS OF AMNIOCENTESIS

To date, there have been three large collaborative studies that have evaluated genetic amniocentesis. The Na-

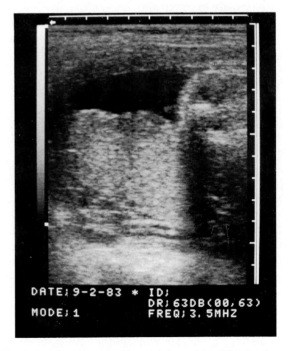

Fig. 7. Anterior placenta with no obvious sight at this level.

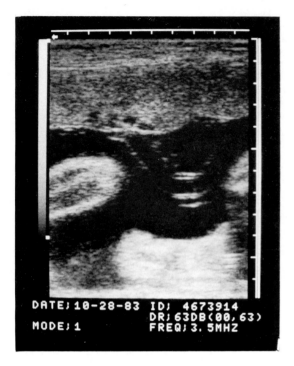

Fig. 8. Posterior placenta with adequate amounts of amniotic fluid.

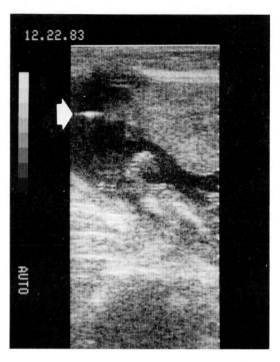

Fig. 9. A fluid pocket seen clear of placenta from the lateral surface of the uterus, (needle tip seen [*arrow*]).

tional Institute of Child Health and Human Development study included 1040 patients and 992 controls.[15] Fetal loss was the same in each group. Immediately after delivery, there was no difference in physical injuries, and at 1 year, developmental examinations could not differentiate between the two groups. In 1977, the Canadian Medical Research Council evaluated 1223 amniocenteses carried out during 1020 pregnancies.[16] They concluded, as did the former study, that the larger the needle used for amniocentesis and the more insertions required to obtain fluid, the greater the complication rate. Once again, fetal loss was no greater than in the control group. The Medical Research Council of Great Britain studied 2428 patients and a group of poorly matched controls.[22] Fetal loss was increased and occurred in 1 to 1½ percent in the subjects undergoing amniocenteses. One recent study showed a fetal loss of 16 per 1000 in experienced hands.[23] Although a dry tap occasionally occurred during the second trimester, a repeat ultrasound and attempt at amniocentesis may be rewarded with success. It has been our own personal practice not to puncture the uterus more than twice in any one day. Fortunately, we rarely have to puncture it even twice.

If blood contaminates the amniotic fluid obtained, cell growth may be impaired from a second trimester sample,[24,25] and the lecithin–sphingomyelin ratio in the later half of the pregnancy may become un-

reliable.[26] The importance of culture failures as a complication of second trimester amniocentesis has been greatly reduced in recent years. Golbus et al.[27] have reported a culture failure rate of only 1.7 percent on the first attempt in over 3000 amniocenteses. The

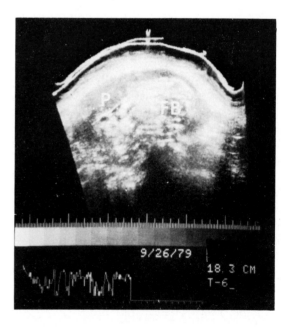

Fig. 10. Transverse scan of a fetus with intrauterine growth retardation. Note marked oligohydramnios. FB, fetal body. P, placenta.

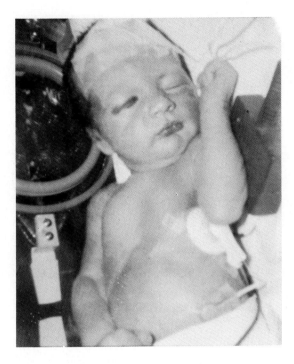

Fig. 11. Newborn infant with a right eyelid laceration secondary to a traumatic amniocentesis.

recent experiences at the Los Angeles County/USC Medical Center, Children's Hospital of Los Angeles, the Mayo Clinic, and the Genetics Institute have demonstrated an even lower culture failure rate when fluid was obtained by one of the authors.

TABLE 1
Complications of Amniocentesis

I. Failed Attempt
  A. Dry tap
  B. Bloody tap
  C. Failure of cell growth
II. Fetal
  A. Spontaneous abortion
  B. Spontaneous fetal death
  C. Trauma
  D. Exsanguination
  E. Infection
  F. Amniotic fluid leak
  G. Complete rupture of the membranes
  H. Premature rupture of the membranes
  I. Placental hematoma
  J. Subchorionic hematoma
III. Maternal
  A. Infection
  B. Premature labor
  C. Rectus hematoma
  D. Abruptio placenta
  E. Rh sensitization
  F. Death

Needle puncture of the fetus was reported from our institution in 1976 by Broom et al.[28] It is estimated that this complication may occur in 1 to 3 percent of second trimester amniocenteses.[29] Although most fetal punctures are without long-lasting sequelae, there have been reports of temporary neurologic damage[29] and gangrene of a fetal limb.[30] As a result, the possibility of fetal trauma should be mentioned during the counseling session prior to amniocentesis. We believe, however, that this complication should be significantly reduced with the use of the direct ultrasound-guiding technique.

Reports of fetal injury after third trimester amniocentesis have included pneumothorax, fetal abdominal puncture with liver or splenic trauma,[31] and myocardial penetration with cardiac tamponade.[32] Even the brain and central nervous system have been involved.[31] Cross and Maumenee[33] reported a case of ocular trauma secondary to amniocentesis. We are aware of other cases of ocular trauma, some of which fortunately have had operative correction that has restored sight.[34] Although maternal death has been reported from infection after amniocentesis, the incidence of amnionitis when strict attention to asepsis is adherred to, is less than 1/1000.[15,16] We are aware of a case of bacterial endocarditis following amniocentesis: this occurred in spite of strict attention to asepsis.

The incidence of amniotic fluid leakage per vagina after amniocentesis is reported to be between 1 and 1½ percent.[15,16] In our experience, this number appears high.

Fetal bleeding has been reported to occur in approximately 2 to 3 percent of amniocenteses. Mennutti and others[23] have demonstrated an elevation of the α-fetoprotein following amniocentesis in up to 14 percent of cases. This may represent evidence for fetal maternal bleeding. Umbilical cord laceration is one etiology of fetal hemorrhage that could rapidly be fatal. When bloody amniotic fluid is obtained during the third trimester amniocentesis, its origin should be determined. One can perform a Kleihauer Betke test or an Apt test, which will determine the origin of the fetal blood. If it is fetal, heart rate monitoring should be initiated. A tachycardia followed by a bradycardia with intermittent decelerations is presumptive evidence of significant fetal hemorrhage, and delivery is indicated.[34,35]

Others have identified the laceration in the cord and the stream of blood projecting from the cord on ultrasound guidance. If the fetus is found to be immature and a bloody tap is identified, careful in-hospital evaluation with continuous fetal monitoring should be carried out in order to prevent intrauterine fetal death. Fetal death and other vascular injuries have been reported after second trimester amniocentesis;[35] however, the incidence of this complication appears to be rare. Fetal activity[36,37] may be affected by amniocentesis. In addition, uterine contractility[38] appears to increase after third trimester amniocentesis. The normal fetal response is heart rate acceleration. This appears to be a valuable indicator of fetal well being. A pathologic response or lack of accelerations or decelerations is associated with a higher incidence of fetal distress.[39,40] Premature labor must be considered as a complication of amniocentesis.[41] Although Terramo and Sipinen[42] have noted an increased incidence of spontaneous rupture of fetal membranes dependent upon site of amniocentesis, others have not.[43] This may be explained by Terramo and Sipinen's mean time from amniocentesis to ruptured membranes of 22.9 days. This appears to include those cases of ruptured membranes that occurred at a time when it would otherwise have been expected. Maternal rectus,[41] placental and subchronic hematomas,[44] as well as abruptio placenta,[45] have all been previously reported. Figure 12 illustrates a rectus hematoma that developed immediately after second trimester amniocentesis.

Fetal/maternal hemorrhage after amniocentesis has been reported by a number of investigators.[11,46] In our own unpublished study, these data have been substantiated. Additionally, we have found that, in a group of patients at risk for Rh sensitization, there is almost a threefold increase in patients becoming sensitized following amniocentesis.[17] Therefore, we have recommended the use of Rh immune globulin, 150 to 300 μg following amniocentesis in unsensitized women. Because of the further chance of antibody enhancement, we now recommend a booster dose at 28 weeks in those patients receiving the Rh immune globulin at the time of a second trimester amniocentesis. Other investigators have not agreed with this viewpoint.[47] Direct fetal death has been observed following genetic amniocentesis in as high as 3/2000 in 1 series.[35] In our own experience, we have been fortunate in not observing this phenomenon. Occasionally, however, we have observed what appears to be a cardiac standstill, at which time we place the patient on her side: in one instance, after revisualization, to our relief, cardiac activity was present.

The rate of complications has clearly been shown to be a product of one's experience. Hecht[48] has shown that the fewer amnioceteses performed by the operator, the greater the chance of spontaneous abortion or other complications. It is, therefore, our recommendation that amniocentesis be carried out by a select group of people trained both in amniocentesis and ultrasound. In this fashion, the hand-to-eye coordination will allow for an ideal procedure at a minimum risk for the patient.

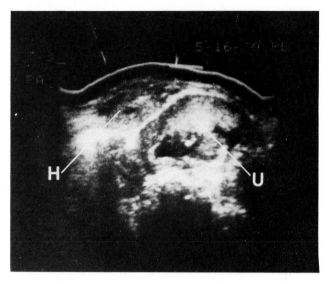

Fig. 12. Transverse scan after amniocentesis at 16 weeks of gestation. A rectus hematoma (H) impinging upon the uterus (U).

This chapter has outlined the authors' experiences with ultrasound as an aid to diagnostic amniocentesis in the second and third trimesters of pregnancy. The technique that has been developed permits a skilled physician to obtain the desired information safely and quickly. With thoughtful regard for the complications that might ensue, knowing when not to attempt a difficult amniocentesis becomes as important as understanding when the procedure is indicated.

REFERENCES

1. Scrimgeour JB: Amniocentesis: Technique and complications, in Emery AEH (ed): Antenatal Diagnosis of Genetic Disease. Baltimore, Williams & Wilkins, 1973, pp 11–39
2. Bevis DCA: Composition of liquor amnii in haemolytic disease of newborn. Lancet 2:443, 1950
3. Hytten FE, Lind T: Diagnostic Indices in Pregnancy. Basel, Ciba-Beigy, 1973, pp 95–116
4. Gluck L, Kulovich MV, Borer RC Jr, et al: Diagnosis of the respiratory distress syndrome by amniocentesis. Am J Obstet Gynecol 109:440, 1971
5. Chandra P, Nitowsky HM, Marion R, et al: Experience with sonography as an adjunct to amniocentesis for prenatal diagnosis of fetal genetic disorders. Am J Obstet Gynecol 133:519, 1979
6. Nelson MM: Antenatal sex determination, in Emery AEH (ed): Antenatal Diagnosis of Genetic Disease. Baltimore, Williams & Wilkins, 1973, pp 58–68
7. Platt LD, Manning FA, Lemay M: Real time B-scan directed amniocentesis. Am J Obstet Gynecol 130:700, 1978
8. Crandon AJ, Peel KR: Amniocentesis with and without ultrasound guidance. Br J Obstet Gynaecol 86:1, 1979

9. Levine SC, Filly RA, Golbus MS: Ultrasonography for guidance of amniocentesis in genetic counseling. Clin Genet 14:133, 1978

10. Kerenyi TD, Walker B: The preventability of "bloody taps" in second trimester amniocentesis by ultrasound scanning. Obstet Gynecol 50:61, 1977

11. Bartsch FK, Lundberg J, Wahlstrom J: The technique, results and risks of amniocentesis for genetic reasons. J Obstet Gynaecol Br Commonw 81:991, 1974

12. Platt LD, DeVore GR, Gimovsky ML: Failed amniocentesis: The role of membrane tenting. Am J Obstet Gynecol 144:733, 1982

13. Mennuti MT, Brummond W, Crombleholme WR, et al: Fetal–maternal bleeding associated with genetic amniocentesis. Obstet Gynecol 55:48, 1980

14. Robinson A, Bowes W, Droegemuller W, et al: Intrauterine diagnosis: Potential complications. Am J Obstet Gynecol 116:937, 1973

15. The NICHD National Registry for Amniocentesis Study Group: Midtrimester amniocentesis for prenatal diagnosis: Safety and accuracy. JAMA 236:1471, 1976

16. Simpson NE, Dallaire L, Miller JR, et al: Prenatal diagnosis of genetic disease in Canada: Report of a collaborative study. Can Med Assoc J 115:739, 1976

17. Hill LM, Platt LD, Kellogg B: Rh sensitization after genetic amniocentesis. Obstet Gynecol 56:459, 1980

18. Bovicelli L, Michelacci L, Rizzo N, Orsini LF, Pilu G, Montacuti V, Bacchetta M, Pittalis MC: Genetic amniocentesis in twin pregnancy. Prenatal Diagnosis 3:101, 1983

19. Palle C, Andersen JW, Tabor A, Lauritsen JG, Bang J, Philip J: Increased risk of abortion after genetic amniocentesis in twin pregnancies. Prenatal Diagnosis 3:83, 1983

20. Simmoni G, Brambati B, Danesino C, Rossella F, Terzoli GL, Ferrari M, Fraccaro M: Efficient direct chromosome analyses and enzyme determinations from chorionic villi samples in the first trimester of pregnancy. Hum Genet 63:349, 1983

21. Gassner CP, Paul RH: Laceration of umbilical cord vessels secondary to amniocentesis. Obstet Gynecol 48:627, 1976

22. Chayen S: An assessment of the hazards of amniocentesis. Br J Obstet Gynaecol 85:2:1, 1978

23. Mennuti MT, DiGaetano A, McDonnell A, Arnold BS, Cohen W, Liston RM: Fetal-maternal bleeding associated with genetic amniocentesis: Real-time versus static ultrasound. Obstet Gynecol 62:26, 1983

24. Leschot NJ, Treffers PE, Verjaal M, et al: Prenatal diagnosis of congenital malformations in 500 pregnancies. Eur J Obstet Gynaecol Reprod Biol 9:13, 1979

25. Young PE, Matson MR, Jones OW: Amniocentesis for antenatal diagnosis: Review of problems and outcomes in a large series. Am J Obstet Gynecol 125:495, 1976

26. Hallman M, Kulovich M, Kirkpatrick E, et al: Phosphatidylinositol and phosphatidyglycerol in amniotic fluid: Indices of lung maturity. Am J Obstet Gynecol 125:613, 1976

27. Golbus MS, Loughman WD, Epstein CJ, et al: Prenatal genetic diagnosis in 3000 amniocenteses. N Engl J Med 300:157, 1979

28. Broome DL, Wilson MG, Weiss B, et al: Needle puncture of fetus: A complication of second-trimester amniocentesis. Am J Obstet Gynecol 126:247, 1976

29. Karp LE, Hayden PW: Fetal puncture during midtrimester amniocentesis. Obstet Gynecol 49:115, 1977

30. Lamb MP: Gangrene of a fetal limb due to amniocentesis. Br J Obstet Gynaecol 82:829, 1975

31. Creasman WT, Lawrence RA, Thiede HA: Fetal complications of amniocentesis. JAMA 204:949, 1968

32. Berner HW, Seisler EP, Barlow J: Fetal cardiac tamponade: A complication of amniocentesis. Obstet Gynecol 40:599, 1972

33. Cross HE, Maumenee AE: Ocular trauma during amniocentesis. Letter to the Editor. N Engl J Med 287:993, 1972

34. Gabbe SG, Nelson LM, Paul RH: Fetal heart rate response to acute hemorrhage. Obstet Gynecol 49:247, 1977

35. Young PE, Matson MR, Jones OW: Fetal exsanguination and other vascular injuries from midtrimester genetic amniocentesis. Am J Obstet Gynecol 129:21, 1977

36. Hill LM, Platt LD, Manning FA: Immediate effect of amniocentesis on fetal breathing and gross body movements. Am J Obstet Gynecol 135:689, 1979

37. Platt LD, Lenke R, Sipos L: Amniocentesis in the second trimester: The effect on fetal movement. Am J Obstet Gynecol 140:758, 1981

38. Linzey EM, Freeman RK: Fetal monitoring: Antepartum fetal monitoring. Yearbook Obstet Gynecol 1978, pp 85–110

39. Ron M, Yaffe H, Sadovsky E: Fetal heart rate response to amniocentesis in cases of decreased fetal movements. Obstet Gynecol 48:456, 1976

40. Harrigan JT, Marino JF: Fetal heart rate reaction to amniocentesis as an indicator of fetal well-being. Am J Obstet Gynecol 132:49, 1978

41. Schwarz RH: Amniocentesis. Clin Obstet Gynecol 18:1, 1975

42. Teramo K, Sipinen S: Spontaneous rupture of fetal membranes after amniocentesis. Obstet Gynecol 52:272, 1978

43. Gordon HR, Deukmedjian AG: Suprapubic vs periumbilical amniocentesis. Am J Obstet Gynecol 122:287, 1975

44. Picker RH, Smith DH, Saunders DM, et al: A review of 2,003 consecutive amniocenteses performed under ultrasonic control in late pregnancy. Aust NZ J Obstet Gynaecol 19:83, 1979

45. Bennett MJ: The technique and complications of amniocentesis. S Afr Med J 46:1545, 1972

46. Queenan JT, Adams DW: Amniocentesis: A possible immunizing hazard. Obstet Gynecol 24:530, 1964

47. Hensleigh R: Preventing rhesus isoimmunization. Am J Obstet Gynecol 146:749, 1983

48. Hecht F: The physician as a risk factor in mid trimester amniocentesis. Letter to the Editor. N Engl J Med 306:1553, 1982

49. Isenberg S: Personal communication

29 | Sonography of Trophoblastic Diseases

Arthur C. Fleischer
Howard W. Jones III
A. Everette James, Jr.

Sonography has an important role in the evaluation of patients with gestational trophoblastic disease. Gestational trophoblastic diseases (GTD) are a group of disorders that are thought to result from a combination of male and female gametes whereas non-gestational trophoblastic disease such as testicular or ovarian choriocarcinoma do not involve a gestational event. Trophoblastic neoplasms arise from the trophoblastic elements of the developing blastocyst and thus retain certain inherent characteristics such as invasive tendencies and the ability to synthesize human chorionic gonadotropin (hCG).

Gestational trophoblastic disease has been classified in a variety of ways according to either its histopathologic or clinical manifestations. The multiple classification schemes have probably contributed to confusion among obstetricians and sonologists concerning the sonographic categorization of these diseases. In this chapter, the sonographic features of the various types of gestational trophoblastic diseases are presented relative to the most widely accepted schema for pathologic and clinical classifications (Table 1).

The role of sonography in gestational trophoblastic disease is greatest in establishing the diagnosis of hydatidiform mole.[1] A characteristic sonographic appearance of hydropic villi occurs with most molar pregnancies. Sonography is considered an important adjunctive test to serial β-hCG assays in malignant trophoblastic disease since the size of the tumor and the presence of distant metastases can be ascertained.[2]

This chapter discusses and illustrates the various sonographic appearances of gestational trophoblastic diseases according to their pathologic and clinical ap-

pearance. Since the sonographic features of an invasive mole and choriocarcinoma are similar, they will be presented under the same heading. Accordingly, the discussion portion of this chapter will be divided into the two major categories of GTD—molar pregnancies, and invasive mole and choriocarcinoma. Although it may be difficult to differentiate the various pathologic types of gestational trophoblastic disorders by their sonographic features alone, the combination of clinical, laboratory, and sonographic findings can usually specify the type and extent of trophoblastic disease that is present.

CLASSIFICATION SCHEMES

Histopathologic

There are presently two different classification schema for gestational trophoblastic disease (Table 1). The older, histopathologic scheme divides trophoblastic disease into hydatidiform mole, invasive mole (chorioadenoma destruens), and choriocarcinoma. Hydatidiform mole is characterized by marked edema and enlargement of the chorionic villi, which is the characteristic that allows sonographic identification. This is accompanied by disappearance of the villous blood vessels and proliferation of trophoblast (or "trophoblastic cells") that line the villi (Fig. 1). Although moles with an abundantly proliferative trophoblast have a greater likelihood of being malignant, it is not possible to accurately predict on the basis of histologic appearance the malignant potential of a given mole. Approximately 20 percent of complete moles are followed by

TABLE 1
Classification Schemas for Gestational Trophoblastic Disease

Pathologic	Clinical

Hydatidiform mole
    Complete
    Partial
    With coexistent fetus
	Benign trophoblastic disease

Invasive mole
    (chorioadenoma destruens)
	Malignant, nonmetastatic
	    trophoblastic disease

Choriocarcinoma	Malignant, metastatic trophoblastic disease

Adapted from Jones Jr H: Gestational trophoblastic disease, in Jones III H, Jones S (eds), Novak's Textbook of Gynecology, 10th ed., Baltimore, Williams and Wilkens, 1981, pp 659–689.

malignant sequelae of invasive mole or choriocarcinoma.[3] The histopathologic classification of hydatidiform mole has not proven to be an accurate prognostic indication to select the 20 percent of patients with a molar pregnancy who will subsequently develop malignant disease.[4]

Invasive mole is the term given to trophoblastic invasion into the myometrium of the uterus. Edematous villi within the myometrium are apparent on microscopic inspection of the tissue. Histologically, there is abundant trophoblastic proliferation with hemorrhage and necrosis of the myometrium. Since hysterectomy is rarely used in the treatment of gestational trophoblastic disease today, the diagnosis of an invasive mole is rarely made at surgical pathology.

Choriocarcinoma is characterized by sheets of highly malignant trophoblast with no villous structures (Fig. 2). It is a widely metastatic lesion that accounts for 5 percent of all gestational trophoblastic diseases.[4] Local pelvic metastases and lung metastases are most common, but liver, brain, kidney, and bowel metastases occur as well.

Clinical

With the advent of hCG monitoring and the use of chemotherapy, the histopathologic classification has been replaced by a more practical clinical classification of gestational trophoblastic disease. This divides patients into a benign and malignant category. The malignant disease category is further subdivided into metastatic and nonmetastatic groups. Patients with a pathologic diagnosis of choriocarcinoma or invasive mole are considered in the malignant category since these tumors are almost always structured in a malignant fashion and require therapy. On the other hand, patients with the pathologic diagnosis of a hydatidiform mole may be classified as benign or malignant depending upon their clinical course.[2]

Clinical experience has further identified a group of high-risk patients within the metastatic group.[5,6] Thus, patients with brain or liver metastases, β-hCG levels of greater than 40,000 mIU/ml prior to therapy, an interval of more than 4 months between pregnancy and therapy, and failure of prior chemotherapy are usually separated into a special high-risk category. These patients require especially diligent radiologic and sonographic evaluation and follow-up.

MOLAR PREGNANCIES

Pathogenesis and Clinical Aspects
The pathogenesis of hydatidiform mole has remained a subject of considerable speculation for many years. Recently, however, the work of Kajii and Ohama demonstrated that hydatidiform mole results from the fertilization of an "empty egg"; that is, an ovum with no active chromosomal material.[7] The chromosomes of the sperm, finding no chromosomal complement from the ovum, reduplicate themselves, resulting in

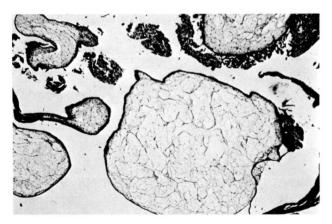

Fig. 1. Microscopic appearance of hydatidiform mole. Note the enlarged avascular edematous villi with a thin rim of proliferative trophoblastic cells.

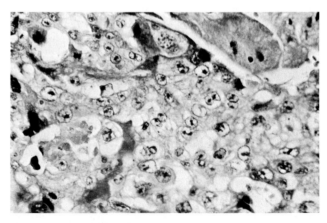

Fig. 2. Choriocarcinoma. Under high magnification, sheets of pleomorphic trophoblastic cells are seen. There are no villi.

a 46XX mole. There are no fetal parts or chorionic membrane associated with this situation, which is called a "complete mole" or "classic mole." Complete moles have varying degrees of trophoblastic proliferation and may be either benign or malignant. Malignant gestational trophoblastic disease may follow a mole or be associated with a spontaneous abortion, ectopic pregnancy, or full term pregnancy.

Some hydatidiform moles may contain a small complement of fetal structures such as a placenta with membranes. This is classified as a "partial mole." Such cases usually involve some edema of the villi but relatively little trophoblastic proliferation. Although malignancy has been reported, "partial moles" are almost always benign.[8] The fetus in such cases usually has significant congenital anomalies and a triploid karyotype.[9] Two chromosomes are of paternal origin and the third is of maternal origin.[10] About two-thirds of triploid fetuses are XXY and one-third are XXX.[11]

Morphologically similar, but much less common than the partial mole, a fetus can coexist with a complete mole. This disorder is thought to result from molar degeneration of one conceptus of an identical twin pregnancy, with the other conceptus developing into a fetus and placenta.[12] In these patients, a fetus and normal placenta can usually be identified as opposed to a partial mole where a normal placenta is not present.

Hydropic degeneration of the placenta may have a similar sonographic appearance to a complete or partial mole but, histologically, is not associated with trophoblastic proliferation. The villi in hydropic degeneration of the placenta are swollen and edematous thus resembling abnormal trophoblastic tissue. Hydropic degeneration may be seen in 20 to 40 percent of placentae from abortuses.[3]

Clinically, a molar pregnancy is first considered in the differential diagnosis of a patient who presents with severe preeclampsia prior to 24 weeks' gestation, a uterus that is too large for dates, and first trimester bleeding. Occasionally, the patient may notice grape-like vesicles passed per vaginum which are diagnostic of this condition. The bleeding may be so intense as to result in shock. The uterus is frequently too large for dates in patients with this condition. However, if significant expulsion of molar tissue has occurred prior to sonographic examination, the uterus may be normal size or even too small for dates.

Theca lutein cysts are frequently encountered in patients with a molar pregnancy. The actual incidence of these cysts with molar pregnancy described in reported series ranges from 18 to 37 percent.[13,14] When compared to clinical examination, sonography can more accurately assess the presence or absence of these cysts (Fig. 3).[15] In one large series, theca lutein cysts

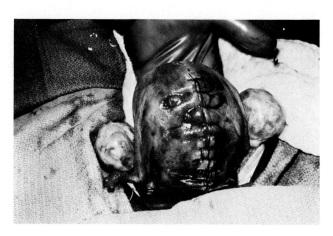

Fig. 3. Bilateral theca lutein cysts in a patient who has undergone hysterotomy for evacuation of a hydatidiform mole.

were detected clinically in 10 percent of patients with a molar pregnancy compared to 37 percent found by sonography.[14] The presence or absence of theca lutein cysts does not seem to be an accurate predictor of later development of an invasive mole or choriocarcinoma.[14]

Laboratory findings for molar gestations are usually diagnostic. Human chorionic gonadotropin, specifically the beta subunit, is usually abnormally elevated in molar gestations and invasive trophoblastic disease. This assay in not foolproof, since it can be spuriously elevated in twin gestations or not significantly abnormal in an occasional molar pregnancy.[16]

The treatment of molar pregnancies typically involves suction curettage (dilatation and evacuation, or D&E). A chest radiograph should be obtained in order to exclude the possibility of metastatic disease. After D&E, serial β-hCGs are obtained in order to follow the activity and presence of remaining trophoblastic tissue. The serum level of this glycoprotein hormone should return to normal 10 to 12 weeks after evacuation.[17] Although theca lutein cysts, if present prior to D&E, should regress with successful treatment of molar pregnancy, the presence or absence of these cysts should not be taken as reliable indications of the presence or activity of residual disease.[18] Sonography does have an important role in these patients in which the β-hCG rises, since it can detect the presence or absence of intrauterine pregnancies, which may occur after D&E. Fetal heart tones may be absent in patients with molar gestations due to intrauterine fetal demise. Approximately 2 percent of molar gestations will have a coexistent fetus.[19]

Sonographic Features

The sonographic appearance of a hydatidiform mole is quite distinctive.[1] In most cases, a sonographic pattern arising from molar tissue consists of echogenic

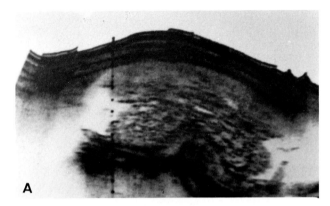
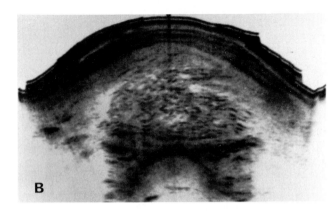

Fig. 4. Hydatidiform mole. **A.** Longitudinal, midline; **B.** Transverse, 10 cm above symphysis pubis. These images demonstrate the typical appearance of a hydatidiform mole. Intrauterine contents have a vesicular texture arising from the numerous hydropic villi. The sonolucent areas in the region of the uterine fundus and lower uterine segment probably represent areas of remaining amniotic cavity that the molar tissue has not occupied. (*Reprinted with permission from Fleischer A, James AE: Introduction to Diagnostic Sonography. New York, Wiley, 1980.*)

intrauterine tissue that is interspersed with numerous punctuate sonolucencies. Irregular sonolucent areas may occur secondary to internal hemorrhage or an area of unobliterated uterine lumen (Figs. 4A,B,5,6,7).

The sonographic appearance of a hydatidiform mole varies according to the gestational duration and the size of the hydropic villi.[20] For instance, hydatidiform moles that occur from 8 to 12 weeks typically appear as homogeneously echogenic intraluminal tissue, since the villi at this stage have a maximum diame-

ter of 2 mm (Figs. 8,9). As the hydatidiform mole matures to 18 or 20 weeks, the vesicles have a maximum diameter of 10 mm, which is readily delineated on sonography (Figs. 10,11).[21]

As opposed to the complete mole, partial molar pregnancy, hydatidiform mole coexistent with fetus and hydropic degeneration of the placenta are associated with the presence of a fetus or fetal parts. Although it may be difficult to differentiate between a partial molar pregnancy and a complete mole with

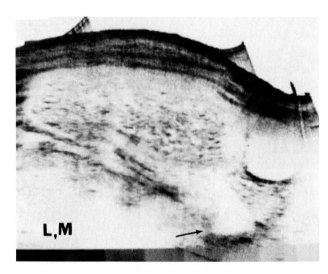

Fig. 5. Hydatidiform mole with theca lutein cyst (longitudinal, midline). There is a cystic mass (*arrow*) associated with the hydatidiform mole. This mass represents a theca lutein cyst, which is encountered in approximately one-third of patients with a hydatidiform mole. These cysts are frequently bilateral and multiloculated. Their size is greatest when hCG production is maximal, which usually occurs between 16 and 22 weeks' gestation (*Reprinted with permission from Fleischer A, James AE, Krause D, et al: Radiology 126:215, 1978.*)

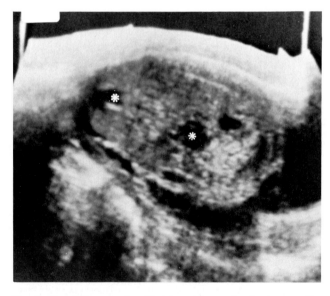

Fig. 6. Hydatidiform mole with internal hemorrhagic degeneration (longitudinal, 2 cm to right of midline, white on black format). Within this hydatidiform mole, there are sonolucent irregular areas representing hemorrhagic internal degeneration (*asterisk*). These are frequently encountered in hydatidiform moles when they reach maximal size.

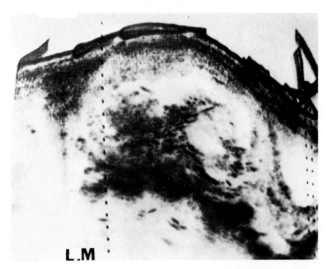

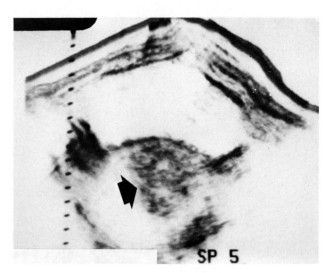

Fig. 7. Hydatidiform mole with hemorrhagic degeneration (longitudinal, midline). The internal contents of the uterus are markedly irregular without a characteristic echo pattern. At surgery, there was a marked internal hemorrhagic degeneration and only scattered areas of remaining molar tissue within the uterus. This image demonstrates the extent of hemorrhagic internal degeneration that one may encounter in hydatidiform moles.

Fig. 8. Transverse static sonogram of first trimester molar pregnancy appearing as echogenic tissue (*arrow*) within the uterus. Since the villi are very small at this stage, they are not depicted as individual cystic structures by sonography.

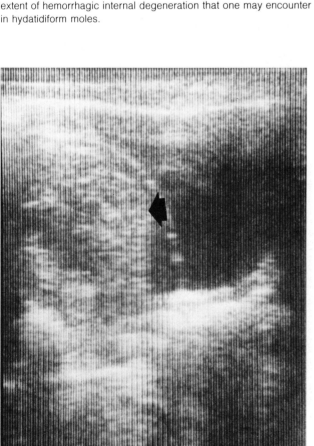

Fig. 9. Sagittal real-time sonogram demonstrating 10- to 12-week uterus that contains echogenic tissue (*arrow*) corresponding to an early hydatidiform mole.

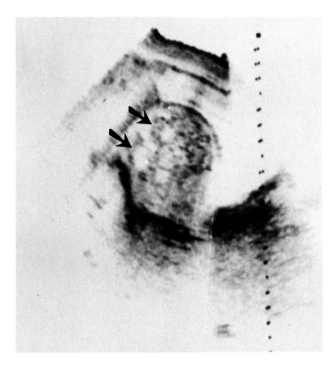

Fig. 10. Longitudinal static sonogram of 10- to 12-week size uterus that contains larger vesicles (*arrows*) arising from molar tissue.

a coexistent fetus on the basis of sonography, these two entities can be differentiated from a complete mole when an identifiable fetus is present (Figs. 12A,B).[12,21,22] In addition, the complete mole with a coexistent fetus typically has a fetus with a separate normal placenta as well as the molar mass. This contrasts with a partial mole in which only a portion of the placenta is normal and the majority of it has a vesicular pattern.

Sonographic Differential Diagnosis

Hydropic degeneration of the placenta associated with incomplete or missed abortions is the most common condition that can simulate the appearance of a molar pregnancy (Figs. 13,14). This is due to the sonographic similarity of a hydropic placenta with marked swelling of the villi to molar tissue. A fetus may or may not be present with hydropic degeneration of the placenta. Serum β-hCG levels are generally lower in hydropic degeneration than in partial or complete moles probably due to the reduced number of functioning trophoblasts.[3]

Technical factors that may be used to improve the ability to distinguish the partial from complete moles or hydropic degeneration have been described.[3] Specifically, detailed examination of the entire intrauterine contents with transducers that are optimally focused to a particular region within the uterus has

been stressed. Using this technique, the typical vesicular texture arising from molar tissue can be correctly distinguished from the tissue texture emanating from retained products of conception or leiomyomata.[3]

Occasionally, the sonographic appearance of a uterine leiomyoma may mimic that of a hydatidiform mole (Fig. 15). However, as illustrated in Chapter 38, uterine leiomyoma typically have a whorled internal consistency which is distinctly different from the vesicular pattern encountered in the hydatidiform mole. They may also contain areas of hyaline and myxomatous degeneration that may simulate the sonographic appearance of hemorrhage within a hydatidiform mole (Fig. 15).[23] We have also encountered some ovarian tumors that contain numerous internal septae that simulate the appearance of a hydatidiform mole (Fig. 16).[24] Patients with this type of mass can usually be distinguished from those with molar pregnancies by clinical and laboratory methods since the β-hCG is not elevated in the nonpregnant conditions.

Finally, patients with retained products of conception with hemorrhage can simulate the sonographic appearance of molar pregnancies. However, one is usually not able to demonstrate a vesicular pattern of the tissue associated with retained products.[3]

Although absolute distinction between the various trophoblastic disorders may not always be possible on the basis of sonography, the sonographic evaluation of these disorders may have clinical importance. Specifically, it is known that the malignant potential of a complete mole is greater than that of a partial mole

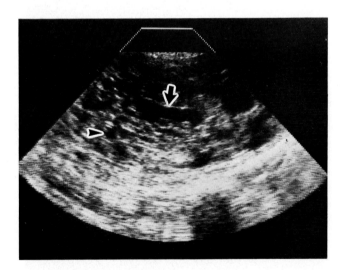

Fig. 11. Transverse real-time sonogram of hydatidiform mole in a patient who was 20 weeks' menstrual age. At this stage of development, hydropic villi (*arrowhead*) measure approximately 12 to 15 mm and are readily detected on sonography. Larger anechoic spaces (*arrow*) correspond to areas of internal hemorrhage.

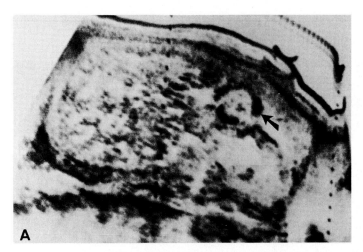
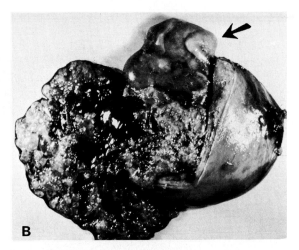

Fig. 12. Hydatidiform mole with 16-week fetus. **A.** Longitudinal, 4 cm to right of midline. This image demonstrates a fetal head (*arrow*) coexistent with molar tissue. Approximately 2 percent of hydatidiform moles may have coexistent fetal growth. When a hydatidiform mole is encountered on sonographic studies, one should exclude the presence of a coexistent fetus since these patients may be managed differently than patients with a hydatidiform mole without fetal growth. **B.** A specimen revealing a 16-week fetus in an amniotic sac (*arrow*) surrounded by vesicular tissue of the hydatidiform mole. The chromosomes of the fetus were XY and the molar tissue is XX; therefore, this type of pregnancy was thought to occur as a result of hydatidiform degeneration of one of the fertilized ova of a biovular twin pregnancy. (*Reprinted with permission from Fleischer A, James AE, Krause D, et al: Radiology 126:215, 1978.*)

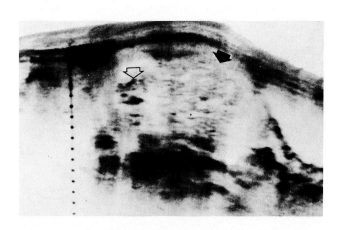

Fig. 13. Hydropic degeneration of the placenta (*large arrow*) encountered in the patient with a missed abortion. The dead fetus is present in the fundal portion of the uterus (*open arrow*).

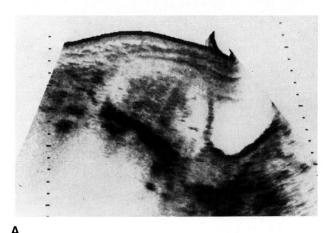

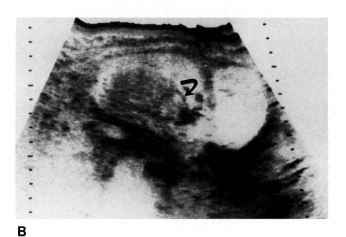

Fig. 14. These sagittal sonograms demonstrate an enlarged uterus which contains echogenic tissue. A dead fetus was present (*arrow*). The placental tissue itself was swollen and contained several hydropic villi. This patient was found to have a missed abortion.

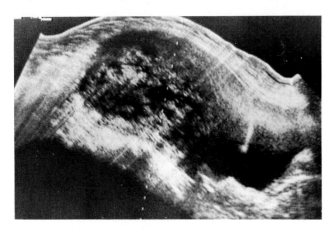

Fig. 15. Degenerated uterine leiomyoma (longitudinal, 2 cm to right of midline, white on black format). The sonographic appearance of this leiomyoma with degeneration mimics that of a hydatidiform mole. A diagnosis should be formulated with the knowledge of the hCG titers. In particular, the beta subunit of the hCG hormone will be markedly elevated in trophoblastic disease, whereas in leiomyomas it should be absent. (*Courtesy of Roger Sanders, M.D.*)

or hydropic degeneration. Thus, the sonographic findings can have a significant clinical impact upon the treatment and management of these disorders.

INVASIVE MOLE AND CHORIOCARCINOMA

Pathogenesis and Clinical Aspects

The majority of patients who develop malignant trophoblastic disease have a history of either molar gestation or missed abortion. Approximately one-fourth of the patients with these diseases will present after having a normal pregnancy or de novo.[25] Histologically, invasive moles differ from choriocarcinoma in the presence of villous structures. Villous structures are present in an invasive mole and usually absent in choriocarcinoma. Both disorders are associated with excessive trophoblastic proliferation.

In general, an invasive mole is first clinically suspected in a patient with a history of evacuation of a hydatidiform mole who presents with continued uterine bleeding or persistently elevated hCG level and/ or persistently enlarged theca lutein cysts.[15] Patients with choriocarcinoma that extends outside the uterus can present for the first time with manifestations of metastatic spread to the lungs, liver, or brain. In the lungs, metastatic choriocarcinoma has a rather specific radiographic appearance of radiodense masses with hazy borders due to hemorrhage around the metastases. The metastates may undergo rapid regression after therapy has been instituted. Since these diseases

are very responsive to chemotherapeutic agents, their sonographic and clinical recognition is imperative.

Sonographic Features

In our experience, tissue from an invasive mole has a similar appearance to the vesicular tissue encountered in molar pregnancies. Specifically, retained trophoblastic tissue typically contains irregular villi that are depicted sonographically as echogenic tissue with scattered punctate sonolucencies (Figs. 17,18). On the other hand, the sonographic appearance of malignant trophoblastic tissue is that of a focal irregular echogenic region within the uterine myometrium (Figs. 19A,B). Irregular sonolucent areas can surround the more echogenic trophoblastic tissue and these correspond to areas of myometrial hemorrhage (Figs. 19–21).

In addition to the echogenic intrauterine areas, sonography is helpful in the detection of theca lutein cysts associated with trophoblastic disease (Figs. 19A,B). These cysts are typically bilateral multiloculated cystic masses that typically measure between 4 and 8 cm in diameter. Sonography has been shown to be a more sensitive examination than physical examination in the detection of these cysts since it may be difficult to palpate a cyst that is displaced high in the pelvis by an enlarged uterus. The presence of theca lutein cysts may be an indication of persistent tropho-

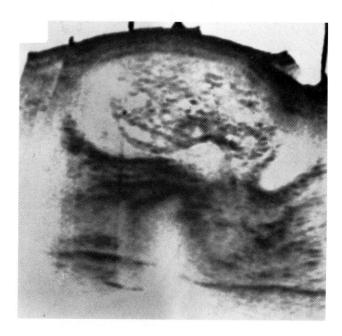

Fig. 16. Papillary serous cystadenoma (longitudinal, 2 cm to left of midline). The sonographic appearance of this multiloculated papillary serous cystadenoma mimics that of a hydatidiform mole. Laboratory tests may be necessary to distinguish an ovarian tumor from a hydatidiform mole. However, since this is an ovarian mass, the uterus could be detected as a separate structure.

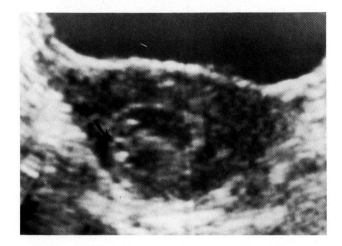

Fig. 17. Retained molar tissue (magnified, transverse, 4 cm above symphysis pubis). The patient presented with elevated hCG levels after spontaneous expulsion of a hydatidiform mole. Molar tissue was demonstrated within the uterus.

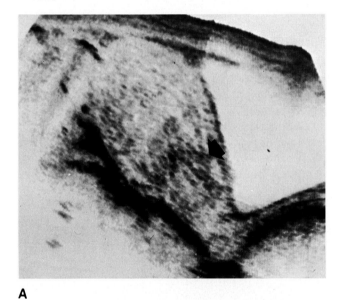

A

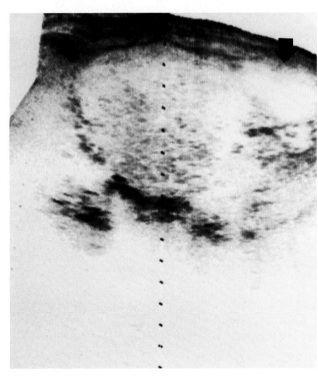

B

Fig. 18. Longitudinal static sonogram of patient 2 weeks after evacuation of molar tissue. **A.** The uterus is persistently enlarged and contains irregular echogenic tissue (*arrow*) that corresponds to persistent trophoblastic tissue. **B.** A theca lutein cyst (*arrow*) was also present in the left ovary.

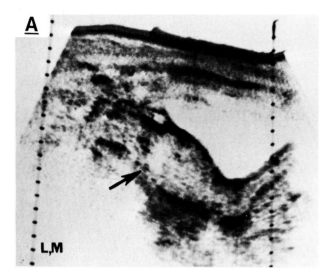
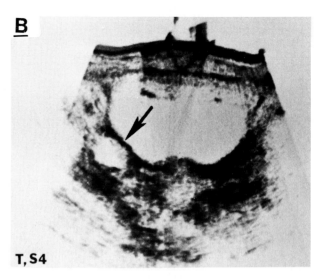

Fig. 19. Chorioadenoma destruens. **A.** Longitudinal, midline. **B.** Transverse 4 cm above symphysis pubis. The patient presented approximately 1 month after dilatation and curettage of a hydatidiform mole with persistent elevation of hCG levels and a persistently enlarged right adnexal mass. In the region of the uterine fundus, there is an irregular sonolucent focus (*arrows*) representing hemorrhage secondary to infiltration of the myometrium by the invasive trophoblastic process. Also, in **B** the right cystic adnexal mass (*arrow*) represented a persistently enlarged theca lutein cyst, indicating continued chorionic tissue activity. (*Reprinted with permission from Fleischer A, James AE, Krause D, et al: Radiology 126:215, 1978.*)

blastic activity since it has been shown that malignant trophoblastic disease develops more commonly in patients with persistent theca lutein cysts than those without.[26] However, since it may take up to 4 months for these cysts to regress after evacuation of a molar pregnancy, their presence or absence during the period of follow-up cannot be taken as an accurate indication of the presence or activity of remaining trophoblastic tissue.[18]

Sonography can be useful, when utilized in combination with serial β-hCG assays, in the evaluation of tumor response to chemotherapy.[25,26] Serial evaluation of tumor volume can be accomplished using sonography and follows closely the diminution in β-hCG values in successfully treated patients.

Sonography also is helpful in evaluation of the liver for metastatic disease in patients with malignant, metastatic trophoblastic disease.[10] Typically, the me-

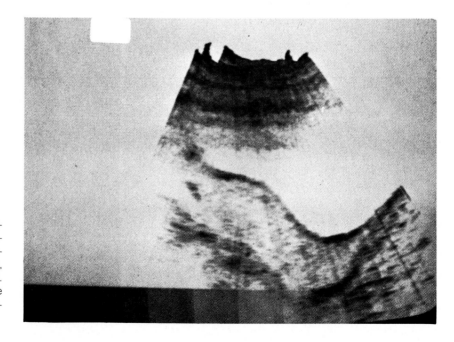

Fig. 20. Choriocarcinoma (longitudinal, midline). This patient presented with right hemiparesis. The cranial computed tomographic scan revealed two frontal metastases. Sonographically, the uterine texture appears grossly normal. Changes in invasive trophoblastic disease may be subtle. Often sonography is only confirmatory to the clinical and laboratory findings.

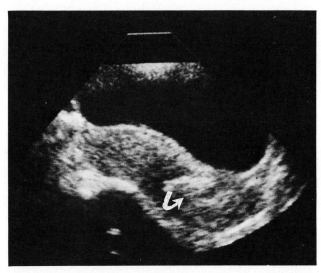

A

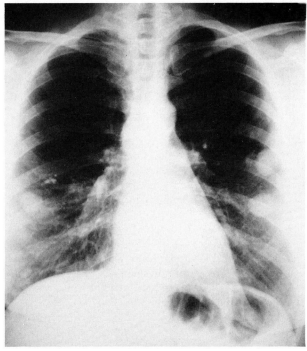

B

Fig. 21. Choriocarcinoma. Longitudinal real-time sonogram of patient with persistent bleeding one month after delivery. **A.** Trophoblastic tumor caused an irregular echogenic area in the lower portion of the uterus (*arrow*); **B.** Metastases to the lungs were already apparent on the chest radiograph.

tastases associated with choriocarcinoma appear as echogenic foci within the liver. The kidneys can also be evaluated for the presence of obstructive uropathy, which is important, not only to rule out metastatic involvement, but because effective chemotherapy often requires adequate renal function.

SUMMARY

As discussed and illustrated in this chapter, sonography has an important role in the evaluation of patients with benign and malignant gestational trophoblastic disease. The sonographic features of hydatidiform mole and its variants are usually diagnostic. If malignant trophoblastic disease is suspected clinically, sonography can be utilized to establish the presence and extent of disease, as well as in the serial evaluation of patients undergoing treatment.

REFERENCES

1. Fleischer A, James A, Krause D, et al: Sonographic patterns in trophoblastic disease. Radiology 126:215, 1978
2. Requard C, Mettler F: Use of ultrasound in the evaluation of trophoblastic disease and its response to therapy. Radiology 135:419, 1980
3. Reid M, McGohan JO: Sonographic evaluation of hydatidiform mole and its look-alike. Am J Roentgenol 140:307, 1983
4. Jones Jr H: Gestational trophoblastic disease, in Jones III H, Jones S (eds), Novak's Textbook of Gynecology, 10th ed., Baltimore, Williams and Wilkins, 1981, pp 659–689
5. Hertig A, Edmundson W: Hydatidiform mole: A pathoclinical correlation of 200 cases. Am J Obstet Gynecol 53:1, 1947
6. Chun D, Braga C, Chow C, et al: Clinical observation on some aspects of hydatidiform moles. J Obstet Gynaecol Br Commonw 71:180, 1964
7. Kajii T, Ohama K: Androgenetic origin of hydatidiform mole. Nature 168:633, 1977
8. Szulman A, Surti J, Berman M: Patient with partial mole requiring chemotherapy. Lancet 1:1099, 1978
9. Szulman A, Surti N: The syndromes of hydatidiform mole. I: Cytogenic and morphologic correlations. Am J Obstet Gynecol 131:665, 1978
10. Szulman A, Surti N: The syndromes of hydatidiform mole. II: Morphologic evaluation of the complete and partial mole. Am J Obstet Gynecol 132:20, 1978
11. Sauerbrei E, Salem S, Fayle B: Coexistent hydatidiform mole and the fetus in the second trimester. An ultrasound study. Radiology 135:415, 1980
12. Munyer T, Callen P, Filly R, et al: Further observations on the sonographic spectrum of gestational trophoblastic disease. J Clin Ultrasound 9:349, 1981
13. Kobayashi M: Use of diagnostic ultrasound in trophoblastic neoplasms and ovarian tumors. Cancer 38:441, 1978

14. Santos-Rasmos A, Forney J, Schwartz B: Sonographic findings and clinical correlations in molar pregnancies. Obstet Gynecol 56:186, 1980
15. Pritchard J, Hellman L (eds): Williams' Obstetrics. New York: Appleton Century Crofts, 1971, p 578
16. Callen P: Ultrasonography in evaluation of gestational trophoblastic disease, in Callen P (ed), Ultrasonography in Obstetrics and Gynecology. Philadelphia, Saunders, 1983, pp 259–270
17. Goldstein D, Berkowitz R, Cohen S: The current management of molar pregnancies. Curr Prob Obstets Gyn 3:1, 1979
18. MacVicar J, Donald I: Sonar in the diagnosis of early pregnancy and its complications. J Obstet Gynaecol Br Commonw 70:387, 1968
19. Jones W, Lauerson N: Hydatidiform mole with coexistent fetus. Am J Obstet Gynecol 122:267, 1975
20. Reuter K, Michlewitz H, Kahn P: Early appearance of hydatidiform mole by ultrasound: A case report. Am J Roentgenol 134:588, 1980
21. Wittmann B, Fulton L, Cooperberg P, et al: Molar pregnancy: Early diagnosis by ultrasound. J Clin Ultrasound 9:153, 1981
22. Naumoff P, Szulman A, Weinstein B, et al: Ultrasonography of partial hydatidiform mole. Radiology 140:467, 1981
23. Rinehart JS, Hernandez E, Rosenshein NB, et al: Degenerating leiomyomata: An ultrasonic mimic of hydatidiform mole. J Reprod Med 26:142, 1981
24. Nelson LH, Fry RJ, Homesely HD, et al: Malignant ovarian tumors simulating hydatidiform mole on ultrasound. J Clin Ultrasound 10:244, 1982
25. Tsai W: Use of sonar in the diagnosis and management of invasive gestational trophoblastic tumors. Int J Fertil 19:227, 1974
26. Requard C, Mettler F: The use of ultrasound in evaluation of trophoblastic disease and its response to therapy. Radiology 135:419, 1980

30 | Sonographic Evaluation of Ectopic Pregnancy

Arthur C. Fleischer
Peter S. Cartwright
David L. DiPietro
A. Everette James, Jr.

Left unrecognized, ectopic pregnancies can result in significant maternal morbidity and mortality. Ectopic pregnancy is now responsible for 26 percent of all maternal deaths.[1] Even though the diagnosis of ectopic pregnancy is frequently considered in women who present with lower abdominal pain and amenorrhea, this entity is missed by the initial examining physician in up to 70 percent of cases.[2] Speedy and accurate diagnosis of patients who are suspected of having ectopic pregnancy is therefore important so that proper management can be instituted.

Ectopic pregnancies are one of the principle causes of female infertility. Once a patient has had an ectopic pregnancy, there is a significant chance of recurrence. Several epidemiologic studies have shown that the incidence of ectopic pregnancies is increasing, which may be a reflection of the increased prevalence of salpingitis. For example, the age-adjusted incidence of ectopic pregnancy rose from 55.5 to 84.2 per 100,000 women in northern California from 1972 to 1978.[3] Nationwide, the number of ectopic pregnancies range from 17,800 in 1970 to 42,000 in 1978. The death rate, however, decreased by 75 percent during this period.[4] The incidence of ectopic pregnancies is greatest in patients with salpingitis or previous tubal surgery. The chance that a tube containing an ectopic pregnancy can be "salvaged" by linear salpingostomy is closely related to the stage at which the ectopic pregnancy is discovered. Therefore, it is most desirable to diagnose an ectopic pregnancy as early as possible.

The recent improvement in the sonographic depiction of adnexal structures with mechanical sector real-time sonography and refinements in the radioimmunoassay (RIA) of the beta subunit of human chorionic gonadotropin (β-hCG) have enhanced the physician's ability to diagnose ectopic pregnancy.[5-9] Although the sonographic findings in ectopic pregnancy can be subtle, a definitive diagnosis of this entity is possible in most cases when the sonographic findings are combined with the results of a single or serial β-hCG assay.[10-12] Most importantly, sonography is useful in the evaluation of patients with suspected ectopic pregnancy in verifying the absence of a viable intrauterine pregnancy.

PATHOGENESIS

The term ectopic pregnancy refers to implantation of the developing zygote outside the endometrial cavity. Ninety-five percent of ectopic pregnancies are tubal, and the majority of these occur in the ampullary or isthmic portions of the oviduct.[10] The remaining 5 percent occur in the abdomen, ovary, cervix, and the retroperitoneal space.

In ectopic tubal pregnancy, the fertilized ovum implants beneath the epithelium of the oviduct to form a fluid-filled gestational sac lined with trophoblastic tissue in the wall of the tube. Since the oviduct has only a thin layer of muscle, the trophoblastic cells that burrow deep into the tubal epithelium distend the oviduct and eventually cause rupture. The gestational sac within the tube of a ruptured ectopic pregnancy is usually surrounded by fluid or blood due to erosion of adjacent vessels. In the vast majority of cases, the separation of the decidua from the wall of the oviduct causes death of the fetus. In rare cases, the fetus may survive an attempt at abortion by reimplantation within the abdomen and reestablishment of the blood supply from the omentum or the mesentery.

Mild uterine enlargement and endometrial hypertrophy are usually present with an ectopic pregnancy and can occasionally be detected clinically. If dilatation and curettage (D&C) is performed on a patient with an ectopic pregnancy, only decidua without chorionic villi will be obtained.

CLINICAL ASPECTS

Several explanations have been proposed to account for the development of an ectopic pregnancy. These include delayed transit of the fertilized zygote secondary to fallopian tube malfunction, obstruction to the passage of the zygote through the oviduct secondary to adhesions from pelvic inflammatory disease, and abnormal angulation of the oviduct relative to the uterine cornu.[10] Prior to the use of antibiotics for pelvic inflammatory disease, tubal inflammation resulted in a much higher incidence of complete tubal closure and sterility. The recent two- to threefold increased incidence of ectopic gestations among pregnant patients has been attributed paradoxically to the use of antibiotics for treatment of tubal inflammation.[13] Antibiotics, although reducing the incidence of sterility, have resulted in more women with an open, but malfunctioning oviduct. The result is an increased incidence of ectopic pregnancy among patients with previous tubal infection. Besides patients who have a history of pelvic inflammatory disease, patients receiving medication for ovulation induction also appear to have a slightly increased incidence of ectopic pregnancy. Once a patient has had an ectopic pregnancy, there is a one in four chance of a recurrence.[10]

The incidence of ectopic pregnancy is between 1 in 100 and 1 in 400 pregnancies.[3,4,14] However, ectopic pregnancy should be considered in the differential diagnosis of any patient presenting with lower abdominal pain because the massive intraperitoneal bleeding associated with rupture of an ectopic pregnancy is such a serious complication.

The most common presenting symptoms of ectopic pregnancy are pelvic pain, which may be mild and intermittent or persistent and severe, and abnormal vaginal bleeding. The clinical symptomatology and routine laboratory findings in ectopic pregnancy are usually not diagnostic by themselves. Abnormal vaginal bleeding is seen in approximately three-quarters

of the patients with ectopic pregnancies and can be confused with other causes of first trimester bleeding such as threatened or spontaneous abortion. However, there is no bleeding or menstrual history that is inconsistent with an ectopic gestation. Vaginal bleeding is statistically more commonly associated with other first trimester conditions such as a threatened spontaneous abortion, cervical polyp, and infection than with an ectopic pregnancy. Diffuse abdominal pain may be present, as may rebound tenderness from peritoneal irritation by free intraperitoneal bleeding.

The presence of an adnexal mass is not specific for the diagnosis of ectopic pregnancy since a mass can occur in many other conditions such as corpus luteum cyst, dermoid cyst, and leiomyomata. In our experience, a palpable adnexal mass is noted in less than one-third of the cases and does not predict whether the gestation has ruptured. Although exceedingly uncommon, the presence of a palpable adnexal mass separate from both ovaries and uterine fundus is highly suggestive of an ectopic pregnancy.

Culdocentesis, the transvaginal aspiration of fluid from the posterior cul-de-sac, remains a valuable diagnostic aid for the evaluation of patients suspected of having an ectopic gestation. The aspiration of nonclotting blood indicates the presence of a hemoperitoneum. However, this finding is not diagnostic of an ectopic pregnancy, since it also may result from a hemorrhagic corpus luteum, complete or incomplete abortion, ovulation, or previous attempts at culdocentesis. In our experience, 70 percent of the patients with an ectopic pregnancy who underwent this procedure had positive taps, and this was one of the key factors resulting in the patient being admitted to the hospital.[15] In only 56 percent of these patients, however, was the tube ruptured; intact tubal pregnancy may produce several liters of hemoperitoneum by bleeding through the fimbriated end of the tube. A negative culdocentesis usually excludes a ruptured tube.

Culdocentesis is quick and safe but does result in some patient discomfort. We have reviewed 18 patients who had an ectopic gestation with sonographic evaluation just before or after culdocentesis to determine if ultrasound may be substituted for culdocentesis. Sonographic scanning accurately predicted the results in 5 of the 11 patients with positive taps. Of the three who had inadequate taps (i.e., *no* fluid obtained), sonographic evaluation correctly predicted the findings of a hemoperitoneum in all three. Sonography has the advantage of being noninvasive. Culdocentesis, however, has the advantage of being extremely rapid and less expensive. The complications resulting from culdocentesis appears to be rare.[15]

Since sonography will show whether there is fluid

in the cul-de-sac, it is suggested that sonography be performed prior to culdocentesis. Performance of sonography prior to culdocentesis is also important since attempted culdocentesis may create cul-de-sac hematoma, which would simulate blood from a ruptured ectopic pregnancy. We have encountered several patients within a negative culdocentesis in whom a cul-de-sac hematoma was observed sonographically. The negative culdocentesis in these patients was probably a result of inability to aspirate clotted blood.

The clinical course of an ectopic pregnancy is related to its site of implantation. The ampullary portion of the oviduct is the most common location for an ectopic implantation. As in other sites, the ectopic pregnancy can expand the oviduct until it ruptures. Complete or partial tubal abortion may also occur, with the contents of the sac extruded through the fimbriated end of the tube into the peritoneal cavity. If the fimbriated end of the oviduct is occluded, hematosalpinx will result. Ectopic pregnancies that occur in the narrow isthmic portion of the oviduct usually distend it eccentrically and, because of the oviduct's small diameter, rupture early in the course of pregnancy.

Ectopic pregnancy in the interstitial portion of the oviduct is uncommon (3 to 4 percent of all ectopic pregnancies) but has the most serious potential complications of all types. Because of its location within the muscular portion of the uterus near the major uterine vessels, the pregnancy can survive until 3 to 4 months' gestation. Then massive bleeding from erosion and profuse bleeding from the uterine arteries and veins can result.

Chronic ectopic pregnancies may occur with hematoma formation in the cul-de-sac. These patients usually present with recurrent, intermittent low-grade fever associated with a palpable solid mass. On physical examination, there is usually a firm pelvic mass that is located in the midline and is difficult to separate from the uterus. Culdocentesis may be negative because the blood in the cul-de-sac is clotted. In very rare cases, the embryo and products of conception will undergo dehydration in situ with the formation of a lithopedian pregnancy.

Other rare sites of implantation include intraabdominal, ovarian, cervical, and extraperitoneal. True advanced abdominal ectopic pregnancies may be difficult to differentiate from normal intrauterine pregnancy; the uterus must be defined separately from the amniotic sac and its contents. Abdominal pregnancies are thought to be the result of reimplantation of an aborted fetus after it aborts out the fimbriated end of the tube and reimplants on the mesentery or omentum. These pregnancies can progress to term without symptoms and first present because of difficulty during the initial stages of labor. Extraperitoneal ectopic pregnancies are quite rare and are probably the result of tubal rupture with abortion of the fetus into the broad ligament. The rupture occurs between the fimbriated end of the oviduct where it is not covered by peritoneum and where the two folds of the broad ligament are loosely opposed. The tubal contents may empty into the soft tissue and mesosalpinx and implant in that region.

BETA hCG ASSAY

Within the last few years, refinements in the radioimmunoassay (RIA) of the beta subunit of human chorionic gonadotropin have enabled the diagnosis of pregnancy as early as 10 days after conception (3½ weeks' menstrual age). Although still not available in all hospitals, this radioimmunoassay has become more widely available as a prepackaged, diagnostic kit.

The beta subunit assay of hCG has become essential to the diagnosis of ectopic pregnancy because of the relatively poor sensitivity of other pregnancy tests, specifically the urine pregnancy test. In one series, the urinary pregnancy test was negative in half of the patients with ectopic pregnancy.[16] This was probably due to the decreased amount of hCG elaborated by an ectopic pregnancy. The urinary pregnancy test (tube or slide) is sensitive to a level of 1 to 15 IU/L of human chorionic gonadotropin. It becomes positive at 4 to 5 weeks after the last menstrual period and can be falsely positive in patients with proteinuria, hematuria, tuboovarian abscess, and certain gynecologic neoplasms and in patients taking aspirins, major tranquilizers, and methadone.[17] Conversely, the beta hCG radioimmunoassay is exquisitely sensitive and specific, and detects chorionic gonadotropin as early as 10 days postconception (3½ weeks' menstrual age). The assay quantitates the beta subunit of hCG since the alpha subunit is shared by other hormones, such as follicle stimulating hormone and luteinizing hormone.

The RIA for the beta subunit of the human chorionic gonadotropin glycoprotein has dramatically improved the obstetrician's ability to detect viable trophoblastic activity associated with early gestations. Using the more sensitive assays, a normal intrauterine pregnancy can be reliably detected 10 days after fertilization (3½ weeks' menstrual age) (Fig. 1A). Various commercial RIA "kits" for β-hCG are available; the better ones have a sensitivity of 1 ng/ml (1 ng/ml = 5 mIU/ml of the 2nd International Standard), and do not cross-react with lutenizing hormone or other nonspecific proteins.

Instead of considering the β-hCG test positive or

402

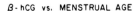

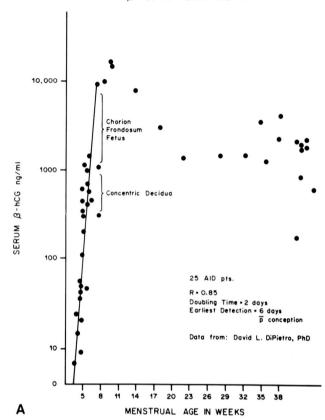

Fig. 1. A. β-hCG in normal pregnancies. Graph depicting levels of β-hCG versus gestational age. β-hCG increases in a linear fashion during the first 10 weeks of pregnancy. By quantitating the β-hCG level, an approximate gestational age can be estimated. From this gestational age assessment, one would expect certain sonographic findings in a normal intrauterine pregnancy. If the β-hCG level is over 6500 mIU/ml, or approximately 1000 ng/ml, a gestational sac should be identified if the pregnancy is intrauterine. The data displayed in this graph was obtained from serial β-hCG levels in 25 patients who underwent artificial insemination by donor. (*Courtesy of David L. DiPietro, Ph.D.*) (*cont.*)

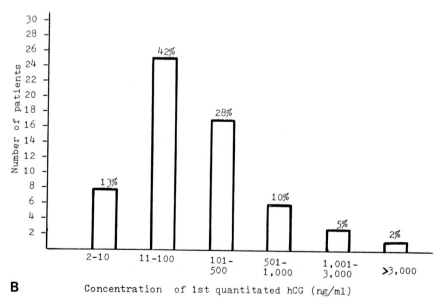

Fig. 1. cont. B. Graph depicting distribution of β-hCG levels at initial clinical presentation of patients with ectopic pregnancy. (*cont.*)

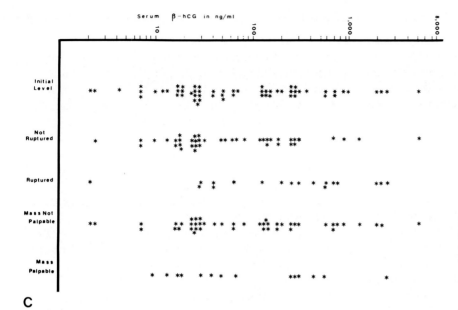

Fig. 1. cont. C. Distribution of β-hCG values in our series of confirmed ectopics divided into those that were unruptured, ruptured, with or without a palpable adnexal mass. (*Adapted from Cartwight P, DiPietro D, personal communication.*) (*cont.*)

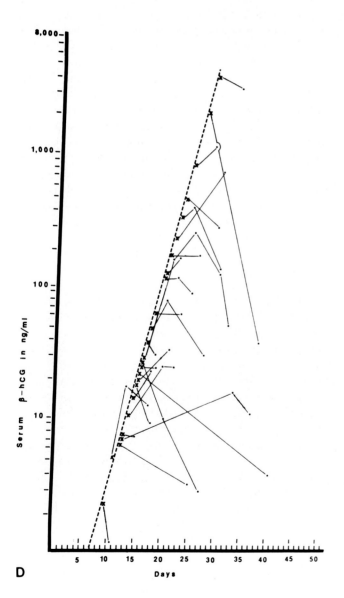

Fig. 1. cont. D. Graph depicting serial β-hCG determinations in 25 patients with an ectopic pregnancy. Most patients with ectopics had β-hCGs that either plateaued or dropped on serial assays. (*Adapted from Cartwright P, DiPietro D, personal communication.*)

negative, the results of this assay should be considered a specific quantity. The amount of β-hCG present can be used to approximate expected gestational duration. The hCG value then, in turn, can be correlated with the presence or absence of certain sonographically apparent developmental "milestones." The sonographic features that are expected to be present at the various β-hCG levels are summarized in Fig. 1A.

Using the assay devised at our institution with the CR 119 reference preparation and the National Institutes of Health (NIH) antiserum, the serum hCG levels in over 200 women with proven ectopic gestation has been evaluated and found to have at least 2 ng/ml of hCG at the time of initial clinical presentation (Fig. 1B).[18] It is essential that accurate assays sensitive to 1 ng/ml be used. The level of hCG in patients with an ectopic pregnancy is characteristically lower than in those with viable gestations at any given gestational age. Figure 1B displays the initial hCG level in 60 consecutive patients with an ectopic gestation. Obviously, the amount of β-hCG present in the initial assay will depend upon when the patient is first examined. Five percent presented with serum levels of 5 ng/ml or less, over half with levels below 100 ng/ml, and all but three were below 1000 ng/ml (Fig. 1B).

By determining the exact serum level of β-hCG, several important facts may be determined. First, the detection of hCG firmly indicates the presence or recent clearance of active trophoblastic tissue (excluding recent hCG injections, or a nongestational neoplasm). Second, the exact level allows a good estimation of the gestational age if the pregnancy is normal. Figure 1A presents the standard serum hCG rise for the first 30 days of a normal gestation with the corresponding sonographic findings. Note the time is "days since conception," which is the gestational age of the pregnancy. The menstrual age is normally 14 days more than the gestational age, but may be exceedingly inaccurate if a delay in ovulation occurred or if there has been accompanying abnormal uterine bleeding. The normal hCG progression is such that for the first 30 days the level doubles about every 2 days, although some viable gestations have been described that show doubling times of 5 to 7 days.

A "discriminatory" hCG zone has been defined for the discrimination of normal (viable) intrauterine pregnancies from ectopic pregnancies.[18] This zone lies between 6000 and 6500 mIU/ml. The absence of an intrauterine gestational sac in conjunction with an hCG value above this discriminatory level signifies the presence of ectopic pregnancy in the majority of cases. The absence of an intrauterine gestational sac associated with hCG value below the discriminatory zone can either be associated with an early intrauterine pregnancy or an ectopic pregnancy. It has, therefore, been

suggested that if the initial sonographic features cannot distinguish between an intrauterine and extrauterine pregnancy, the sonographic examination should be repeated when the value would be expected to be 6500 mIU/ml.[19] For example, if a nondiagnostic sonogram is obtained in a patient whose beta subunit assay is 2000 mIU/ml, repeat examination in 5 days should be able to discriminate between an intrauterine and ectopic pregnancy, since at this point in time, an intrauterine pregnancy should exhibit a concentric and well-defined choriodecidua.

The amount of β-hCG produced with an ectopic pregnancy is usually less than a viable intrauterine pregnancy of the same gestational duration. This may be a result of a less extensive trophoblastic proliferation in an ectopic pregnancy or a difference in implantation in the tube and the endometrium. In addition to being abnormally low, the β-hCG levels in ectopic pregnancies do not progress in a similar rate as viable intrauterine pregnancies. Serial β-hCG assays in patients with ectopic pregnancies usually disclose a lack of normal doubling of the hCG or a decline in the value. This same set of values can occur in patients with nonviable intrauterine pregnancies, however.

There has been a report describing a statistical difference in β-hCG levels in unruptured and ruptured ectopic pregnancies. It was postulated that active and viable ectopic chorionic tissue is more likely to produce high levels of β-hCG and cause rupture. The difference in β-hCG could not be attributed to differences in gestational age either.[20] The experience at our institution does not corroborate this data since there was a wide variation in β-hCGs in the patients who had unruptured or ruptured ectopic pregnancies (Fig. 1C).[21]

Figure 1C presents data collected at our institution and correlates sonographic findings with serum β-hCG levels for 35 patients with ectopic gestation.[22] It has been observed that patients with levels above the discriminatory zone had an "empty" uterus (no decidual changes) by sonographic scanning, while six patients had pseudogestational sacs and levels below this zone.

In our experience, the gestational sac can only rarely be discerned when hCG levels were below 1000 ng/ml. The lack of uterine changes makes an early intrauterine pregnancy just as likely as an ectopic pregnancy. The presence of an adnexal mass in a patient with a β-hCG less than 1000 ng/ml, even with fluid in the cul-de-sac, is still compatible with a viable intrauterine pregnancy and a hemorrhagic corpus luteum. Although knowledge of the hCG level at the time of sonographic evaluation is likely to help distinguish a pseudogestational sac from a viable gestation, there are still many patients that present with serum hCG levels so low that if the gestation is normal, it would not be seen on sonography. In this case, repeating sonography in 1 week may delay the diagnosis. One might postulate that rupture could occur in this interim.

Serial determinations of hCG levels have proven useful for patients in whom the sonographic findings are nondiagnostic. Figure 1D shows the hCG progression in 25 clinically stable patients with an ectopic gestation. The first known value is arbitrarily placed on the standard line, and subsequent values plotted accordingly. It is apparent that most patients had levels that plateaued or fell during the period of preoperative evaluation. This plateau or fall is diagnostic of nonviability when it occurs while levels are below 1000 ng/ml, and at least 48 hours apart. It does not distinguish the nonviable intrauterine gestation from the ectopic, but it does allow one to make appropriate management decisions. It is also apparent from Fig. 1D that some ectopic pregnancies may produce early rises in hCG levels that are identical to normal gestations. This rise quickly falls off, however, and is found only while hCG levels are low and the pregnancy presumably still very early.

By plotting serial hCG values on the standard line presented in Fig. 1A, one may evaluate gestational viability while levels are below the discriminatory zone without knowing the menstrual history or calculating doubling times. Patients showing a plateau or fall while levels are 1000 ng/ml or less have a nonviable gestation and intervention is warranted. Those having an abnormal rise, but no plateau or fall may have a viable gestation.

Serial β-hCG assays appear to be a promising method for the discrimination of ectopic from viable intrauterine pregnancies. However, further experience with this assay is needed in order to evaluate whether there is a range of normalcy of β-hCG variations for a particular gestational age that must be known before this technique becomes widely utilized in clinical practice. Another limitation results from the limited number of hospitals that can accurately assay this glycoprotein. The cost of this assay is approximately $25.00, permitting its use in a serial fashion.

SONOGRAPHIC SCANNING TECHNIQUE, INSTRUMENTATION

Mechanical sector, real-time sonography is recommended for evaluation of the adnexal structures in patients with suspected ectopic pregnancies. The mechanical sector type real-time transducers are favored over linear array real-time transducers in that the mechanical sector type affords better delineation of the adnexal structures than the linear array scanner. Access through the bladder is simpler. The mechanical sector scanner can be more easily obliqued to optimize images of the adnexal structures. If only static scanning is available, longitudinal and transverse sonograms should be performed with a 3.5-MHz transducer with long to medium internal focus.

When one examines a patient with possible ectopic pregnancy, it is important to document any fluid within the cul-de-sac, pericolic recesses, or perihepatic spaces. Therefore, in addition to the pelvis, a survey of the midabdomen concentrating on the pericolic recesses and subhepatic spaces, should be performed in any patient suspected of having an ectopic pregnancy to exclude the presence of intraperitoneal blood.

TABLE 1
Sonographic Findings in Ectopic Pregnancy

	Unruptured	Ruptured
"Diagnostic" features	1. Absence of intrauterine gestational sac bordered by two layers of decidua	1. Absence of intrauterine gestational sac bordered by two layers of decidua
	2. Extrauterine, extraovarian adnexal mass	2. Extrauterine, extraovarian adnexal mass
	3. Fetal motion by real time or fetal heart tones by Doppler exam in extrauterine gestational sac	3. Fetal motion by real time or fetal heart tones by Doppler exam or fetal parts emanating from extrauterine gestational sac
"Suggestive" features	4. "Enlarged" uterus with thick, echogenic endometrium	4. Blood or organized clot in cul-de-sac, or pericolic recesses
		5. "Enlarged" uterus with thick, echogenic endometrium

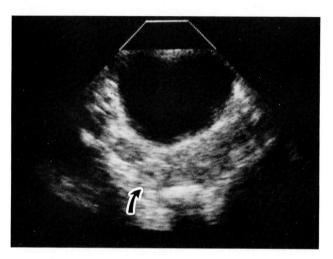

Fig. 2. There is a right adnexal mass (*arrow*) between the uterus and right ovary. The mass has an echogenic rim and small center and represents an unruptured ectopic pregnancy within the right fallopian tube.

SONOGRAPHIC DIAGNOSIS

The sonographic findings that may be encountered in patients with ectopic pregnancy are summarized in Table 1. The sonographic signs are divided into those that are considered "diagnostic" and those thought to be "suggestive." The sonographic diagnosis of an ectopic pregnancy can be made with greater confidence if more than one sonographic sign is present.

Because the size of the ectopic pregnancy can be small (less than 1 cm in size), its sonographic detection as an adnexal mass is variable. In most patients with an unruptured ectopic pregnancy, an adnexal mass separate from the ovary that has a small anechoic center can be identified (Fig. 2).[23] Rarely, fetal heart motion can be detected within the ectopic gestational sac which arises from a live fetus. In addition, the uterus in patients with an ectopic pregnancy typically has an echogenic endometrium, a sign of a decidual thickening associated with ectopic pregnancy (Fig. 3).

Most importantly, sonography is useful in demonstrating the presence or absence of an intrauterine pregnancy in those patients suspected of having an ectopic pregnancy. The more recent widespread utilization of the β-hCG RIA has resulted in presentation of patients for sonographic evaluation earlier in their pregnancy. Thus, one is faced with the difficult task of distinguishing an early intrauterine pregnancy from an ectopic pregnancy before an embryo can be delineated.

Recent studies have reported the utility of careful evaluation of the intrauterine decidual changes in the discrimination of early intrauterine pregnancy from the decidual transformation associated with ectopic pregnancies.[24] These sonographic features of the decidua can be helpful in distinguishing an intrauterine pregnancy from an ectopic pregnancy prior to sonographic depiction of the embryonic pole.[19] Specifically, two concentric rings of decidua (the double decidual sac) can be identified in an early intrauterine pregnancy if detailed images of the intrauterine contents can be

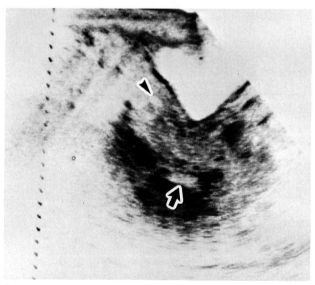

A

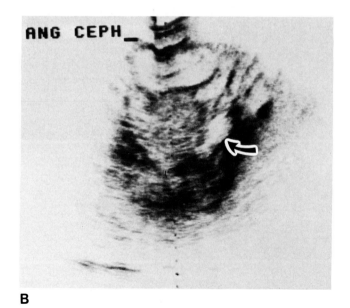

B

Fig. 3. Longitudinal **(A)**, and transverse **(B)** static sonograms demonstrating a fusiform left adnexal mass representing a ruptured ectopic pregnancy (*curved arrow*). On the longitudinal sonogram, a small amount of blood was present in the cul-de-sac (*arrow*). In addition, there is fluid within the interine lumen (*arrowhead*), probably resulting from bleeding from separation of the decidual cast.

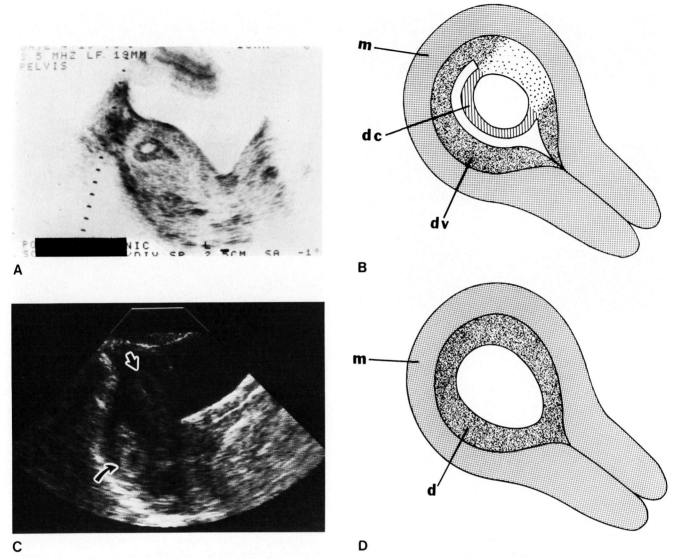

Fig. 4. Sonographic depiction of the decidua in early intrauterine and extrauterine pregnancies. **A.** Longitudinal real-time sonogram of early (4 week) intrauterine pregnancy prior to sonographic depiction of an embryo. Two layers of decidua surround the developing gestational sac. **B.** Diagram of the two decidual layers that can be seen in an early intrauterine pregnancy. The innermost ring of decidua surrounds the developing gestational sac and represents the decidua capsularis (dc). The thickened endometrium forms the decidua vera (dv). (m = myometrium). **C.** Longitudinal real-time sonogram of a ruptured ectopic pregnancy (*curved arrow*) associated with a decidual cast (*arrow*) in the uterus. The decidual cast is composed of only one layer. **D.** Diagram of the decidual cast that is associated with an ectopic pregnancy (d = decidua; m = myometrium).

obtained (Fig. 4). The two concentric rings of decidua correspond to the decidua capsularis that borders the gestational sac and the decidua vera that surrounds the decidua capsularis and developing gestational sac. In contrast to the two concentric rings of decidua that can be identified in an early intrauterine pregnancy, the decidual cast of an ectopic pregnancy has only one layer of decidua. A central anechoic area within the decidua cast usually is the result of separation of the decidua and bleeding. A double decidual sac can occasionally be mimicked by separation of the decidua

from the myometrium prior to expulsion of a decidual cast associated with an ectopic pregnancy.

A double decidual sac can also be encountered in patients with or incomplete abortion (Figs. 5A,5B). In these patients, the double decidua is accentuated by the bleeding that occurs around the gestational sac. This appearance has also been reported in one patient with an ectopic pregnancy when the decidual cast was in the process of being shed.[19]

If a double decidual sac is not seen, one probably should rely upon assessment of gestational viability

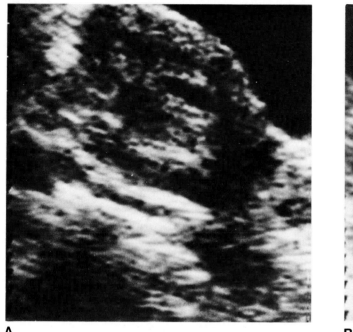

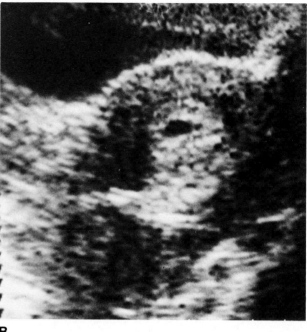

A   B

Fig. 5. Longitudinal **(A)** and transverse **(B)** real-time sonograms of patient with adnexal mass and concentric decidual layers within the uterus. An ectopic pregnancy was thought to be less likely than an intrauterine pregnancy with a corpus luteum cyst on the basis of the double decidual layers. The patient was found to have separation of the decidual layers secondary to an incomplete abortion.

as determined by serial hCGs. In a recent series, approximately 6 percent of the patients with a single decidual layer had a viable intrauterine pregnancy. The consequences of performing a D&C on a patient with a single decidual layer who has a viable intrauterine pregnancy should make one cautious in interpreting this sonographic sign as definitive of an ectopic pregnancy. When possible, the sonographic findings should be correlated with serial β-hCG assays in order to assess gestational viability or the presence of an ectopic pregnancy.

In addition to the finding of a double decidua, or intrauterine pregnancies, in pregnancies greater than 5 weeks, localized thickening of the choriodecidua corresponding to the chorion frondosum should be present in early intrauterine pregnancies and not in ectopic pregnancies. An embryo should be detected in pregnancies greater than 6 week's menstrual age.

The sonographic detection of the double decidua is highly dependent upon the resolution of the scanner used and the scanning ability and experience of the individuals who perform the examination. For example, if the transducer that is used is not focused at the proper depth, it is doubtful that the double decidual layers will be documented, even if present. We, therefore, advocate the use of mechanical sector scanners with transducers that are optimally focused at the region of interest. In addition, evaluation of the patient

with a fully distended bladder is advocated since this places the uterus and its contents nearly horizontal to the beam, thus allowing evaluation of this structure with axial rather than lateral resolution.

Besides meticulous sonographic evaluation of the uterus and adnexa, one should carefully evaluate the cul-de-sac for the presence of intraperitoneal blood in patients suspected of having an ectopic pregnancy. The presence of blood within the cul-de-sac in a patient who is pregnant most frequently indicates the presence of a ruptured ectopic pregnancy (Fig. 6). One should realize that blood within the cul-de-sac can occasionally result from attempts at culdocentesis (Fig. 7). We therefore recommend sonographic evaluation of the patient with a suspected ectopic pregnancy prior to attempts at culdocentesis. If a massive amount of hemorrhage has occurred, blood can be identified not only in the cul-de-sac, but also in the pericolic recesses and perihepatic spaces.

The sonographic appearance of intraperitoneal blood varies from anechoic to hypoechoic, probably depending upon the amount of organization that has occurred within the clot. Unclotted blood is typically anechoic and becomes more echogenic as it organizes. An organized hematoma can become anechoic after fibrinolysis has occurred.

The adnexal mass arising from an ectopic pregnancy can be associated with a corpus luteum. A corpus

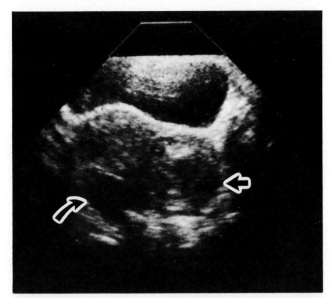

A

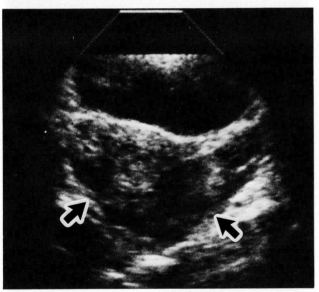

B

Fig. 6. A. Transverse real-time sonogram demonstrating complex left adnexal mass (*arrow*) which is associated with fluid in the cul-de-sac (*curved arrow*). This patient has a ruptured left tubal pregnancy with blood in the cul-de-sac. **B.** Transverse sonogram of patient with ruptured ectopic pregnancy. Posterior to the uterus is some moderately echogenic material (*arrows*) that corresponds to clotted blood within the cul-de-sac secondary to hemoperitoneum from a ruptured ectopic pregnancy.

luteum can be differentiated from an adnexal mass resulting from an ectopic pregnancy by its location within the ovary and more rounded configuration (Fig. 8). Identification of the location of a corpus luteum can be used to indicate the probable side of the ectopic pregnancy. In over half of the cases, the ectopic pregnancy will be within the tube on the ipsilateral side to the corpus luteum.

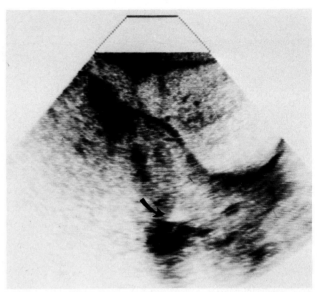

Fig. 7. A small amount (3 to 4 cc's) of fluid (*curved arrow*) was present in the cul-de-sac after culdocentesis was performed on this patient. If possible, it is best to delay culdocentesis until after the sonographic examination, since blood produced by the procedure mimics the sonographic findings of hemoperitoneum secondary to a ruptured ectopic pregnancy.

The sonographic diagnosis of an interstitial ectopic pregnancy rests primarily with recognition of an eccentrically placed gestational sac that still appears to be within the outline of the uterus (Figs. 9 and 10).[19] The amount of uterine wall surrounding the gestational sac in an interstitial ectopic pregnancy is usually thinner than that seen in a gestational sac within a bicornuate uterus (Fig. 10). In some cases, however, it may be difficult to differentiate an interstitial ectopic pregnancy from a gestational sac within a bicornuate uterus. In such patients, sonographic evaluation of the kidneys may be helpful since there is an association of unilateral renal agenesis with duplication anomalies of the uterus.

The sonographic diagnosis of an abdominal ectopic pregnancy involves recognition of the extra-uterine location of the gestational sac and fetus or an unusual fetal position (Figs. 11A-E).[25-27] In early intra-abdominal pregnancies, the uterus is typically bulbous and enlarged and the gestational sac and fetus are identified in the lower portion of the peritoneal cavity. Sonographic diagnosis of a more advanced abdominal ectopic pregnancy may be difficult. Blood or fluid may be present in the paracolic recesses or hepatorenal pouch (Fig. 11D). The only sonographic sign that can be recognized might be an unusual fetal position or placental location and the inability to trace the confines of the uterus surrounding the fetus and placenta. One should be careful not to mistake an intrauterine preg-

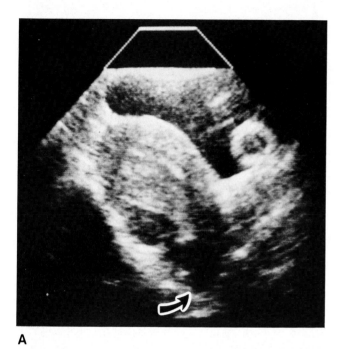

A

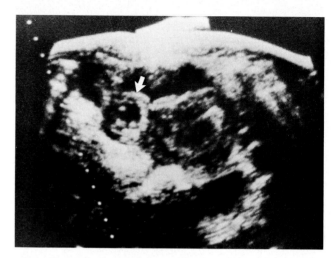

Fig. 9. Interstitial ectopic pregnancy (transverse static sonogram, 4 cm above symphysis, pubis). There is an eccentrically located gestational sac within the uterine outline (*arrow*). Its unusual location suggested an interstitial ectopic pregnancy. (*Courtesy of Thomas Lawson MD and Charles C Thomas Publishers.*)

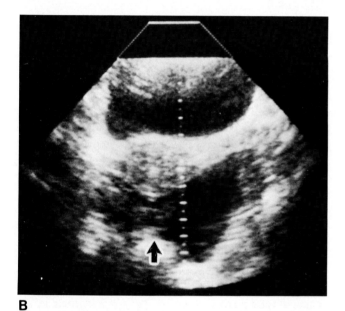

B

Fig. 8. Longitudinal **(A)** and transverse **(B)** of a ruptured corpus luteum cyst (*arrow*) that simulates the appearance of a ruptured ectopic pregnancy. The cul-de-sac blood (*arrow*) crossed the midline and, therefore, was thought to be intraperitoneal. A Foley catheter is present within the urinary bladder. The β-hCG assay confirming that the patient was not pregnant, therefore was of the upmost importance in correctly distinguishing this entity from a ruptured ectopic pregnancy.

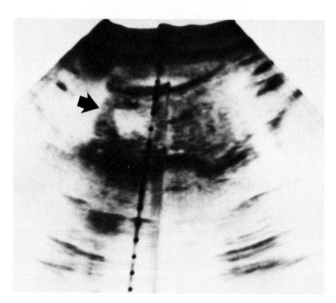

Fig. 10. Transverse static sonogram of patient with an interstitial (cornual) ectopic pregnancy (*arrow*). The eccentric location of the gestational sac and apparent lack of border between the uterus and mass was suggestive of a cornual pregnancy. (*Courtesy of Dean Birdwell, RDMS*)

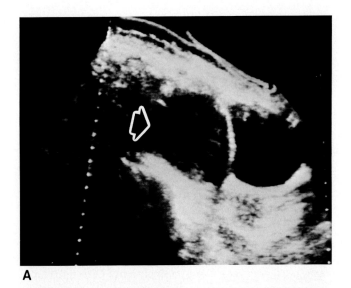

A

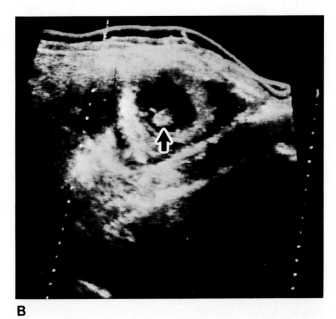

B

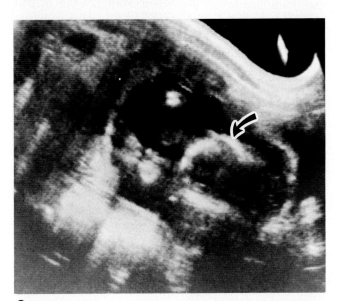

C

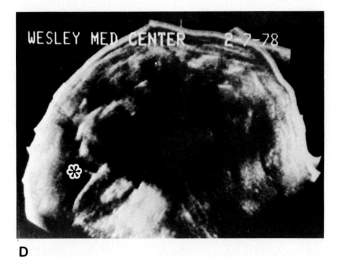

D

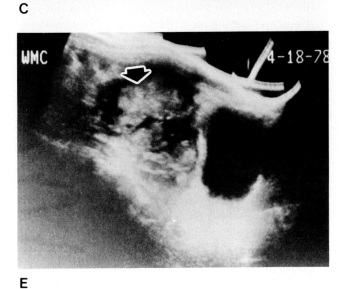

E

Fig. 11. Abdominal ectopic pregnancies. **A.** Longitudinal sonogram of patient with abdominal ectopic pregnancy demonstrating enlarged uterus (*arrow*) without gestational sac or decidual proliferation. **B.** Longitudinal sonogram of same patient performed 6 cm to the right of midline demonstrating well-defined gestational sac surrounded by intact choriodecidua. The fetus (*arrow*) demonstrated fetal heart motion and fetal motion. The ectopic gestational sac was located within the lower peritoneal cavity, on top of the right iliopsoas muscle. **C.** Longitudinal static sonogram of patient presenting with severe abdominal pain during second trimester. The fetal head (*arrow*) is adjacent to a normal-sized uterus. Since it was prospectively detected that the shape of the "uterus" was abnormal, an abdominal ectopic pregnancy was considered. (*Courtesy of Brad Reeves, M.D.*) **D.** Transverse static sonogram of same patient demonstrating fluid (*) in the hepatorenal pouch and perihepatic spaces. **E.** Longitudinal sonogram of same patient after removal of a fetus demonstrating retained placenta (*arrow*). In most abdominal pregnancies, the placenta is not removed due to the possibility of prolonged bleeding and inability to separate the placenta from the bowel or mesenteric attachments.

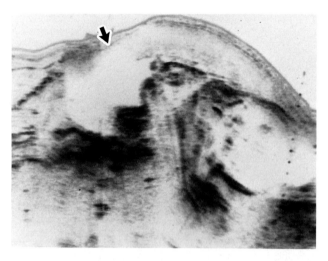

Fig. 12. Intrauterine pregnancy with very thin fundal myometrium (*arrow*) which might be confused with an abdominal ectopic pregnancy. However, in this case, a separate uterus could not be identified, leading one to suspect an intra- rather than extrauterine pregnancy.

nancy that has a very thin uterine wall surrounding it for an abdominal ectopic pregnancy (Fig. 12).

The rarest types of ectopic pregnancy are cervical and ovarian. Probably because of their rarity, these types of ectopic pregnancy are usually not prospectively diagnosed.[28,29] They appear as a complex mass near the cervix or ovary. It is conceivable that ovarian

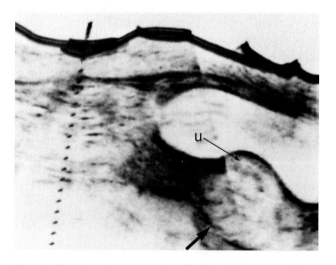

Fig. 13. Chronic ectopic pregnancy (longitudinal, 3 cm to right of midline). This patient presented with intermittent fever and a palpable pelvic mass. The patient denied any episode of lower abdominal pain. Adjacent to the uterus (u), a moderately echogenic mass was identified (*arrow*). The uterus is displaced anteriorly by the mass. This is the most common appearance of a chronic ectopic pregnancy. Chronic ectopic pregnancies usually result from rupture of an ectopic pregnancy with subsequent hematoma formation.

ectopic pregnancies could mimic the appearance of a corpus luteum hematoma.

Chronic ectopic pregnancies appear typically as moderately echogenic masses which are adjacent to the uterus (Fig. 13). They result from previous rupture of an ectopic pregnancy with hematoma formation.[30]

DIFFERENTIAL DIAGNOSIS

There are a variety of conditions that may mimic the sonographic features of an ectopic pregnancy. However, when one combines the sonographic features with the results of either single or serial β-hCG the differential diagnosis can be narrowed considerably. A discrepancy between β-hCG levels and sonographic features most frequently occurs in patients with nonviable intrauterine pregnancies. If, for example, the patient is expected to be 8 or more weeks pregnant and does not demonstrate intact choriodecidua and an embryo or fetus and the β-hCG are less than expected and falling, a nonviable intrauterine pregnancy is most likely present.

One of the most difficult entities to distinguish from an ectopic pregnancy is a corpus luteum cyst or hematoma. A hemorrhagic corpus luteum cyst may appear as a complex adnexal mass and may be associated with intraperitoneal blood if rupture has occurred (Fig. 8). In most corpus luteum cysts, in our experience, the hypoechoic mass can be identified to be located within the ovary, whereas an ectopic pregnancy can be defined separately from the uterus and ovary. One should be aware that corpus luteum cysts can be associated with early intrauterine pregnancies and elevated β-hCG values.

Ectopic pregnancy is commonly encountered in patients with a hydro- or pyosalpinx, and it is unlikely that one will detect coexistent ectopic pregnancies in these patients. In this situation, laparoscopy should not be discouraged when there is a suspected ectopic pregnancy and a preexisting hydro- or pyosalpinx or tuboovarian abscess. Ectopic pregnancies can also be encountered in patients with other adnexal masses (Figs. 14D and 15).

Other conditions that might mimic ectopic pregnancy include a normal intrauterine pregnancy in a retroflexed uterus, and other complex adnexal masses, such as endometriomas that contain clotted blood. A patient with an intrauterine pregnancy within a retroflexed uterus can usually be distinguished sonographically from an ectopic pregnancy by careful analysis of the location of the gestational sac relative to the uterine fundus (Fig. 16). Although most patients with endometriosis have fertility disorders, the presence of

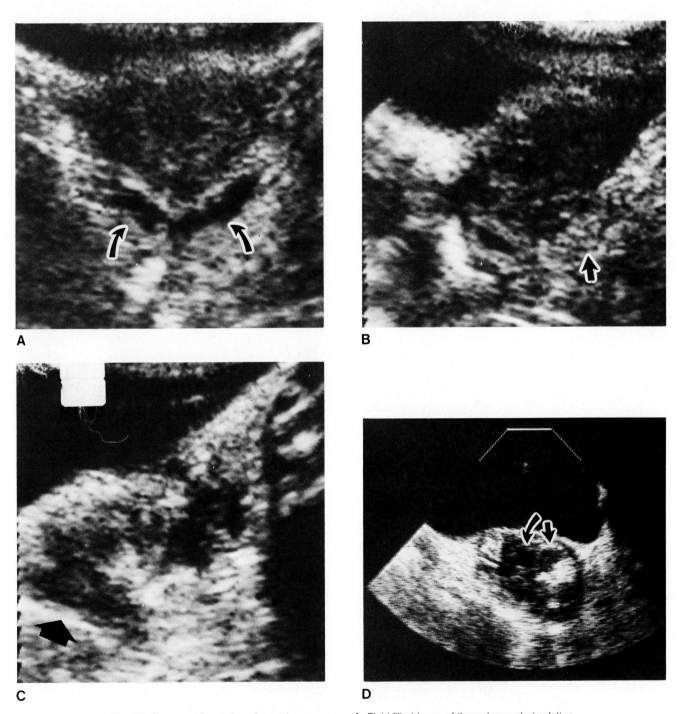

Fig. 14. Sonographic mimics of ectopic pregnancy. **A.** Fluid-filled loops of ileum (*arrows*) simulating bilateral fusiform adnexal masses. **B.** Approximately 2 second later, the portion of the bowel to the left of midline (*arrow*) has contracted. **C.** Five seconds later the entire bowel segment (*arrow*) has contracted. **D.** Transverse real-time sonogram showing a complex mass (*arrow*) which is surrounded by hypoechoic areas. This patient had an ectopic pregnancy (*curved arrow*) and dermoid cyst (*arrow*).

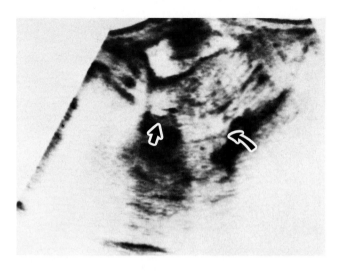

Fig. 15. Transverse sonogram of patient with known pelvic inflammatory disease. A complex right adnexal mass (*arrow*) associated with fluid in the cul-de-sac (*curved arrow*) is present. Based on these sonographic findings, an ectopic pregnancy could not be excluded. The β-hCG assay confirmed the lack of a pregnancy; the complex adnexal mass corresponded to a tuboovarian abscess.

this condition does not exclude the possibility of a coexistent ectopic pregnancy. Therefore, one should obtain appropriate laboratory tests, specifically a β-hCG, if an ectopic pregnancy might be present.

Fluid-containing small bowel loops may mimic the complex adnexal masses encountered in ectopic pregnancy. Real-time sonography can be used to demonstrate typical changes in bowel configuration associated with peristalsis of fluid-filled bowel (Figs. 14A,B, and C).

Although there have been a few case reports of patients with an ectopic pregnancy coexistent with an

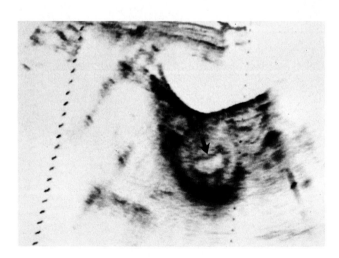

Fig. 16. Longitudinal static sonogram of an early intrauterine pregnancy within a retroflexed uterus. The fundus of this uterus is directed posteriorly. Within the uterus is an intact gestational (*arrow*).

intrauterine pregnancy, this condition is exceedingly rare, with a reported incidence of between 1 in 16,000 and 1 in 30,000 pregnancies.[14,31] However, the incidence is increasing and some have suggested that heterotopic pregnancy may occur as frequently as 1 in 7000.[35,36] It does, however, appear to be most frequently encountered in patients undergoing ovulation induction and also has been encountered in patients with a persistent adnexal mass after spontaneous or elective abortion.[14,32]

CONCLUSION

In summary, it is believed that the combined use of β-hCG assay(s) and mechanical sector real-time sonography should result in detection of the vast majority of patients with an ectopic pregnancy. The combined use of these two modalities has markedly improved the detection of patients with ectopic pregnancies and will contribute to a decreased mortality and morbidity from this disorder.[33,34]

REFERENCES

1. Tancer M, Delke L, Veridiano N: A fifteen year experience with ectopic pregnancy. Surg Gyn Ob 152:179, 1981
2. Breen J: A 21-year survey of 654 ectopic pregnancies. Am J Ob Gyn 106:1004, 1970
3. Shiono P, Harlap S, Pellegrin F: Ectopic pregnancies: Rising incidence rates in Northern California. Am J Public Health, 72:173, 1982
4. Rubin G, Peterson H, Dorfman S, et al: Ectopic pregnancy in the United States 1970 through 1978. JAMA 249:1725, 1983
5. Laing F, Jeffrey R: Ultrasound evaluation of ectopic pregnancy. Radiol Cl NAM 20:383, 1982
6. Schoenbaum S, Rosendorf L, Kappelman N, et al: Gray scale ultrasound tubal pregnancy. Radiology 127:757, 1978
7. Maklad N, Wright C: Gray scale ultrasonography in diagnosis of ectopic pregnancy. Radiology 126:221, 1978
8. Lawson T: Ectopic pregnancy: Criteria and accuracy of ultrasonic diagnoses. Am J Roentgenol 131:153, 1978
9. Brown TW, Filly RA, Laing FC, et al: Analysis of ultrasonic criteria in the evaluation of ectopic pregnancy. Am J Roentgenol 131:967, 1978
10. Conrad M, Johnson J, James AE Jr: Sonography in ectopic pregnancy, in Sanders R, James AE (eds), Ultrasonography in Obstetrics and Gynecology. New York, Appleton-Century-Crofts, 1977, pp 113–121
11. Kadar N, DeVore G, Romero R: Discriminary hCG zone: Its use in sonographic evaluation for ectopic pregnancy. Obstet Gynecol 58:156, 1981
12. Kadar N, Romero R: The timing of a repeat ultrasound examination in the evaluation for ectopic pregnancy. J Clin Ultrasound 10:211, 1982

13. Kleiner G, Roberts T: Current factors and causation of tubal pregnancy: A prospective clinical pathologic study. Am J Obstet Gynecol 99:21, 1967
14. Glebatis D, Janerich D: Ectopic pregnancies in upstate New York. JAMA 249:1730, 1983
15. Cartwright P: Culdocentesis and ectopic pregnancy. (submitted for publication)
16. Schwartz R, DiPietro D: Beta hCG is a diagnostic aid for suspected ectopic pregnancy. Obstet Gynecol 56:197, 1980
17. Jacobsen E, Rothe D: False positive hemaglutination inhibition tests for pregnancy with intra-ovarian abscess. Int J Gyn Ob 17:307, 1980
18. DiPietro D: Ectopic pregnancy: Interpreting hCG levels. Lab Manag 43, 1981
19. Nyberg D, Laing F, Filly F, et al: Ultrasonic differentiation of the gestational sac of early intrauterine pregnancy from the pseudogestational sac of ectopic pregnancy. Radiology 146:755, 1983
20. Ackerman R, Deutsch S, Krumholtz B: Levels of human chorionic gonadotropin in unruptured and ruptured ectopic pregnancy. Obstet Gynecol 60:13, 1982
21. Cartwright P, DiPietro D: Personal communication
22. Cartwright P, DiPietro D: Ectopic pregnancy: Change in serum hCG concentrations. Obstet and Gynecol 63:76, 1984
23. Fleischer A, Boehm H, James AE Jr: Sonographic evaluation of ectopic pregnancies, in Sanders R, James AE (eds), Principles and Practice of Ultrasonography in Obstetrics and Gynecology. New York, Appleton-Century-Crofts, 1980, pp 277–290
24. Bradley W, Fiske C, Filly R: The double sign of early intrauterine pregnancy: Use in exclusion of ectopic pregnancy. Work in progress. Radiology 143:223, 1982
25. Allibone G, Fagan C, Porter S: The sonographic features of intra-abdominal pregnancy. J Clin Ultrasound 9:383, 1981
26. Kurtz A, Dubbins P, Wagner R, et al: Problems of abnormal fetal position. JAMA 247:3251, 1982
27. Graham D, Johnson T, Sanders R: Sonographic findings in abdominal pregnancies. J Ultra Med 1:71, 1982
28. Raskin MM: Diagnosis of cervical pregnancy by ultrasound: A case report. Am J Obstet Gynecol 130:234, 1978
29. Laughlin C, Lee T, Richards R: Ultrasonographic diagnosis of cervical ectopic pregnancy: A case report. J Ultra Med 2:137, 1983
30. Rogers W, Shaub M, Wilson R: Chronic ectopic pregnancy: Ultrasonic diagnosis. J Clin Ultrasound 54:257, 1977
31. Penkava R, Bohling J. Ultrasound demonstration of combined ectopic and intrauterine pregnancy: A case report. Am J Roentgenol 132:1012, 1979
32. Berger M, Taymor M: Simultaneous intrauterine and tubal pregnancies following ovulation induction. Am J Obstet Gynecol 113:812, 1972
33. Brenner P, Roy F, Mitchell D: Ectopic pregnancy: A study of 300 consecutive surgically treated cases. JAMA 243:673, 1980
34. Burbrow M, Bell H: Ectopic pregnancy: A sixteen year survey of 905 cases. Obstet Gynecol 20:500, 1962
35. Reece EA, Petrine RH, Simons MF, et al: Combined intrauterine and extrauterine gestation: A review. Am J Obstet Gynecol 146:323, 1983
36. Hann LE, Bachmann DL, McArdle CR: Coexistent intrauterine and ectopic pregnancy: A reevaluation. Radiology 152:151, 1984

31 | Sonography in Induced Abortion

David Graham
Roger C. Sanders
Theodore M. King

Since the Supreme Court decision legalizing abortion, pregnancy termination has become one of the most common procedures performed in gynecologic practice. It is estimated that in the United States each year, there are more than one million pregnancy terminations.[1]

The method of termination performed is dependent on the gestational age of the pregnancy at the time of the procedure. Up to approximately 14 menstrual weeks, the method of choice is transcervical aspiration. After 14 weeks, the size of the fetus makes this procedure more hazardous and alternative methods must be used. The two most commonly performed midtrimester termination procedures are dilatation and evacuation (D&E), where the cervix is dilated and the fetus morcellated and extracted, and instillation procedures, where a transabdominal amniocentesis is performed and an agent such as hypertonic saline, urea, or prostaglandin $F_{2\alpha}$ injected to induce labor. These procedures may be preceded by insertion of laminaria into the cervix to make subsequent dilatation of the cervix easier (Fig. 1). The risk of complications from elective pregnancy termination appear to increase with increasing gestational age.[2] Midtrimester abortion is associated with an increased incidence of retained products of conception and/or endometritis. D&E may be associated with uterine perforation.

Ultrasound is of value in the patient who requests pregnancy termination or following such a procedure in a number of well-defined situations.[3-5]

1. Dating the pregnancy, most commonly because there is a discrepancy in the uterine size and menstrual dates.
2. Diagnosis of coexistent pelvic masses such as uterine fibroids, adnexal masses, or uterine anomalies that might make determination of gestational age more difficult or that may interfere with the termination procedure (Fig. 2).
3. Localization of a coexistent intrauterine device.
4. Guidance for amnioinfusion or curettage procedures.
5. Diagnosis of complications of termination such as uterine perforation, uterine, or pelvic infection and retained products of conception.

ESTIMATION OF GESTATIONAL AGE

The estimation of gestational age in the first and second trimesters has already been discussed in depth in other chapters (see Chapters 9, 10). In the first trimester, this is most accurately performed with a crown-rump length while in the second trimester, biparietal diameter and femur length measurements are more useful.

Gestational age assessment may be necessary because of a discrepancy between the uterine size and the menstrual dates under the following circumstances:

1. Unknown or uncertain menstrual history, since 20 to 40 percent of patients have unknown or uncertain menstrual history[6,7] or a significant discrepancy between menstrual dates and the uterine size palpated on examination.

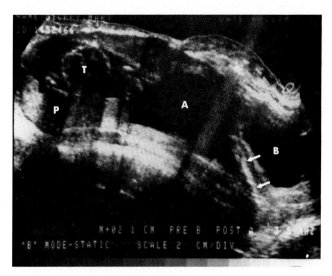

Fig. 1. Laminaria in cervix. A longitudinal midline scan of the uterus performed after insertion of laminaria shows the linear echogenicity produced by this foreign object. Placenta, P; fetal thorax, T; amniotic fluid, A; maternal bladder, B.

2. Coexistent uterine mass or fibroids that make clinical estimation of gestational age inaccurate, usually leading to overestimation of gestational age. Assignment of an incorrect gestational age may lead to an inappropriate procedure being carried out, with a potential for unnecessary complications.
3. Multiple pregnancy, usually diagnosed because of a uterine size significantly large for dates. Where amnioinfusion techniques are to be performed, both sacs need to be tapped separately.

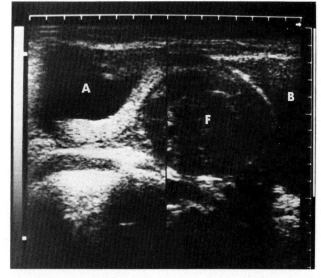

Fig. 2. Fibroids in second trimester. A longitudinal midline real-time sonogram showing a large lower uterine fibroid (F). The location of this fibroid would prevent "blind" lower midline amniocentesis. Amniotic fluid, A; maternal bladder, B.

4. Uterine anomalies such as bicornuate uterus, may make clinical uterine size estimation more difficult, may mimic an adnexal mass and may interfere with the termination procedure.
5. Coexistent adnexal masses will not only interfere with clinical evaluation but may also lead to an inappropriate choice of termination procedure or may lead to more serious consequences such as attempts at aspiration of or infusion of abortifacient into the adnexal mass (Fig. 3).
6. Extrauterine pregnancy, in a number of patients who present for pregnancy termination, an extrauterine pregnancy may be suspected clinically at the initial examination or after the procedure when only scanty tissue is obtained and histology shows no evidence of chorionic villi. Since follow-up may be difficult or impossible in a significant number of patients after pregnancy termination has been performed, it is very important to make the diagnosis as soon as possible.
7. The patient is not pregnant—on initial examination, the uterus is found to be normal size and it may be suspected that the patient is either not pregnant or has had an incomplete or complete spontaneous abortion.
8. Fetal death in utero—where fetal death has already occurred, subsequent spontaneous abortion will be expected and attempts at elective termination, especially with an inappropriate type of procedure may be avoided.
9. Fetal anomalies (see Chapters 14–20)—in unusual circumstances, a fetal anomaly may lead to polyhydramnios or oligohydramnios and so cause incorrect gestational age estimation. While it might not be important to know that the fetus has an anomaly when the procedure is performed, it would be important to know the type of anomaly present to allow counseling about subsequent pregnancies.
10. Trophoblastic disease (see Chapter 29)—trophoblastic disease will often lead to an inappropriately large fundal height. It is very important to diagnose this condition prior to attempting any type of procedure so that appropriate initial and adjunctive therapy may be initiated.
11. In the uncooperative or obese patient, ultrasound may provide the only reliable way of assessing gestational age because of difficulty in clinical estimation of uterine size.

Where the uterine size and menstrual dates are compatible with dates, then gestational age assessment may be needed

1. where the pregnancy is near 14 weeks to determine the type of procedure to be performed; and

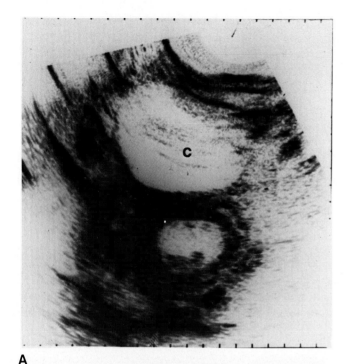

A

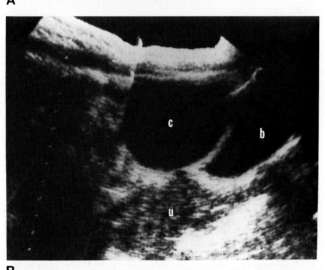

B

Fig. 3. A. Preabortal sonogram. **B.** Postabortal sonogram. In this patient following a first trimester termination pregnancy, it was thought at the postabortal examination that the uterus remained enlarged. The postabortal sonogram, however, shows a large cyst (c) anterior to the uterus (u), maternal bladder (b). Retrospective evaluation of the preabortal sonogram showed that what was considered to be bladder was actually the cyst (c).

2. where uterine size and dates are near the limit where pregnancy termination may be legally performed.

In evaluating some patients, e.g., the uncooperative young adolescent, the mentally retarded, or where obesity makes examination suboptimal, ultrasound

may be the only way in which a reliable estimation of the pregnancy may be obtained.

DIAGNOSIS OF COEXISTENT PELVIC MASS

The presence of a coexistent mass, most often uterine anomalies or an adnexal mass such as corpus luteum cyst may not only interfere with gestational age assessment but might also interfere with the performance of the procedure (Fig. 2). (See Chapter 33.) Uterine fibroids in particular may be quite large and may further enlarge with the pregnancy leading to a significant miscalculation of gestational age. Their size or location may interfere with aspiration procedures, dilatation and evacuation and amnioinfusion techniques, while after the procedure, retained products of conception may be a problem. Where amnioinfusion techniques are used, a theoretical possibility is the injection of the mass rather than the uterus, with possible adverse consequences.

LOCALIZATION OF A COEXISTENT INTRAUTERINE DEVICE

While the intrauterine device (IUD) provides significant protection against pregnancy, there is a failure rate of 2 to 3 per 100 women-years.[8] Where a patient presents with symptoms of pregnancy and a history of having an IUD in place, several possibilities exist. The patient may have an IUD in place either in a normal or abnormal position, together with an intrauterine pregnancy, or may have an extrauterine pregnancy and an intrauterine IUD (see Chapter 41).

In the patient having a termination procedure, ultrasound allows confirmation that the device is indeed intrauterine and allows easier removal of the device when it is in an abnormal location (Fig. 4).

GUIDANCE OF AMNIOINFUSION OR CURETTAGE PROCEDURES

In the majority of patients, the performance of a curettage or an amnioinfusion technique is without any complications. However, curettage procedures may be made more difficult by problems such as uterovaginal anomalies (Fig. 5), or uterine fibroids. Where there is difficulty encountered in entering the uterine cavity, intraoperative real-time ultrasound may be of great help in visualizing both the endometrial cavity and the curette and therefore reduce the possibility of uterine perforation (Fig. 6).

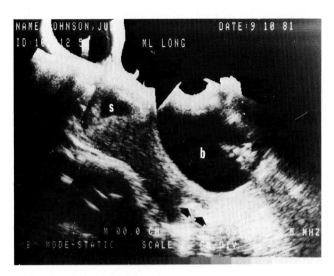

Fig. 4. Abnormal location of IUD. A longitudinal scan of the uterus at 7 weeks' gestation shows the gestational sac (s) at the uterine fundus. In the area of the cervical canal is seen a linear echogenicity due to a malpositioned copper IUD (*arrows*). Initial attempts at removal prior to the sonographic localization were unsuccessful. Maternal bladder, b.

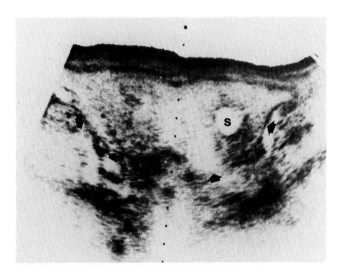

Fig. 5. Bicornuate uterus and pregnancy. In this transverse sonogram, the uterus is seen to have the broadened shape of a bicornuate uterus (*arrows*). In the left horn is seen a gestational sac (s). Such uterine anomalies may make uterine curettage more difficult.

Amnioinfusion techniques may be made more difficult by multiple pregnancy, uterine fibroids, uterine anomalies, transient myometrial contractions, patient obesity, and lateral displacement of the uterus. The value of ultrasound in performing amniocentesis in midtrimester for genetic purposes has been well documented[9-11] and is of equal value in abortion procedures.

DIAGNOSIS OF COMPLICATIONS OF TERMINATION

Although in the majority of patients, pregnancy termination is performed easily and without adverse consequence, there are a number of well-recognized complications to pregnancy termination. Curettage procedures are associated with risks of cervical injury, uterine perforation, retained products of conception and postabortal endometritis.[2]

Uterine perforation may be recognized intraoperatively by the appearance of omentum or bowel at the cervical os (Fig. 7) or may not be recognized until postabortally by the development of a mass adjacent to the uterus, compatible with a cul-de-sac or broad ligament hematoma or abscess (Fig. 8). Ultrasound is of value in recognizing these complications when they are suspected postprocedure by the presence of a pelvic mass separate from the uterus. A pelvic hematoma will be visualized as a predominantly cystic mass, often with internal echoes. If this hematoma becomes in-

fected, then the appearances may change with irregular, ill-defined borders and crossing of tissue planes.

Occasionally, an adnexal mass which was undetected at the time of the procedure may be palpated for the first time at the postprocedure examination (Fig. 3). In those patients who are examined sonographically before completion of a procedure to determine the existence of any abnormalities present, an incidental finding may be the visualization of the laminaria tents that are used to prepare the cervix for dilatation. Laminaria are usually sticks of dried seaweed that are placed in the undilated cervix. After a number of hours, they gradually swell by the absorption of water from sur-

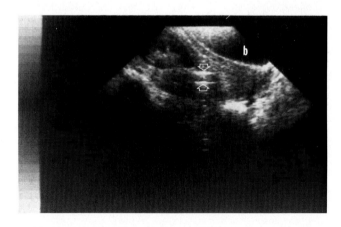

Fig. 6. Curette in uterus (operative sonogram). Longitudinal sector scan study of the lower portion of the uterus in a 9-week pregnancy. A suction curette (*arrows*) is seen in the lower uterine segment.

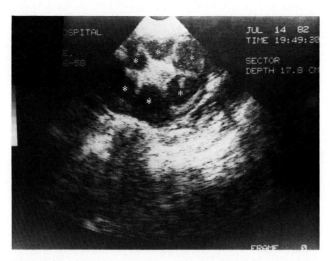

Fig. 7. Bowel loops in uterus following uterine perforation. In this sonogram following a mid-trimester determination, several cystic masses (*) are seen within the uterus and represent bowel in the uterus following uterine perforation. (*Picture courtesy of P. Dunner, M.D. and E. Lipsit, M.D.*)

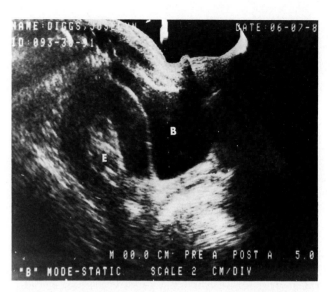

Fig. 9. Retained products of conception. A longitudinal midline scan of the uterus following a suction abortion shows a central collection of echoes (E) in the endometrial cavity, compatible with retained products of conception and/or blood. Maternal bladder, B.

rounding tissues and dilate the cervix, reducing the likelihood of trauma from subsequent mechanical dilatation. Sonographically, laminaria will appear as strong linear echogenicities in the endocervical canal (Fig. 1).

Retained products of conception may complicate both curettage and amnioinfusion techniques. In the first trimester procedure, retained products will be visualized sonographically as inhomogeneously increased endometrial echoes (Fig. 9). However, both re-

tained products of conception and endometrial blood have a similar appearance and may not be differentiated sonographically.[3,12] Nevertheless, where sonography shows well-defined narrow endometrial echoes, one may be reasonably confident that there are no significant retained products of conception.

In mid-trimester amnioinfusion procedures, the placenta is not uncommonly retained, necessitating postprocedure curettage in a number of patients.

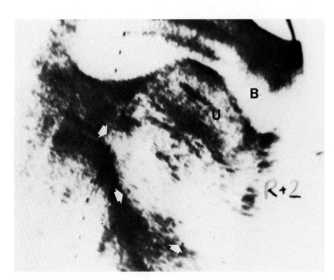

Fig. 8. Cul-de-sac hematoma. Longitudinal midline sonogram showing a large and complex mass (*arrows*) posterior to the uterus (u) and representing a hematoma occurring secondary to uterine perforation.

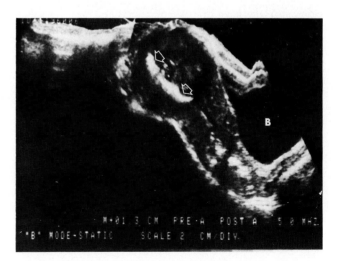

Fig. 10. Retained placenta following mid-trimester abortion. A longitudinal scan of the pelvis following a urea-prostaglandin termination showing a bulbous enlargement of the uterine fundus with nonhomogeneous increased echoes (*arrows*) in the endometrial cavity due to retained placental tissue.

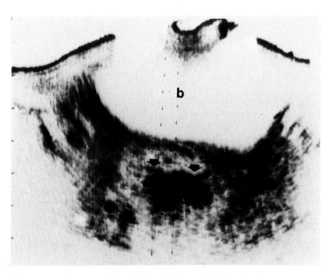

Fig. 11. In utero gas formation with retained products of conception. A transverse section of the uterus following a pregnancy termination shows a densely echogenic area (*arrows*) with distal shadowing due to gas forming organisms in retained products of conception. Maternal bladder, b.

Where curettage produces what appears to be an insufficient amount of tissue, sonograpy will indicate both the amount of tissue retained and its location, allowing directed curettage. Retained placental tissue following mid-trimester abortion causes the uterine fundus to have a somewhat bulbous appearance, with an inhomogeneous collection of echogenic material in the endometrial cavity (Fig. 10).

Where retained products of conception have not been recognized and infection has supervened, then the sonographic appearances may change. With infection with gas-forming organisms, there may be visualization of densely echogenic areas within the endometrial cavity, with distal shadowing or "tornado" formation from intrauterine gas (Fig. 11).

REFERENCES

1. Center for Disease Control. Abortion Surveillance, 1978. Atlanta, Georgia, Nov 1980
2. Grimes D, Cates W: Complications from legally-induced abortion. Obstet Gynecol Surv 34:183, 1979
3. Stone M, Elder MG: Evaluation of sonar in the prediction of complications after vaginal termination of pregnancy. Am J Obstet Gynecol 120:890, 1974
4. Sanders RC, Curtin MJ, Tapper AJ: Ultrasound in the management of elective abortion. Am J Roentgenol 125:469, 1975
5. Atienza MF, Burkman RT, Wight DJ, et al: Ultrasonography in the management of induced abortion, in Sanders RC, James AE (eds), Ultrasonography in Obstetrics and Gynecology, 1st ed. New York, Appleton-Century-Crofts, 1977
6. Campbell S: The assessment of fetal development by diagnostic ultrasound. Br Med J 2:730, 1974
7. Dewhurst DJ, Beazley JM, Campbell S: Assessment of fetal maturity and dysmaturity. Am J Obstet Gynecol 113:14, 1972
8. Second Report on Intrauterine Contraceptive Devices. U.S. Dept. of Health, Education, & Welfare. Food and Drug Administration. The Medical Device and Drug Advisory Committee on Obstetrics and Gynecology, 1978
9. Kerenyi TD, Walker B: The preventability of "bloody taps" in second trimester amniocentesis by ultrasound scanning. Obstet Gynecol 50:61, 1977
10. Chandra P, Nitowsky HM, Marion R, et al: Experience with sonography as an adjunct to amniocentesis for prenatal diagnosis of fetal genetic conditions. Am J Obstet Gynecol 133:519, 1979
11. Nolan GH, Schmickel RD, Chantaratherakitti P, et al: The effect of ultrasonography on midtrimester genetic amniocentesis complications. Am J Obstet Gynecol 140:531, 1981
12. Sanders RC: Postpartum diagnostic ultrasound, in Sanders RC, James AE (eds), Ultrasonography in Obstetrics and Gynecology, 1st ed. New York, Appleton-Century-Crofts, 1980

32 | Fetal Death

Roger C. Sanders

Bleeding and abdominal cramps are relatively commonplace problems in the first trimester of pregnancy. Such symptoms can be due to an eroded cervix or cervical polyp, but are often due to an abortion that is threatened or in progress. Several entities associated with pregnancy have a similar clinical presentation; a different management can be determined with the aid of ultrasound.[1] Clinical problems with distinctive sonographic appearances in the first trimester of pregnancy can be differentiated into:

1. Threatened abortion
2. Inevitable abortion
3. Incomplete (spontaneous) abortion
4. Blighted ovum
5. Missed abortion
6. Complete spontaneous abortion

Distinction between some of these entities is somewhat "theologic"[2] since inevitable abortion, incomplete spontaneous abortion, blighted ovum, and missed abortion are all treated in the same fashion with dilatation and curettage. The critical distinction from a clinical viewpoint is between (a) a threatened abortion with a viable fetus, (b) a dead or nonexistent fetus with retained products of conception, and (c) spontaneous abortion with no retained products of conception. However, since the distinction between incomplete spontaneous abortion, blighted ovum, and missed abortion may have some value in determining the genetic cause of habitual abortion these entities will be described in some detail.

THREATENED ABORTION

"Threatened abortion" is a term used to describe a first trimester pregnancy associated with vaginal bleeding with a live fetus. Several investigators have found ultrasound to be helpful in threatened abortion in showing a viable as opposed to a dead fetus. The appropriate clinical management is then one of expectancy.[1,3] Many patients with a "threatened abortion" have a live but sick fetus (Fig. 1). Ultrasonically, the principal features suggesting a poor prognosis are relative fetal inactivity and lack of expected growth of the gestational sac even though fetal heart movement can be seen resulting in a disproportion between fetal size and sac size[4] and a poor sac outline. The fetal pulse may be slow.[5] Decreased fetal movement, however, may be seen on a temporary basis in the normal fetus.[6] If no spontaneous movements are seen over prolonged observation but the fetal heart beat is present, the prognosis is grave.[7]

Patients with a clinical question of threatened abortion are generally put on bed rest or given Dilalutin in the hope that the fetus will survive. However, in many instances fetal death subsequently ensues and therapeutic abortion is appropriate. Ultrasound is the best means of monitoring fetal viability and reassuring the mother that the fetus is still alive.

Several comparisons of the diagnostic accuracy of estrogen excretion versus ultrasound have been made. Prior to 1975 estriol assay was found to be superior.[3] Today, real-time ultrasound provides reliable diagnosis of a viable or nonviable fetus.[8] Some viable fetuses

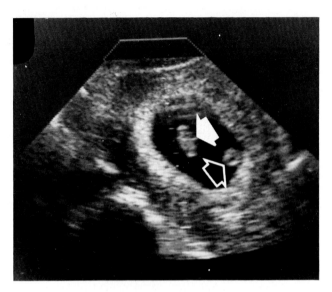

Fig. 1. Normal gestational sac in which the fetus (*solid arrow*) and the yoke sac (*open arrow*) can be seen. Note the relatively well defined trophoblastic reaction.

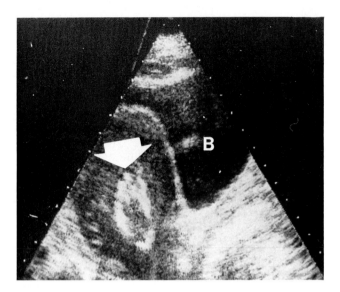

Fig. 2. Retained products of conception with an irregular echogenic circular structure (*arrow*) within the uterus. This could either be blood or fetal parts. B = bladder.

subsequently abort, however.[9] Estriol correlation with fetal prognosis is less than ideal[5]; ultrasound is now considered to be the most accurate technique.[10-12] A qualitative human chorionic gonadotropin (hCG) combined with real-time fetal heart monitoring is conclusive evidence of fetal viability or nonviability.[10]

INCOMPLETE ABORTION

An incomplete abortion is considered to be present when some of the products of conception (e.g., a portion of the fetus or placenta) remain within the uterus even though the majority of the pregnancy has been expelled. It can be difficult to decide whether some products of conception remain within the uterus if groups of central echoes without recognizable fetal parts are seen (Fig. 2). This problem is dealt with in greater detail in Chapter 34.

INEVITABLE ABORTION

Inevitable abortion refers to a situation in which the gestational sac and fetus are present within the uterus but have become detached from the implantation site and will be spontaneously aborted within the next few hours. The sac will be located in the lower uterine segment or even, rarely, in the vaginal canal (Fig. 3). Occasionally one may see a fetus that is in the process of being aborted. A gestational sac will be visible containing an immobile fetus and the cervix will be dilated.

If the cervix becomes dilated in the first or second trimester, abortion is inevitable.[13] As a rule, the aborting sac will be surrounded by a crescentic sonolucent zone representing blood between the trophoblastic tissue and the myometrium. Occasionally there will be internal echoes within the sac forming a fluid–fluid level (presumed to represent blood). An examination after a relatively short period (an hour or two) will show the disappearance of the aborting sac because it has been expelled.

Patients with first trimester bleeding apparently had a significantly higher percentage of lower implantation sites (25.8 percent) versus controls (4.8 percent); however, patients with the lower implantation site had a similar abortion rate to those with a high implantation site.[14] Presumably in earlier studies sacs were observed while they were traveling down the uterine cavity[14] in the process of being aborted.

BLIGHTED OVUM

A "blighted ovum" is an anembryonic pregnancy: a gestational sac is present but is empty. The fetus is absent or so small that it cannot be seen ultrasonically; it may have actually disappeared and not be found at pathology. There are several ultrasonic signs of a blighted ovum.[15] The gestational sac is too small for dates. Often the size difference is substantial, e.g., a 15-week pregnancy with reliable dates may be found to contain a gestational sac of approximately 8- to 9-week size. The gestational sac may have an unusual shape, sometimes assuming a flattened configuration

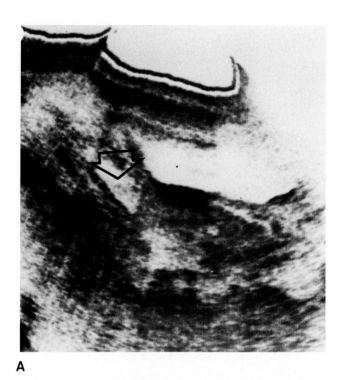 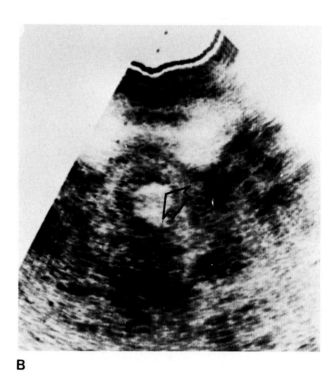

A   **B**

Fig. 3. A. Longitudinal. **B.** Transverse. This uterus contains a gestational sac which is in the process of being aborted. A fluid-filled level (*arrow*) can be seen within the gestational sac. The echo-free area in the region of the cervix represents blood which is leaking around the aborting sac. A repeat sonogram two hours later showed no evidence of intrauterine gestational sac.

(Fig. 4). However, an odd shape may be due to compression by the bladder, a leiomyoma, or a myometrial contraction. The thickness of the trophoblastic reaction (the rind) around the gestational sac in blighted ovum is variable, some areas being normal and others thin.

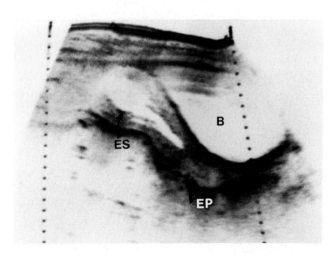

Fig. 4. Longitudinal scan of patient with gestational sac of approximately 12 weeks. The gestational sac is compressed in configuration. There is an inadequate decidual reaction around the gestational sac. The appearance resembles that of a "tennis racquet." ES, empty sac; EP, extruding products in the cervix; B, bladder. (*Courtesy of A. Everette James, MD*)

The gestational sac rind may be incomplete or overall poorly developed (Fig. 5). It is usual in the normal pregnancy to see one portion of the sac thickening to become the placenta at about the 8th week. This thickening is usually absent in blighted ovum.

Conclusive ultrasonic evidence of blighted ovum sometimes exists. The gestational sac can be measured and correlated with the table prepared by Kobayashi et al.[16] The sac may be at a stage at which a fetus should be seen (the fetal pole is seen from 6 to 7 weeks on) (Fig. 5). If it is 8 or 9 weeks by size and a thorough search has been made with real time for a fetal pole and none has been found, one can then assume that a blighted ovum exists. A reliable sign of fetal death with or without a fetus is the presence of a fluid–fluid level or of internal echoes in the gestational sac (Figs. 6,7). This is probably a consequence of intrasac bleeding. Further suggestive evidence of fetal death in the first trimester is a sonolucent gap between the gestational ring and the myometrium extending more than three-fourths of the way around the sac (Fig. 8). This is more than the separation between gestational sac and endometrial cavity that occurs as a normal variant and has been termed an "implantation bleed" (Fig. 9) (see Chapter 24). It also differs from the second sonolucent area seen with an incompletely visualized twin gestational sac (Fig. 10).

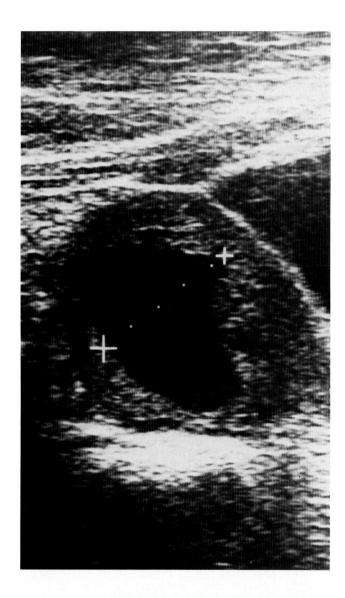

Fig. 5. Blighted ovum. Poorly defined gestational sac that is too large for the uterus. No fetal pole was seen. Note the feeble trophoblastic reaction.

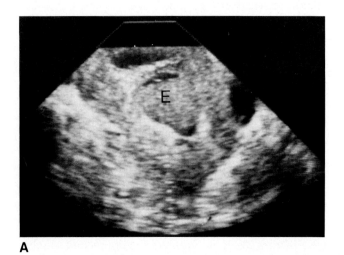

A

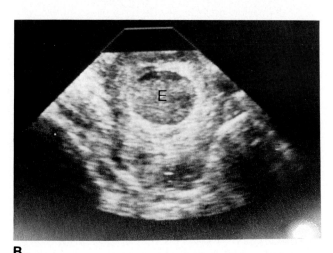

B

Fig. 6. A. Longitudinal and **B.** transverse. Impending abortion. There is a fluid–fluid level within the sac due to echogenic blood (E).

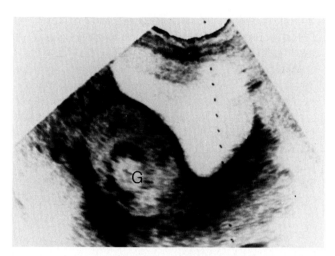

Fig. 7. Blighted ovum. Sac (G) containing low-level echoes due to blood.

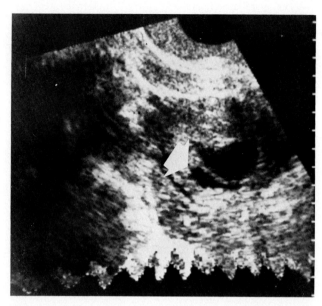

Fig. 9. "Implantation bleed" around the gestational sac. The sonolucent area (*arrow*) proved to be of no pathological significance.

A problem exists if the gestational sac has a measurement consistent with a 5- to 7-week size postmenstrual age. Unless a fluid–fluid level is present or a gap between sac and myometrium is seen prior to the visualization of the fetal pole, no reliable means of differentiating a blighted ovum from a gestational sac of less than 7-week size exists. If the shape and rind of the sac are abnormal, the likelihood of a blighted ovum is strong but not overwhelming. A helpful sign of a blighted ovum is a disproportion between gestational sac and the uterine size. The uterus in a blighted

ovum may involute at a faster rate than the gestational sac so that the sac, although small, occupies a disproportionately large amount of the uterine outline (Fig. 5). Should one be uncertain whether or not a blighted ovum exists because the sac size is less than 8 weeks, a follow-up study should be advised. Failure of the gestational sac to increase in size by over 75 percent in the course of a week is an indication of blighted ovum.[17] The gestational sac diameter increases rapidly during the first trimester at a rate of approximately 0.48 cm per day from the 40th through the 80th day.[18]

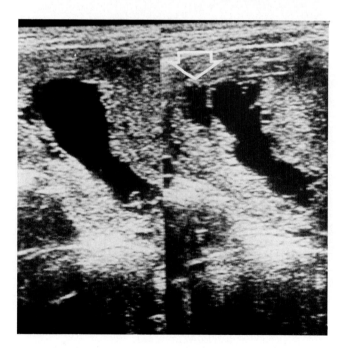

Fig. 8. Blighted ovum. Poorly defined irregular trophoblastic reaction. Note the space between the sac and the myometrium near the fundus (*arrow*). This sac aborted shortly thereafter.

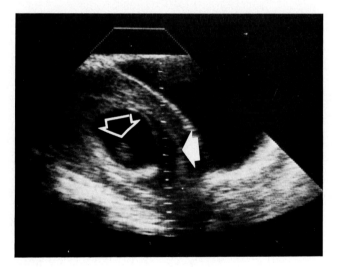

Fig. 10. Twin gestational sacs. A fetal pole (*open arrow*) can be seen within one sac. A portion of a second sac (*closed arrow*) can be seen surrounding the lower portion of the sac.

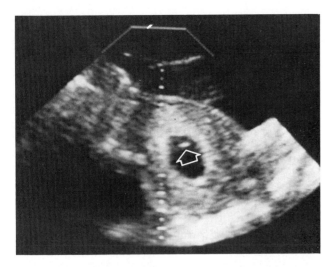

Fig. 11. Blighted ovum. Although this sac has a well defined border, only a yoke sac (*open arrow*) can be seen. No fetal pole was identified and this pregnancy later spontaneously aborted.

The yolk sac is quite often seen with modern real-time equipment in association with small fetuses of 6- to 7-week size (see Chapters 4 and 8). This is a normal finding (Fig. 1). However, if a yolk sac is seen without visualization of the fetus, this is a bad sign and almost inevitably indicates that a blighted ovum is developing (Fig. 11). This unusual finding has been of clinical value when the sac size has been such that a fetal pole might not be present because the gestational age is still less than 7½ weeks.

The development of a blighted ovum is particularly likely in multiple pregnancy. It is known that a proportion of twin pregnancies fail in the first trimester (see Chapter 24). The difference between a viable and nonviable gestational sac is seen in Figure 12. Note the irregular gestational sac outline to the abnormal pregnancy. A repeat sonogram 2 weeks later shows only one surviving sac. Another situation with increased likelihood of blighted ovum development is a malformed uterus (Fig. 13).

MISSED ABORTION

"Missed abortion" is a term generally used to describe a fetus still present in the amniotic sac but immobile and sometimes so deformed by the maceration that takes place after death that it no longer has the shape of a fetus (Fig. 14). However, the term is also used for fetuses that are essentially normal in appearance but without evidence of fetal heart or limb motion. A missed abortion generally occurs at a later stage than a blighted ovum, frequently between 10 and 14 weeks after menstruation. The uterus is small for dates but placental development has occurred. The fetus may

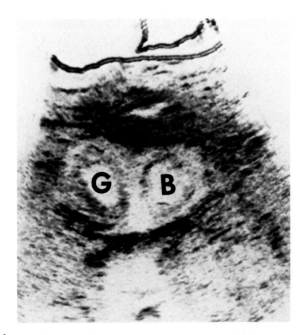

A

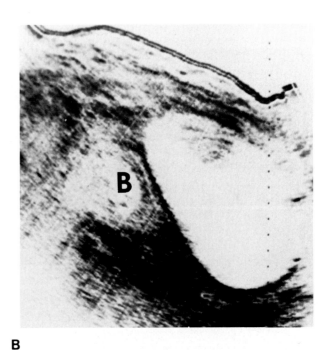

B

Fig. 12. A. Transverse section of twin gestational sacs at the fundus of the uterus. One sac (G) has a normal outline and is viable. The sac on the left (B) is smaller and poorly outlined. **B.** Longitudinal section through poorly outlined sac (B). Two weeks later a repeat sonogram showed only one sac remaining in the uterus.

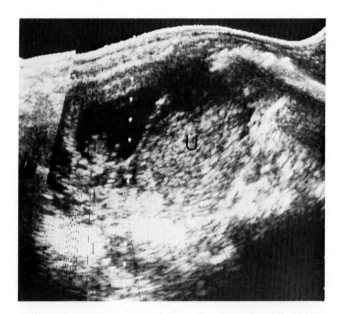

Fig. 13. Bicornuate uterus (U) with gestational sac. Note the eccentric position of the gestational sac. Such pregnancies are at increased risk of spontaneous abortion.

be much smaller than expected for the gestational sac size. It is essential that a high-quality real-time unit be used to make the diagnosis; otherwise a false positive diagnosis of fetal death may occur with a viable pregnancy. In one series using a gray scale B-scan unit, four false positive diagnoses of missed abortion were made based on an irregular sac shape and a misshapen fetus.[19] As already mentioned, the distinction between missed abortion, blighted ovum, and incomplete spontaneous abortion is largely academic since all are treated by curettage.

Often the placenta in a missed abortion is unduly large and dominates the ultrasonic appearances (Figs. 14,15). The placenta may show "hydropic" changes at pathology suggestive of hydatidiform mole.[20] Indeed it is widely accepted that a hydatidiform mole originates in a missed abortion[21] (Fig. 16). Fibroids can also mimic the findings seen with missed abortion and hydatidiform mole (Fig. 17).

SPONTANEOUS ABORTION

Spontaneous abortion represents a situation in which the fetus and the gestational sac have been aborted with the passage of blood clots. If the fetus does abort and the mother passes material vaginally, a definite diagnosis of spontaneous abortion can be established if the material is inspected by an obstetrician. Should, as is commonly the case, the mother dispose of the material without showing it to the doctor, it is usually

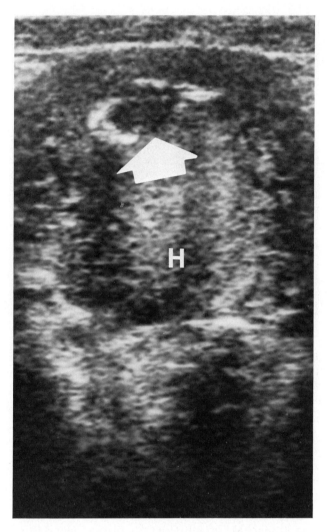

Fig. 14. Missed abortion. The fetus (*arrows*) has a strange deformed appearance. Note the large size of the placenta, which is hydropic (H).

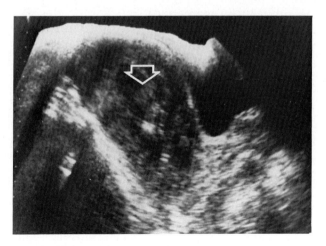

Fig. 15. Missed abortion with somewhat coarse acoustical pattern. The deformed fetal pole can just be seen (*arrow*).

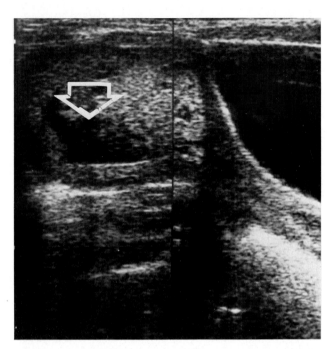

Fig. 16. Hydatidiform mole with a sonolucent space (*arrow*) within, presumably due to blood. The appearances are similar to those seen with missed abortion.

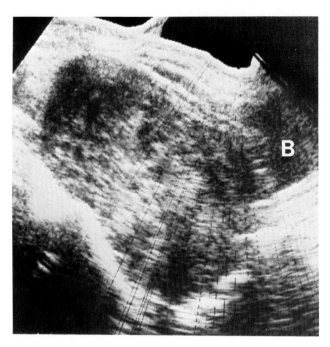

Fig. 17. Fibroid uterus mimicking the appearances of missed abortion or of hydatidiform mole. B = bladder.

uncertain whether a complete or incomplete spontaneous abortion has occurred. The role of ultrasound in such patients is to determine whether retained products of conception persist within the uterus. Sonographically if abortion is complete, the uterus contains a few small central groups of echoes or a central line representing a decidual reaction. There is no evidence of a gestational sac or any other products of conception. To be confident that no retained products are present, one should see a uterus of completely normal shape and an endometrial cavity lining that is slim and of normal configuration (see Chapter 34). Such a finding can substantially reduce inpatient time by making a dilatation and curettage unnecessary in patients in whom it is clinically uncertain whether or not a miscarriage has been complete.[22]

INCOMPLETE SPONTANEOUS ABORTION

Diagnosis of retained products of conception when part or most of the fetus has been aborted is difficult. This entity is described in considerable detail in Chapter 34 but at this early stage of pregnancy a clear-cut decision can be made that the fetus is viable or that there are no retained products of conception present if the uterus is entirely empty and normal in size and shape. A distinction between blood clot and some retained products of conception is generally impossible. The

presence of retained products of conception is supported by evidence of acoustical shadowing within the uterine cavity in the absence of instrumentation indicating either retained bone or gas due to infection. A large clump of echoes within the endometrial cavity, particularly if it is located at the fundus, should be viewed with great suspicion (Fig. 2).

The use of ultrasound in this complex problem can substantially reduce inpatient stay[22] by showing that continued therapy is pointless if the fetus is dead and that evacuation is appropriate.

FETAL DEATH IN SECOND AND THIRD TRIMESTER

A number of ultrasonic techniques exist for the diagnosis of fetal death in the second and third trimesters. The best known and most used technique is Doppler monitoring of the fetal heart (Chapter 6). Failure to find the fetal heart sound with Doppler is often considered diagnostic of fetal death. However, in clinical practice the test is not that reliable. Therefore, patients are referred for real-time examination to confirm fetal death, particularly under the following conditions: (a) an obese mother, (b) an anterior placenta, (c) an early pregnancy, and (d) an inexperienced Doppler examiner. In a small proportion of the cases in which the fetal heart cannot be heard by Doppler, real-time techniques will reveal a normal fetus. In particular, a false positive diagnosis of fetal death may be made by Doppler when the fetal heart rate approximates that of the mother such as in conditions of fetal heart block or fetal distress.[23] Because of the potential for a false positive diagnosis of fetal death, Doppler techniques should be used only for screening purposes. For definite confirmation, real-time ultrasound evidence of fetal death is necessary.

There is an increased risk of fetal death where the mother has chronic hypertension, diabetes mellitus, or where erythroblastosis fetalis, an umbilical cord accident, a fetal anomaly, infection, or premature rupture of membranes is present. Fifty percent of the time the cause of fetal death is not diagnosed. An ultrasonic effort to identify a fetal anomaly should be made; repeated miscarriages may be explained by the presence of a genetically determined fetal anomaly.

Real-time ultrasound today represents the preferred method of diagnosing fetal death.[24] Fetal movement first becomes obvious at 6 to 7 weeks depending on the quality of the real-time system. The limbs can be seen as tiny buds shooting out from the side of the soft tissue sphere that represents the body of the fetus. The fetus remains in the dependent portion of the gestational sac until approximately 12 to 13 weeks. Absence of evidence of fetal heart movement is reliable evidence of fetal death; however, fetuses in which there is evidence of fetal heart movement may not show fetal motion.

Fetal heart movement becomes obvious on real time earlier than evidence of fetal limb movement can be seen at about 6 to 7 weeks. One sees flickering within the body of the fetus at a rapid rate. The fetal heart movement differs in rate and rhythm from the random movement of nearby echogenic structures influenced by changes in maternal respiration and position. The absence of fetal heart motion is a better indication of fetal death than fetal movement, for the fetus may be relatively immobile and yet alive. The fetus should be evaluated by more than one examiner. A videotape should be obtained if the patient is obese or there is any uncertainty about the diagnosis. If fetal life is seen, recording a simultaneous M-mode tracing of the fetal heart provides excellent documentation that the fetus was viable at the time of the study.

Studies have documented the accuracy of real time in discriminating between fetal life and death. Out of 399 fetuses of a total of 440 examinations, only 1 false positive diagnosis was made.[25] These results, obtained in 1977, should be better with the high-quality real-time systems available today.

SLOW SCAN FOR FETAL HEART MOVEMENT

If one does not possess a real-time instrument, a B-scan version of a real-time study of the fetal heart can be obtained using a technique described by Scheer and Nubar.[26] The fetal heart is located by scanning the fetal trunk and is aligned in a longitudinal fashion. The fetal heart is then scanned very slowly so that a number of fetal cardiac pulsations will occur during the time that the transducer is over the fetal heart. If the fetus is alive, a serrated pattern derived from the movement of the septum will be seen within the fetal heart (Fig. 18). If fetal death is present, the various cardiac chambers will be seen. Absence of filling of the fetal bladder and visualization of the fetal aorta are also reported to be features suggestive of fetal death.

A variety of techniques based on older ultrasonic instruments can give evidence that the fetal heart is beating, such as B-scan with Doppler,[27] vaginal Doppler,[25] or fetal echocardiography.[7,28] These cumbersome techniques have been rendered obsolete by real-time ultrasound.

SONOGRAPHIC SIGNS OF FETAL DEATH

B-scan ultrasound represents a suboptimal method of diagnosing death; a number of late ultrasound signs are seen.[27,29,30] Some nonspecific signs of fetal death are helpful. With fetal death, growth ceases and the biparietal diameter measurements repeated from one week to the next either remain the same or decrease. However, absent growth need not indicate fetal death and may be seen in a viable fetus experiencing intra-

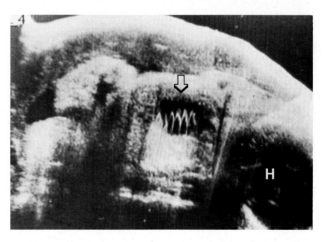

Fig. 18. Longitudinal section. Cephalic presentation. A serpiginous series of lines in the mid-thorax (*arrow*) represents the heart scanned very slowly so that the pulsations of the heart can be seen. H, head.

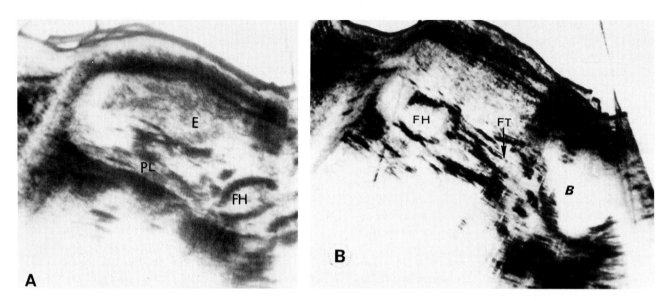

Fig. 19. A. Longitudinal section of a 30-week fetus that had been dead for at least 2 weeks. The fetal anatomy is markedly distorted. Note the oblong fetal head (FH), absence of the normal thoracic echoes and extra echoes (E) within the amniotic fluid due to macerated skin. The placenta (PL) lies posteriorly. **B.** Longitudinal section of a fetus that died at 25 weeks. A flattened fetal head (FH) can still be seen. Spinal column connects the fetal head to the compressed fetal trunk (FT). B, bladder.

uterine growth retardation. Definite decrease in head size is highly suggestive of fetal death but is sometimes seen if one of the examinations is performed with poor technique. A shape change may herald fetal death; the development of dolicocephaly may precede fetal demise.[31]

B-scan signs of fetal death depend on the time at which death occurred in relation to the examination and the stage of pregnancy at which the examination was performed. These signs vary in reliability. If the fetus grows at less than the normal rate and dies before the 20th to 25th week of pregnancy, the macerated fetus may have an appearance resembling a missed abortion rather than fetal death (Fig. 14).

Growth may be so poor that a gestational sac may still appear to be present with a distorted fetal pole without recognizable structure. A similar appearance may be seen if the fetus remains within the uterus for a long period of time after death (over 2 weeks). Limbs, thorax, and head all collapse and form a barely recognizable structure (Fig. 19). Since the fetal echoes are clustered and compact, the findings may resemble those of a dermoid or uterine neoplasm. The uterus may decrease in size following fetal death.

The process of fetal dissolution with fetal death may be seen in a dramatic and abbreviated form when a hyperosmotic solution is infused into the uterus to induce an elective abortion and labor does not ensue. Within 24 hours the amniotic cavity is filled with echoes. These are so uniform that they can be confused with a hydatidiform mole.

If the fetus dies in the late second or third trimester other B-scan signs of fetal death are seen. Unfortunately, none of these more specific signs are present within the first 48 hours after death. When fetal death takes place, amniotic fluid penetrates the fetal epidermis and underlying tissues with subsequent epidermal separation, protein breakdown, and the creation of new tissue–fluid interspaces. These early changes are evidenced in an alteration of the acoustic characteristics of the fetus itself. Later changes include the appearance of echoes in the amniotic fluid due to separation of tissue fragments from the fetus. Within 2 to 4 days after fetal death definite fetal skin edema develops[32] (Fig. 20). The amount of fetal edema is generally in the range of 5 to 8 mm if death has been present more than 5 days although early cases may show a 2 and 3 mm thickness. Fetal scalp edema may be seen in live fetuses in association with diabetes mellitus (Chapter 23) and erythroblastosis fetalis (Chapter 21) and other causes of fetal hydrops.

Gas in the fetus is occasionally detected on radiographic studies following fetal death. Such gas can be seen ultrasonically (Fig. 21). There will be a strong echo within the fetus with acoustic shadowing behind the fetus.[33] Unexpected inability to view the posterior aspect of the fetus should be a signal for the performance of an abdominal radiograph which will reveal gas in the fetal vascular system. When the fetus has been dead for a relatively long period, midline echoes derived from the falx cease to be detectable.[27] Actual overlapping of the fetal skull bones (ultrasonic Spal-

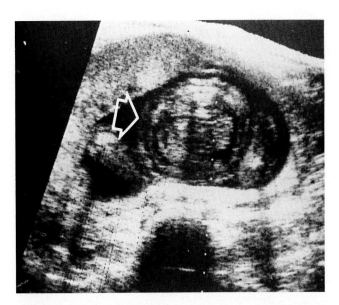

Fig. 20. Fetal death. Note the skin thickening around the fetal trunk (*arrow*).

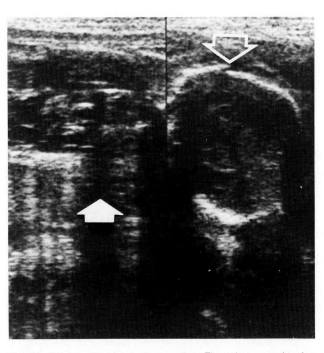

Fig. 21. Fetal death. Longitudinal section. There is an overlapping of the fetal skull (Spalding's sign) (*open arrow*). Gas in the fetal heart created the acoustical shadowing originating in the trunk (*arrow*).

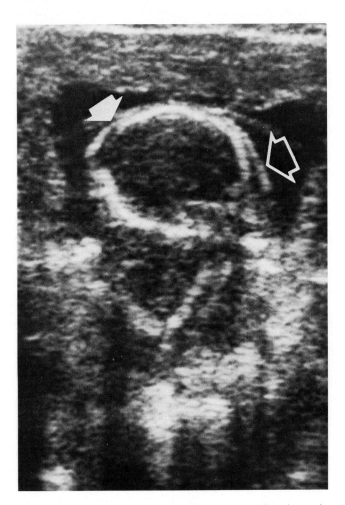

Fig. 22. Fetal death with positive Spalding's sign (*closed arrow*). Note the flattened shape of the head and the evidence of skin thickening (*open arrow*).

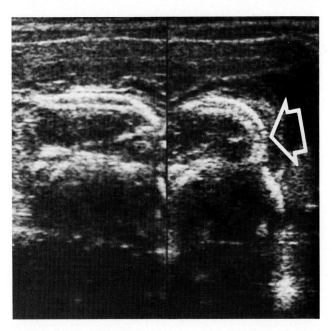

Fig. 23. Grossly deformed fetal position due to fetal death. The fetal neck is acutely angled (*arrow*).

dings sign) is a late ultrasonic feature of fetal death (Figs. 21,22). Such overlapping may be seen in normal fetuses if an examination is performed during labor. Trunk changes also occur in fetal death. Dead fetuses adopt strange positions; they can be curled up, hyperflexed (Fig. 23), or flattened. A coarse appearance to the outline of the thorax due to the development of subcutaneous edema has been described.[29]

Unfortunately, although reliable, these signs are not seen until the fetus has been dead at least 48 hours. Real-time scanning unquestionably represents the preferred ultrasonic technique for the diagnosis of fetal death.

REFERENCES

1. Levi S, Hechtermans R, L'Hermite-Baleriaux M: Etablissement du pronostic de la menace d'avortement spontané. J Gyn Obst Biol Repr 2:155, 1973
2. Hobbins J, Berkowitz R, Winsberg F: Ultrasonography in Obstetrics and Gynecology. Baltimore, Williams & Wilkins, 1983
3. Duff G: Prognosis in threatened abortion: A comparison between predictions made by sonar, urinary hormone assays and clinical judgment. Br J Obstet Gynaecol 82:858, 1975
4. Martoni M, Pedersen JF: Fetal growth delay in threatened abortion. Paper presented at the World Federation of Ultrasound in Medicine and Biology, Brighton, England, 1982
5. Jouppila P: Diagnostics in threatened abortion. A study by ultrasonic, clinical, hormonal and histopathological methods. Ultrasound Med 3A:595, 1976
6. Reinold E: Clinical value of fetal spontaneous movements in early pregnancy. J Perinat Med 1, 1973
7. Robinson HP: Detection of fetal heart movement in the first trimester of pregnancy using pulsed ultrasound. Br Med J 4:466, 1972
8. Eriksen PS, Philipsen T: Prognosis in threatened abortion evaluated by hormone assays and ultrasound scanning. Obstet Gynecol 55:435, 1980
9. Asokan S, Niijensohn E, Patel V, et al: High resolution real time ultrasound in threatened vs missed abortion in the first trimester of pregnancy. Paper presented at the Radiological Society of North America, Chicago, 1981
10. Jouppila P, Huhtaniemi I, Tapanainen J: Early pregnancy failure: Study by ultrasonic and hormonal methods. Obstet Gynecol 55:42, 1980
11. Yuen BH, Livingston JE, Poland BJ, et al: Human chorionic gonadotropin, estradiol, progesterone, prolactin, and B-scan ultrasound monitoring of complications in early pregnancy. Obstet Gynecol 57:207, 1981
12. Anderson SG: Management of threatened abortion with real-time sonography. Obstet Gynecol 55:259, 1980
13. Sarti D, Sample WF, Hobel CJ, et al: Ultrasonic visualization of a dilated cervix during pregnancy. Radiology 130:417, 1979
14. Smith C, Gregori C, Breen J: Ultrasonography in threatened abortion. Obstet Gynecol 51:2, 1978
15. Donald I, Morley P, Barnett E: The diagnosis of blighted ovum by sonar. J Obstet Gynaecol Br Commonw 79:304, 1972
16. Kobayashi M, Hellman L, Cromb E: Atlas of Ultrasonography. New York, Appleton-Century-Crofts, 1972
17. Robinson H: The diagnosis of early pregnancy failure by sonar. Br J Obstet Gynaecol 82:849, 1975
18. Defoort P, Van Eyck J, De Schryver O, et al: Gray scale ultrasound for the investigation of early pregnancy. Europ J Obstet Gynec Reprod Biol 8:9, 1978
19. Dessaive R, de Hertogh R, Thomas K: Correlation between hormonal levels and ultrasound in patients with threatened abortion. Gynecol Obstet Invest 14:65, 1982
20. Buschi AJ, Brenbridge NAG, Cochrane JA, et al: Hydropic degeneration of the placenta simulating hydatidiform mole. J Clin Ultrasound 7:60, 1979
21. Szulman AE, Surti U: The syndromes of hydatidiform mole: Cytogenetic and morphologic correlations. Am J Obstet Gynecol 131:665, 1978
22. Drumm J, Clinch J: Ultrasound in management in clinically diagnosed threatened abortion. Br Med J 2:424, 1975
23. Hutson JM, Fox HE: Real-time ultrasonography for the differential diagnosis of intrapartum fetal death. Am J Obstet Gynecol 142:8, 1057, 1982
24. Platt LD, Manning FA, Murata Y, et al: Diagnosis of fetal death in utero by real-time ultrasound. Obstet Gynecol 55(2):191, 1980
25. Levine SC, Filly RA: Accuracy of real-time sonography in the determination of fetal viability. Obstet Gynecol 49:475, 1977
26. Scheer K, Nubar JC: Rapid conclusive diagnosis of intrauterine fetal death. Am J Obstet Gynecol 128:907, 1977
27. Piiroinin O: Features in ultrasonic B-scan after fetal death in last two trimesters. Ann Chir Gynaecol Fenn 63:194, 1974
28. Jouppila P, Piiroinen O: Ultrasonic diagnosis of fetal life in early pregnancy. Obstet Gynecol 46:616, 1975
29. Gottesfeld KR: The ultrasonic diagnosis of intrauterine fetal death. Am J Obstet Gynecol 108:623, 1070
30. O'Malley BP, Salem S: Ultrasonic diagnosis of intrauterine fetal death. J Can Assoc Radiol 27:273, 1976
31. Ford KB, McGahan JP: Cephalic index: Its possible use as a predictor of impending fetal demise. Radiology 143:517, 1982
32. Weill F, Heroit G, Colette C, et al: Un signe tomoechographique de la mort foetale. La Presse Medicale 9:52, 1971
33. Weinstein BJ, Platt LD: The Ultrasonic appearence of intravascular gas in fetal death. J Ultrasound Med 2:451, 1983

33 | Sonographic Evaluation of Pelvic Masses and Maternal Disorders Occurring During Pregnancy

Arthur C. Fleischer
Frank H. Boehm
A. Everette James, Jr.

The atraumatic and biologically innocuous nature of diagnostic sonography makes it an excellent modality for the evaluation of pelvic masses that occur during pregnancy. The apparent lack of biologically significant changes at diagnostic power output levels allows serial examination of patients with pelvic masses for assessment of growth or enlargement with little fear of untoward effects.[1,2] Information obtained by diagnostic sonography concerning the size, location, and internal consistency of a pelvic mass can be very helpful in the management of these patients (Table 1). Since sonography can accurately assess the gestational age of the pregnancy, it is also utilized to determine the optimal time for surgical intervention if clinically indicated. In addition, the sonographic data concerning the location and mobility of a pelvic mass is helpful in determining the mode of delivery.

The patient who is seen during pregnancy with a pelvic mass presents a special problem for the obstetrician. Any type of invasive diagnostic procedure can disturb the pregnancy and potentially cause premature labor. It is frequently difficult or impossible to establish the size and extent of the mass that occurs during pregnancy by physical examination alone. In general, obstetricians usually adopt a conservative approach when dealing with a gravid patient with a pelvic mass that they consider to be benign, less than 6 cm in diameter (such as a corpus luteum cyst), and that does not appear to enlarge or endanger the pregnancy.[3] This approach is followed since corpus luteum cysts, one of the most common types of pelvic mass encountered in pregnancies, is expected to regress by 14 to 15 weeks. If a

mass is greater than 6 cm in diameter and appears to enlarge during pregnancy, surgical intervention is usually indicated. Of all types of masses that can be encountered during pregnancy, the most common one to exhibit enlargement is the ovarian cystadenoma.[4]

Because of its accurate portrayal of the internal consistency of a pelvic mass encountered during pregnancy, the information obtained by sonography may be sufficient to specify the type of pelvic mass present, thereby allowing conservative management. Although not completely diagnostic, the sonographic finding of a completely sonolucent mass with well-defined and thin borders and distal acoustical enhancement is highly suggestive of the diagnosis of a benign cyst. If operative intervention is deemed necessary, the sonographic examination has a significant role in establishing the exact duration of gestation. The obstetrician usually prefers to explore patients with pelvic masses during the second trimester since at this time there is the least likelihood of inducing premature labor by surgical intervention.

Some pelvic masses become clinically evident for the first time during pregnancy when an enlarged uterus makes the mass more readily palpable. Other pelvic masses that occur during pregnancy come to the attention of the obstetrician because of the pain they produce or because they compromise normal labor. Pain during pregnancy associated with a pelvic mass may be an indication that torsion around a pedicle has occurred, that there has been extensive internal hemorrhagic degeneration, that the mass has caused extrinsic compression of other pelvic organs, or that

TABLE 1
Sonographic Features of Some Common Pelvic Masses Occurring with Pregnancy

Mass	Sonographic Features
Uterine	
Leiomyoma	Mildly echogenic to moderately echogenic depending on ratio of smooth muscle to collagen and presence and type of degeneration
	Intramural leiomyoma identified within the uterine outline
	Subserosal pedunculated leiomyoma can appear separate from uterus; attachment to the uterus can be delineated
Extrauterine	
Dermoid cyst	Complex to echogenic appearance depending on internal composition
	Frequently located anterior to uterine fundus
Mucinous cystadenoma	Predominantly cystic mass with septations
Serous cystadenoma	Frequently cystic
Corpus luteum cyst	Echogenic if contains organized clot
	Sonolucent if contains resorbed blood
Theca lutein cyst	Bilateral, multiloculated masses
	Frequently associated with molar gestation
Other	
Abscess	Predominantly cystic with internal echoes arising from pus, cellular debris, and gas
Pelvic kidney	Reniform shape with central echogenic interface arising from renal pelvis

rupture of the mass has occurred. Appendicitis is another cause of acute abdominal pain in a gravid patient and is a significant complication because of potential spread of the infection to the gravid uterus.

SCANNING TECHNIQUE

Since masses that are fixed within the pelvis have an increased incidence of rupture when labor ensues, assessment of the mobility of a mass is an important quality to assess sonographically. The mobility of a mass can be determined by scanning the patient before and after voiding or in various positions such as the right and left posterior oblique or decubitus or Trendelenburg positions. If a mass is not attached to the peritoneum or bladder wall, it should change in position relative to the symphysis pubis after these maneuvers have been performed. Conversely, if it is fixed, no change in position will be apparent.

Real-time scanning can be used to survey for associated disorders such as loculated ascites or obstructive uropathy. It can also be used to evaluate the mobility of the internal contents of a mass when the scan is performed in a variety of patient positions.

PELVIC MASSES OCCURRING DURING PREGNANCY

Pelvic masses that occur during pregnancy are discussed according to their approximate frequency of occurrence.

Solid Masses

The uterine leiomyoma or "fibroid" is one of the most common pelvic masses encountered during pregnancy. Leiomyomas consist of collagen and smooth muscle components in various proportions. Although most fibroids remain about the same size during pregnancy, they may enlarge since their growth is stimulated by estrogen.[5] Those fibroids that demonstrate rapid enlargement may outgrow their blood supply, resulting in infarction and necrosis. Leiomyomata may compromise the ability of the uterus to contract effectively, thus producing uterine dyskinesia and sometimes uterine inertia. If a leiomyoma lies in the lower uterine segment, it may prevent vaginal delivery altogether. Spontaneous abortion and intrauterine growth retardation may also occur more frequently with fibroids.[5] Patients with multiple leiomyomata tend to have a higher incidence of complications than those with a single tumor.[5]

Sonographically, leiomyomas are variable in appearance, ranging from minimally echogenic masses to complex masses with areas of cystic degeneration to masses that are diffusely echogenic (Figs. 1A,1B). The concentric arrangement of connective tissue and smooth muscle can be recognized sonographically as rounded concentric masses (Fig. 1A). As in the nongravid patient, uterine leiomyomas may be either within the uterine wall (intramural) or subserosal and pedunculated. The echogenicity of the leiomyoma depends on the ratio of smooth muscle to collagen as well as the presence and type of degeneration. Hyaline and cystic degeneration appear as areas of sonolucency within a leiomyoma whereas areas of calcific degeneration appear as highly echogenic foci with distal acoustical shadowing. If the leiomyoma consists primarily of smooth muscle, it may appear sonolucent. The differentiation of leiomyoma from cystic masses depends upon the lack of distal acoustical enhancement seen in leiomyomata that consist primarily of smooth muscle. Intramural leiomyomas frequently cause nodular

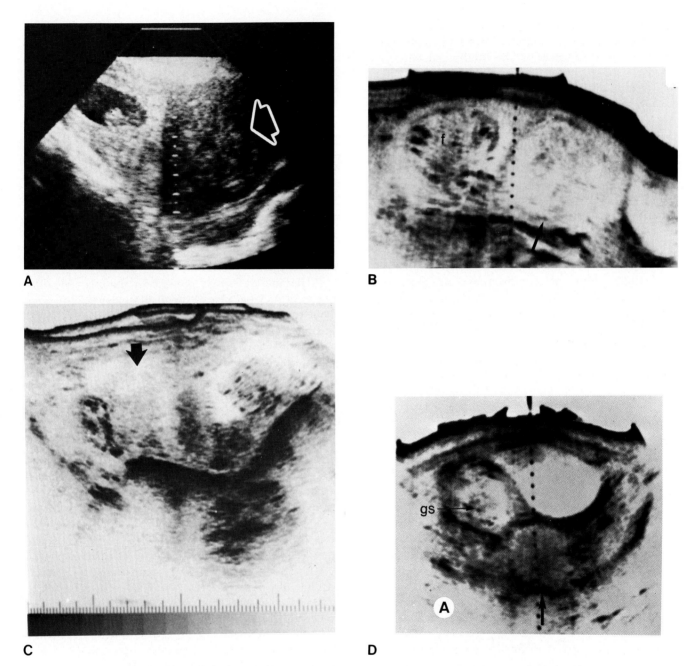

Fig. 1. Solid masses. **A.** Modified real-time sonogram of patient with large leiomyoma (*arrow*) and 13 week pregnancy. The whorled configuration of the internal structure of the fibroid can be identified. **B.** Intramural leiomyoma associated with a 20-week pregnancy (longitudinal, 4 cm to left of midline). This mildly echogenic mass involving the anterior portion of the lower uterine segment (*arrow*) was found to be an intramural leiomyoma. These masses frequently appear as mildly echogenic and can demonstrate internal hyaline, cystic, or calcific degeneration (see Chapter 38 on sonographic evaluation of uterine disorders). The 20-week fetus (f) was imaged transversely in the region of the fetal abdomen. (*Reprinted with permission from Fleischer, James, Krause, Millis: Radiology 126:215, 1978.*) **C.** Transverse static sonogram of thickened uterine wall (*arrow*) simulating the appearance of a fibroid. This area was thinner on a repeat sonogram 30 minutes after the initial study. **D.** Hemorrhagic corpus luteum cyst (transverse, 3 cm above symphysis pubis). Associated with this first trimester pregnancy is an echogenic mass in the midline (*arrow*). This mass represented a corpus luteum cyst that contained organized clot, which is demonstrated by its echogenic appearance. When the contents of a corpus luteum cyst undergo liquefaction, a sonolucent appearance will be seen. These masses are normally encountered in the first trimester of pregnancy and will later regress. An intact gestational sac is also demonstrated (gs) in this patient. (*Reprinted with permission from Fleischer, James: Introduction to Diagnostic Sonography, New York, Wiley, 1980.*)

enlargement of the uterus. A pedunculated leiomyoma may appear as an extrauterine mass. In some cases, however, its attachment to the uterus can be delineated.

A contracted portion of the uterus can simulate the sonographic appearance of uterine leiomyoma (Fig. 1C). Differentiation between these two entities can be facilitated by repeat examination of the patient with a suspected contracted portion of the uterus. On a repeat examination 15 to 30 minutes after the initial study, a contracted portion of the uterus typically becomes thin and regular whereas the mass created by a uterine leiomyoma remains unchanged. As described previously, the mobility of a pedunculated leiomyoma can be confirmed by scanning the patient in various positions. The separation between the leiomyoma and the myometrium or placenta is shown on most sonograms as a boundary between soft tissue of two different echogenicities (Figs. 1A,B). Leiomyomas tend to be less echogenic than the normal myometrium.[6]

Occasionally, a bicornuate uterus with a non-gravid horn may simulate the sonographic findings of a leiomyoma, but the "pseudomass" created by the bicornuate uterus tends to have the same texture as the remaining portion of the uterus (Fig. 4F). A solid ovarian tumor, such as adenocarcinoma, can simulate a pedunculated leiomyoma except that a solid ovarian tumor should be defined as being extrinsic to the uterus. Masses created by large cervical tumors can also mimic the sonographic appearance of a cervical fibroid.[7] Broad ligament hematomas or cystic masses with organized clots may also appear as solid masses.

In summary, leiomyomas are one of the most common pelvic masses encountered during pregnancy. They frequently are associated with uterine dyskinesia.[5] Fibroids occurring during pregnancy appear sonographically as mild to moderately echogenic lesions either within (intramural) or attached to the uterus (pedunculated, subserosal) and may show evidence of cystic, calcific, or hyaline degeneration.

Cystic Masses

Cystic masses associated with pregnancy are easily delineated by sonography.[8] If they are pedunculated, torsion can occur causing acute abdominal pain. As in other pelvic masses that occur during pregnancy, it is important to assess their mobility or fixation (Figs. 2A,B).[9] Cystic masses that are found to be fixed in the lower uterine segment may rupture during pregnancy and necessitate a cesarean section.[3]

As mentioned previously, corpus luteum cysts can be found in normal intrauterine pregnancies and usually regress by 12 to 15 weeks (Figs. 2C,D). Occasionally, these cysts will persist past the first trimester and

may reach a size of 10 cm in diameter. If they contain organized clot, an echogenic appearance may be encountered (Figs. 1D,2E). Usually, the blood within a corpus luteum cyst becomes resorbed, which results in a sonolucent appearance (Figs. 2A,B).

In a recently completed study, it was found that the majority of completely cystic masses associated with pregnancy resolved before term.[8] These cysts most likely represented corpus luteum cysts and, therefore, should exhibit significant diminution in size by 16 to 18 weeks. Cystic masses that persist after this time should be followed with serial sonographic examinations. In this series, those cystic masses that did not regress included a mucinous cystadenomas, benign cystic teratoma, paraovarian cyst, benign cystic teratoma, and tuboovarian abscess.[8]

Dermoid cysts may present for the first time during pregnancy because of the displacement of the mass from the pelvis by the enlarged gravid uterus. Sonographically, dermoid cysts have a wide spectrum of sonographic appearances, ranging from totally sonolucent to complex, predominantly solid masses. Dermoid cysts can appear as cystic masses although this is not their most characteristic appearance. More commonly, dermoid cysts appear as a complex mass with echogenic components (Figs. 3A,B).[10]

Mucinous and serous cystadenomas are other cystic masses that occur during pregnancy. Mucinous cystadenomas tend to have internal separations which are easily recognized by sonography (Figs. 2F,G,J,K). Although rare, ascites associated with this type of mass may indicate concomitant malignancy as seen in Figures 2L and 2M. Ascites associated with pregnancy may also be due to cirrhosis or severe toxemia.

Other cystic masses that occur during pregnancy include the paraovarian cyst and theca lutein cyst. Paraovarian cysts range from a few centimeters in size to pelvoabdominal in dimension (Fig. 2H,I). They arise from a mesoovarium and are separate from the ovary. Theca lutein cysts are frequently encountered in patients with molar pregnancies but also can be encountered in a variety of conditions that result in fetal hydrops.[11,12] They can also be encountered in patients with a multiple pregnancy. It is thought that theca lutein cysts are caused by elevated levels of human chorionic gonadotropin associated with fetal hydrops.[11] Theca lutein cysts typically regress after delivery .

Complex Masses

As the term implies, these masses contain both fluid and solid components and demonstrate a sonographic appearance consisting of both sonolucent and echogenic textures. The most common mass in this category

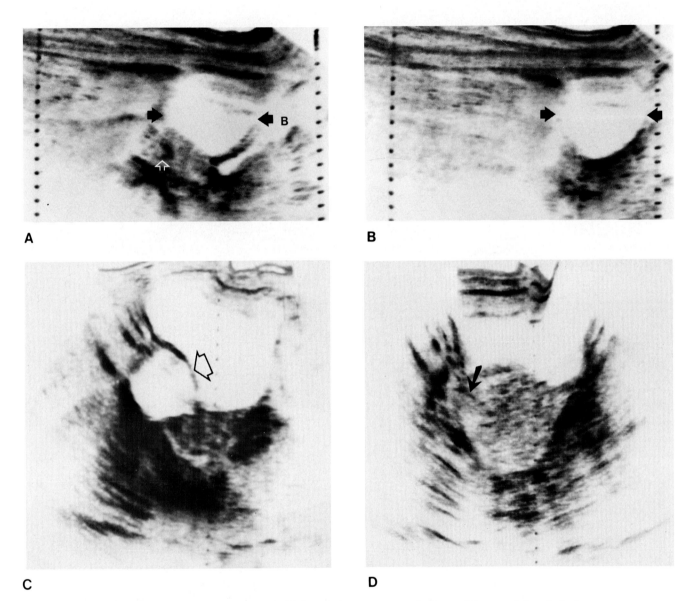

Fig. 2. Cystic masses associated with intrauterine pregnancy. **A.** Corpus luteum cyst (longitudinal, midline). There is a large cystic mass associated with an early first trimester intrauterine pregnancy (*arrows*). The gestational sac is not well demonstrated on this image (*open arrow*). B, bladder. **B.** Mobility of corpus luteum cyst after voiding (longitudinal, midline, post-void). The mass moves approximately 5 cm toward the symphysis pubis after voiding. This demonstrates the mobility of the mass. If the mass was fixed to the anterior abdominal wall or pelvic peritoneum, the mass would not demonstrate this degree of movement. It is an important parameter to evaluate since fixed masses associated with pregnancy have an increased tendency to rupture during labor. Most corpus luteum cysts contain liquefied products. **C.** Transverse static sonogram of corpus luteum cyst (*arrow*) in an 11-week pregnancy. **D.** Same patient as in **C** at 16 weeks demonstrating involution of the corpus luteum cyst (*arrow*) (*cont.*).

440

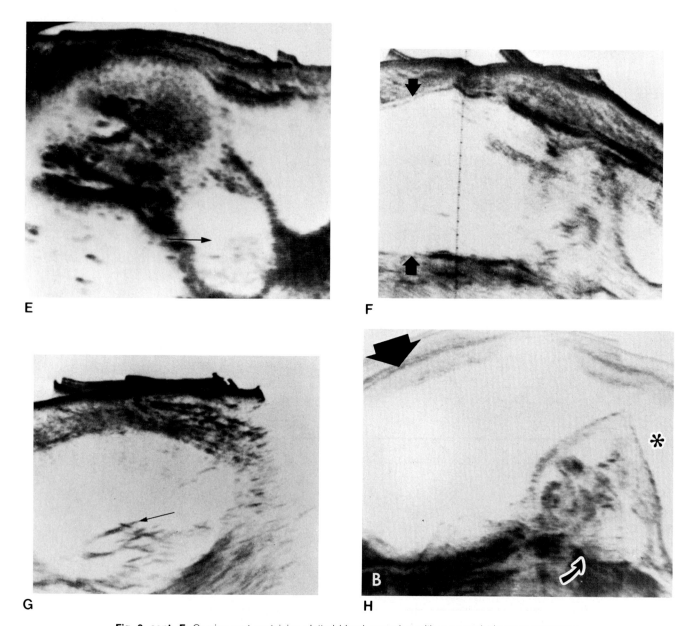

E

F

G

H

Fig. 2. cont. E. Ovarian cyst containing clotted blood occurring with a second trimester pregnancy (longitudinal, midline). Within the cystic mass is moderately echogenic material which forms an internal interface (*arrow*). The echogenic material represented clotted blood within an ovarian cyst. (*Courtesy of Roger Sanders, MD*) **F.** Mucinous cystadenoma associated with 12-week intrauterine pregnancy (longitudinal, midline). There is a large cystic pelvoabdominal mass anterior and superior to the uterine fundus. The mass is delineated to best advantage on the sonogram 3 cm to the left of midline. **G.** Mucinous cystadenoma with 12-week intrauterine pregnancy (longitudinal, 6 cm to left of midline). This cystic pelvic mass associated with the 12-week intrauterine pregnancy contains several thin septations (*arrows*) demonstrated on sonography. An appearance such as this suggests the diagnosis of mucinous cystadenoma. The patient was operated upon during the second trimester; the mass was removed and the pregnancy progressed to term. Surgical intervention is usually performed during the second trimester since the likelihood of inducing premature labor is least during this stage of pregnancy. **H.** Longitudinal static sonogram of large cystic mass (*arrow*) superior to a gravid uterus (*curved arrow*) and maternal urinary bladder (*). The upper portion of the mass is not included on this image. This represented a paraovarian cyst which was successfully removed during the second trimester of pregnancy (*cont.*).

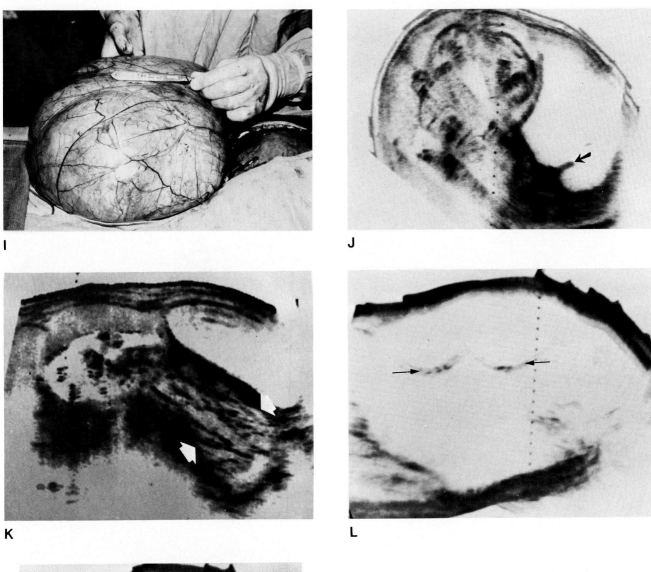

Fig. 2. cont. I. Picture of paraovarian cyst at surgery. **J.** Transverse static sonogram of term intrauterine pregnancy with a large cystic mass. There is a single, thin, regular septation (*arrow*) within the mass that proved to be a mucinous cystadenoma. **K.** Longitudinal static sonogram of predominately cystic, septated mass (*arrows*) posterior to the lower uterine segment. This corresponded to a cystadenoma. **L.** Mucinous cystadenocarcinoma associated with third trimester pregnancy (longitudinal, 8 cm to left of midline). There is a large, predominantly cystic abdominal mass which contains thin internal septations. **M.** Ascites associated with mucinous cystadenocarcinoma (transverse, 6 cm below xyphoid). Bilateral ascitic fluid collection (a) is demonstrated. The right kidney (*curved arrow*) appears to be displaced medially. The gravid uterus is surrounded by ascitic fluid. The presence of ascitic fluid was not apparent on physical examination but is seen well on ultrasound study. Sonography is a sensitive detector of ascitic fluid. (*Reprinted with permission from Fleischer, James: Introduction to Diagnostic Sonography. New York, Wiley, 1980.*)

442

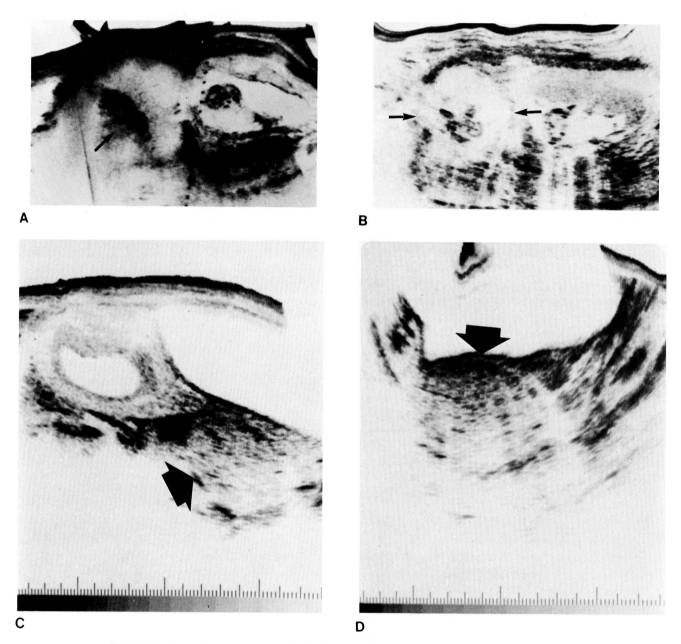

Fig. 3. Complex pelvic masses associated with intrauterine pregnancy. **A.** Dermoid cyst containing calcified foci associated with intrauterine pregnancy (longitudinal, 4 cm to right of midline). There is a complex mass anterior to the uterine fundus which contains a focus of highly echogenic material (*arrow*). This corresponded to radiographically demonstrable calcifications. Dermoid cysts associated with pregnancy are frequently located anterior to the uterine fundus, particularly if they are pedunculated. (*Courtesy of Bill Willson, MD.*) **B.** Dermoid cyst without calcification associated with intrauterine pregnancy (transverse, 3 cm above symphysis pubis). There is a complex mass to the right of the gravid uterus (*arrows*). The mass contains echogenic components which can be seen with dermoid cyst. (*Courtesy of Dean Birdwell, RDMS*). **C.** Longitudinal static sonogram of 11-week pregnancy with echogenic mass (*arrow*) posterior to the lower uterine segment. **D.** Transverse sonogram through lower uterine segment of patient depicted in **C.** to its echogenic nature, this mass (*arrow*) was correctly identified as a dermoid cyst.

is the dermoid cyst, which is frequently encountered in asymptomatic individuals for the first time during pregnancy. Dermoids usually contain sebum and ectodermal elements which produce moderate- to high-level echoes within predominantly cystic masses. The calcified content can be identified as high-level echoes with distal acoustic shadowing within these lesions (Fig. 3A).[10] The sebum within a dermoid cyst can be very echogenic, making it difficult to delineate the posterior wall of the mass (Figs. 3C,D).[13] Such a mass can simulate gas-filled loops of bowel and not be recognized sonographically. If the clinical management of the patient will be altered by establishment of the presence of a dermoid cyst and the sonographic examination does not convincingly demonstrate this type of mass, a single radiograph of the pelvis can be obtained. The radiographic findings of dermoids include the demonstration of teeth, radiolucency, or mural calcification.[14] Dermoid cysts usually come to the attention of the obstetrician because of pain secondary to torsion but usually do not prohibit normal delivery. There has been one report of a cystadenoma that impacted within the pelvis and may have contributed to uterine rupture.[15]

Pregnancy can rarely be found associated with pelvic inflammatory disease and other intraabdominal abscesses. The sonographic appearance of pelvic inflammatory disease is discussed in Chapter 40. Intraabdominal abscesses usually appear as moderately well-defined, predominantly anechoic masses that contain internal echoes. The echoes usually arise from cellular debris, pus, or gas within the abscess (Fig. 5E). Rarely, an abscess will appear as an echogenic mass but usually exhibits distal acoustical enhancement.[16] Heavier inflammatory fluid can layer in a dependent portion of the mass resulting in gravity dependent internal interface. Since it is of great importance to recognize an abscess concomitant with an intrauterine pregnancy, additional studies, such as supine and upright radiographs or needle aspiration of the mass, may be indicated. Of the complex pelvic masses that are encountered in a gravid patient, abdominal abscess is a most important entity to establish since systemic toxicity to the mother and fetus can develop if this entity remains unrecognized.

Other Masses

One should be aware of several normal structures that, when displaced by the enlarged gravid uterus, may become clinically apparent or produce symptoms. Specifically, normal structures such as pelvic kidneys, bicornuate uteri, or "wandering spleens" may be detected serendipitously or may produce symptoms first in the gravid patient. Masses associated with a molar pregnancy are discussed in Chapter 29.

It is important to demonstrate a pelvic kidney in a gravid patient since a pelvic kidney may occasionally obstruct the birth canal or sustain injury during delivery.[17] Pelvic kidneys appear as fusiform masses with a central echogenic interface corresponding to the fat surrounding the renal pelvis (Figs. 4A,4H). They are typically located near the sacral promontory. One should carefully examine both renal fossa if a pelvic kidney is suspected. In a patient with a horseshoe kidney, both kidneys will be abnormally low in position, whereas in a patient with a solitary pelvic kidney, the opposite kidney should be in normal position (Figs. 4A–4C).

The nongravid horn of a bicornuate uterus can simulate the sonographic appearance of a leiomyoma. Typically, the endometrium in the nongravid horn becomes thickened during pregnancy, allowing sonographic differentiation from a leiomyoma (Fig. 4F). If a patient is encountered with a bicornuate uterus, one should scan both kidneys since there is an increased incidence of renal agenesis with this uterine malformation.[8]

Other normal structures that may simulate masses in the pregnant patient include the "wandering spleen" and fecal-filled colon (Fig. 4G). An ectopic spleen appears as a moderately echogenic mass and is typically located superior to the uterine fundus. On the other hand, a fecal-filled colon appears as a tubular mass with high level echogenicity along its proximal border. Another structure that can become enlarged during pregnancy is the ureter. A dilated ureter is best delineated on modified longitudinal scans performed in the plane of the iliopsoas muscle. The dilated ureter appears as a tubular structure measuring between 1 and 1.5 cm outer-to-outer diameter. Its insertion into the maternal urinary bladder as well as its continuity can usually be documented with a hydronephrotic renal collecting system.

Maternal Disorders

Sonography is helpful in the evaluation of the gravid patient who presents with nonspecific abdominal disorders (Figs. 5B–5E).[19,20] For instance, sonography can be used to detect cholelithiasis and its complications in the gravid patient (Fig. 5A). A transducer that utilizes only a small scanning surface, such as a mechanical sector real-time scanner, is helpful in evaluation of the gallbladder in gravid patients. The pancreas is more difficult to delineate in pregnancy due to the protuberant abdomen of pregnant women in the mid and late trimester.

Sonography may be used in the initial workup of gravid patients who are suspected of having a vascular aneurysm. The splenic, hepatic, and renal vessels can be delineated with real-time sonography. Further

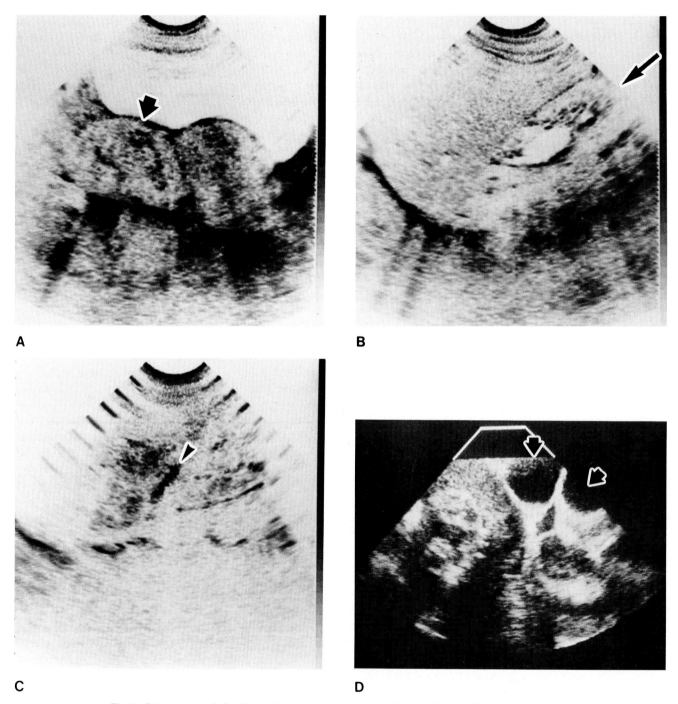

Fig. 4. Other masses. **A.** Sagittal real-time sonogram demonstrating a left pelvic kidney (*arrow*) superior to the enlarged uterine fundus in a 10-week pregnancy. **B.** Same patient as in **A** and imaged in a sagittal plane in the right upper quadrant demonstrating normotopic position of right kidney (*arrow*). **C.** Same patient as in **A** and **B** as imaged in the sagittal plane near the left iliac fossa. Gas within the lumen of the splenic flexure of the colon can be identified within the left renal fossa. **D.** Transverse sonogram of patient with distended, fluid-filled loops (*arrows*) of small bowel in the left upper quadrant (*cont.*).

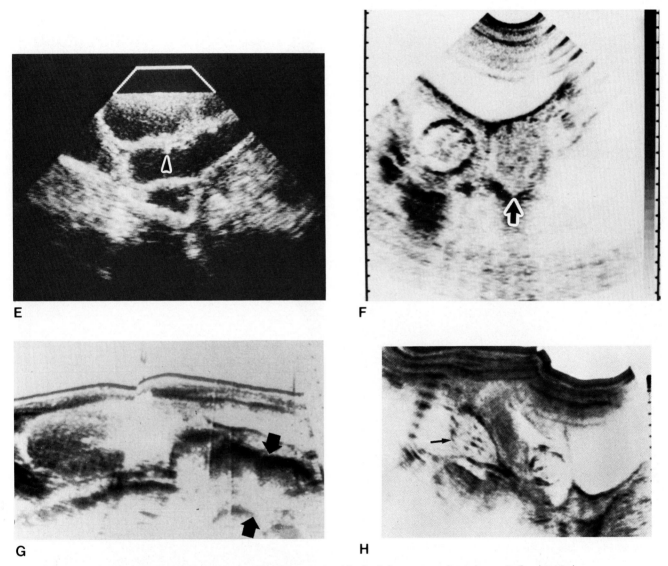

E

F

G

H

Fig. 4. cont. E. Longitudinal sonograms obtained in the left upper quadrant demonstrating haustral markings (*arrowhead*) of the distended fluid-filled bowel. This patient had obstruction of the rectosigmoid colon due to adhesions. **F.** Transverse real-time sonogram through lower uterine segment of bicornuate uterus demonstrating non-gravid left uterine horn (*arrow*) and fetal head in lower uterine segment of right uterine horn. **G.** Fecal material simulating pelvic mass with second trimester pregnancy (longitudinal, midline). The rectum is filled with feces and appears as an ill-defined, tubular mass which is highly echogenic at its proximal border. (*Courtesy of Roger Sanders, MD.*) **H.** Ectopic kidney associated with second trimester pregnancy (longitudinal, midline). There is a reniform-shaped mass posterior to the gravid uterus representing an ectopic kidney (*arrow*). (*Courtesy of Dean Birdwell, RDMS.*)

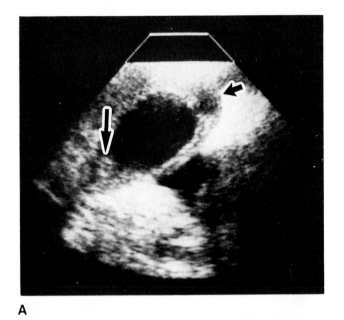

A

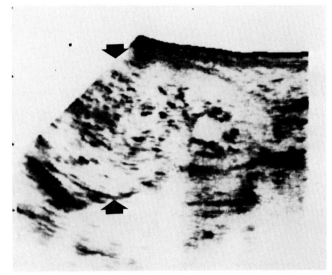

B

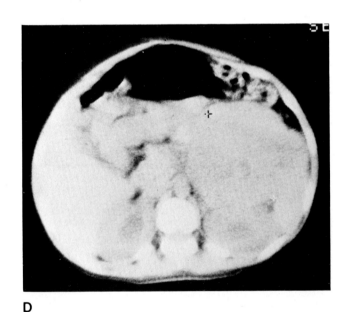

C

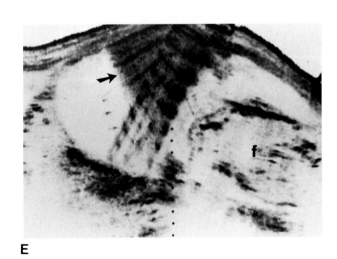

D

E

Fig. 5. Maternal disorders. **A.** Calculous cholecystitis in gravid patient. The uterine fundus demonstrates a thickened wall (*arrow*) which corresponded to a gangrenous portion of the gallbladder. A stone (*large arrow*) was present within the neck of the gallbladder. **B.** Prone static sonogram of gravid patient demonstrating hypernephroma (*arrow*) in the upper pole of the left kidney. **C.** Large solid mass (*arrow*) superior to the left upper pole in hypertensive patient at 26 weeks. The left kidney is slightly hydronephrotic. (*Courtesy of Neil Wolfman, MD.*) **D.** Limited CT scan of obtained through mass (delineated by +s) demonstrating that it is well circumscribed. This represented a pheochromocytoma. This mass was excised at 26 weeks and the patient became normotensive. **E.** Intra-abdominal abscess associated with intrauterine pregnancy (f, fetus) (longitutinal, 2 cm to left of midline). There is a complex mass anterior to the uterus which contains highly echogenic material (*arrow*). The patient was on steroid treatment for Crohn's disease and experienced sporadic fever prior to her admission. Movement of the gas within was documented on realtime scanning.

evaluation may include either conventional arteriography or digital subtraction angiography.

Abnormally distended fluid-filled bowel secondary to obstruction of an ileus in a gravid patient can be recognized (Figs. 4D,E). The haustral or mucosal folds of bowel can be identified, thus distinguishing distended fluid-filled bowel from other fusiform cystic masses.

SUMMARY

Ultrasonography is very useful in evaluating pelvic masses associated with pregnancy. In most cases, sonography should be the initial diagnostic examination performed, followed, if necessary, by other radiologic studies.

REFERENCES

1. Baker M, Dalrymple G: Biological effects of diagnostic ultrasound: A review. Radiology 126:479, 1978
2. Azimi F, Bryan P, Marangola J: Ultrasonography in obstetrics and gynecology: Historical notes, basic principles, safety considerations, and clinical applications, in Critical Reviews in Clinical Radiology and Nuclear Medicine. Cleveland, OH, CRC, 1976, pp 153–166
3. Pritchard J, Hellman L (eds): Williams' Obstetrics. New York, Appleton-Century-Crofts, 1975, pp 653-654
4. Beischer N, Buttery B, Fortune D, Macafee C: Growth and malignancy of ovarian tumors in pregnancy. Aust NZ J Obstet Gynecol 11:208, 1971
5. Sanders R, Nelson M, Cavalieri R, Graham D: Myomas in pregnancy discovered by sonography. (In preparation)
6. Hassani S, Bard R: Ultrasonic changes of uterine fibroids during pregnancy. Presented at AIUM, San Diego, 1978
7. Mack L, Gottsfeld K, Johnson M: Ultrasonic evaluation of a cervical mass in pregnancy; Case report. J Clin Ultrasound 9:49, 1981
8. Nelson M, Cavalieri R, Graham D, Sanders R: Cysts in pregnancy discovered by sonography: A prevalence study. (In preparation)
9. Bezjian A, Caretero M: Ultrasonic evaluation of pelvic masses in pregnancy. Clin Obstet Gynecol 20:325, 1977
10. Fleischer A, James A, Millis J, et al: Differential diagnosis of pelvic masses by gray scale sonography. Am J Roentgenol 131:469, 1978
11. Filliming P, McLeary R: Non-immunologic fetal hydrops with theca lutein cyst: A case report. Radiology 141:169, 1981
12. Caspi E, Schreyer B, Burkovsky: Ovarian lutein cysts in pregnancy. Obstet Gynecol 42:388, 1978
13. Guttman P: In search of the elusive benign cystic teratoma: "Tip of the iceberg sign." J Clin Ultrasound 5:403, 1977
14. Zakin D: Radiological diagnosis of dermoid cysts of the ovary. Obstet Gynecol Surv 31:165, 1976
15. Dystocia caused by abnormalities of the generative tract, in Hellman C, Pritchard L (eds), Williams' Obstetrics, 14th ed. New York, Appleton-Century-Crofts, 1971, p 928
16. Subramanyam B, Balthazar E, Raghavendra B, et al: Ultrasound analysis of solid appearing abscesses. Radiology 146:487, 1983
17. Anderson G, Rice G, Harris B: Pregnancy and labor complicated by pelvic ectopic kidney abnormalities: Review of literature. Obstet Gynecol Surg 4:737, 1949
18. Fried A, Oliff M, Wilson E: Uterine anomalies associated with renal agenesis: Role of gray scale sonography. Am J Roentgenol 131:973, 1978
19. Anderson J, Lee T, Nagel N: Ultrasound diagnosis of a non-obstetric disease during pregnancy. Obstet Gynecol 48:359, 1976
20. Fleischer A, Boehn L, James AE: Sonography and radiology of pelvic masses and other maternal disorders. Obstetrical Radiology. Semin Roentgenol 17:172, 1982

34 | Postpartum Sonography

Beatrice L. Madrazo

INTRODUCTION

The value of sonography during pregnancy is well established. We have found ultrasound useful in the postpartum period to assess the uterine cavity for retained products of conception and endometritis. In post-cesarean section patients, the abdominal wall and uterine scar can be evaluated for complications such as abscesses and hematomas.

The postpartum period (or puerperium) refers to the 6 to 8 weeks following delivery of a fetus. The most common life-threatening complications during puerperium are hemorrhage, infection, and thromboembolism.[1] Prior to the antibiotic era, approximately 150 per 100,000 women in the puerperal period died, mainly from sepsis. In spite of antibiotics and other advances, maternal mortality is still high and is reported to be 30 to 40 per 100,000 deliveries.[1]

Postpartum hemorrhage due to uterine atony is controlled with oxytocic drugs, which induce uterine contraction. Uterine curettage is sometimes necessary to remove retained products of conception responsible for uterine hemorrhage. Surgical uterine manipulations during the puerperium are associated with a high risk of complications, such as further hemorrhage, uterine perforation, and chronic pelvic infection.[2]

Thromboembolic episodes are frequent during the puerperium, and have been attributed to vascular stasis and the hypercoagulable state of the puerpera.[3,4] Invasive methods of diagnosis such as phlebography are frequently necessary to establish the presence of thrombosis of pelvic veins. Deep venous thrombosis of the lower extremities has been diagnosed by im-

pedance phlebography with an overall diagnostic accuracy of 95.6 percent.[5]

In 1973, Malvern and Campbell reported a series of 40 patients, with postpartum bleeding evaluated with sonography, but they were discouraged by a 17 percent false positive rate.[6] These authors were utilizing bistable equipment with its inherent limitations.

This chapter deals with the usefulness and limitations of sonography in the evaluation of the puerpera. Since the postpartum pelvis differs in appearance from the nonpregnant and pregnant pelvis, a section is devoted to the normal sonographic appearance of the postpartum pelvis. Subsequent sections deal with normal events of the puerperium, as well as with common problems of the puerperium and their management.

NORMAL SONOGRAPHIC ANATOMY

Uterus

The uterus undergoes biochemical and physiologic changes during pregnancy to ensure adequate nutrition to the developing fetus. At the cellular level, changes in the composition of the pregnant uterus are brought about by hormones (luteal and placental), as well as by the stretching effect exerted by the growing fetus. After delivery, pregnancy-induced, uterine changes gradually disappear since both hormonal and mechanical factors have ceased.[7]

Following delivery of the fetus and elimination of the amniotic fluid and placenta, the uterus rapidly contracts and descends from its subxyphoid position to a level just above the umbilicus. It also attains a

449

TABLE 1
Normal Sonographic Parameters of the Postpartum Uterus

Parity	No. of Patients	Normal Values	Uterine Size (cm)			End. Cavity (cm) AP Thickness	Uterine Wall (cm)
			L	AP	W		
Primipara	11	Mean	19.8	8.4	10.9	0.89	3.9
		Range	(16.5–25)	(7–10)	(8.5–14)	(0.5–1.2)	(3–5)
Multipara	14	Mean	21.2	9	12.1	0.98	5.0
		Range	(19–22)	(7–11)	(9–13.5)	(0.5–1.3)	(4.1–6.5)

slightly dextroverted position, referred to as "physiologic right torsion of the uterus."[7]

Table 1 lists the sonographic parameters of the postpartum uterus of 25 normal postpartum patients who underwent spontaneous vaginal delivery.[8] Sonograms were obtained during the first 3 days following delivery. Uterine size was slightly less in primipara than multipara. The separation of the endometrial cavity walls (AP thickness) varied from 0.5 to 1.3 cm without focal areas of greater separation. The uterine walls had a homogenous medium intensity echogenicity and averaged 3 to 6.5 cm in thickness. Prominent myometrial vessels could be seen within the uterine walls.

The puerperal uterus is ovoid in shape. For an adequate sonographic evaluation of the postpartum pelvic cavity, distention of the urinary bladder is needed for the following reasons:

1. The uterine cavity becomes perpendicular to the sound beam due to the anteflexed position of the puerperal uterus. Bladder distention stretches the uterus, enabling a good display of the uterine cavity.
2. Display of the adnexa and cul-de-sac is possible once gas-filled bowel loops are displaced out of the pelvic cavity by the distended urinary bladder.

Figures 1 and 2 illustrate the normal sonographic appearance of the puerperal uterus.

Broad Ligaments

This double reflection of the parietal peritoneum extends from the pelvic side walls to the lateral surfaces of the uterus on each side. These ligaments extend

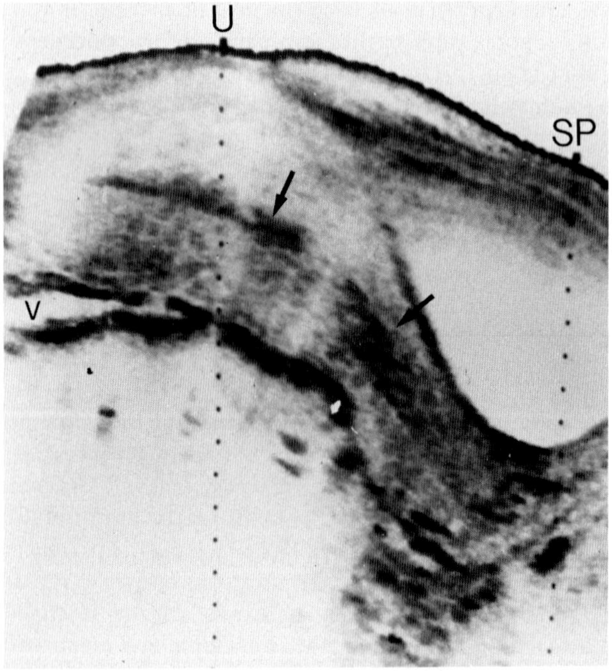

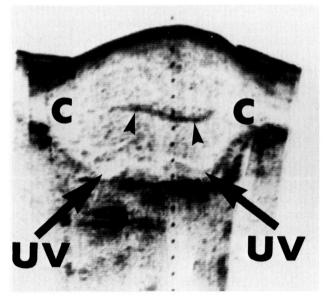

Fig. 1. Longitudinal sonogram of the normal postpartum uterus displays the uterine cavity as a high-intensity central linear echo (*arrows*). The uterine walls generate medium-intensity, homogeneous echoes. Posterior to the uterus, the distal portion of the great vessels and/or their branches can be seen (V). SP, symphysis pubis; U, umbilicus.

Fig. 2. Transverse sonogram of the normal postpartum uterus at the level of the uterine fundus. The linear central echo represents the uterine cavity (*arrowheads*). The uterine cornua (C) are seen, which represent the superior most aspect of the broad ligaments. Prominent uterine vessels (UV) are seen on the posterior uterine wall.

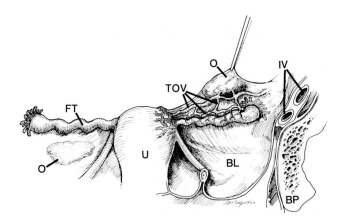

Fig. 3. Artist's rendition of the broad ligaments as seen in the coronal plane. U, uterus; BL, broad ligament; FT, fallopian tube; TOV, tuboovarian vessels; O, ovary; IV, iliac vessels; BP, bony pelvis.

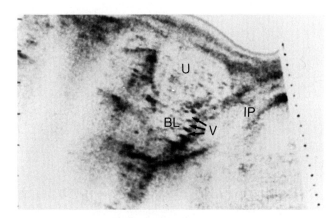

Fig. 4. Longitudinal sonogram to the right of midline displays the lateral margin of the uterus (U) overlying a portion of the broad ligaments (BL). Normally engorged vessels are seen within the broad ligament (V). The iliopsoas muscle is also portrayed (IP).

caudally to the pelvic floor, forming the infundibulo-pelvic ligament, which divides the pelvis into two fossae, namely the vesicouterine and the rectouterine. The broad ligaments contain loose areolar tissue, the fallopian tubes, the uterine artery and vein, the ovarian artery (distal portion), parametrium, and round ligament. The ovaries are peritonealized and are attached to the posterior surface of the broad ligament.[9] The superior most aspects of the broad ligaments are referred to as "the uterine cornua."

Due to their small size, the broad ligaments are not consistently imaged while scanning the nonpregnant uterus. During pregnancy, the broad ligaments distend to accommodate the increase in uterine size and blood supply. Although seen infrequently in postpartum sonograms, it is important to correctly identify the broad ligaments and their components and to not confuse them with an abnormality. Figures 3 through 5 illustrate the appearance of these uterine ligaments in the postpartum period.

Ovaries

In a review of 150 postpartum sonograms, the ovaries could not be identified in a single case. The ovaries might be extrapelvic in position during the puerperium as they become displaced by the large uterus. Adjacent gas-filled bowel loops may obscure their sonographic depiction.

Cul-de-Sac

In our series of 25 normal postpartum patients evaluated with sonography, only one patient was considered to have free-fluid in the cul-de-sac. We have no experience in uncomplicated post cesarean-section patients and therefore cannot comment on the presence or absence of findings in the cul-de-sac in this patient population.

UTERINE INVOLUTION

Immediately after delivery, the uterus weighs 1000 to 1100 g, and, as mentioned previously, the fundus lies just above the umbilicus. Due to the rapid uterine involution in the early postpartum period, within 1 week after delivery, the uterus weighs 500 g and lies midway between the symphysis pubis and umbilicus (Fig. 6).

Van Rees et al. assessed uterine involution in 40 patients with gray scale sonography, and determined that the uterine area decreased 31 percent in the 1st week, 48 percent in the 2nd and 3rd weeks, and 18 percent after the 21st day.[10]

Uterine involution is easily and accurately assessed by clinical examination. Sonography may play a complimentary role in assessing uterine involution in those patients in whom an adequate clinical pelvic examination is not possible due to pain, recent surgery, or obesity.

POSTPARTUM HEMORRHAGE

Approximately 500 ml of blood are lost during delivery when episiotomies are performed. An additional 90 ml of blood are lost in the first 2 hours postpartum. Any additional blood loss in excess of 500 ml is considered postpartum hemorrhage.[9]

In a series of 10,000 deliveries reported by Dewhurst in 1966, postpartum hemorrhage occurred in 1 percent of patients.[11] At our institution, there was a 1.5 percent incidence of postpartum hemorrhage in 3822 deliveries.[8] Vorherr reports an incidence of 4.5 percent.[7]

Following separation of the placenta from the ma-

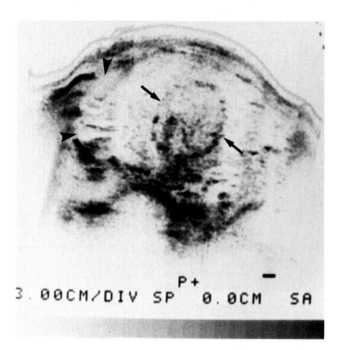

3.00CM/DIV SP P+ 0.0CM SA

Fig. 5. Transverse sonogram displays the puerperal uterus. A placental fragment is retained within the cavity (*arrows*). The right broad ligament is well displayed (*arrowheads*).

ternal decidua spongiosa, a slightly raised residual crater measuring approximately 10 × 7 cm is present along the inner surface of the uterus.[9] Bleeding is initially controlled as the contracting uterus compresses the uterine vessels. A series of local events takes place during the healing process of the uterine wound:

> thrombi develop within the lumen of the uterine vessels, followed by intimal thickening and infiltration of the vessel walls, fibrin and connective-tissue are deposited and finally hyalinization and obliteration of the vessel walls occur.

During healing of the placental site, a copious exudate is discharged through the vagina. This is referred to as "lochia." The total amount of postpartum lochial secretions is 200 to 500 ml. If the healing process of the uterine wound is altered by extraneous factors, such as infection or incomplete uterine involution, postpartum hemorrhage will result.

Table 2 lists the risk factors predisposing towards postpartum hemorrhage.

Postpartum hemorrhage can result from uterine or extrauterine factors. The two most common causes of postpartum uterine bleeding are (1) uterine atony and (2) retained products of conception.

1. *Uterine atony* refers to failure of the uterus to contract following delivery, resulting in copious bleeding from the placental site. In a series of 89 patients

TABLE 2
Postpartum Bleeding—Predisposing Factors

Uterine overdistention (large fetus, multiple pregnancy, hydramnios)
Multiparity
Malnutrition
Toxemia of pregnancy
Prolonged labor
Rapid delivery
Intrauterine manipulations
General anesthesia
Use of estrogens to suppress lactation
Blood coagulopathy

with postpartum bleeding reported by Dewhurst, 66 percent of the cases were due to uterine atony.[11]

The clinical diagnosis of uterine atony is made when both postpartum hemorrhage and flaccid uterus are present. Patients in our hospital suspected of having uterine atony are given a therapeutic trial of intravenous oxytocin and external uterine massage. If bleeding continues, sonography is utilized to exclude the presence of retained products of conception within the uterine cavity.

We have found no significant difference in the size or shape of the uterus in patients with uterine atony as compared to those with a normal postpartum uterus.[8] Therefore, in a patient with postpartum uterine bleeding and a normal postpartum sonogram, the most likely cause for the hemorrhage is uterine atony.

2. *Retained products of conception*—incomplete elimination of the products of conception will lead to uterine hemorrhage since the uterine cavity will remain expanded, and bleeding continues at the previous site of placental attachment.

Retained products of conception have a variable sonographic appearance, depending on what has been retained in the uterine cavity (placental fragments, blood clots, membranes, and so on), as well as their degree of necrosis at the time of scanning. Table 3 lists common sonographic findings seen with retained placental fragments. Figures 5 and 7 illustrate their appearance.

Extrauterine causes of postpartum bleeding include lacerations (cervical, vaginal, and perineal) and hematomas (pelvic soft tissues, broad ligament, etc.).

TABLE 3
Sonographic Appearance of Retained Placental Fragments

1. Round or oval echogenic intracavitary tissues
2. Stippled echo pattern
3. High-intensity foci with associated acoustical shadowing
4. Fluid within the uterine cavity

Uterine Involution Post Partum

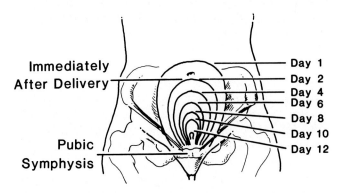

Fig. 6. Schematic representation of the uterine fundal height in the first 12 days of the puerperium.

Figure 8 is of a patient who developed a broad ligament hematoma after cesarean section.

PUERPERAL INFECTION

Puerperal infection is suspected when the patient experiences elevated body temperatures of 100.4°F (38°C) or more on two consecutive days, not including the first day of fever.[1]

Infection accounts for 6 to 8 per 100,000 maternal deaths. Endometrial infection develops in 3 to 4 percent of women following delivery. The incidence of endometritis in post-cesarean section patients is 13 to 27 percent.[1] Predisposing factors to puerperal infections are listed in Table 4.

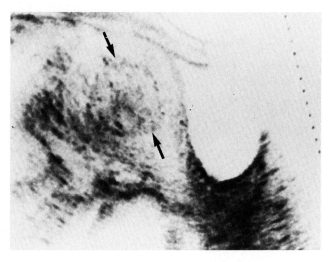

Fig. 7. Longitudinal sonogram of the uterus displays a 6 × 7 cm retained placental fragment in the uterine cavity (*arrows*).

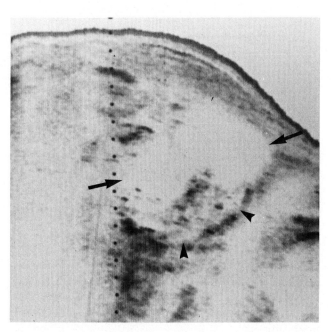

Fig. 8. Broad ligament hematoma. Longitudinal sonogram to the left of the uterus displays a sharply circumscribed anechoic collection within the broad ligament (*arrows*). The areolar tissue, fallopian tube and vascular structures of the broad ligament are displaced posteriorly (*arrowheads*).

The most common route of infection into the uterine cavity is through the vagina. The vaginal milieu of nonpregnant and pregnant females is acid, due to the production of lactic acid by the normal Dorderlein bacilli. This acidity prevents many pathogens from proliferating in the vagina.

Once there is rupture of the amniotic membranes, microorganisms readily ascend from the vagina into the amniotic cavity. Chorioamnionitis can be found in 50 percent of patients with membranes ruptured for longer than 24 hours.[1]

After delivery, the vagina becomes alkaline due to the neutralizing effects of the amniotic fluid, blood,

TABLE 4
Puerperal Infections—Predisposing Factors

Poor nutrition and hygiene
Anemia
Vaginitis—cervicitis
Coitus late in pregnancy
Toxemia
Premature or early rupture of membranes
Prolonged labor and frequent vaginal examinations during labor
Intrapartum maternal and fetal monitoring
Cesarean section
Lacerations (spontaneous or operative vaginal delivery)
Manual removal of placenta
Retention of secundines

TABLE 5
Sonographic Findings in Patients with Endometritis

	Number of Patients
Dilated uterine cavity with echogenic tissues	10
Dilated uterine cavity with fluid	10
Dilated uterine cavity with fluid and gas	2
Gas within the uterine cavity	3
Normal uterine cavity with fluid in the cul-de-sac	3
Normal sonograms (false negatives)	6
Total	34

and lochia. The vaginal lactobacilli are also decreased in the puerperium. This alkalinity of the vagina favors bacterial growth, and microorganisms ascend into the uterine cavity invading the uterine wound. The thrombosed uteroplacental vessels provide a good culture site outside the uterine cavity; parametritis, septic pelvic thrombophlebitis, and pelvic, as well as generalized, peritonitis may result.

Puerperal infections are caused by anaerobic bacteria in 70 percent of cases and by aerobic microorganisms in 30 percent. A large number of puerperal infections are caused by a mixed flora. The most common pathogens in cases of endometritis are anaerobic and aerobic streptococci, bacteroides, *Escherichia coli,* and pyogenic streptococci.[1] In mild to moderate intrauterine infections, blood cultures are usually negative. Clinically it is difficult to distinguish between endometritis and urinary tract infection.

Table 5 lists the sonographic findings in 34 patients with proven endometritis. Figures 9 and 10 illustrate the sonographic findings in endometritis.

Endometritis can result both from retention of products of conception and contamination of the uterine cavity by microorganisms from the vagina. The sonographic findings of retained products of conception and endometritis overlap. Of interest are the six patients listed in Table 5 with normal sonograms and clinical endometritis. These patients were treated with antibiotics, but curettage was not performed. We presume that a certain degree of inflammation and exudation has to be present within the uterine cavity before separation of the cavity walls occurs and the process becomes apparent sonographically. Milder forms of endometritis are not detectable sonographically.

Certain microorganisms produce gas, which is readily identified by sonography. Gas-forming organisms frequently present in cases of endometritis include *E. coli* and *C. perfringens* (Welchii). The former is a common pathogen in human infections. The latter may cause endotoxin shock and death. When evaluating the uterus for endometritis, it is important to perform sonograms prior to dilatation and curettage. Air can be introduced into the uterine cavity during surgical manipulations. However, if gas is present within the endometrial cavity and no manipulations have been performed, endometritis with gas formation is present.

In cesarean section patients, infections may develop in the uterine incision and in the abdominal wall incision. Burger et al. reported on the variable sonographic appearance of the uterine incision of cesarean section.[12] They concluded that the appearance was related to local tissue reaction, as well as to the type and amount of suturing material utilized. In our experience, it is normal to see a small, rounded area

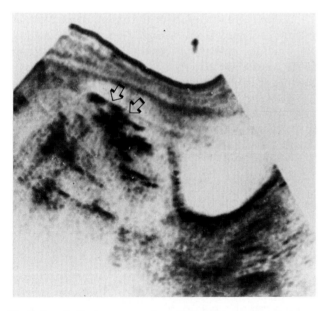

Fig. 9. Longitudinal sonogram of a patient with proven *E. coli* endometritis. Interrupted high-intensity, linear echoes in the uterine cavity with associated "ring down" are due to intracavitary gas collections (*arrows*).

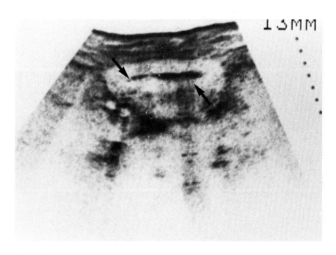

Fig. 10. Transverse sonogram of a patient with proven endometritis. Gas and fluid are present within the uterine cavity (*arrows*).

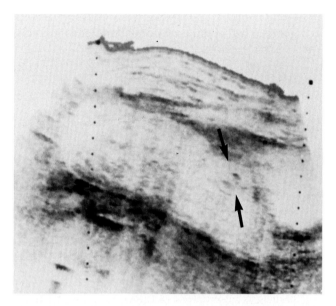

Fig. 11. Longitudinal sonogram of an asymptomatic post-cesarean section patient. The normal uterine scar is seen in the lower uterine segment (*arrows*).

within the anterior uterine wall, at the level of the uterine segment, during the first week after cesarean section (Fig. 11). Usually, the uterine incision area contains strong echoes generated by the suturing material and medium-intensity echoes surrounding it. Small seromas or hematomas may develop in the uterine incision, but in a febrile patient, any fluid collection in

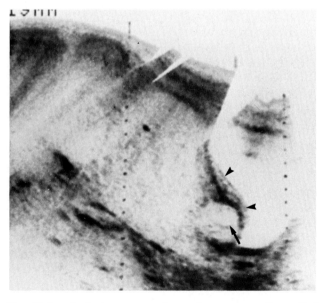

Fig. 12. Longitudinal sonogram of a post-cesarean section patient with an abscess of the uterine scar. A 1 cm anechoic collection is present (*arrow*). Inflammation of the adjacent bladder wall is seen (*arrowheads*).

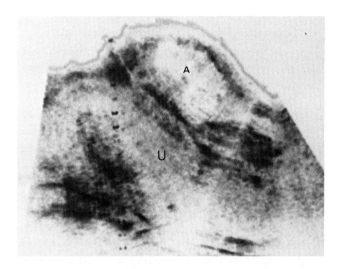

Fig. 13. A large abscess is present in the abdominal wall incision following a cesarean section. U, uterus.

the uterine incision is suspicious for an abscess (Fig. 12). Evidence of strong echoes with associated acoustical shadowing usually represents an abscess with gas formation.

Abdominal wall disorders, although superficial in location, may be difficult to detect clinically due to tenderness to palpation. Induration of the abdominal wall due to edema may also make it difficult to assess. Abdominal wall collections can be easily demonstrated by sonography. Seromas, hematomas, and abscesses have a similar sonographic appearance. In a febrile, postcesarean patient, abdominal wall collections should be drained. Figure 13 illustrates an abdominal wall abscess.

THROMBOEMBOLIC EPISODES IN THE PUERPERIUM

Venous stasis, changes in the blood clotting factors, and alterations in the vessel wall predispose to intravascular clotting of blood. An increased incidence of thromboembolic episodes during pregnancy and the puerperium is well recognized.[13] Throughout pregnancy there is venous stasis of the pelvis and lower extremities. Extensive studies have confirmed the hypercoagulable state of the pregnant and puerperal female.[13] Anaerobic streptococcus is a common cause of thrombophlebitis.[10,13] The incidence of thrombophlebitis during pregnancy, varies between 0.018 and 0.29 per 100 deliveries.[13]

Impedance phlebography has been successfully utilized to assess the deep veins for thrombosis.[5] Thrombosis of deep pelvic uterine, and ovarian veins is difficult to diagnose clinically, although computed tomography and sonography may play a role in the detection of ovarian vein thrombophlebitis. In one instance an echogenic mass inferior to the right kidney was shown at computed tomography to represent a thrombosed ovarian vein.[14]

Puerperal ovarian vein thrombophlebitis was first described by Austin in 1958.[15] In 1971, Brown reviewed 20 cases previously reported and added 16 cases of his own. He reported an incidence of 1 case per 569 deliveries, or an incidence of 0.18 percent.[3] The main factors contributing to the development of puerperal ovarian vein thrombophlebitis are stasis in the ovarian vein as its flow suddenly decreases in the puerperium, the hypercoagulable state of the postpartum patient, and infection. Clinical features of ovarian vein thrombophlebitis include lower abdominal pain, nausea, vomiting and fever that usually starts on the second or third postpartum day. The enlarged and tortuous ovarian veins can enlarge to 2 to 8 cm in diameter exceeding that of the inferior vena cava.[3]

Careful examination of the patient may reveal a ropelike mass, which extends lateral and cephalad from the uterine cornua. The right side is most frequently involved, although left-sided or bilateral involvement can occur. This condition can be mistaken for appendicitis, ovarian torsion, pelvic abscess, broad ligament hematoma, and volvulus of the bowel. Anticoagulation therapy can be instituted to prevent embolization. One-third of patients with ovarian vein thrombophlebitis develop septic pulmonary emboli.[3]

Radiographic evaluation may reveal the presence of an ileus. Cases diagnosed by sonography have not been reported, although awareness of this condition and knowledge of the anatomy of the ovarian veins may allow the sonographic diagnosis. Shaffer et al. reported a case of ovarian vein thrombophlebitis, diagnosed by computed tomography.[16]

CONCLUSIONS

The significant contribution made by sonography to the management of postpartum complications is the noninvasive assessment of the uterine cavity for retained products of conception and infections. Mild forms of endometritis may not be detectable on sonograms.

Ultrasound may have a future role in the detection of puerperal pelvic and ovarian vein thrombophlebitis as combined use of gray scale and Doppler sonography becomes more widespread.

REFERENCES

1. Vorherr H: Puerperal genitourinary infection, in Sciarra (ed), Gynecology and Obstetrics. Philadelphia, Harper and Row, 1982, vol 2, chap 91, pp 1–29
2. Rome RM: Secondary post-partum hemorrhage. Br J Obstet Gynecol 82:289, 1975
3. Brown TK, Mannick RA: Puerperal ovarian vein thrombophlebitis—A syndrome. Am J Obstet Gynec 109:263, 1971
4. Montalto NJ, Bloch E, Malfetano JH, et al: Postpartum thrombophlebitis of the ovarian vein. Obstet Gynecol 34:867, 1969
5. Pearson DLC, Creasman WT: Diagnosis of deep venous thrombosis in obstetrics and gynecology by impedance phlebography. Obstet Gynecol 58:52, 1981
6. Malvern J, Campbell S, May P: Ultrasonic scanning of the puerperal uterus following secondary post-partum hemorrhage. J Obstet Gynecol Br Commonw 80:320, 1973
7. Vorherr H: Puerperium: Maternal involutional changes—Management of puerperal problems and complications, in Sciarra (ed), Gynecology and Obstetrics. Philadelphia, Harper and Row, 1982, vol 2, chap 90, pp 1–44
8. Lee CY, Madrazo BL, Drukker BH: Ultrasonic evaluation of the postpartum uterus in the management of postpartum bleeding. Obstet Gynecol, 58:227, 1981
9. Gray H: Anatomy of the Human Body, 29th ed. Philadelphia, Lea & Febiger, 1973
10. Van Rees D, Bernstine RL, Crawford W: Involution of the postpartum uterus: An ultrasonic study. J Clin Ultrasound 9:55, 1981
11. Dewhurst CJ: Secondary postpartum hemorrhage. J Obstet Gynecol Br Commonw 73:53, 1966
12. Burger NF, Dararas B, Boes EGM: An echographic evaluation during the early puerperium of the uterine wound after cesarean section. J Clin Ultrasound 10:271, 1982
13. Villasanta U: Thromboembolic disease in pregnancy. Am J Obstet Gynecol 93:142, 1965
14. Wilson PC, Lerner RM: Diagnosis of ovarian vein thrombophlebitis by ultrasonography. J Ultrasound Med 2: 187, 1983
15. Austin OG: Massive thrombophlebitis of the ovarian vein. Am J Obstet Gynecol 72:428, 1956
16. Shaffer PB, Johnson JC, Bryan D, et al: Diagnosis of ovarian vein thrombophlebitis by computed tomography. J Comp Assist Tomogr 5:436, 1981

35 | Principles of Differential Diagnosis of Pelvic Masses by Sonography

Arthur C. Fleischer
Stephen S. Entman
Lonnie S. Burnett
A. Everette James, Jr.

It has taken several years of clinicopathologic correlation for the specificity and clinical utility of sonography for the evaluation of patients with pelvic masses to become established.[1-3] The recent improvements in the resolution and imaging flexibility of real-time systems has enhanced sonographic examination of normal and abnormal pelvic structures.

Although the role of sonography relative to computed body tomography varies from institution to institution, sonography remains an excellent modality for the initial evaluation of a patient with a pelvic mass.[4] Computed tomography remains the modality of choice for evaluation of tumor infiltration or recurrence such as that associated with cervical carcinoma or the detection of lymphadenopathy associated with gynecologic neoplasms.[5-7]

Sonography has an important role in the evaluation of a patient with a suspected or palpable pelvic mass. The list below summarizes features of a pelvic mass that are clinically relevant and that can be determined by sonography:

1. Confirming the presence or absence of a mass.
2. Determining the organ of origin and anatomic relationship of the mass to other organs.
3. Evaluating the size, consistency, and contour of a mass.
4. Demonstrating the involvement of other organs by the mass.
5. Delineating the presence or absence of ascites and/ or other metastatic lesions.

Because of the nonspecificity of the sonographic features of most pelvic masses, one should fully evaluate these parameters rather than endeavoring to formulate a specific diagnosis. Rather than mentioning all of the possibilities in a certain diagnostic category, the individual interpreting the sonogram should be able to narrow the diagnostic possibilities to one or two of the most probable entities based on sonographic features and clinical findings (Table 1).[8]

DIAGNOSTIC CRITERIA

The gamuts for the sonographic differential diagnosis of pelvic masses presented here are based on specific sonographic criteria for the evaluation of pelvic masses (Fig. 1). These criteria are adapted from the more general scheme for the sonographic evaluation of soft tissue masses by gray scale sonography proposed by Kossoff et al.[9] The following criteria used for evaluation of pelvic masses were adopted because of reliability and clinical relevance:

1. Origin, size, and location of pelvic mass.
2. Internal consistency
3. Definition of walls
4. The presence or absence of ascites or other metastatic lesions

Although all the major criteria are useful for the proper sonographic diagnosis of a pelvic mass, the size and location of the mass are of primary importance. These evaluations will determine to some extent the surgical approach as well as the postoperative management. Consequently, it is helpful to relate the location of a mass in relation to the uterus. Since the determina-

TABLE 1
Sonographic Differential Diagnoses of Pelvic Masses*

Cystic	Complex	Solid
Completely cystic	Predominately cystic	Uterine
Physiologic ovarian cysts	Cystadenomas	Leiomyoma (sarcoma)
Cystadenomas	Tuboovarian abscess	Endometrial carcinoma,
Hydrosalpinx	Ectopic pregnancy	sarcoma
Endometrioma	Cystic teratoma	
Paraovarian cyst		
Hydatid cyst of Morgani		
Multiple	Predominately solid	Extrauterine
Endometriomas	Cystadenoma (carcinoma)	Solid ovarian tumor
Multiple follicular cysts	Germ cell tumor	
Septated		
Cystadenoma (carcinoma)		
Mucinous		
Serous		
Papillary		

* Based upon most common appearance.

tion of the presence of infiltration of the tumor into surrounding structures may be difficult to evaluate by sonography alone, additional radiographic studies such as barium enema, and computed tomography may be required in selected patients.[4]

The internal consistency of a pelvic mass is portrayed well by sonography and can be utilized in formulating a differential diagnosis. The clinical utility of this parameter is illustrated by the fact that cystic masses that are less than 5 cm in diameter are generally benign, whereas complex masses that contain irregular septations and/or solid components have a high likelihood of being malignant.[10] Establishment of the cystic nature of a pelvic mass by sonography may allow clinical observation of the mass rather than its surgical removal.

Sonography can depict the thickness and regularity of the wall of a pelvic mass. Masses with thick and/or irregular walls usually represent tumors or inflammatory masses. Whether or not the tumor has spread past the capsule of mass is difficult to determine by sonography. The presence of ascites with a mass usually indicates that peritoneal spread has occurred. The ascites may result from peritoneal irritation or disruption of lymphatic return.

Once a pelvic mass is delineated, the sonographer should examine certain areas that may manifest changes associated with a gynecologic malignancy. Specifically, the cul de sac, pericolic, and perihepatic spaces should be examined for the presence of ascitic fluid, the liver parenchyma evaluated for the presence of metastatic foci, the peritoneal surfaces and omentum for evidence of tumor implants, and the kidneys for obstructive uropathy (Table 2).[4]

The remainder of the chapter is divided into a discussion of those parameters of a pelvic mass that have clinical relevance.

Size and Location

The size of a pelvic mass may rarely suggest a particular diagnosis but is not usually helpful in the differential diagnosis of a pelvic mass. This is due to the fact that almost every pelvic mass, if given time, will enlarge and present as a pelvoabdominal mass. Only a few pelvic masses, such as ovarian mucinous cystadenomas, consistently attain a pelvoabdominal size. Conversely, some tumors, such as the ovarian fibroma or Brenner tumor, rarely enlarge over 5 cm.

Whether a mass is unilateral or bilateral assists in the differential diagnosis because some conditions, such as polycystic ovary disease, tend to be bilateral. About 15 percent of patients with serous cystadenomas or cystic teratomas will have bilateral masses.[1]

The location of a pelvic mass should be documented with scans obtained in at least two planes. Additional scans can be performed oblique to the transverse or longitudinal planes when delineation of the mass is incomplete using routine scanning planes. For example, on one plane, some masses may appear to be separate from the uterus but, on another, may prove to be an extension of the uterus. A fully distended bladder can displace an adnexal mass out of the pelvis. Consequently, some masses may be missed if the area above the bladder is not examined.[11]

According to definition, adnexal masses are those that are confined to the pelvis and involve either the oviduct or ovary. The term "adnexal" is occasionally used interchangeably with the term "pelvic" and has

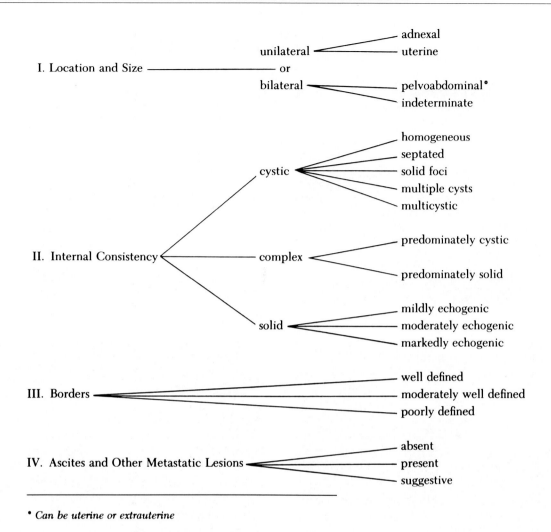

* *Can be uterine or extrauterine*

Fig. 1. Criteria for sonographic categorization of pelvic masses.

acquired a more general definition to imply a mass that involves the fallopian tubes and ovaries and is outside of the uterus and within the pelvis. Except for the pedunculated leiomyoma, uterine masses can usually be identified as being contiguous with the uterine outline.

Since some pelvoabdominal masses can simulate an abdominal mass sonographically, the pelvic component should be clearly delineated before a diagnosis is made. Abdominal masses that enlarge in a caudad direction can be distinguished by their apparent displacement of bowel from pelvic masses that enlarge

TABLE 2
Additional Views Needed When a Pelvic Mass Is Found

1. Cul de sac, paracolic recesses for fluid.
2. Kidneys for obstructive uropathy.
3. Liver for metastases.
4. Subdiaphragmatic area, peritoneum and omentum for metastases.

in a cephalad direction (Fig. 2A). Gas-filled bowel loops appear as an echogenic area on either side of the mass, which is associated with a mottled, incomplete, or "dirty" acoustical shadow. Fluid-filled bowel loops that result from fluid ingestion for bladder distension may appear as rounded anechoic pelvic masses on pelvic sonography (Figs. 3A,B).[12] The characteristic peristaltic motion of fluid-filled bowel loops, however, is readily depicted on real-time scanning.

The uterus serves as a reference point for describing the location of a mass within the pelvis. It is usually identified by its relatively echogenic endometrial interface and contiguity with the vagina.[13]

Some solid masses that are adjacent to the uterus are often indistinguishable from the uterus and produce the "indefinite uterus" sign (Fig. 2B). This sign refers to an apparent enlargement of the uterine outline by a solid mass whose border is sonographically indistinct from the uterus.[14]

Occasionally, it will be difficult to localize large

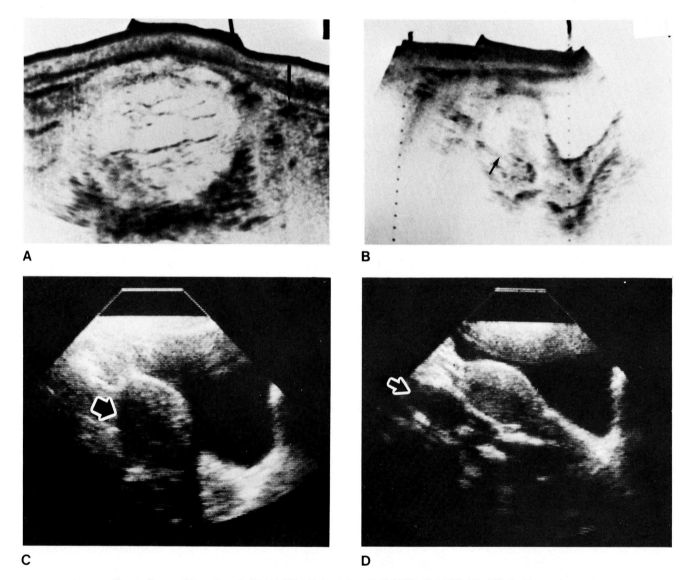

Fig. 2. Size and Location. **A.** Bowel displacement (longitudinal, 6 cm to left of midline). A complex, predominantly cystic mass that contains solid component and thin septations is seen. Its intraabdominal retroperitoneal location is implied by the fact that the mass resulted in bowel displacement inferiorly (*arrow*). Bowel loops demonstrate a high degree of echogenicity with a mottled distal acoustical shadowing. This is due to the scattering effect of gas and contents within bowel loops. In the distinction between abdominal and retroperitoneal masses, generally masses that arise from the pelvis tend to displace bowel along their superior aspect. **B.** "Indefinite uterus sign" (longitudinal, midline). There is a solid mass adjacent to the uterine fundus (*arrow*). The proximity and similar echo pattern of the mass in comparison with the uterus creates apparent enlargement of the uterine outline or the "indefinite uterus sign." This circumstance is often associated with diagnostic interpretative error. If this situation is encountered, transverse, longitudinal, and oblique scans should be performed in an attempt to delineate if the mass is separate from the uterus. This "indefinite uterus" sign frequently occurs with hematomas adjacent to the uterus and solid mass lesions such as this ovarian teratoma. **C.** Sagittal real-time sonogram of patient with fever of unknown origin. There was suggestion of a hypoechoic, ill-defined mass (*arrow*) posterior to the uterus on this scan. **D.** Same patient as in **C** after water distension of the rectum and rectosigmoid colon (*arrow*). No retrouterine masses were identified.

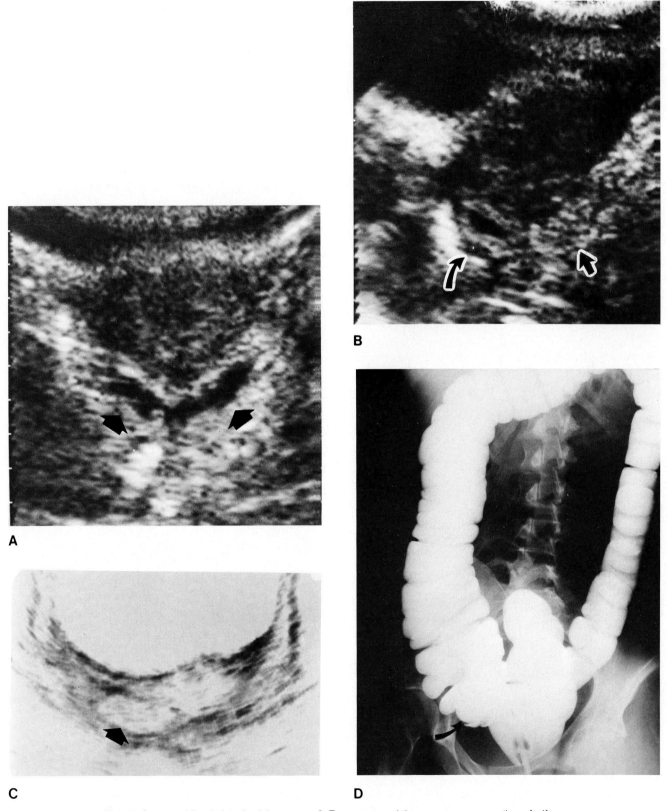

Figs. 3. Sonographic mimics of pelvic masses. **A.** Transverse real-time sonogram suggesting a fusiform retrouterine mass (*arrows*) in patient who ingested water for urinary bladder distension. **B.** Same patient, 1 to 2 seconds later. A portion of the bowel has contracted (*straight arrow*) while a portion remains distended (*curved arrow*). Therefore, the previously identified fusiform structure represented a transiently distended small bowel. **C.** Transverse static sonogram suggesting presence of solid right adnexal mass (*arrow*). **D.** Radiograph from barium enema of patient in **C** shows a low-lying cecum (*curved arrow*). The mass observed on sonography was due to a fecal-filled cecum (*cont.*).

462

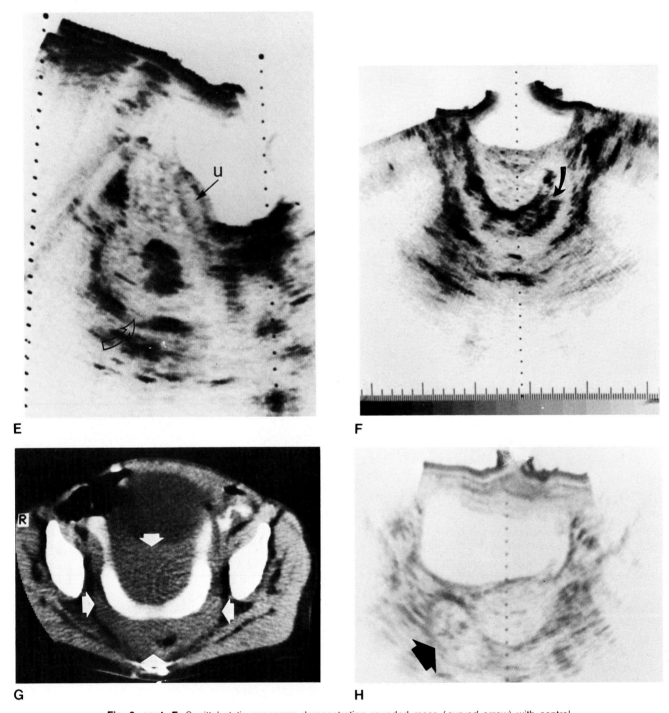

Fig. 3. cont. E. Sagittal static sonogram demonstrating rounded mass (*curved arrow*) with central echogenicity posterior to uterus (u). **F.** Transverse static sonogram of same patient showing mass with central echogenic core (*arrow*). **G.** Computed tomogram of patient in Figure 3E showing extensive thickening of ileal wall (*arrow*) secondary to lymphoma. **H.** Transverse static sonogram demonstrating a solid right adnexal mass (*arrow*). This represented fat that had herniated through the broad ligament. (*Courtesy of M. Louis Weinstein, MD.*)

pelvic masses in relation to the uterus due to their distortion of normal pelvic landmarks. Masses that cannot be adequately localized should be considered "indeterminate" in location. Masses that do not represent gynecologic disorders, such as gastrointestinal tract tumors, can occasionally be clinically, radiographically, and sonographically confused with a pelvic or pelvoabdominal mass (Figs. 3A–C).[15] In these cases, a contrast gastrointestinal series is helpful for further evaluation of the mass.

Water distension of the rectum and rectosigmoid is helpful when it is difficult to determine whether or not a pelvic mass might be spuriously created by bowel (Figs. 2C,D).[16] In addition, this technique may be helpful in delineation of tumor spread in the bladder in patients with carcinoma of the cervix.[17]

Internal Consistency

Before the introduction of gray scale image processing, sonographic studies using conventional bistable B-mode methods could only characterize masses into those that were cystic, complex, and solid.[18] However, the development of gray scale sonography enabled subtle differences in soft tissue textures to be demonstrated, thereby making possible more specific sonographic diagnoses.[9] For example, when gray scale sonography is utilized, cystic masses can be divided into those that are homogeneously cystic, septated, or those in which a soft tissue focus can be identified. Complex masses can be similarly divided according to their overall internal pattern, i.e., complex, predominantly solid mass, or complex, predominantly cystic mass. Solid masses can be divided into those that are mildly, moderately, or markedly echogenic. Since the echogenicity of a solid mass is related to its collagen content, recognition of the relative echogenicity of a solid mass is helpful in establishing a differential diagnosis.[19] Low-level internal echoes can arise from cholesterol crystals and cellular debris.[20]

As is true for cystic masses outside the pelvis, the sonographic characteristics of a cystic mass within the pelvis consist of an echo-free center, well-defined boundaries, and, because of good through transmission, distal acoustical enhancement (Fig. 4A). If these characteristics are not observed, an alternative diagnosis should be considered. This concept is illustrated in Figure 4B, in which a hypoechoic pelvic mass was considered atypical for a cystic mass since there was no posterior acoustical enhancement. This mass was found to represent lymphomatous metastases to the ovary. The mass consisted of a homogenous, densely cellular mass with little or no intervening stroma.

Solid masses are characterized sonographically by

their echogenic appearance. Their borders may be either well or poorly defined. The echogenicity of a solid mass seems to be related to the amount, arrangement, and elasticity of its stromal components (interstitial or collagenous framework), and its degree of degeneration and vascular supply.[19] For example, lymphomatous masses tend to be almost entirely sonolucent and can even be confused occasionally with cystic pelvic masses (Fig. 4B). This sonolucency is probably related to the characteristic lack of stromal elements within a highly cellular lymphomas. Leiomyomata, conversely, are usually moderately echogenic, which is probably because of their dense arrangement of connective tissue and smooth muscle fibers (Fig. 4C). The variation in echogenicity seen within leiomyomata may be related to their relative proportion of fibrous tissue and smooth muscle as well as their degree and type of degeneration. Sebum within a dermoid cyst, organized clot, pus, and cellular debris can produce echoes within a cystic mass (Figs. 4D,E).[20,21] A linear echogenic interface that is gravity dependent can be observed to change if the patient is scanned in a right or left posterior oblique position (Fig. 4G).

Irregular and disorganized solid material within a pelvic mass suggests neoplastic rather than benign growth (Fig. 4F).[10] This type of pattern may be observed in papillary adenocarcinomas. Irregular areas of cystic degeneration within a solid mass may also create this type of sonographic pattern. In general, the more solid components within a complex mass, the greater likelihood it is malignant. The determination of benign or malignant properties of a mass, however, can only be reliably made at pathologic examination.

Borders of a Mass

Irregular borders of a mass suggest a neoplastic or inflammatory process. In contrast, a thickened wall that is regular can be the result of vascular congestion secondary to torsion of a mass around its pedicle.

Cystic masses usually possess a smooth border due to the compression of surrounding soft tissue as fluid accumulates within them, whereas infiltrating neoplasms or inflammatory masses exhibit an irregular and sometimes indistinct sonographic border (Fig. 4A). As an example, Figure 5B demonstrates a solid ovarian adenocarcinoma that had infiltrated into the bladder wall, as evidenced by a markedly irregular border and indistinct mass–soft tissue interface.

Similarly, slight irregularity in the wall of an anechoic mass should not be considered indicative of a pathologic process (Figs. 5C–E). Irregular thickening of a wall must be differentiated from layering of cellular debris along the dependent wall, which may also

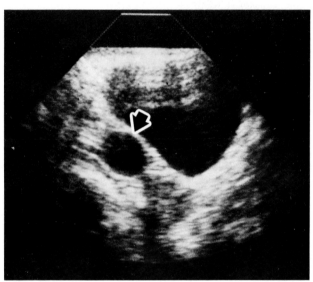

A

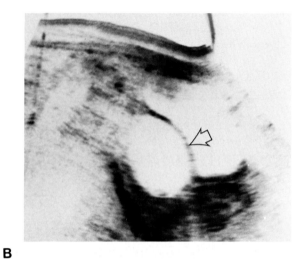

B

Fig. 4. Internal consistency parameters. **A.** Follicular cyst depicted as a completely cystic adnexal mass with well-defined, smooth borders. **B.** Lymphoma (longitudinal, 3 cm to right of midline). The lymphomatous mass demonstrates a sonolucent texture (*open arrow*). This appearance probably reflects the lack of interstitial tissue within the highly cellular lymphomas. **C.** Intramural leiomyoma (longitudinal, midline). There is a mass located within the uterine outline depicted as an area of diminished echogenicity along the posterior aspect of the myometrium (*white arrow*). The intrauterine location of leiomyoma is also confirmed by its proximity to the endometrial lumen (*black arrow*). The echogenic appearance of the endometrium observed during menstruation can be utilized to locate the position of the mass relative to the uterus (*Courtesy of Roger Sanders, MD*) (*cont.*).

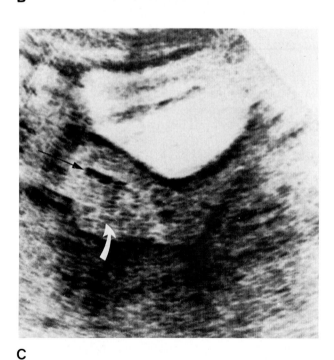

C

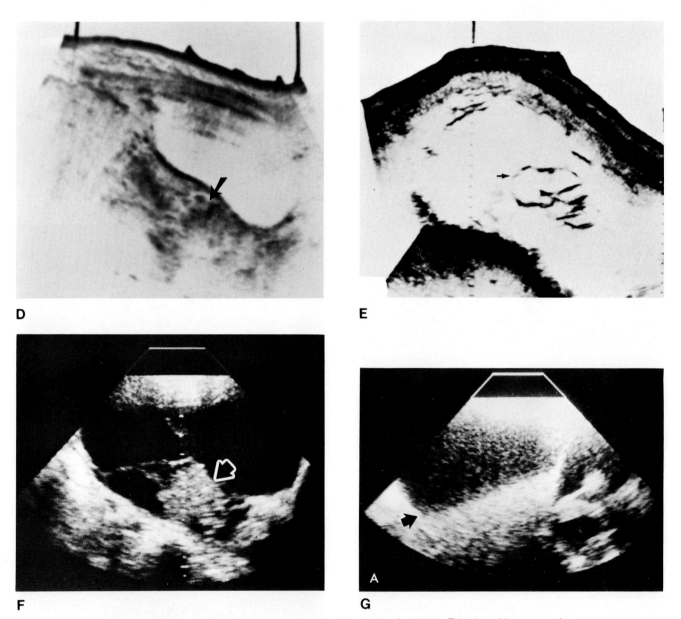

Fig. 4. cont. D. Dermoid cyst (longitudinal, 3 cm to right of midline). This dermoid cyst contains echogenic components (*arrow*) which represent sebaceous material. The echogenicity of the sebum within the cyst hampers delineation of the posterior aspect of the mass. This feature is commonly encountered in evaluation of dermoid cysts that contain a large amount of sebum and has been referred to as the ''tip of the iceberg'' effect.[9] (*Reprinted with permission from Fleischer A, James E: Introduction to Diagnostic Sonography. New York, Wiley, 1980.*) **E.** Predominantly cystic, septated, pelvoabdominal mass (longitudinal, 2 cm to right of midline). This predominantly cystic mass contains thin internal septations. **F.** Longitudinal real-time sonogram demonstrating solid component (*arrow*) and septations within pelvoabdominal mass that was found to be a cystadenocarcinoma. **G.** Longitudinal real-time sonogram of complex, pelvoabdominal mass containing layering material. This layer (*arrow*) was created by less echogenic serous fluid and heavier cellular debris within this papillary cystadenocarcinoma.

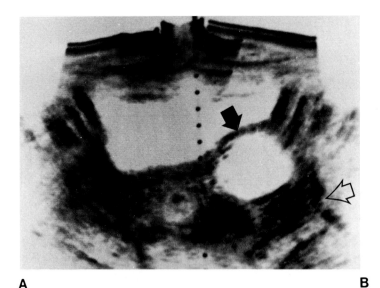

A

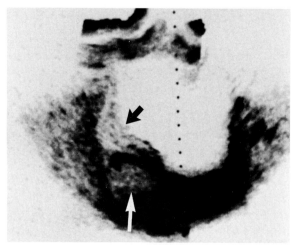

B

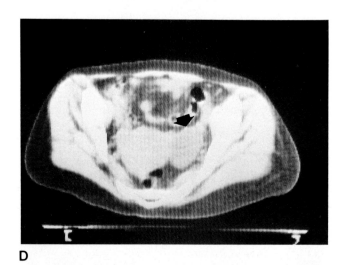

C

D

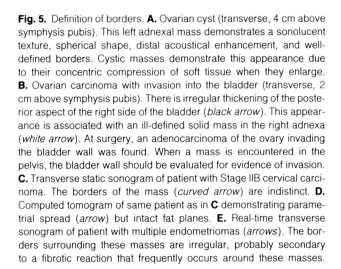

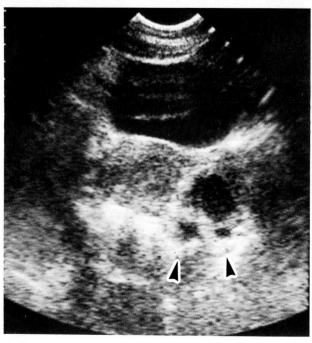

E

Fig. 5. Definition of borders. **A.** Ovarian cyst (transverse, 4 cm above symphysis pubis). This left adnexal mass demonstrates a sonolucent texture, spherical shape, distal acoustical enhancement, and well-defined borders. Cystic masses demonstrate this appearance due to their concentric compression of soft tissue when they enlarge. **B.** Ovarian carcinoma with invasion into the bladder (transverse, 2 cm above symphysis pubis). There is irregular thickening of the posterior aspect of the right side of the bladder (*black arrow*). This appearance is associated with an ill-defined solid mass in the right adnexa (*white arrow*). At surgery, an adenocarcinoma of the ovary invading the bladder wall was found. When a mass is encountered in the pelvis, the bladder wall should be evaluated for evidence of invasion. **C.** Transverse static sonogram of patient with Stage IIB cervical carcinoma. The borders of the mass (*curved arrow*) are indistinct. **D.** Computed tomogram of same patient as in **C** demonstrating parametrial spread (*arrow*) but intact fat planes. **E.** Real-time transverse sonogram of patient with multiple endometriomas (*arrows*). The borders surrounding these masses are irregular, probably secondary to a fibrotic reaction that frequently occurs around these masses.

466

simulate the finding of an irregular cyst wall. Again, this can be excluded by scanning the patient in various oblique positions in order to assess the mobility and separate the debris from the wall of the mass.

Metastatic Disease

Real-time sonography allows more complete and accurate evaluation of the presence of metastases in patients with malignant pelvic masses. With aggressive clinical management, patients with ovarian cancer survive longer, and the sonographer and sonologist will encounter more patients with metastatic disease to the liver.[22] Cystic metastases can be seen in patients with metastatic squamous cell carcinoma of the cervix as well as patients with advanced ovarian carcinoma (Fig. 6A). In general, intrahepatic metastases associated with ovarian carcinoma are hypoechoic (Figs. 6B,C).

After a pelvic mass is identified, survey scans of the cul de sac, pericolic and perihepatic recesses, liver, and kidney are recommended (Table 2). Excretory urography may be needed to differentiate obstructive uropathy due to compression by a pelvic mass from infiltration and involvement of the ureter itself. A barium enema is needed to detect extension or involvement of bowel by a pelvic mass.[23] Some pelvic disorders such as endometriosis can implant on the bowel serosa. This abnormality cannot be reliably depicted by sonography.

Although the presence of loculated ascites is usually associated with metastatic ovarian disease, it may also be associated with inflammatory processes (Figs. 6D,E,F). In those patients with advanced ovarian carcinoma, loculated ascites occurs when surface implants adhere, creating blind spaces and fixating bowel.[22] Loculated ascites may also be the result of an inflammatory process such as rupture of a tuboovarian abscess. In these patients, loculated ascites occur secondary to adhesions restricting the location of bowel loops. Occasionally one encounters low-level, gravity-dependent echoes suspended within ascitic fluid (Fig. 6G). This has been observed in patients with bloody ascites.[24]

Bowel involvement by tumor is best documented by upper and lower gastrointestinal series.[23,25] Computed tomography is more accurate than sonography for the detection of lymphadenopathy associated with gynecologic neoplasms.[26] Peritoneal implants greater than 2 cm appear as solid masses adjacent to the peritoneal wall. They are best delineated by sonography, particularly when ascites is present (Figs. 6H,I). Diffuse thickening of the omentum can also occur as the result of tumor infiltration (Fig. 6J).

GENERAL COMMENTS

The noninvasive, atraumatic, and seemingly nontoxic qualities of sonography make it particularly desirable for the evaluation of patients presenting with a pelvic mass that is thought to be benign.[4] Sonography provides direct evaluation of the size, location, extent, and internal consistency of a pelvic mass. The information obtained by sonography is complementary to other radiographic studies, such as barium enema, excretory urogram, or computed tomography, for the complete evaluation of a patient prior to surgical intervention. When "conservative" management is deemed appropriate, serial sonographic examinations can be performed to assess the enlargement or regression of a mass.

Although the sonographic appearance of pelvic masses is, in general, nonspecific, the diagnostic accuracy for establishing the presence, extent, and internal consistency of a pelvic mass by pelvic sonography is estimated to be over 90 percent.[3] Certain pelvic masses, such as dermoid cysts, exhibit a spectrum of sonographic appearances depending on their internal composition.[21] Conversely, a few pelvic masses demonstrate a more or less specific sonographic appearance, such as the predominantly cystic, septated pattern of a mucinous cystadenoma.

Prediction of whether or not a mass is benign or malignant according to its sonographic appearance is only moderately reliable. This determination is still the domain of the gynecologic surgeon and pathologist. If ascites is demonstrated with a pelvic mass, however, it is frequently a sign of malignancy. Ascites is usually the result of peritoneal secretions incited by tumor implants. Exceptions to this rule occasionally occur, such as the association of ascites with ovarian fibromas (Meigs' syndrome). Cystic masses that contain an irregular, solid component are usually malignant rather than benign. However, if the mass is cystic and the borders are smooth and well defined, it is most likely benign.

The number of false positive and false negative sonograms in pelvic mass assessment has been estimated to be less than 5 percent.[1] The majority of errors in the sonographic evaluation of pelvic masses can be attributed to poor scanning technique (improper transducer angulation or gain settings), lesions that are below the scanning resolution of the equipment (less than 2 cm), or misinterpretation of bowel or pelvic masses. Soft tissue masses with acoustic properties similar to the surrounding soft tissues can also be difficult to delineate sonographically. This concept is illustrated by the cystic ovarian teratoma whose sebum and solid

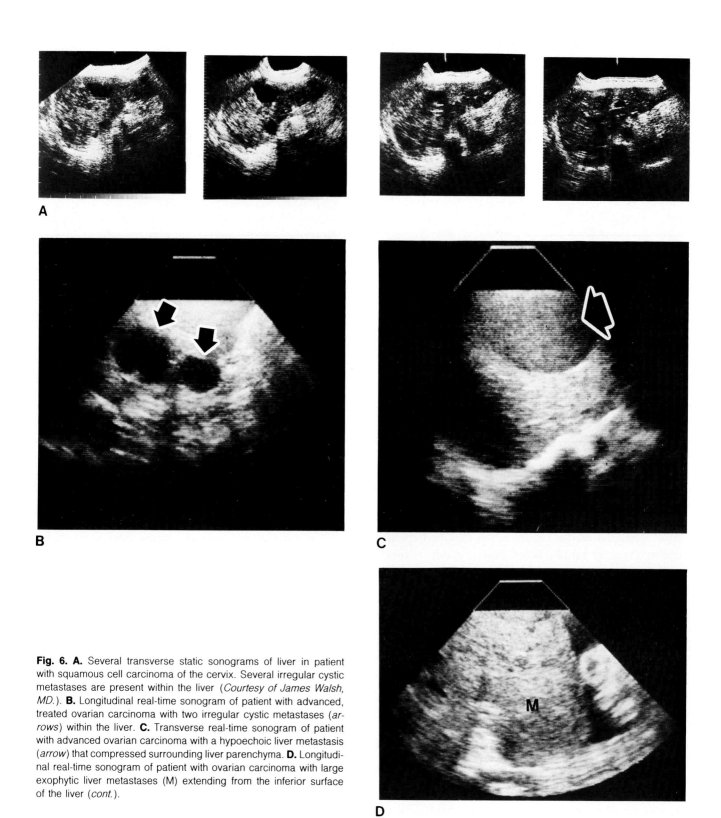

A

B

C

D

Fig. 6. A. Several transverse static sonograms of liver in patient with squamous cell carcinoma of the cervix. Several irregular cystic metastases are present within the liver (*Courtesy of James Walsh, MD.*). **B.** Longitudinal real-time sonogram of patient with advanced, treated ovarian carcinoma with two irregular cystic metastases (*arrows*) within the liver. **C.** Transverse real-time sonogram of patient with advanced ovarian carcinoma with a hypoechoic liver metastasis (*arrow*) that compressed surrounding liver parenchyma. **D.** Longitudinal real-time sonogram of patient with ovarian carcinoma with large exophytic liver metastases (M) extending from the inferior surface of the liver (*cont.*).

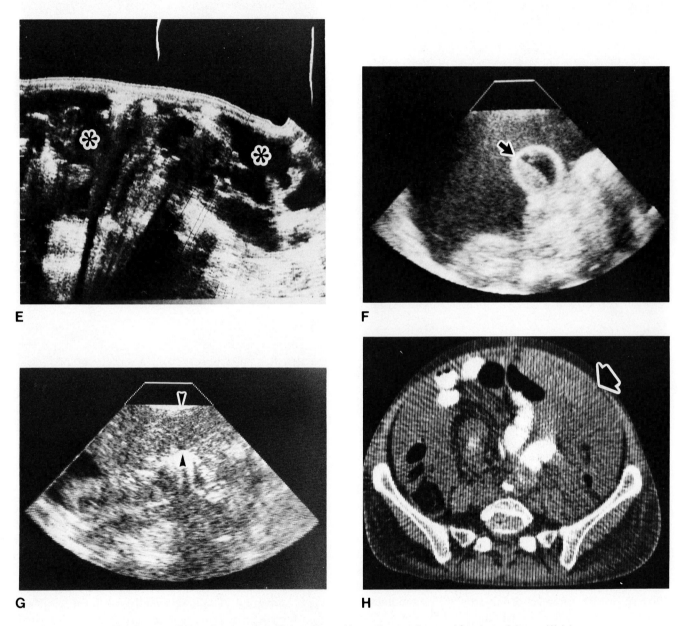

E

F

G

H

Fig. 6. cont. E. Loculated ascites (*) in patient with ovarian carcinoma. (*Courtesy of James Walsh, MD.*) **F.** Transverse real-time sonogram demonstrating "bloody" ascites, as depicted by low level echoes suspended within ascitic fluid. There is a sludge layer (*arrow*) within the gallbladder. **G.** Longitudinal real-time sonogram showing a large peritoneal implant (*arrow*) delineated by echogenic, gas containing bowel. **H.** Computed tomography of same patient as in **G.** The peritoneal implant was not as readily depicted on CT as on sonography (*cont.*).

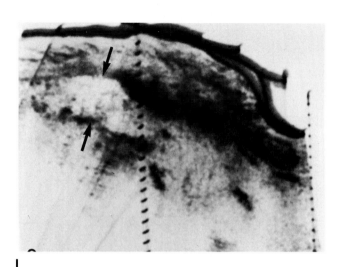

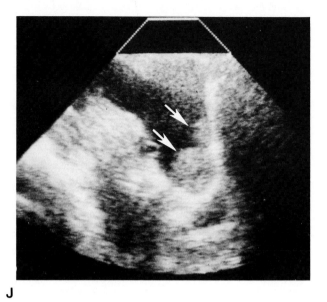

I   J

Fig. 6. cont. I. Omental band (longitudinal, 4 cm to right of midline). There is a moderately echogenic band of tissue adjacent to the anterior aspect of the peritoneum. This represents an omental band which results from a neoplastic infiltration of the omentum by carcinomatous processes. This is commonly associated with ovarian carcinoma and is another sign of malignancy. **J.** Longitudinal real-time sonogram depicting serosal implants (*arrows*) superior to the dome of the urinary bladder in a patient with advanced ovarian carcinoma.

components produces an ill-defined area of echogenicity that can be interpreted as a loop of gas-filled bowel (Fig. 4D).

Although the sonographic appearance of bowel is nonspecific, there are several patterns that suggest bowel loops. Fluid-filled loops of bowel appear as fusiform sonolucent structures.[17] A change in configuration during peristalsis can be documented using real-time sonography. Proximal small bowel that is distended with fluid can be identified because the mucosal folds appear as short linear echoes projecting into the lumen from the bowel wall. Similarly, haustral sacculations are seen in the ascending and transverse colon when it is fluid filled. Collapsed bowel that contains mucus and gas frequently exhibits a "bull's-eye" pattern. This pattern consists of an echogenic core with a sonolucent halo. Normal bowel demonstrates a bull's-eye pattern whose halo is symmetrical to the central echogenic core and can be documented to change in configuration with peristalsis. The bull's-eye pattern observed in bowel tumors and related conditions as a thick halo and the echogenic core tends to be eccentrically located. Abnormal peristalsis of the involved bowel segment can be observed using real time of the particular bowel segment involved.[17] The sonolucent halo in pathologic bull's-eye patterns is two to three times greater in size than the echogenic core and tends to be eccentric. This pattern has been observed in a variety of neoplastic and inflammatory conditions that have in common thickening of the bowel wall. These entities include adenocarcinoma of the bowel, intussusception, lymphoma, hemorrhage, and Crohn's disease.[17]

CONCLUSION

Sonography is a useful diagnostic technique in the evaluation of pelvic masses, particularly when they occur during pregnancy (Chapter 33). Comparisons of the clinical efficacy of computed tomography to sonography in the evaluation of the pelvic mass reveals that although the two modalities may be complementary, sonography depicts equally well the clinically pertinent features of a pelvic mass.[23] However, computed tomography can depict spread of the tumor into the retroperitoneal areas better than sonography because of its ability to detect invasion and involvement of the bony structures in the pelvis. In addition, computed tomography can demonstrate nodal enlargement associated with a mass better than sonographic examination.[26] To date, the determination of whether or not a pelvic mass is benign or malignant can only be established by pathologic examination. The impetus for the future development of gynecologic sonography will probably be directed toward the detection of subtle parenchymal changes as the first sign of pathologic changes within the pelvic organs. Current equipment improvements make it likely that significant progress will be made in visualizing these subtle changes.

REFERENCES

1. Fleischer A, James AE Jr, Millis J, et al: Sonographic differential diagnosis of pelvic masses. Am J Roentgenol 131:469, 1978
2. Walsh J, Taylor K, Rosenfield A, et al: Gray scale ultrasound in 204 proven gynecologic masses: Accuracy and specific diagnostic criteria. Radiology 130:391, 1979
3. Lawson T: Diagnosis of gynecologic pelvic masses by gray scale ultrasonography: An analysis of specificity and accuracy. Am J Roentgenol 128:1003, 1977
4. Fleischer A, Walsh J, Jones H, et al: Sonography of pelvic masses: Method of examination and role relative to other imaging modalities. Radiol Clin N Am 20:347, 1982
5. Coulam C, Julian C, Fleischer A: Clinical efficacy of CT and ultrasound in the evaluation of gynecologic pelvic tumors. Appl Radiol 11:79, 1982
6. Meire G, Lee J, Stanley R, et al: Accuracy of computed tomography in detecting ultra-abdominal and pelvic lymph node metastases from pelvic cancers. Am J Roentgenol 131:675, 1978
7. Sanders R, McNeil B, Finberg H, et al: A prospective study of computed tomography and ultrasound in the detection and staging of pelvic masses. Radiology 146:439, 1983
8. Towne B, Mahour G, Woolley M, et al: Ovarian cysts and tumors in infancy and children. J Pediatr Surg 10:311, 1975
9. Kossoff G, Garrett W, Carpenter D, et al: Principles and classification of soft tissues by gray scale echography. Ultrasound Med Biol 2:89, 1976
10. Meire H, Forrant P, Guha T: Distinction of benign from malignant ovarian cysts by ultrasound. Br J Obstet Gynecol 85:893, 1978
11. Kurtz A, Ashman F, Dubbins P, et al: Ultrasound evaluation of palpable ovarian masses: Comparison of filled and partially emptied urinary bladder technique. Appl Radiol 11:101, 1982
12. Sukov R, Whitcourt M: Rapid oral hydration: A cause of pelvic fluid collections or sonography. J Clin Ultrasound 9:115, 1981
13. Callen P, DeMartini W, Filly R: The central uterine cavity echo: A useful anatomic sight in the ultrasonographic evaluation of the female pelvis. Radiology 131:187, 1979
14. Bowie J: Ultrasound of gynecologic pelvic masses: The indefinite uterus and other patterns associated with diagnostic error. J Clin Ultrasound 55:323, 1977
15. Schnur P, Symmonds R, Williams T: Intestinal disorders masquerading as gynecologic problems. Surg Obstet Gynecol 128:1016, 1969
16. Kurtz H, Rubin C, Kramer F, et al: Ultrasound evaluation of the posterior pelvic compartment. Radiology 132:677, 1980
17. Fleischer A, Muhletaler C, James AE Jr: Real-time sonography of the bowel, in Winsburg F, Coopersburg P (eds), Real-time Ultrasonography, Clinics in Ultrasound. New York, Churchill-Livingstone, 1982
18. Morley P, Barnett W: Use in ultrasound in diagnosis of pelvic mass. Br J Radiol 43:602, 1970
19. Fields S, Dunn F: Correlation of the echographic visualization of tissue with biological composition in physiologic state. J Acoust Soc Am 54:809, 1973
20. White E, Filly R: Cholesterol crystals as the source of both diffuse and layered echoes in a cystic ovarian tumor. J Clin Ultrasound 8:241, 1980
21. Sandler M, Silver T, Karo J: Gray-scale ultrasonic features of ovarian teratomas. Radiology 131:705, 1979
22. Pawling M, Shawker T: Abdominal ultrasound in advanced ovarian carcinoma. J Clin Ultrasound 9:435, 1981
23. Gedgaudas R, Kelvin F, Thompson W, et al: The value of the pre-operative barium enema examination in the assessment of pelvic masses. Radiology 146:609, 1983
24. Edell S, Gefter W: Ultrasonic differentiation of types of ascitic fluid. Am J Roentgenol 133:111, 1979
25. Requard C, Mettler F, Wicks J: Preoperative sonography of malignant ovarian neoplasms. Am J Roentgenol 137:79, 1981
26. Walsh J, Amendola M, Konerding K, et al: Computed tomographic detection of pelvic and inguinal lymph-node metastases from primary and pelvic malignant disease. Radiology 137:157, 1980

36 | The Ovarian Mass

Patricia Morley
Ellis Barnett

Ultrasonic imaging is one of the major diagnostic procedures used in the assessment of pelvic pathology. The basic examination technique was initially described in 1958 by Donald[1] and has since been elaborated and expanded by numerous contributors.[2-20] Its success is dependent on the accurate demonstration of pelvic morphology, combined with acoustic tissue differentiation of identified mass lesions. Useful information can be provided in a significant proportion of clinical disorders, but it must be emphasized that a specific diagnosis is not always possible on the basis of echographic features alone. Serious diagnostic errors will be made unless all available clinical information is taken into consideration, and even then a definitive diagnosis is not always possible.

EXAMINATION TECHNIQUE

The pelvic soft tissue structures are examined by direct contact scanning through the abdominal wall using static scanners or high-resolution real-time systems. Radial scanning systems have also been designed that can examine the ovaries and parametria,[7,8,21] the transducer being inserted either into the rectum or vagina. This technique has not become generally accepted even though it may display diagnostic information difficult to demonstrate by abdominal scanning.

For detailed visualization of pelvic structures the urinary bladder should be fully distended. Adequate filling is usually achieved by a water load given orally to the patient 1 to 2 hours prior to the examination, although occasionally diuretics or retrograde filling of

the bladder through catheterization may be necessary. Assessment of pelvic pathology should not be made sonographically without definite identification of the bladder (Fig. 1). Failure to ensure this criteria can result in major diagnostic errors, and if there is any doubt about the location of the bladder even after voiding, a catheter should be introduced, the bladder emptied, and the scan repeated. The distended bladder displaces the small bowel out of the pelvis and permits clear visualization of soft tissue detail; it also acts as an important anatomic reference point. At the same time, variations in the appearance of the bladder wall and outline can be studied, and the mobility of a mass can be assessed as the bladder fills. A mobile mass will be pushed up into the lower abdomen; an impacted or fixed mass will remain in the pelvis (Fig. 2).

In the patient with reasonable bladder capacity, transducers of 5.0 MHz with a medium or long internal focus are usually employed. In those patients who are obese or have a reduced bladder capacity it may be necessary to use 3.5 MHz to obtain diagnostic information from the posterior pelvis. Radial scanning systems use transducers of 3.5 or 5.0 MHz with a short focus, which give excellent soft tissue detail in the lesser pelvis.

With abdominal scanning detailed sectional information is obtained using linear, sector, or compound scans; a relatively low sensitivity is employed, high sensitivity tending to obliterate soft tissue detail and exaggerate artifacts. Swept gain settings also are critical for definition of soft tissue planes such as the pelvic floor musculature. However, to examine areas of specific interest in detail sector scans using varying sensi-

473

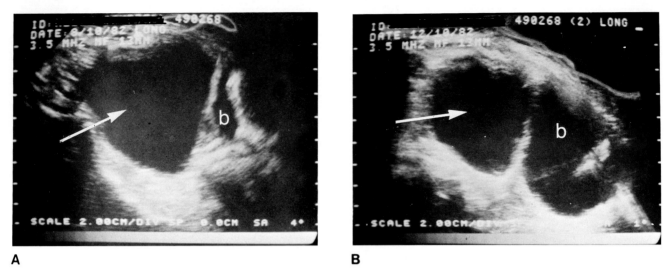

Fig. 1. A. Incompletely filled bladder. There is a large unilocular cystic mass filling the pelvis. The bladder contains a very small volume of urine and is seen caudad to the cyst. **B.** Repeat examination with fully distended bladder. The cyst has been displaced upwards into the lower abdomen. The diagnosis of a unilocular mobile ovarian cyst was confirmed at laparotomy. (Serous cystadenoma.) [b—Bladder.]

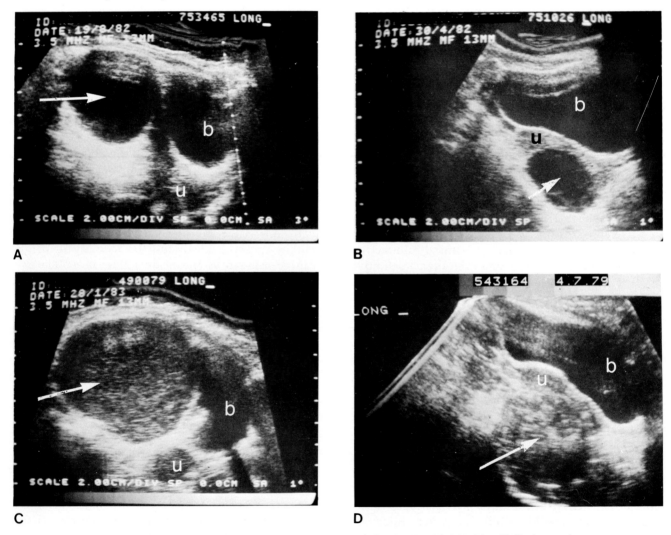

Fig. 2. A. Mobile cystic mass displaced out of the pelvis by the distended bladder. (Follicular cyst.) **B.** Cystic mass impacted in the pelvis. It lies behind the bladder and uterus. (Serous cystadenoma twisted around edematous fallopian tube.) **C.** Mobile solid mass displaced into the lower abdomen by the bladder. The uterus is seen posteriorly. (Cystadenofibroma.) **D.** Solid mass impacted in the pelvis behind the bladder and uterus. (Ovarian fibroma.) [b—Bladder, u—Uterus.]

tivity give the truest representation of the acoustic characteristics of the underlying tissues. Scans should be carried out with meticulous care in both longitudinal and transverse planes, with clear demonstration of normal anatomy. Variations in the shape, size, and position of the pelvic organs are noted, as well as the presence of any abnormal soft tissue mass.

In many cases, particularly in patients presenting with possible pelvic malignancy and those who are being monitored after diagnosis, the ultrasonic examination must be extended to include the urinary tract, the liver, the paraaortic area, omentum, gut and the peritoneal cavity—this is sometimes referred to as the panabdominal examination.

THE NORMAL PELVIS

A knowledge of normal ultrasonic pelvic anatomy is essential for interpretation of pathological change. The distended bladder has a characteristic outline that is usually symmetric, although in a transverse section the lateral wall may be displaced by the colon. The uterus is outlined behind the bladder, with normal ovaries lying laterally on either side. The uterine fundus, body, and cervix are routinely identified and the position of the vagina and rectum defined. The development of improved resolution systems has resulted in the visualization of more detailed pelvic soft tissue anatomy. The ovaries are identified in a high proportion of premenopausal and perimenopausal women and normal physiologic variations recognized.[21-24] The postmenopausal ovary can also be located using high resolution sector scanning systems.[25] The proximal portion of the fallopian tube and the round ligaments of the uterus may be demonstrated. The rectus abdominus, ilio psoas, obturator internus, and pelvic floor muscles are commonly displayed and in a detailed pelvic examination an attempt should be made to identify these structures. Arteries can be recognized from their pulsation—this is more easily seen using real-time systems, though A- and M-mode techniques are also employed.[26] The slightly dilated ureter may be outlined adjacent to the bladder and it may also be seen as it crosses anterior to the iliac artery adjacent to the ovary. The normal ureters and ureteric orifices may be seen using intravesical radial scanning systems.[27] System resolution does not as yet permit visualization of normal size pelvic lymph nodes and the bowel does not present a constant echo pattern. Specific segments of colon can not be consistently recognized except by use of a water enema, though the rectosigmoid junction may be identified when gas distended. Loops of small bowel are recognized by their peristaltic activity, which

is easily seen with real-time systems. When a transverse scan is extended around the outer aspect of the trunk, the pelvic bones, femoral heads, and trochanters can be included in the display as well as the gluteal muscle mass. Though no attempt is made to define these structures routinely it is a technique that can be usefully applied to radiotherapy planning procedures. The ultrasonic appearance of the major pelvic viscera and soft tissue planes has been fully described and the reader is referred to relevant texts on the subject.[6,15,26,28-30] (See Chapter 7.)

THE NORMAL OVARIES

The ovary lies on the posterior surface of the broad ligament inferior to the fallopian tube. It lies in the ovarian fossa near the lateral wall of the pelvis and is closely related to the ureter, the internal iliac vessels posteromedially, and the external iliac vessels anterolaterally. It is supported by the infundibulopelvic ligament and the uteroovarian ligament. On the transverse pelvic scan the ovaries are located in the angle formed by the lateral wall of the full bladder, the iliopsoas muscle, and the lateral pelvic wall (Fig. 3). They usually lie approximately at the level of the uterine fundus. The appearance of the normal ovary is discussed in detail in Chapter 7.

With the development of high-resolution real-time systems the normal ovaries can usually be located by careful scanning. Using static scanners identification of the ovaries may be more difficult. Failure to identify both ovaries should not necessarily be considered as abnormal; the left ovary in particular can be difficult to demonstrate, as it may be obscured or displaced upwards by the colon. It should be noted that during pregnancy the ovaries are carried superiorly with the expanding uterus and that postpartum the ovary may return to a site other than described as its normal anatomic position.

Hackelöer[26] has attempted to define a reference plane to differentiate the ovary from the lateral part of the uterus, particularly an ovary without any internal cystic structure. He identifies the ovarian vessels in the infundibulopelvic ligament and the mesovarium using a combination of B-mode, A-mode and TM-mode to localize the pulsatile vessels. The internal iliac artery passes beneath the ovary and this may also be identified. However, the position of the ovary is variable to the internal iliac artery but stable to the vessels in the infundibulopelvic ligament, and the latter should be used as the reference plane.

The normal ovary is an ovoid structure measuring approximately 20 × 30 × 20 mm, although it can mea-

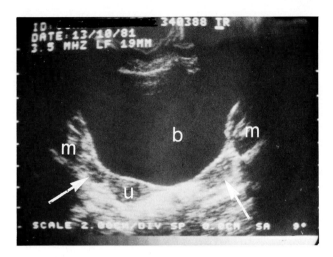

Fig. 3. Normal ovaries. Transverse section at the level of the uterine fundus defining both ovaries lying in the angle formed by the bladder, the iliopsoas muscle and lateral pelvic wall. [b—Bladder, u—Uterus, m—Muscle.]

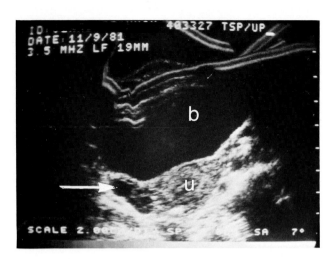

Fig. 4. Small retention cyst in the right ovary. Though these cysts are commonly asymptomatic this subject presented with pelvic pain. [b—Bladder, u—Uterus.]

sure up to 50 mm in any one axis. The surface of the ovary is covered by the germinal epithelium, a single layer of cuboidal cells that is continuous with the mesothelium of the peritoneum. Under the germinal epithelium there is a condensed layer of fibrous tissue called the tunica albuginea. The ovary has a cortex and a medulla. Follicles originate in the ovarian cortex, the medullary portion consists of blood vessels, lymphatics, nerves, connective tissue, and remnants of the Wolffian body precursors. When an ovary is sectioned a number of ripening follicles are visible to the naked eye, the smaller follicles and oogonia are not visualized. These larger follicles are demonstrated on the pelvic ultrasonogram.

Ovarian size can be measured from the ultrasonogram with reasonable accuracy[28] and ultrasonic measurements compare favorably with those obtained by pelvic pneumography[31] and at laparoscopy or laparotomy. Ovaries are considered to measure less than one-half the size of the normal uterus as seen on the pelvic pneumogram and if greater than 30 mm in two axes they are considered enlarged. More accurate measurements are obtained by assessing the surface area (maximum 8.8 cm²); the uterine-to-ovarian ratio, that is the ratio of the maximum diameter of the fundus to the longitudinal diameter of the ovary (normal range is 1.5 : 1.8); and the ovarian volume, calculated by the formula, length times width times thickness divided by 2 (normal range is 1.8 to 5.7 cm³, mean is 4.0 cm³).[22,32,33] Normal limits of size for prepubertal ovaries are also known[6,24] and the diameter and volume of the postmenopausal ovary has been assessed.[25] Ovarian enlargement is seen with cysts, cystic tumors, solid tumors, ovarian haematoma, and more rarely massive odema of the ovary.

When menstruation commences the ovaries enlarge and vary in size depending on the phase of the menstrual cycle. Between them the ovaries usually produce one mature ovum per menstrual cycle. This develops as the follicle, which ruptures approximately midcycle, releasing the ovum into the peritoneal cavity. The remaining lining cells of the follicle develop into a corpus luteum that degenerates towards the end of the menstrual cycle into a fibrous scar, the corpus albicans. After ovulation follicle retention cysts may develop with a normal size limit of 20 mm (Fig. 4). Less commonly, the corpus luteum may persist with cyst formation. If pregnancy occurs the corpus luteum enlarges progressively for some months to reach a maximum size at about 8 to 10 weeks.

Physiologic changes in the ovaries can be monitored by sonography (see Chapter 37). This technique was first described by Kratochwil[21] and Hackelöer.[22] Kratochwil and Hackelöer also monitored patients on ovarian stimulation therapy, with Kratochwil demonstrating the development of follicles. When stimulation was successful and when patients were not responding ovarian enlargement could be shown. Hackelöer measured the size and number of follicles, predicting ovulation and relating follicle size with blighted ova. The physiologic changes seen in the ovary and techniques of follicular monitoring are discussed in Chapter 37.

SCREENING TO EXCLUDE OVARIAN MASS LESIONS

Ultrasound may be used as a relatively coarse screening technique to exclude ovarian pathology. With improved resolution systems and particularly with real-time sector scanners the ovaries can be demonstrated in a high proportion of pre- and perimenopausal women, but postmenopausal ovaries remain difficult to define. However, system resolution and mass consistency may limit the detectable lesions to those greater than 1 or 2 cm. With obese patients or those with restricted bladder capacity and when the ovary cannot be demonstrated, exclusion of a small ovarian mass is not possible. It is therefore not feasible to definitely exclude ovarian pathology by ultrasonic examination even though the larger mass is readily identified. Infiltrative lesions may also cause diagnostic difficulties, as inflammatory and postoperative reaction may produce changes similar to the infiltrating neoplasm. Interval assessment is often required to assess minor variations in the pelvic soft tissues.

Currently the diagnosis of ovarian cancer is a matter of chance. By the time it has been diagnosed ovarian cancer has in more than 60 to 70% of patients spread beyond the ovary.[34] It has been reported that the chance of detecting an ovarian neoplasm during routine pelvic examination in an asymptomatic patient is 1 in 10,000. One diagnostic sign of early ovarian cancer in the postmenopausal woman is the palpation of what represents a normal-sized ovary in the premenopausal woman. Barber states that all such palpable lesions prove to be new growths, not necessarily malignant but not functional or dysfunctional.[34] Goswamy, Campbell, and Whitehead[25] are screening a large group of asymptomatic perimenopausal women to try and detect early ovarian cancer. Normal values for ovarian diameter and volume are being established in different age groups and identified mass lesions are assessed by laparoscopy or laparotomy. The value of this technique

as a screening procedure has not as yet been established.

DIFFERENTIAL DIAGNOSIS

An ultrasonic examination is usually employed to confirm the clinical diagnosis of an ovarian mass, to determine its size, and to assess its consistency. Before the ultrasonic diagnosis of an ovarian mass can be considered, the mass must be defined as being separate from the uterus and bladder. This can be achieved only by using the full bladder method of pelvic examination (Fig. 5). By acoustic analysis the identified pelvic or abdominal mass lesions are divided into two major groups—fluid-filled and solid. The common fluid-filled pelvic lesions include the ovarian and parovarian cysts, endometrial cysts, cystic ovarian tumors, parasitic cysts, lymphocysts, retroperitoneal cysts, tuboovarian abscess, hydrosalpinx, ectopic pregnancy, pelvic abscess, and pelvic hematocele, as well as fluid-filled loops of bowel and the distended atonic bladder. Many of these are discussed in other chapters of this book (see Chapters 30, 35, and 40). Solid mass lesions commonly encountered are the enlarged uterus, ovarian tumors, retroperitoneal tumors, infiltrative intestinal tumors, bladder tumors, enlarged lymph glands, the pelvic kidney, and impacted feces. In patients with gross abdominal distension primary pathologic enlargement of other abdominal organs should also be considered in the diagnosis, as well as the possible presence of ascites (Fig. 6).

The ultrasonic appearance of the ovarian mass is discussed in this chapter, but for details of the echo-

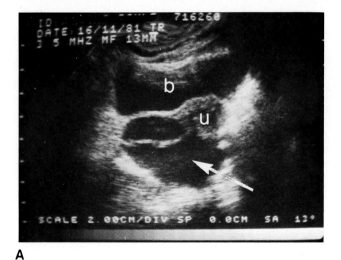

A

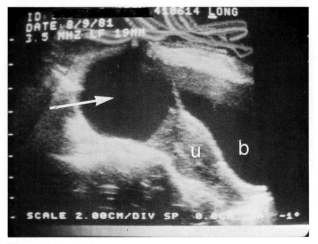

B

Fig. 5. A. Mobile cystic mass lying above the uterus and bladder. (Mucinous cystadenoma.) **B.** Impacted septated cyst lying behind the bladder and uterus. (Mucinous cystadenoma.) [b—Bladder, u—Uterus.]

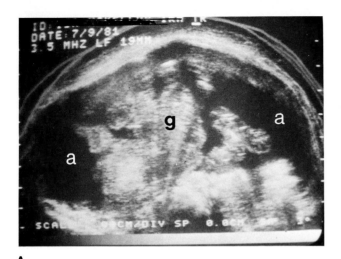

A

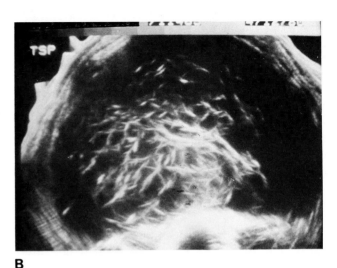

B

Fig. 6. Abdominal distension. **A.** Gross ascites. The ascitic fluid lies laterally in the peritoneal cavity. Segments of gut are seen centrally. **B.** Large ovarian cyst. The cyst fills the abdomen, it is complex containing numerous thin septa. (Mucinous cystadenoma.) [a—Ascites, g—Gut.]

graphic features and ultrasonic differentiation of other lesions mentioned above the reader is referred to Chapters 33, 35, and 40 and to other texts on the subject.[15,35-38] Table 1 correlates ultrasonic signs with ovarian pathology.

THE CYSTIC OVARIAN MASS

Cysts are easily identified on the pelvic scan and have characteristic ultrasonic features. The outline of a cyst is clearly defined and the mass is fully transonic, strong echoes being returned from the distal wall. Echoes are frequently identified within the cyst arising from septa, mucin, blood, pus, dermoid elements, or malignant tissue (Figs. 7A–I).

Septa are typically displayed by high-intensity echoes and are usually thin and linear, varying in num-

ber and complexity. If thickened septa are demonstrated the possibility of malignancy should be considered. Thick mucin can produce recordable echoes but is not commonly seen at normal sensitivity settings, though with high sensitivity fine echoes may be recorded. The appearance of blood within a cyst depends on the degree of organization. Echoes are not commonly identified from recent hemorrhage, but medium-intensity echoes can be seen with diffuse organizing hemorrhage. Organized clot is clearly defined as a solid area within the cyst.[39] It can be mistaken echographically for malignant tissue, and a small cyst filled with organized thrombus may appear to be homogeneously solid. Pus is sometimes seen as a collection of discrete fine echoes similar to organizing hemorrhage and there may also be associated loss of definition and thickening of the cyst wall. A more detailed discussion of pelvic inflammatory disease and

TABLE 1
Ovarian Masses

Morphology	Type	Diagnostic Features
A. Single cysts	Follicular cyst	Thin walled, unilocular, may be associated with fibroids, endometrial hyperplasia, long-term hormone administration. Can be estrogenic.
	Corpus luteum cyst	Small, unilocular. May be associated with pregnancy. Hemorrhage may occur and leakage or rupture.
	Parovarian cyst	Thin walled. May be large; occasional septum. Sometimes pedunculated.
	Serous cystadenoma	Variable size. Can be large with occasional septum.

TABLE 1 (*continued*)

Morphology	Type	Diagnostic Features
B. Multiple cysts	Endometriosis	Usually small, in cul de sac, or behind fundus. Often bilateral. Fixation, hemorrhagic contents and thick walls.
	Theca lutein cysts	Associated with hydatidiform mole and choriocarcinoma though may rarely be seen in normal pregnancy.
	Polycystic ovaries	Small, thin walled cysts. Bilateral or unilateral ovarian enlargement.
	Pelvic inflammatory disease	Irregular thick walls; fixation. Thick septa.
C. Complex cysts	Cystic teratoma	Solid areas; septa; "fluid levels"; axial or bilateral.
	Mucinous cystadenoma	Can be very large, multiple thin septa: occasionally solid elements.
	Clear cell tumor	May contain hemorrhagic material.
	Cystadenofibroma	Small, multilocular. Rarely malignant. Can cause hyperoestrinism.

	Malignant cysts
	  Cystadenocarcinoma
	  Endometrioid carcinoma
	  Clear cell carcinoma
		Complex solid areas in cyst. Thick septa. Fixation. Loss of definition. Ascites.

	Infarcted cyst	May have no specific features. Thickened walls, hemorrhagic debris.
	Secondary tumor	Complex cyst. Fixation.
D. Solid mass	Cystic teratoma	Homogeneously solid when filled with hair and sebaceous material.
	Fibroma	Acoustically absorbent. Homogeneously solid. Associated ascites. Commonest tumor found in Meig syndrome. Usually unilateral.
	Brenner tumor	Large, often unilateral, may be estrogenic.
	Solid teratoma	Commoner in childhood and adolescence. Solid with complex echo pattern. May be malignant.
	Granulosa–theca–luteal cell tumor	Can be estrogenic, usually solid but may be cystic. Granulosa cell tumors often locally recurrent.
	Arrhenoblastoma	Virilizing tumor: may be malignant.

	Primary solid malignant tumors
	  Endometrioid carcinoma
	  Clear cell carcinoma
	  Dysgerminoma
	  Arrhenoblastoma
	  Choriocarcinoma
	  Endodermal sinus tumor
	  Papillary adenocarcinoma
		Poorly defined mass, variable consistency, fills pelvis.

	Secondary tumor	Bilateral. If unilateral commoner on right side.

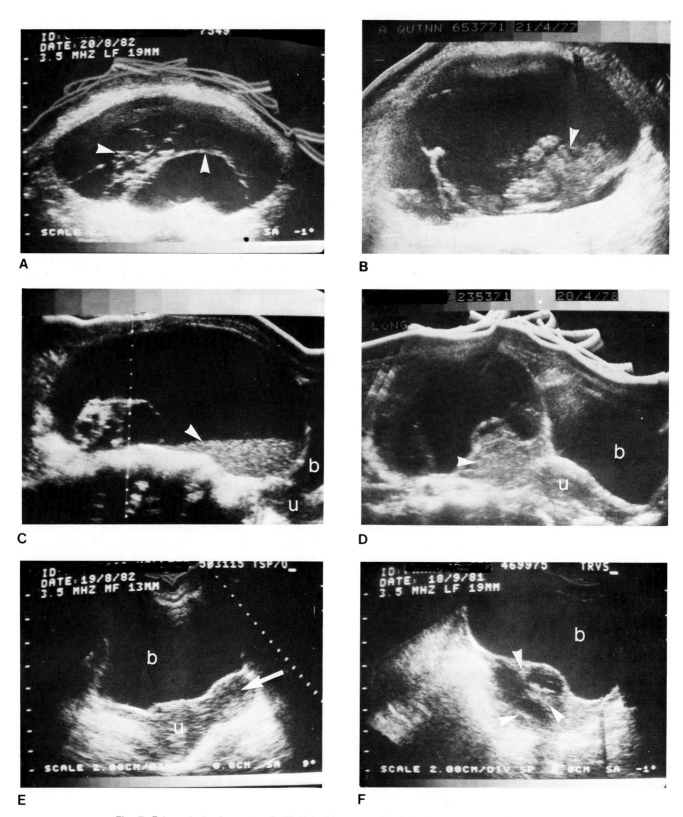

Fig. 7. Echoes in benign cysts. **A.** Multiple thin septa. (Mucinous cystadenoma.) **B.** Thick mucin. Septa are also present. (Mucinous cystadenoma.) **C.** Organized blood forming a fluid level. Slightly thickened septa are also seen in this section. (Adenocarcinoma.) **D.** Organized blood clot in an infarcted cyst. **E.** Organized clot in a corpus luteum cyst. The cyst appears homogeneously solid. **F.** Infected cyst. The cyst is complex with thickened fibrotic walls (*cont.*). [b—Bladder, u—Uterus.]

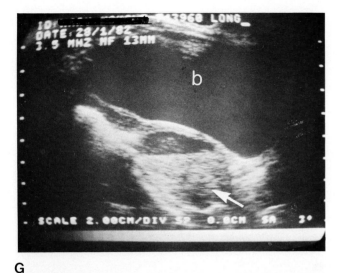

G

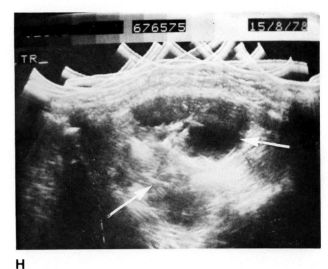

H

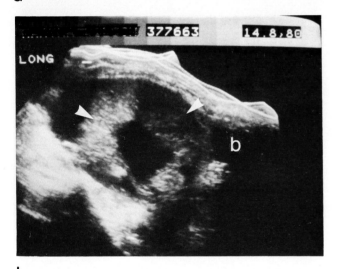

I

Fig. 7. cont. Echoes in benign cysts. **G.** Dermoid cyst. Typical "fluid level" appearance seen in some dermoid cysts. **H.** Infarcted cyst. The cyst appears complex with loss of definition of outline due to extravasation of blood into the cyst wall. **I.** Solid tissue—this cyst was complex and contains large areas of solid material. (Mucinous cystadenoma.) [b—Bladder.]

ovarian abscess appears in Chapter 40. The appearance of dermoid elements is extremely variable depending on the type of tissue present (see page 495). "Fluid levels" may sometimes be present, or a complex septate pattern may be seen, giving the appearance of compartments within the cyst. Solid areas are common and may cast an acoustic shadow. A dermoid cyst full of hair and sebaceous material is evenly echogenic. Malignant tissue is discussed in the next section but it should be noted that the appearance of an infarcted cyst when there is extravasation of blood into the cyst wall may be very similar to that of a complex malignant ovarian mass.

FEATURES SUGGESTIVE OF MALIGNANCY IN A CYSTIC MASS

The following echographic features are more frequently associated with malignant cysts but are not specifically diagnostic of malignancy. Malignant tissue may be seen as bizarre solid projections from the cyst wall, as grossly thickened septa, or solid replacement of loculations. A complex internal structure with solid areas that may originate from the cyst wall or from septa is sometimes indicative of malignant change. However, very complex multiseptate cysts, even with solid areas, may be histologically benign. If there is gross infiltration of tumor through the cyst capsule definition of the cyst wall can be impaired. When this infiltration is very advanced the outline of the cyst may be completely lost. Minimal loss of definition is difficult to assess, however, as a poor scanning technique can produce a similar appearance. Fixation in the pelvis may be the only echographic evidence of infiltration through the cyst wall into the pelvis. This is assessed by the full bladder technique but is not always a reliable diagnostic sign. Although ascites is sometimes seen in association with benign cysts it is more commonly a feature of malignancy. (Figs. 8A–I.)

482

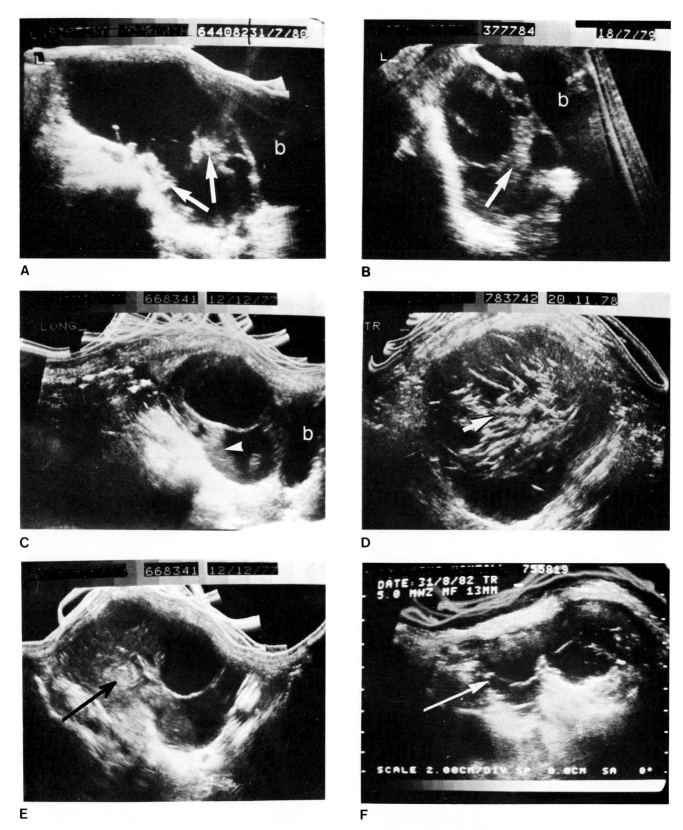

Fig. 8. Features associated with malignant cysts. **A.** Bizarre solid projections from the cyst wall (cystadenocarcinoma). **B.** Grossly thickened septa. (Secondary ovarian tumor.) **C.** Solid replacement of loculations. (Cystadenocarcinoma.) **D.** Complex internal structure. (Cystadenocarcinoma.) **E.** Solid areas (Cystadenocarcinoma.) **F.** Loss of definition of the cyst wall. (Cystadenocarcinoma.) (*cont.*) [b—Bladder.]

G

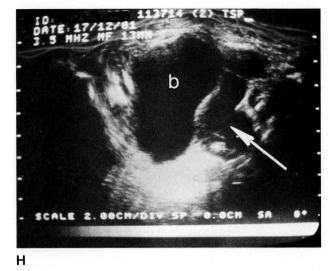

H

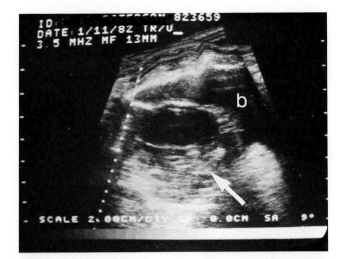

I

Fig. 8. cont. Features associated with malignant cysts. **G.** Loss of definition of the cyst wall with associated pelvic fixation. (Cystadenocarcinoma. Residual tumor.) **H.** Fixation of the cyst in the pelvis. There is displacement of the bladder laterally to the right. (Cystadenocarcinoma.) **I.** Associated ascitic fluid. The cyst that contains solid material is seen posteriorly in the lesser pelvis with a small volume of free fluid anteriorly. (Papillary adenocarcinoma.) [b—Bladder, g—Gut, a—Ascites.]

THE SOLID OVARIAN MASS

Like all solid lesions, a solid ovarian mass contains echoes but there is a wide variation in their reflectivity. The mass outline is not usually as clearly defined as that of a cyst, and small solid tumors may prove difficult to detect as they merge with the pelvic soft tissue echoes (Fig. 9A). Benign lesions are usually acoustically homogeneous and are often relatively solid, requiring low frequencies or high sensitivity to obtain echoes from their distal surface (interface). They are usually acoustically similar to or "harder" (less transonic) than uterine fibroids (Figs. 9B,2D).

ULTRASONIC FEATURES ASSOCIATED WITH SOLID MALIGNANT TUMORS

The soft vascular malignant mass exhibits increased transonicity (through transmission) when compared with a benign solid tumor. Very friable tumors can be penetrated by higher ultrasonic frequencies, they are "acoustically soft." Relatively high level echoes are returned from the tumor and the internal pattern shows patchy variations in texture due to changes in consistency, areas of necrosis being represented by low-amplitude echoes or cystic spaces. There is loss of definition of tumor outline, the mass fills the pelvis and the outline of the tumor merges with the pelvic soft tissues, the uterine outline may be impossible to define. There is usually obvious fixation of the mass in the pelvis. As with the cystic ovarian tumors, ascites occurs more commonly in association with malignant than with benign tumors (Figs. 10A–E).

With any ovarian mass that is possibly malignant the ultrasonic examination should be extended to the remainder of the abdomen to assess possible tumor dissemination. This is discussed in greater detail in the section on advanced ovarian carcinomatosis.

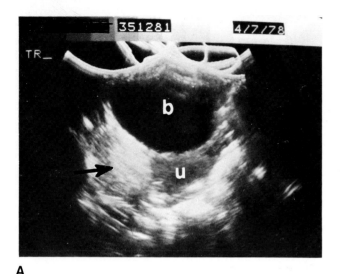
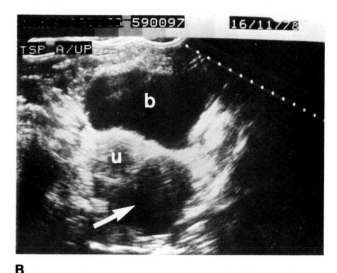

Fig. 9. The solid benign ovarian mass. **A.** Solid ovarian tumor. The acoustic density of the mass is similar to that of the pelvic connective tissue. (Dermoid cyst.) **B.** Solid ovarian tumor with an acoustic density lower than that of the pelvic connective tissue and the uterus. (Ovarian fibroma.) [b—Bladder, u—Uterus.]

COMMONLY ENCOUNTERED OVARIAN MASS LESIONS

Although the ultrasonic appearance of many ovarian masses does not permit a specific diagnosis, there are often identifying features that may be highly suggestive in a particular case (Table 1). Features typical of the commonly encountered ovarian cysts and tumors are discussed below. Tuboovarian abscess and ovarian pregnancy are described in Chapters 40 and 30, respectively.

ENDOMETRIOSIS

Endometriosis is the term used to describe the presence of endometrial glands or stroma in abnormal locations. Internal endometriosis or adenomyosis refers to abnormal endometrium within the myometrium and is discussed in Chapter 36. In external endometriosis, tissue identical to the endometrium is found at a distance from the uterus. It occurs most commonly in the ovary, the wall of the fallopian tube, or the broad ligament, in the posterior cul de sac and rectovaginal septum. Other more rare sites include the umbilicus, laparotomy scars, bladder, and bowel, and more distant sites such as the lungs, pleura, and limbs. External endometriosis is most commonly seen in the third and fourth decade. It is principally a disease of active reproductive life, and its clinical manifestations varies with the distribution of the endometrial lesions and their functional activity. The foci of endometrium usually undergo cyclic menstrual changes and hemorrhage can occur. They enlarge to form nodules that coalesce and may cause dense fibrous adhesions. Involved ovaries become enlarged by cystic spaces known as "chocolate cysts" or "endometriomas."

With pelvic endometriosis symptoms may be absent; when they do occur severe dysmenorrhoea and pelvic pains result from intrapelvic bleeding and peritoneal adhesions. Symptoms regress if pregnancy occurs. When the tubes and ovaries become involved sterility results. Clinically the features are very similar to chronic salpingitis and this must be considered in the differential diagnosis.

Echographically pelvic endometriosis presents a very broad spectrum and the appearance is not specific. There may be no detectable ultrasonic abnormality. Sandler and James[40] describe demonstrable lesions as being cystic or mixed or solid and consider the solid pattern as difficult to differentiate from ovarian carcinoma. The appearance of endometriosis and adenomyosis has also been reported by Walsh et al.[19] Endometriotic cysts are usually small, measuring between 2 and 5 cm (chocolate cysts), though larger cysts, up to 20 cm in diameter, may develop (endometriomata). The cysts are frequently multiple and bilateral and are typically located behind the fundus of the uterus and in the pouch of Douglas. The cyst walls may be thickened and hemorrhagic debris can sometimes be identified. Fixation of the cysts occur in association with pelvic adhesions (Figs. 11A–E). Rarely endometriomas may occur during pregnancy and the diagnosis should be considered when predominantly cystic masses are found in pregnant patients with a previous history of infertility.[41]

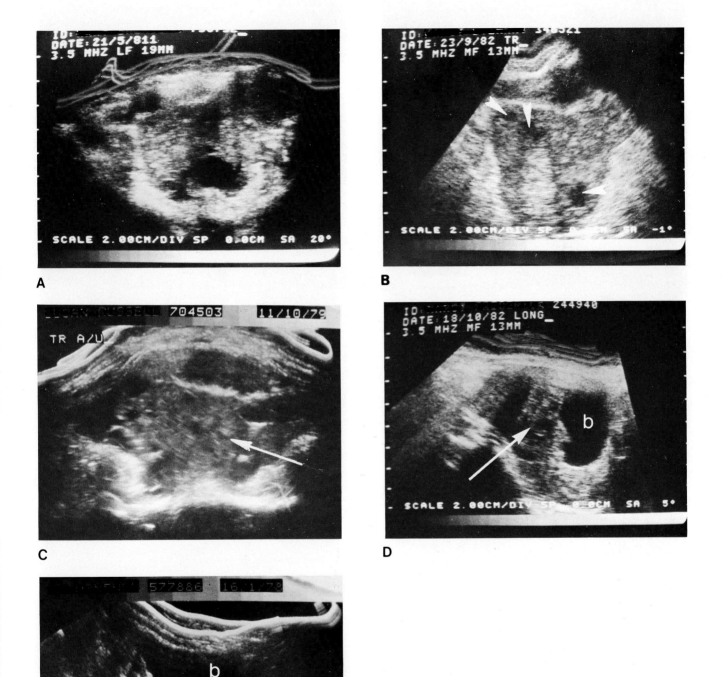

Fig. 10. The solid malignant ovarian mass. **A.** Increased through transmission. Complex mass filling the pelvis with minimal acoustic attentuation. (Cystadenocarcinoma.) **B.** Variation in texture. Solid mass with areas of cystic degeneration. (Adenocarcinoma.) **C.** Loss of definition of outline. Huge complex mass filing the lower abdomen. (Mixed mesodermal tumor.) **D.** Fixation. Solid mass adherent to the posterior wall of the pelvis. (Adenocarcinoma.) **E.** Associated ascites. Homogeneous pelvic mass with ascites. (Papillary adenocarcinoma.) [b—Bladder, a—Ascites.]

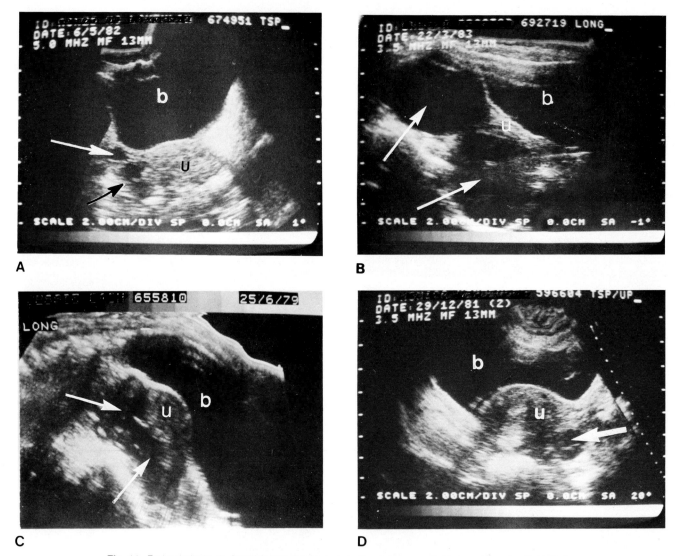

Fig. 11. Endometriosis. **A.** Small endometriotic cysts in the right ovary. **B.** Endometriomata. **C.** Multiple endometriotic cysts behind the fundus of the uterus. **D.** Endometriotic cysts involving the left ovary and containing hemorrhagic debris. There were associated pelvic adhesions. [b—Bladder, u—Uterus.]

HEMATOMATA OF THE OVARY

Hematomata of the ovary may be seen in endometriosis, with hemorrhage into either a follicular cyst, a corpus luteum, or a small serous cyst and with ovarian pregnancy. "Chocolate" or "tarry" cysts are usually considered to be associated with endometriosis, but it is also a term used to describe any ovarian hematoma (Figs. 7D,12).

MASSIVE EDEMA OF THE OVARY

This is a rare condition seen in young females and was originally described in 1969 by Kalstone, Jaffe, and Abel.[42] Patients present with lower abdominal pain

and a tender adnexal mass. Ultrasonically the ovary has been described as hypoechoic with slightly increased through transmission.[43] The edema of the ovary is caused by incomplete torsion of the mesovarium without associated hemorrhage or infarction. It more commonly affects the right ovary.

BROAD LIGAMENT OR PAROVARIAN CYSTS

The parovarian is a vestigal remnant of the Wolffian body and lies in the broad ligament between the tube and the hilum of the ovary. In the adult female, the main duct is known as Gartners duct, the blind outer end of the duct forming small cystic structures known

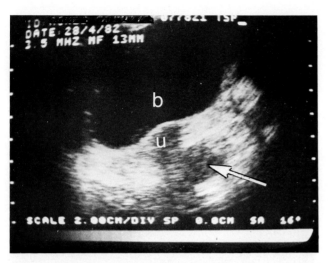

Fig. 12. Ovarian hematoma. Hemorrhagic cyst containing organized blood clot. (Simple cyst.) [b—Bladder, u—Uterus.]

as the Hydatids of Morgagni. Cysts may develop from the main ducts, the Hydatids of Morgagni or from any subsidiary tubules. The latter tend to be small and multiple, whereas the cysts of the main duct can be quite large. They cause pelvic symptoms when large or if pedunculated and torsion occurs. Clinically the cysts in the broad ligament are difficult to separate from the uterus. Those encountered echographically are usually thin walled and fairly large, measuring up to 15 or 18 cm. When pedunculated they are mobile and can rise out of the pelvis; others remain located deep in the pelvis adjacent to the uterus. Occasionally a thin septum is seen, although the majority are unilocular. They are similar in appearance to larger follicular cysts and serous cystadenomas.

FUNCTIONAL CYSTS OF THE FOLLICLE AND CORPUS LUTEUM

Follicular Cysts
Follicles enlarge normally up to approximately 15 mm and when the ovum dies the follicle involutes. Cysts are so common as to be virtually physiologic variants and originate in unruptured follicles or in follicles that have ruptured and sealed immediately. They tend to regress spontaneously and are rarely seen more than 1 year after the menopause. They may be single but are usually multiple. They are also usually small, measuring 10 to 20 mm in diameter, and rarely exceed 100 mm. When they are small with atrophic lining cells, they are of no clinical significance. Rarely an increased production of estrogen can be associated with these cysts, which may stimulate endometrial hyperplasia and prolonged irregular bleeding. They are sometimes associated with uterine fibroids and larger

cysts may be seen in patients undergoing long-term hormone administration. Some degree of follicular cyst formation is a relatively common finding at operation in women who have no apparent symptoms related to the cysts. Sometimes multicystic ovaries are associated with dysmenorrhoea, menstrual irregularity, dyspareunia, and pelvic discomfort. Echographically, solitary follicular cysts are thin walled and unilocular, and the smaller single cyst cannot always be differentiated from other small fluid-filled adnexal masses, such as a hydrosalpinx (see Chapter 40). The larger cysts are similar in appearance to small serous cystadenomas and to parovarian cysts (Figs. 4,13A–D). Polycystic ovaries are discussed on page 489.

Corpus Luteum Cyst
The normal corpus luteum measures approximately 12 to 17 mm and is formed after rupture of the follicle. It increases in size until the 22nd day of the menstrual cycle and then regresses slowly. This is known as the corpus luteum of menstruation. The corpus luteum of pregnancy enlarges progressively and reaches maximum size, about 30 mm, at around 8 to 10 weeks. It is concerned with embedding and development of the ovum during the first months of pregnancy. Corpus luteum cysts can develop from either the corpus luteum of menstruation or the corpus luteum of pregnancy (see Chapter 33). They are often asymptomatic although they can be associated with menorrhagia and a clinically palpable mass. Occasionally the corpus luteum of menstruation continues to produce hormones; clinically there is amenorrhoea, a slightly enlarged uterus, and a unilateral cystic swelling. Sometimes these cysts rupture and cause intraperitoneal hemorrhage, the clinical features being very similar to an ectopic pregnancy.

The cysts can be demonstrated echographically. They are small, unilateral, and thin walled (Fig. 14A). The possibility of a cyst developing in the corpus luteum of pregnancy should be considered if there is associated menstrual irregularity and the uterus then carefully examined for an early gestation. If hemorrhage has occurred into the cyst without rupture, solid contents may be present (Figs. 7E, 14B). With hemorrhage and rupture, free fluid may be identified in the cul de sac. These hemorrhagic cysts cannot be differentiated from ectopic pregnancy with any degree of confidence and laparoscopy is usually clinically indicated.

Theca Lutein Cysts
These are special types of cysts usually associated with hydatidiform mole and choriocarcinoma (see Chapter 29). They may rarely, however, be associated with a normal pregnancy.[44] The cysts are multiple and bilateral and may be several centimeters in diameter (Fig.

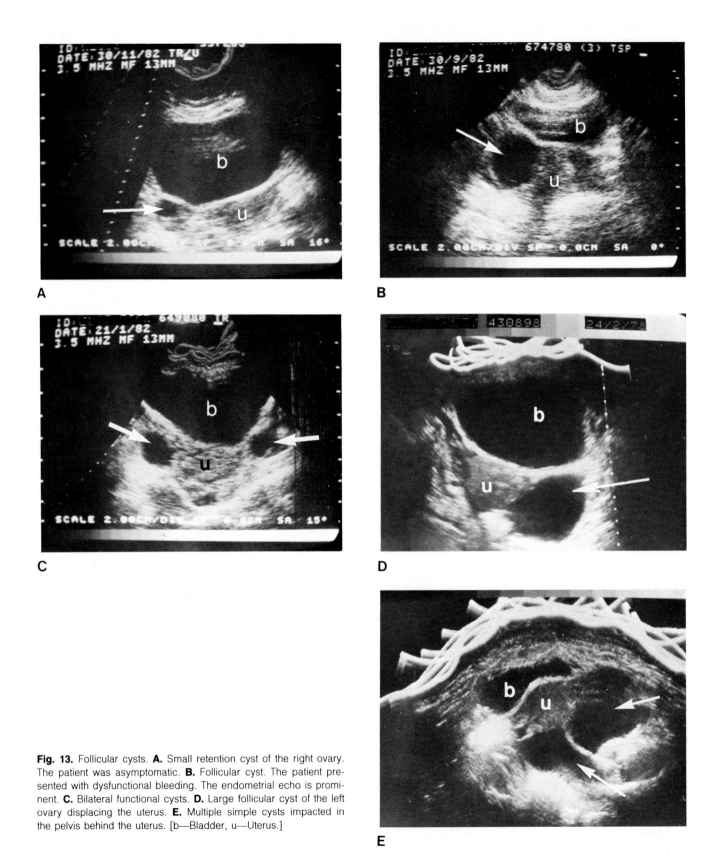

Fig. 13. Follicular cysts. **A.** Small retention cyst of the right ovary. The patient was asymptomatic. **B.** Follicular cyst. The patient presented with dysfunctional bleeding. The endometrial echo is prominent. **C.** Bilateral functional cysts. **D.** Large follicular cyst of the left ovary displacing the uterus. **E.** Multiple simple cysts impacted in the pelvis behind the uterus. [b—Bladder, u—Uterus.]

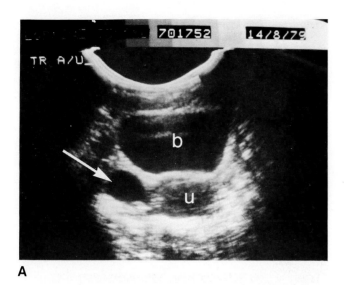
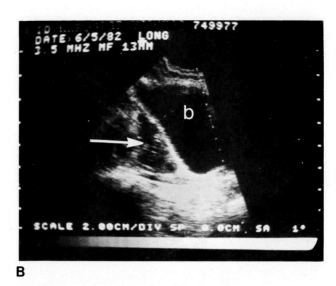

Fig. 14. Corpus luteum cysts. **A.** Corpus luteum cyst of the right ovary. The diagnosis was confirmed at laparoscopy. **B.** Hemorrhagic corpus luteum cyst causing persistent pelvic pain. [b—Bladder, u—Uterus.]

15). They can be clearly outlined echographically. The cysts involute when the source of gonadotropin is removed by elimination of the mole or excision of the choriocarcinoma.

POLYCYSTIC OVARIAN SYNDROME

Stein Leventhal Syndrome

The classic Stein Leventhal syndrome was first described in 1935.[45] This syndrome is seen in women in their late second or early third decade. It is character-

ized by hirsuitism, menstrual irregularity, reduced fertility or sterility, and bilateral cystic ovaries (Fig. 16). The ovaries are described as being large and white; the cysts are small, rarely exceeding 5 mm in diameter, and consist of multiple cystic follicles of varying size. Variants of the classic syndrome have since been described with hirsuitism, oligomenorrhoea, obesity, and menstrual irregularity. Polycystic ovaries may also be associated with Cushing syndrome, basophilic pituitary adenoma, post-pill amenorrhoea, and virilizing ovarian or adrenal tumors,[46,47] and they may be linked with endometrial carcinoma in women under 40 years

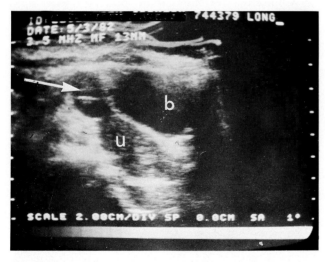

Fig. 15. Theca lutein cyst. The cyst was demonstrated in association with a rise in serum gonadotropin following previous evacuation of a hydatidiform mole. There is also an abnormal area of increased density in the uterus. [b—Bladder, u—Uterus.]

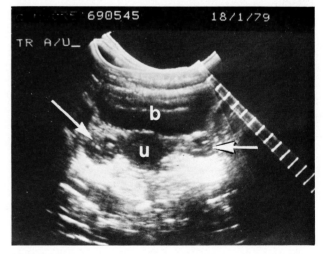

Fig. 16. Polycystic ovaries. Bilateral cystic ovaries in association with other features of the Stein Leventhal syndrome. Both ovaries are significantly enlarged and contain multiple cystic follicles. [b—Bladder, u—Uterus.]

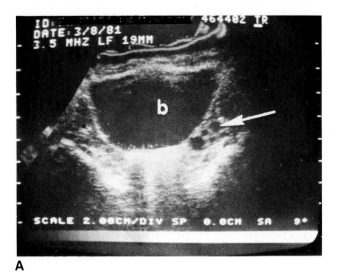
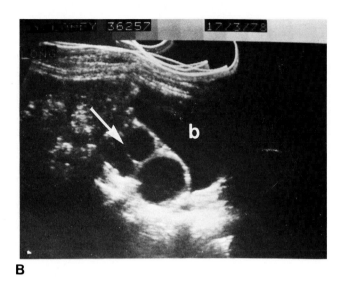

A   **B**

Fig. 17. Unilateral polycystic ovaries. **A.** Multiple small follicular cysts of the left ovary. **B.** Large cyst involving the left ovary. Histologically these were follicular cysts and serous cystadenoma. [b—Bladder, u—Uterus.]

of age. Ovaries of prepubertal girls may appear morphologically similar[24] and polycystic ovaries can be seen without any of the clinical signs or symptoms.[33]

The ovaries are 2 to 5 times their normal size; the enlargement is symmetric with cyst formation. The cysts vary in size and are best demonstrated by high-resolution real-time systems, being more difficult to display with static scanners. There have been several studies of this syndrome by ultrasound. Swanson, Saverbrei, and Cooperberg[33] surveyed a group of 863 patients and found 2.5 percent had evidence of polycystic ovaries. The volume of the ovaries varied from 6 to 30 cm³ and hirsuitism, obesity, and menstrual irregularity was seen in 50 percent—none were infertile. The cysts varied in number from 6 to 16 and their diameter varied from 2 to 6 mm. Parisi et al.[32] looked at a group of 78 patients with amenorrhoea, oligopolymenorrhoea, hirsuitism, obesity, and sterility and found nine patients with polycystic ovaries—four of these were confirmed at operation and were shown to have micropolycystosis with bilateral follicular cystoatresia. The ovaries were large and white with a sclerosed surface. The surface area varied from 12 to 22 cm² and the uterine ovarian ratio was 0.8 to 1.0.

Other Types of Polycystic Ovaries

Polycystic ovaries unaccompanied by features of the above syndrome are not uncommon. They are usually unilateral and the cysts slightly larger and are both follicular and luteal in origin. (Figs. 11A,13E,17A,B). It is possible to observe changes with menstruation. There may be no associated symptoms or there may be dysmenorrhoea, menstrual irregularity, dyspareunia, and pelvic discomfort. They may be found in association with pelvic inflammation, endometriosis, uterine myomata, metropathia hemorrhagica, and may occur following ovarian stimulation by pituitary preparation and chlomiphene.

OVARIAN HYPERSTIMULATION

This syndrome is usually associated with therapy for infertility. It has also been described in patients with hydatidiform mole, chorioepithelioma, multiple pregnancies, and single pregnancy.[48]

Clinically overstimulation may produce mild symptoms of abdominal heaviness, swelling, and pain. Ovarian cystic enlargement occurs and these cysts can be easily demonstrated ultrasonically (Fig. 18).[49,50] Severe symptoms are rare but may occur, the syndrome being associated with ascites, hydrothorax, shock, and thromboembolic phenomena.

PRIMARY TUMORS OF THE OVARY

Tumors of the ovary are a common form of neoplasm in women. Many are highly aggressive and they cause a high proportion of fatalities among female genital tract malignancies. There are a wide variety of types and their classification differs depending on whether the criteria employed are based on macroscopic appearance, microscopic appearance, clinical behavior, or histogenesis. In 1971 the World Health Organization (WHO) developed a classification based on morpho-

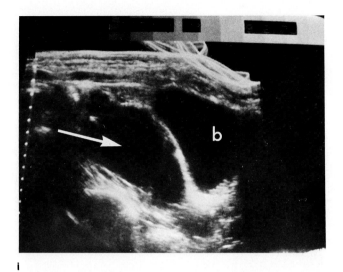
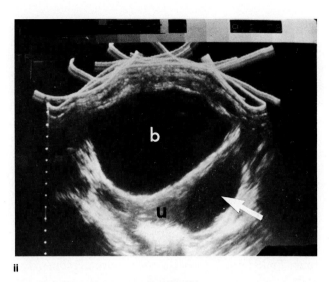

Fig. 18. Large left-sided clomiphene induced cyst. i. Longitudinal. ii. Transverse. [b—Bladder, u—Uterus.]

logic criteria that is now generally employed.[34,51] The histopathologic classification of epithelial tumors adopted by the WHO corresponds with that proposed by the International Federation of Gynaecology and Obstetrics (FIGO).

Some ovarian tumors are functionally active. The ovarian stroma can differentiate into the various cells of the follicle such as the granulosa and theca interna cells. Granulosa cell tumors and thecomas may have a strong estrogen effect; the cystadenofibroma and Brenner tumor also sometimes exhibit estrogen activity. Virilizing tumors that secrete androgens may also occur, the arrhenoblastoma being the typical example (Table 2).

Ovarian tumors tend to produce the same general clinical picture. Many, particularly the simple cysts, produce no symptoms until they are large enough to cause obvious abdominal distension. When very large, pressure symptoms include abdominal discomfort, vomiting, flatulence, and dyspnea. Pain may develop if there are adhesions to the parietal peritoneum, impaction in the pelvis with urine retention, or if torsion occurs. The rate of growth of even benign tumors can be rapid, though on the whole rapid growth suggests

malignancy. The development of ascites also produces an increase in abdominal distension. Occasionally malignant tumors may cause amenorrhoea; this is more likely to occur if they are bilateral. Simple cysts even when unilateral may cause menstrual irregularity. Clinical features suggesting malignancy are bilateral tumors, ascites, a semisolid consistency, edema of one leg, pain of sacral nerve distribution, rapid growth, immobility, and the palpation of hard nodules in the cul de sac.

Complications most likely to occur are torsion, rupture, and infection. Torsion with hemorrhagic infarction produces pain and tenderness with extravasation of blood into the wall of the tumor. Rupture can occur spontaneously and may pass unnoticed, though pain may result from acute peritoneal irritation. Infection is most likely to develop in the puerperium or result from associated salpingitis, appendicitis, or diverticulitis. These complications are difficult to diagnose echographically. With rupture, fluid can be identified in the cul de sac or the paracolic gutters if there is significant spillage of cyst contents. With torsion, there may be no identifiable sonographic change, though occasionally there is some loss of definition of the cyst structure, presumably due to edema. Hemorrhage into the cyst can only be identified when the blood becomes organized. A hemorrhagic infarcted cyst can have very similar ultrasonic characteristics to a semisolid malignant tumor or cystic tumor (Fig. 7H). None of these complications can be diagnosed with any degree of confidence from the ultrasonogram alone.

The classification of ovarian tumors is complex and there is often a multiplicity of terminology. The

TABLE 2
Hormone Producing Cysts and Tumors

Estrogenic	Androgenic
Follicular cyst	Arrhenoblastoma
Granulosa cell tumor	Leydig cell tumor
Thecoma	
Cystadenofibroma	
Brenner tumor	

more commonly encountered primary ovarian tumors are discussed in the following sections under five main headings. A specific diagnosis cannot always be made echographically, as different tumors have similar acoustic features. The ultrasonologist will, however, encounter many of these tumors and some knowledge of their clinical behavior is of value. The ultrasonic features typical of cystic and solid ovarian tumors as well as the common characteristics associated with benign and malignant lesions are discussed in a previous section of this chapter (Table 1). Benign tumors include the cystic teratoma, fibroma, thecoma, cystadenofibroma, and Brenner tumor. Tumors that are potentially malignant include all tumors of epithelial origin, the solid teratoma, granulosa cell tumor, and arrhenoblastoma. Endodermal sinus tumors, choriocarcinoma, dysgerminoma, and endometrioid tumors are usually malignant.

TUMORS OF THE SURFACE EPITHELIUM AND OVARIAN STROMAL ORIGIN

The large majority of tumors fall into this group. They may be benign, borderline, or malignant, and vary in size from relatively small to massive tumors filling the pelvis and much of the abdomen. Most are cystic but some are solid. Papillary projections are seen in the cystic tumors which become more prominent with aggressive tumors, eventually solidifying some of the cystic spaces.

Serous Cystadenomas

See Figures 1, 2B, and 19A. These are thin walled cysts with an occasional septum. These cysts may be small or as large as 15 to 20 cm in diameter, and occasionally they can be very large, filling much of the abdomen. They may be bilateral, though this can be overlooked echographically, as the second cyst may be mistaken for a loculus of the first. Benign cysts rarely show solid papillary ingrowths and ascites is uncommon though, rarely, free fluid is present in a histologically benign tumor when the cyst has ruptured with spillage of its contents into the peritoneum. Serous cystadenomas and cystadenocarcinomas account for about 30 percent of ovarian tumors. They are seen in the 20- to 50-year-old age group and the ratio of benign to malignant is approximately 1:9.

Serous Cystadenocarcinomas

See Figures 8 and 19B. These tumors account for 60 percent of carcinomas of the ovary. Complex solid ar-

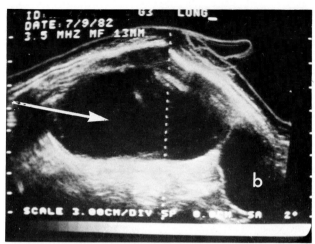

A

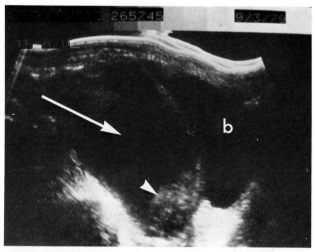

B i

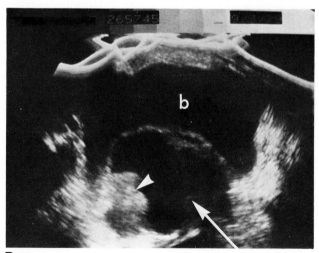

B ii

Fig. 19. Serous cystodenoma: serous cystadenocarcinoma. **A.** Large mobile unilocular cyst. (Serous cystadenoma.) **B.** Large fixed cyst with some solid elements. The uterus is not demonstrated. i. Longitudinal. ii. Transverse. (Serous cystadenocarcinoma.) [b—Bladder.]

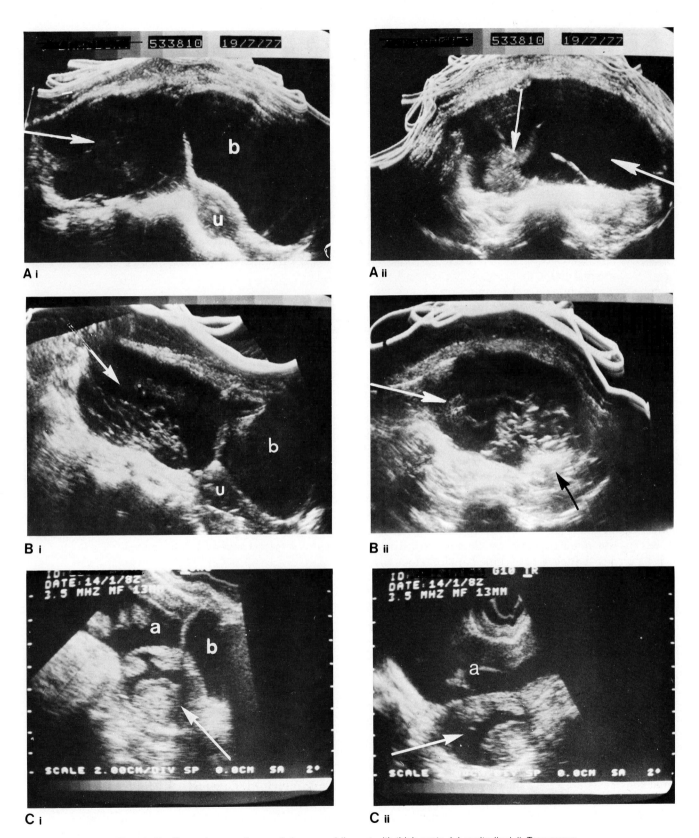

Fig. 20. Papillary adenocarcinoma. **A.** Large mobile cyst with thick septa. i. Longitudinal. ii. Transverse. **B.** Complex cyst with loss of definition of the posterior side wall. i. Longitudinal. ii. Transverse. **C.** Cyst with solid areas fixed in the pelvis. There is associated ascites. i. Longitudinal. ii. Transverse. [b—Bladder, u—Uterus, a—Ascites.]

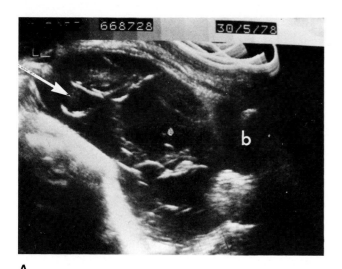

A

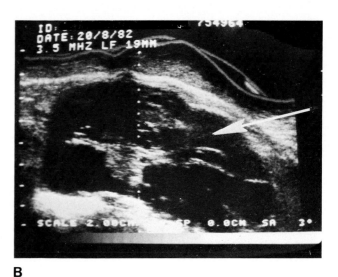

B

Fig. 21. Mucinous cystadenoma and cystadenocarcinoma. **A.** Mucinous cystadenoma. Large impacted complex cyst filling the pelvis and lower abdomen. **B.** Stage I mucinous cystadenocarcinoma. Large mobile cystic mass extending from the pelvis to above the umbilicus. [b—Bladder.]

eas develop within the cyst, and as they spread by infiltration through the capsule into the pelvis there may be loss of capsular definition and fixation that can be seen ultrasonically. Surface implantation of papillary growth also occurs, causing associated ascites. There is often early spread to lymph nodes, with involvement of the paraaortic, mediastinal, and sometimes the supraclavicular nodes. Patients with enlarged supraclavicular lymph nodes may be referred for ultrasonic examination of the pelvis if histology of the nodes suggest an ovarian primary. Serous cystic tumors have a greater tendency to become papillomatous than mucinous cystic tumors and the papillary cystadenocarcinoma is usually classified under serous tumors.[51] However, mucinous tumors may have similar characteristics and cannot be distinguished from the serous cystadenocarcinoma (Figs. 20A–C).

Mucinous Cystadenomas

See Figures 5A, 5B, 6B, 7, and 21A. These are less common and account for about 20 percent of ovarian neoplasms. The benign-to-malignant ratio is 7:1. They can become very large and are multilocular. The septa are thin and may be very complex; they may also contain solid elements but be histologically benign. Benign mucinous cysts are rarely bilateral, and ascites is uncommon. Rupture may occur and cause pseudomyxoma peritoneii, which may appear ultrasonically similar to ascites. Occasionally in these mucinous tumors nodules of a dermoid cyst or a Brenner tumor are found in the wall of a cystic space.

Mucinous Cystadenocarcinomas

See Figures 7, 8, and 21B. These are rarer than their serous counterpart. They are difficult to assess echographically, as many benign mucinous cysts have a complex internal structure. The presence of bilateral tumors, solid areas within the cyst and associated evidence of capsular infiltration, fixation, and loss of definition, are highly suspicious features. Ascites is often detectable. Mucinous cystadenocarcinomas do not usually produce a solid frozen pelvis, nor do they frequently metastasize to lymph nodes.

Pseudomyxoma Peritonei

See Figure 22. Metastases from or rupture of a cystadenocarcinoma can give rise to pseudomyxoma peritonei. The peritoneal cavity becomes filled with a mucinous material resembling the cyst contents. Multiple tumor implants are encountered on the serosal surface and there are extensive adhesions producing matting of the abdominal contents. The mucinous material resembles ascitic fluid on the echogram but with higher sensitivity fine punctate echoes, and sometimes linear strands, can be identified.[52] Less commonly, rupture of a benign mucinous cyst may cause pseudomyxoma peritonei.

Endometrioid Tumors

See Figures 23A-C. Most endometrioid tumors are malignant. They account for around 15 percent of ovarian cancer. Histologically the epithelium of these tumors resembles the endometrium of the uterus and in approximately one-third of cases there is associated carci-

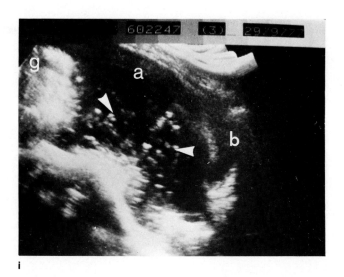
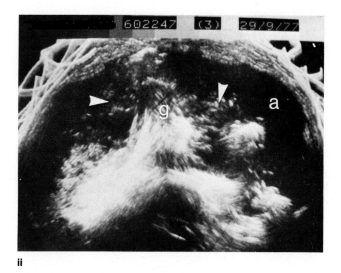

i

ii

Fig. 22. Pseudomyxoma peritonei. Gelatinous material containing punctate echoes is seen in the pelvis and abdomen. The bowel outline is abnormal due to extensive infiltration. i. Longitudinal. ii. Transverse. [b—Bladder, g—Gut, a—Ascites.]

noma of the endometrium. The tumors, which are of moderate size, are either cystic or solid, and the cystic tumors are not usually complex. In about one-third of cases, both ovaries are involved.

Cystadenofibroma

See Figure 2C. This is a variant of the serous cystadenoma. They are usually small, multilocular and have simple papillary processes. These tumors can sometimes give rise to hyperoestrinism. They are rarely malignant.

Clear-Cell (*Mesonephroid*) Tumors

See Figure 24. So called because their cellular structure bears a resemblance to the clear-cell carcinoma of the kidney, clear-cell tumors can be predominantly solid or cystic, and vary from benign to borderline to malignant and are occasionally bilateral. The cysts may contain hemorrhagic, chocolate-colored material. Morphologically similar tumors are sometimes seen in the broad ligament, cervix, or vagina.

Brenner Tumors

See Figure 25. These uncommon, usually solid tumors vary in size from small nodules up to 20 to 30 cm in diameter. They are seen at all ages, from childhood up to old age, with a peak incidence at 40 to 70 years. Brenner elements may be identified histologically in association with a mucinous cystadenoma. Some Brenner tumors have estrogenic hormonal activity.

GERM CELL TUMORS

Dysgerminoma

See Figure 26. This is the ovarian counterpart of the seminoma of the testis. It is relatively rare, accounting for about 1 percent of all ovarian neoplasms and occurs at all ages, with a peak in the second and third decade. The tumor is solid, varying in size from a small nodule up to a large mass that can fill most of the abdomen. All dysgerminomas are considered to be malignant and are highly radiosensitive, so that even those that have spread beyond the ovary can be controlled. Choriocarcinoma can sometimes be found in a dysgerminoma.

Endodermal Sinus Tumor

See Figure 27. This is a highly malignant tumor. It can sometimes develop in association with a teratoma, dermoid cyst, or choriocarcinoma. As well as developing in the ovary it may be found in the sacrococcygeal region and the thorax. It is seen most commonly in young women and is very malignant, with pelvic or abdominal recurrence being found within a few months of excision.

Cystic Teratoma (*Dermoid Cyst*)

See Figures 7A and 28. Dermoid cysts are encountered relatively frequently—they account for about 25 percent of ovarian neoplasms. Their echographic appearance is very variable.[53] Small solid cysts full of sebaceous material and hair can be very difficult to define, as they merge acoustically with the pelvic soft tissues;

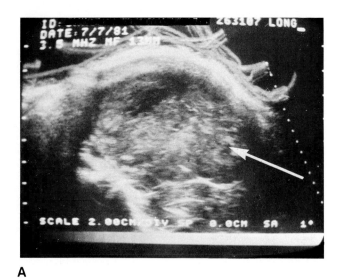

A

B

C

Fig. 23. Endometrioid tumors. **A.** Huge solid pelvic mass. (Mixed mesodermal tumor.) **B.** Infiltrating fixed pelvic mass above the bladder. (Mixed mesodermal tumor involving the uterus and ovaries.) **C.** Large fixed cystic tumor with solid areas. The tumor was adherent to gut, uterus, and peritoneum. (The solid area represents endometrioid carcinoma with squamous metaplasia in a serous cystadenoma.) [b—Bladder.]

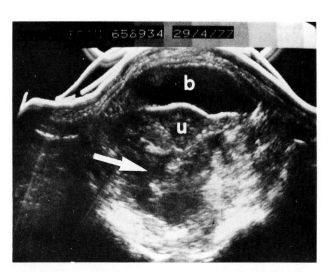

Fig. 24. Clear cell carcinoma. Solid infiltrating mass behind the uterus. [b—Bladder, u—Uterus.]

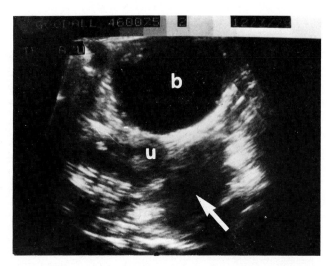

Fig. 25. Brenner tumor. Solid mass lying to the left of the uterus. This tumor had estrogenic activity and was causing postmenopausal bleeding. [b—Bladder, u—Uterus.]

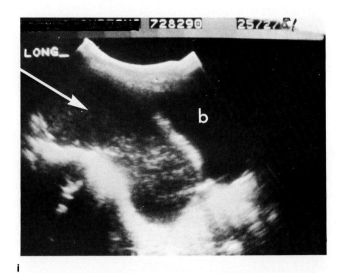

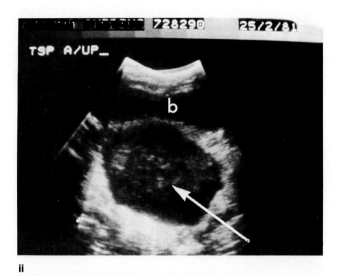

Fig. 26. Dysgerminoma. Huge solid mass filling the pelvis and lower abdomen. The mass is necrotic as there is little acoustic attenuation by the tumor. This tumor presented as abdominal swelling early in the second decade. i. Longitudinal. ii. Transverse. [b—Bladder.]

clinically, they are easily palpable, but ultrasonically they are poorly defined. They may cast an acoustic shadow or displace the lateral bladder wall. The diagnosis of a small cystic teratoma should be considered when an ovarian mass is easily palpated clinically but not defined ultrasonically. The larger cysts may be complex, with solid areas, septa, "compartments," and "fluid levels," or present as a large cystic mass with a small area of solid material. Dental elements cannot be differentiated from other very solid areas that cast an acoustic shadow. Dermoid cysts are usually unilateral and frequently axial though bilateral cysts are not uncommon. They are usually seen in young women

during active reproductive life. They are almost always benign, with only 1 or 2 percent becoming malignant (Fig. 29). They tend to twist more commonly than other ovarian neoplasms.

The *struma ovarii* has a thyroid-like structure. It may form part of a teratoma or occur without associated structures. It is usually regarded as a one-sided development of a particular tissue in a teratoma. Cases in which the tissue predominates with hormonal effect are rare. Ultrasound can be of value in identifying a pelvic lesion in hyperthyroid patients when there is no evidence of a thyroid lesion in the neck.[54] A primary carcinoid tumor may also arise in the wall of a dermoid cyst.

Solid Teratomas
See Figure 30. These are seen mainly in childhood and adolescence. They are usually unilateral though 10 percent are bilateral. Teratomas vary from benign tumors to highly aggressive malignant lesions. Acoustically they are usually a large, reasonably well defined solid mass, with a complex internal echo pattern.

Choriocarcinoma
Though most commonly of placental origin, choriocarcinoma can arise primarily in the ovary, varying in size from a small nodule up to 15 cm mass. They are aggressive tumors and metastasize widely by hematogenous dissemination to other organs and produce high levels of chorionic gonadotropins. Choriocarcinoma sometimes occur in association with a dysgerminoma.

Fig. 27. Endodermal sinus tumor. Large necrotic tumor mass filling the pelvis. There was massive recurrence within 1 year of diagnosis. [b—Bladder.]

498

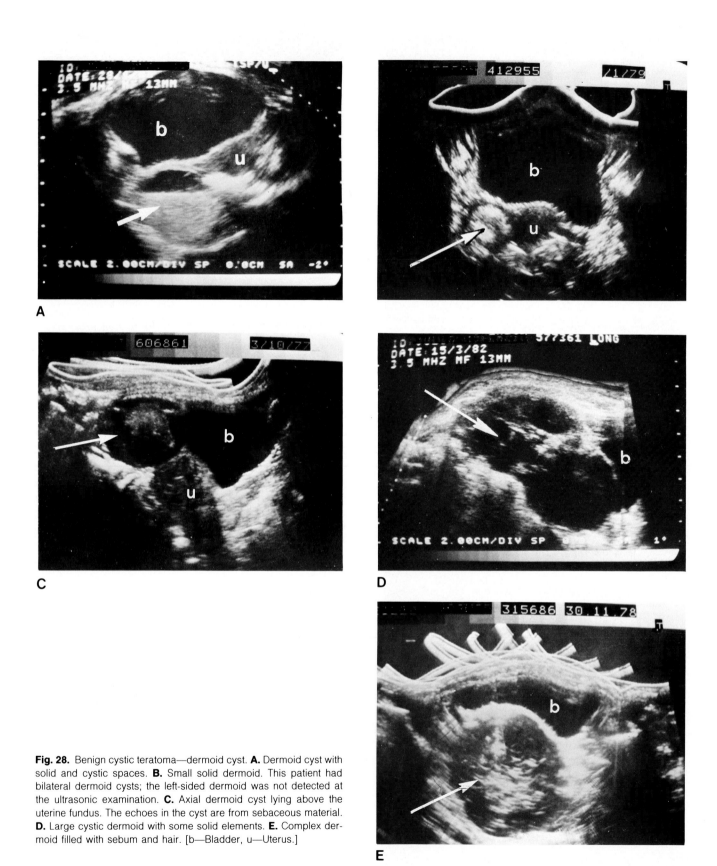

Fig. 28. Benign cystic teratoma—dermoid cyst. **A.** Dermoid cyst with solid and cystic spaces. **B.** Small solid dermoid. This patient had bilateral dermoid cysts; the left-sided dermoid was not detected at the ultrasonic examination. **C.** Axial dermoid cyst lying above the uterine fundus. The echoes in the cyst are from sebaceous material. **D.** Large cystic dermoid with some solid elements. **E.** Complex dermoid filled with sebum and hair. [b—Bladder, u—Uterus.]

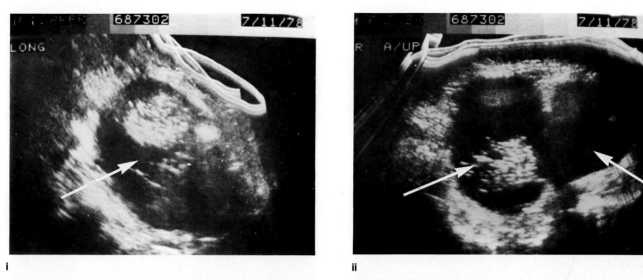

Fig. 29. Malignant dermoid cyst. Bilateral dermoid cysts fixed in the pelvis. The left-sided cyst was histologically benign. The cyst on the right side, which contained some solid elements was malignant. i. Longitudinal. ii. Transverse.

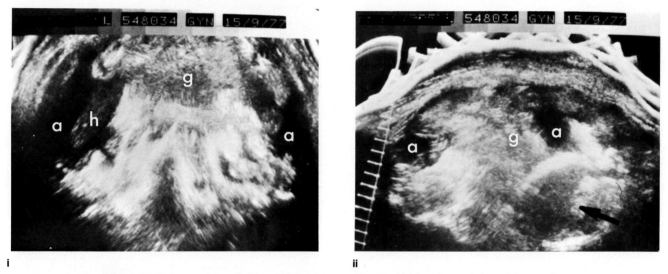

Fig. 30. Malignant teratoma. Solid well-defined tumor with associated ascites and abnormal gut outline due to peritoneal dissemination. i. High Transverse. ii. Low Transverse. [g—Gut, a—Ascites, h—Lung.]

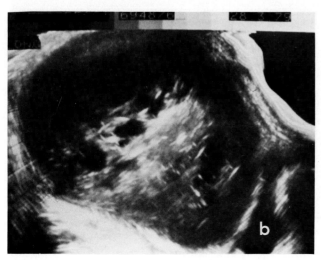

Fig. 31. Granulosa cell, theca luteal cell tumors. Huge fibrothecoma with a complex internal structure. [b—Bladder.]

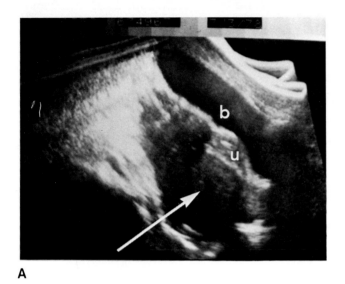

A

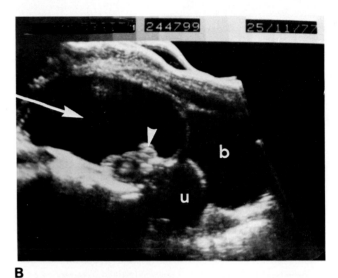

B

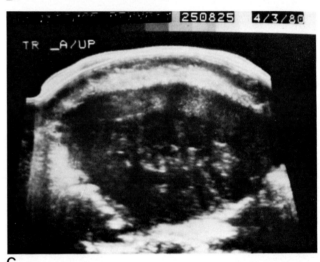

C

Fig. 32. Ovarian fibroma. **A.** Large solid homogeneous tumor impacted in the pelvis behind the uterus and bladder. There is strong acoustic attentuation through the fibroma. **B.** Cystic mass with solid elements above the uterus and bladder. The cystic area contained cream-colored amorphous debris: the solid area was a nodular mass of tissue. **C.** Large ovarian fibroma with a coarse echo pattern and acoustic attentuation. This fibroma was mobile and filled the lower abdomen. [b—Bladder, u—Uterus.]

SEX CORD–MESENCHYME TUMORS

Ovarian tumors included in this group are derived from the sex cord of the embryonic gonad or from the mesenchyme of the ovary. Many of these tumors are functional and have a feminizing effect, though some are virilizing.

Granulosa–Theca–Luteal Cell Tumors

See Figure 31. The tumors in this group are composed of a varying proportion of granulosa cells, theca cells, and luteinized cells. The tumors are usually solid and unilateral and vary from small foci to large well-defined masses up to 30 cm in diameter. Acoustically they contain homogeneous echoes, similar to the uterine fibromyoma. When small they may be difficult to define if of a similar echo density to the pelvic connective tissues. They can occur at any age but the majority

are seen around menopause and are clinically important in that they may produce large amounts of estrogen. In childhood, hyperoestrinism can result in precocious puberty; in adult life, signs and symptoms vary, though in most cases irregular vaginal bleeding is the main feature, and pathologic changes may occur in the breast and in the endometrium. The predominantly granulosa cell group are potentially malignant and are locally recurrent with the same metastatic potential as other forms of ovarian carcinoma.

Arrhenoblastoma (*Sertoli–Leydig Cell Tumor*)

These tumors are important in that they produce masculinization or defeminization, though a small proportion have an estrogenic activity. They occur at all ages but are commonest in the second and third decade. Most are unilateral and solid in consistency—though degeneration may be seen in larger tumors. They are more commonly malignant than the granulosa cell group.

TUMORS DERIVED FROM CONNECTIVE TISSUE

Fibroma and Fibrosarcoma
See Figures 2D, 32A-C. This group of tumors accounts for about 10 percent of ovarian neoplasms. Usually unilateral, they are commonly solid with a diameter between 5 and 10 cm. Sarcomatous change is uncommon. Acoustically they have a consistency similar to a uterine fibromyoma though they may be "harder" or more absorbent, with a low-level homogeneous internal echo pattern. Some may be cystic with solid elements. Differentiation of the solid fibroma of the ovary from the uterine fibromyoma may be difficult unless the tumor can be defined as separate from the uterus.

Clinically these tumors are important in that though benign they are often associated with ascites. Uncommonly there is also hydrothorax. The triad of ovarian tumor, ascites, and hydrothorax is known as *Meigs syndrome.* Cure of the condition by removal of the tumor is a fourth characteristic of the syndrome. This syndrome is not restricted only to the fibroma, though they constitute more than half of the associated ovarian tumors.

MISCELLANEOUS OVARIAN TUMORS

Other primary tumors that may arise in the ovary include the Lipoid cell tumors, ademantenoid tumors, and soft tissue tumors not specific to the ovary.[51]

Lipoid Cell Tumors
See Figure 33. These are usually solid, unilateral, and small. They are well defined and round or oval. Three histologic types are recognized—the Leydig or hilus cell tumor, the adrenal cell tumor, and the luteoma of pregnancy. The Leydig cell tumor has hormonal activity and is usually virilizing.

SECONDARY TUMORS OF THE OVARY

These tumors (Figs. 8B,34) are relatively common. Two main groups contribute to a high incidence—those arising from other pelvic organs and carcinomas originating in the upper gastrointestinal tract. Other primaries include breast, bronchus, and some reticuloendothelial

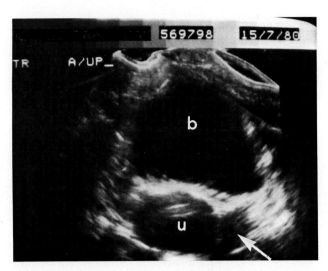

Fig. 33. Hilus cell tumor. Small solid mass to the left of a bulky uterus. The patient presented with virilizing features with severe hirsutism. [b—Bladder, u—Uterus.]

tumors. Primary lymphosarcoma of the ovary is rare; secondary involvement by lymphosarcoma is more commonly encountered. Leukemic infiltration also occurs and the sonographic appearance in childhood has been described.[10,55] *Krukenberg tumors,* originally described as large solid bilateral ovarian tumors, were accepted as being metastases of gastric carcinoma to the ovary, but the term has been expanded to include all ovarian metastases from gastrointestinal primary carcinomas as well as those from the pancreas and biliary tree (Fig. 34C).

Secondary tumors are usually bilateral, but if unilateral tend to be more common on the right side. They are frequently fixed and may be solid or a complex cyst and cannot usually be differentiated from primary ovarian tumors by ultrasound. When bilateral solid ovarian tumors are found at ultrasonic examination the upper abdomen should be scanned for a possible primary tumor.

THE CLINICAL STAGING OF MALIGNANT OVARIAN TUMORS

The prognosis for any patient with an ovarian malignancy depends on the histopathologic type and on the anatomic extension of the tumor when first diagnosed. There is no clear correlation between histologic and clinical malignancy in ovarian tumors. This applies particularly to epithelial tumors, granulosa cell tumors, and virilizing tumors. The International Union against Cancer has adopted a system in which the extent of the primary tumor, the involvement of lymph nodes, and presence of metastasis is considered (T.N.M. System). The International Federation of Gynaecology and Obstetrics recommends a definitive stage grouping as follows:

- Stage I.   Growth limited to the ovaries.
- Stage Ia.   Growth limited to one ovary; no ascites.
    i. No tumor on external surface: capsule intact.
    ii. Tumor present on external surface and/or capsule ruptured.
- Stage Ib.   Growth limited to both ovaries; no ascites.
    i. No tumor on external surface: capsule intact.
    ii. Tumor present on external surface and/or capsule ruptured.
- Stage Ic.   Tumor either Stage Ia or Stage Ib but with ascites present or positive peritoneal washings.
- Stage II.   Growth involving one or both ovaries with pelvic extension.
- Stage IIa.   Extension and/or metastases to the uterus and/or tubes.
- Stage IIb.   Extension to other pelvic tissues, including peritoneum and uterus.
- Stage IIc.   Tumor either Stage IIa or IIb but with ascites present or positive peritoneal washings.
- Stage III.   Growth involving one or both ovaries with widespread intraperitoneal metastases, and/or positive retroperitoneal nodes. Tumor limited to true pelvis with proven histologic malignant extension to small bowel or omentum.
- Stage IV.   Growth involving one or both ovaries with distant metastases. If a pleural effusion is present there must be positive cystology.
- Special category   Cases that are thought to be ovarian carcinoma but where it has been impossible to determine the origin of the tumor.

This stage grouping is based on findings at clinical examination and surgical exploration. It should be noted that cases of germ cell tumors, hormonal-producing neoplasms, and metastic carcinomas are to be excluded from therapeutic statistics on ovarian neoplasms.

The histopathologic classification of common tumors of the ovary are described in textbooks on gynecology, gynecologic pathology, and gynecologic oncology.[34,51]

Ascites

Peritoneal dissemination of tumor is usually accompanied by ascites. Small amounts of ascitic fluid can be most easily detected in the right paracolic gutter, above the liver in the right anterior subphrenic space, or in the posterior pelvis (Fig. 35). However, with pelvic pathology the pouch of Douglas is often obliterated and fluid is seen lateral to and above the bladder. If the pouch of Douglas is clearly defined and ascites is present, the cause of the ascites is less likely to be of ovarian origin (Fig. 34C). Larger accumulations of fluid are easily identified in the lower abdomen, in both paracolic areas and around the liver. Ascites is seen in over two-thirds of Stage III tumors but is not so frequently associated with Stage I and Stage II tumors. However, it must be stressed that large volumes of fluid may be present with benign ovarian tumors (see page 501) and in some early stages of malignancy ascites is generalized, even when the tumor is confined to the pelvis or within the capsule of a cyst. (See Stage Grouping of Primary Carcinoma of the Ovary).

Pleural Fluid

Pleural fluid may also be present in association with benign and malignant ovarian tumors (see page 501). Pleural effusions may be identified by ultrasound; small collections are more easily identified in the right chest (Fig. 36).

Omental and Peritoneal Dissemination

Small disseminated seedlings of tumor cannot be defined, though the presence of ascites infers the diagnosis. Cytologic confirmation of the presence of malignant cells is required for accurate staging, however. Small deposits in the pouch of Douglas are better identified clinically than by ultrasound. Solid localized omental deposits are occasionally defined, but frequently omental spread of tumor, identified at laparotomy, cannot be diagnosed echographically prior to operation or retrospectively on review of the ultrasonic images. Extensive peritoneal involvement with matting of the bowel may be recognized, although in the absence of ascites this can also prove to be a difficult ultrasonic diagnosis. When ascites is present and the bowel is "caked" together the diagnosis is obvious. The outline of the gut and omental echoes is bizarre, often with fluid loculations, and tends to become bound down posteriorly. This is usually seen at an advanced clinical stage, but "free" ascites with apparently normal gut echoes can be present even with extensive intraabdominal dissemination of tumor (Fig. 37).

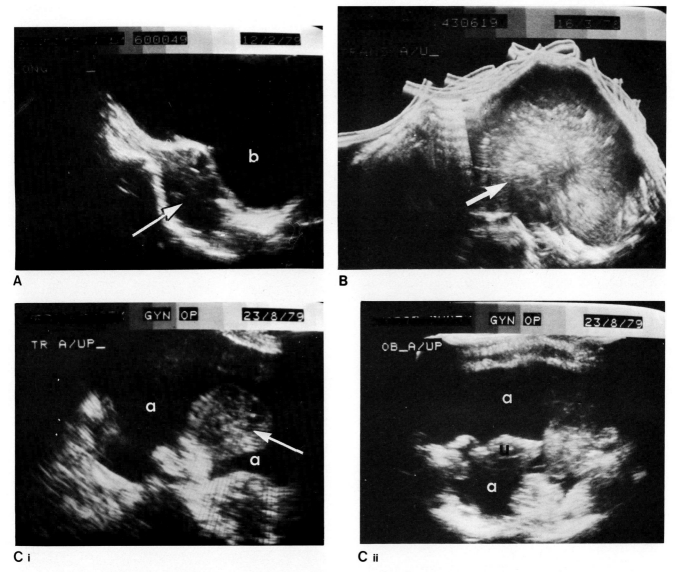

Fig. 34. Secondary tumors of the ovary. **A.** Secondary tumor involving the right ovary from a breast carcinoma. The tumor is solid with variable consistency. **B.** Huge solid ovarian tumor. The patient had massive bilateral tumors histologically mucin secreting adenocarcinoma. The primary tumor was not identified. **C.** Krukenberg tumor involving the left ovary from a gastric carcinoma. There is gross associated ascites. Note that the pouch of Douglas is clearly seen behind the uterus. i. Transverse. ii. Low Transverse. [a—Ascites, b—Bladder, u—Uterus.]

504

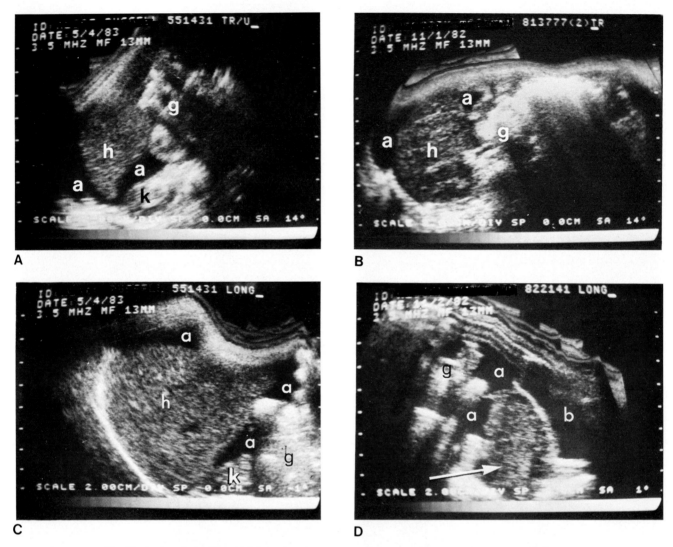

A

B

C

D

Fig. 35. Ascites. **A.** Ascitic fluid in the right paracolic gutter. **B.** Ascitic fluid in the right anterior subphrenic space. **C.** Ascitic fluid in Morrison's pouch and the right anterior subphrenic space. **D.** Ascitic fluid above the bladder. The pouch of Douglas is obliterated by tumor involving the uterus, tubes and ovaries. [b—Bladder, g—Gut, a—Ascites, h—Lung, k—Kidney.]

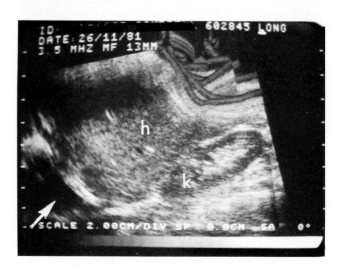

Fig. 36. Pleural effusion. Small pleural effusion in the right costo-phrenic angle. (Stage IV ovarian carcinoma.) [h—Lung, k—Kidney.]

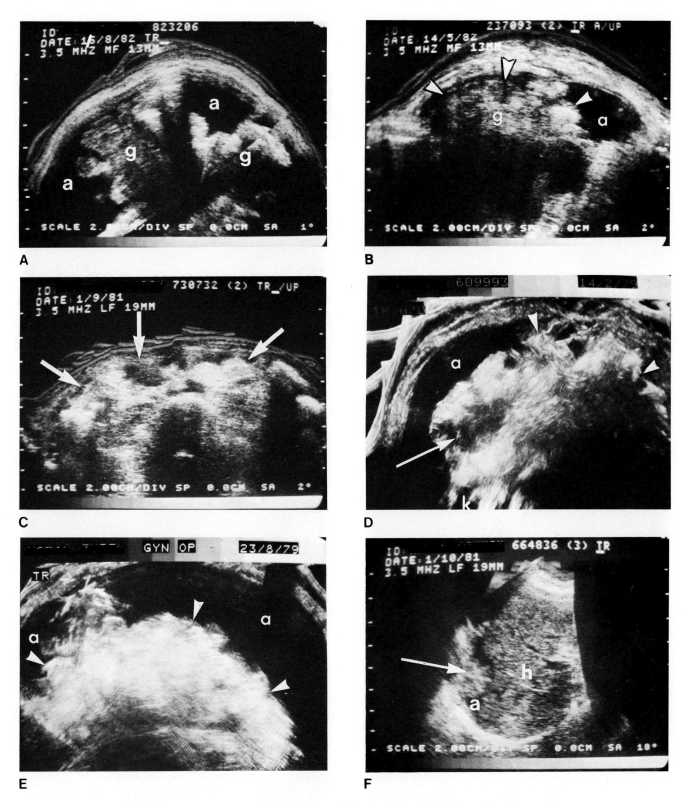

Fig. 37. Peritoneal and omental dissemination. **A.** Ascites without infiltration of bowel or omentum. Segments of bowel float anteriorly and peristatic activity may be seen. **B.** Localized infiltration by tumor with an associated pocket of ascitic fluid. (Stage IV ovarian carcinoma.) **C.** Generalized infiltration without ascites. There is an abnormal pattern with variations in density. (Stage IV ovarian carcinoma.) **D.** Omental tumor deposit with associated generalized infiltration and ascites. (Stage III ovarian carcinoma.) **E.** Advanced peritoneal carcinomatosis. The bowel and omentum are ''caked'' and lie posteriorly in the peritoneal cavity with ascitic fluid anteriorly. (Primary gastric carcinoma with secondary tumor in the ovary.) **F.** Peritoneal deposit adherent to parietal peritoneum in the upper abdomen, lateral to the right lobe of the liver. It is outlined by the ascitic fluid. [a—Ascites, g—Gut, h—Lung, k—Kidney.]

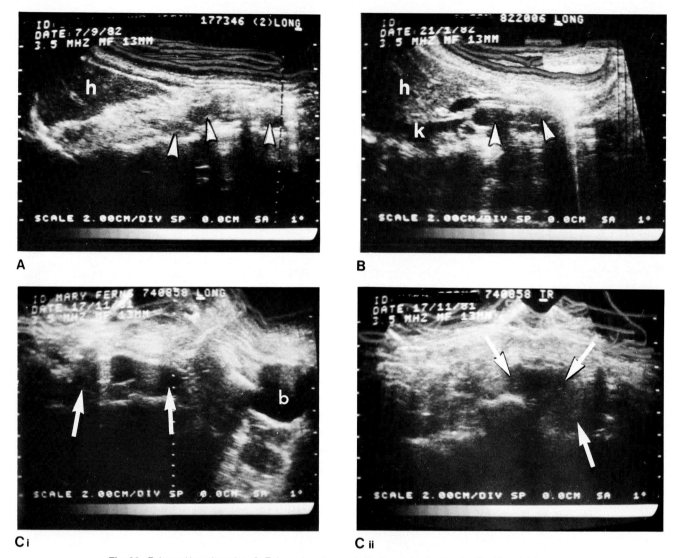

Fig. 38. Enlarged lymph nodes. **A.** Enlarged nodes medial to the abdominal aorta. (Papillary adenocarcinoma.) **B.** Enlarged nodes anterior to the vena cava. (Dysgerminoma.) **C.** Enlarged infiltrated pelvic lymph nodes. (Serous cystadenocarcinoma.) i. Longitudinal. ii. Transverse. [b—Bladder, h—Lung, k—Kidney.]

Paraaortic Lymph Nodes

Unless there is marked abdominal distension the presence of enlarged nodes in the paraaortic chain and porta hepatis may be determined by careful scanning using the aorta and vena cava as anatomic landmarks (Fig. 38). Grossly enlarged nodes are rounded or lobulated and when surrounding the aorta, sometimes obliterate its outline.[35,56,57] Smaller nodes can be seen as more discrete masses in the position of the lymphatic chains in the upper abdomen. Enlarged metastatic pelvic nodes are rarely seen. Involvement of nodes without nodal enlargement is not detectable by ultrasound. In the presence of omental and peritoneal involvement it may be difficult to differentiate enlarged nodes from the matted bowel and omentum, and in many patients

with advanced ovarian carcinoma the paraaortic area is obscured.

The Renal Tract

Both kidneys should be examined for evidence of ureteric obstruction. This is a particularly useful examination in patients with known ovarian carcinoma who are being monitored after laparotomy, as serial scanning may detect progressive obstruction before signs of recurrence or extension of the tumor are clearly evident on the pelvic scan. It is not such a useful sign in the presence of a large pelvic mass, as the obstruction may be due to local compression of the ureters rather than soft tissue involvement by tumor. Rarely bladder involvement may be identified (Fig. 39).

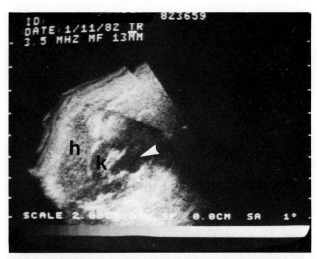

A i

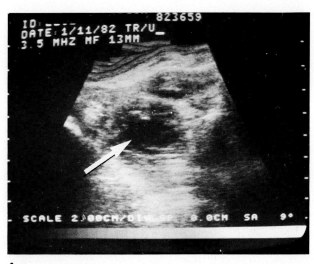

A ii

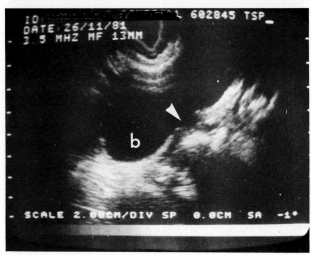

B

Fig. 39. Renal tract involvement. **A.** Right hydronephrosis. Incomplete removal of right-sided ovarian carcinoma with residual infiltrative tumor seen posteriorly in the iliac fossa. The tumor is obstructing the right ureter. i. Transverse. ii. Low Transverse. **B.** Invasion of the bladder wall by residual unresectable tumor. [b—Bladder, h—Lung, K—Kidney.]

Hepatic Metastases

With the introduction of gray scale imaging the assessment of hepatic pathology made a major advance. Intrahepatic metastatic deposits may be detected (Fig. 40) and ultrasound can be used for pretreatment clinical staging or to assess the extent of known liver involvement.[58,59] However, most ovarian carcinomas usually spread by direct extension and hepatic metastases are identified at laparotomy on the surface of the liver. These surface metastases cannot usually be recorded echographically unless large and outlined by the presence of ascites. Large intrahepatic parenchymal metastases are less common, as hematogenous spread occurs, usually at a later stage of the disease. It should also be appreciated that with gross abdominal distension, caused either by ascites or omental tumor, ultrasonic examination of the liver may be technically difficult or impossible.

ULTRASONIC ASSESSMENT OF THE MALIGNANT OVARIAN TUMOR

Diagnosis and Staging Prior to Laparotomy

Ultrasonic features that suggest the possible diagnosis of ovarian malignancy have already been discussed. They include bilateral tumors, complex cysts, solid tissue either within a cyst or a solid pelvic mass, loss of definition of a cyst wall, fixation of a mass, ascites, omental plaques, and hepatic deposits. Unfortunately many of these features are not specifically diagnostic and may be seen in a significant proportion of histologically benign tumors; and a small percentage of malignant tumors have no identifiable features to suggest malignancy.[13] In a retrospective study of 245 histologically benign ovarian cysts, 42 cysts showed evidence of fixation, in 15 there was loss of capsular definition,

12 were complex or contained solid areas, 5 were bilateral and complex, and in 2 there was associated ascites. In a similar study of 106 ovarian carcinomas, 11 had no ultrasonic features to suggest the presence of malignancy (unpublished data).

In a larger series of malignant ovarian tumors reviewed after histologic diagnosis it was found that the ultrasonic examination (59 percent) was only slightly better at arriving at a confident diagnosis of a malignant ovarian tumor than a competent clinical examination by an experienced gynecologist (52 percent). Many of the patients examined were scanned only a few days prior to laparotomy and the ultrasonic examination did not significantly alter patient management. However, in a small number where the clinical diagnosis was incorrect and urgent laparotomy was not considered necessary, ultrasound made a significant contribution by identifying possible malignancy. This group included solid fixed carcinomas diagnosed clinically as impacted uterine fibroids, cystic tumors with a highly complex internal structure, and cases where unsuspected ascites, omental invasion, and liver metastases were identified. There was also a small but significant number of cases where ultrasound detected ovarian tumor that was not clinically palpable.

Further analysis of the malignant tumors in this series suggested that the ultrasonic scan identified features indicating malignancy in a higher proportion of Stage I and Stage II tumors than the clinical examination (54 to 28 percent) whereas with Stage III tumors there was no significant difference (63 percent). However, many of the echographic features considered to be associated with early malignancy were also seen in the histologically benign group of tumors. There is therefore significant overlap in the ultrasonic characteristics of benign tumors and the early stages of malignancy.

Attempts at prospective and retrospective clinical staging of the tumors was found to be too inaccurate to be of significant value except in advanced cases, where the diagnosis and stage was obvious both on clinical examination and on the ultrasonic scans. Local pelvic invasion could not be excluded, omental deposits were not always defined, and in the presence of ascites there was gross overstaging. Obviously ultrasound cannot replace staging laparotomy though it is of use when operative procedures are contraindicated.

It is apparent in its present stage of development that ultrasound does not detect or clinically stage early ovarian carcinoma with an acceptable degree of reliability, though it can alert the clinician to the possible diagnosis, and any mass reported as suspicious warrants closer examination. When a confident ultrasonic diagnosis of ovarian malignancy is made the malignant process is frequently at an advanced stage.

Ultrasound as a Possible Screening Technique for the Detection of Ovarian Cancer

The early diagnosis of ovarian cancer is clinically a matter of chance.[34] Means of early detection are limited at present, and the usually described presenting clinical features are associated with an advanced stage of the disease—early manifestations are vague and insiduous and are often not considered as important.

Clinically a woman over 35 years has a significant risk of developing ovarian cancer, a patient of 40 years with persistent gastrointestinal symptoms that cannot be diagnosed may have early ovarian cancer, and a long history of ovarian imbalance or malfunction may be associated with developing ovarian cancer. When this triad of features is present in a patient it is important to consider the possibility of ovarian cancer.[34]

To date ultrasound and CAT has added little to the early diagnosis. It is possible, however, that the screening procedure being developed by Campbell and Goswamy (page 477) may lead to earlier detection.[26]

MANAGEMENT AFTER DIAGNOSIS

Radiotherapy Planning

Ultrasonic scanning has been used to provide accurate data for radiotherapy planning[60-63] though in many centers CAT is now employed. Ultrasound remains useful in assessing the pelvic mass. By careful examination the size and extension of the tumor is displayed, its depth below the surface measured, and its relationship to normal structures identified. The proposed radiation field can be checked and corrected when necessary (Fig. 41). This technique is discussed in greater detail in Chapter 39.

Long-Term Monitoring

Ultrasound is proving to be of significant clinical value in the long-term management of patients with ovarian carcinoma.[14]

The initial ultrasonic examination should be carried out as soon as practicable after histologic diagnosis in order to obtain a series of baseline recordings. In addition to the histologic report, full operative details should be available at the time of this examination. Particular note should be made of pelvic soft tissue detail, the volume and location of any ascitic fluid, variations in the bowel echoes, the presence of omental deposits and lymph node enlargement, the size and

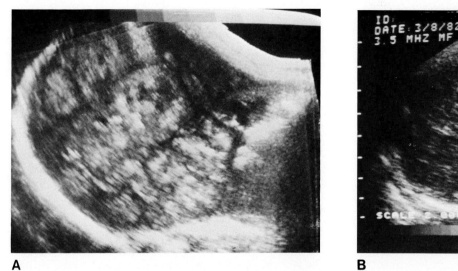
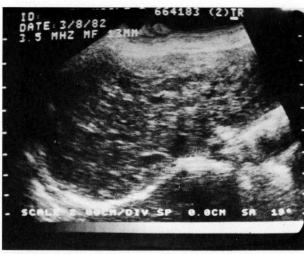

A

B

Fig. 40. Hepatic metastases. **A.** Multiple, large, high-density metastases with areas of central necrosis. **B.** Multiple small low density metastases disseminated throughout both lobes.

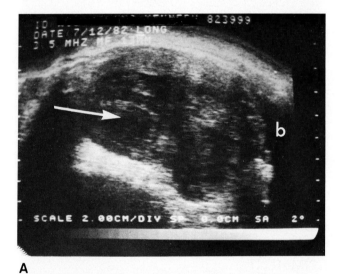
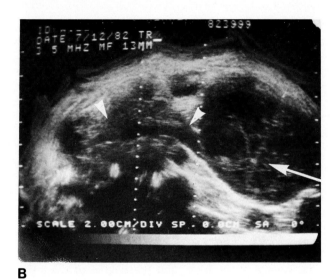

A

B

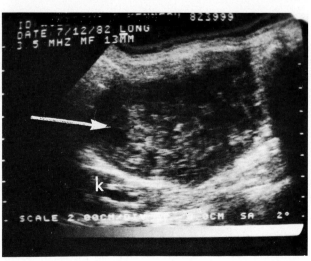

C

Fig. 41. Radiotherapy field check. Extensive tumor (Stage IV) diagnosed at laparotomy with incompletely resected pelvic tumor. Enlarged paraaortic nodes were noted at the time of operation. No scans taken until the patient presented 2 months later for a field check prior to radiotherapy. **A.** Pelvic tumor clinically palpable. **B.** Enlarged infiltrating lymph nodes in upper abdomen not included in planned field which is shown by cm depth markers. In addition there is a large mass of tumor in the left upper quadrant that had not been identified clinically. **C.** Sagittal section of tumor in the left upper quadrant which is compressing the kidney. [b—Bladder, k—Kidney.]

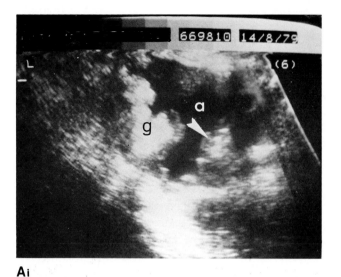

Ai

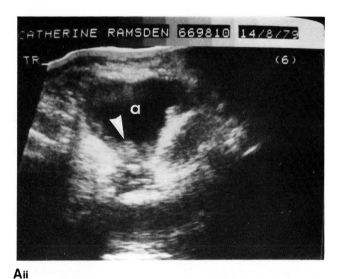

Aii

B

Fig. 42. Monitoring patients after initial diagnosis. **A.** Ascitic fluid and pelvic tumor. Stage III papillary adenocarcinoma diagnosed in November 1977 treated by surgery and chemotherapy. Clinically in remission in August 1979 when ascitic fluid and pelvic tumor recurrence demonstrated at routine ultrasonic examination. i. Longitudinal. ii. Transverse. **B.** Aspiration of ascites for cytologic examination. Stage III ovarian adenocarcinoma diagnosed in November 1979. Treated by surgery and chemotherapy. Vague dyspeptic symptoms developed in September 1980. No clinical or ultrasonic evidence of recurrence until October 1980 when ascites demonstrated. The ascitic fluid was aspirated under ultrasonic control and cytological examination confirmed papillary adenocarcinoma. Further treatment with chemotherapy. Patient well May 1983 (*cont.*). [a—Ascites, g—Gut.]

consistency of the liver, and the degree of dilatation of the renal collecting system. With experience and using high-resolution real-time systems total abdominal examination is a relatively quick procedure and pathologic changes can be recognized.

Interval ultrasonic examination is then employed to monitor relevant changes in the abdominal soft tissues. It is possible to monitor regression of residual tumor or to detect progression or early recurrence before the diagnosis is clinically evident. Where the soft tissue changes are not definitive or if confirmatory evidence of active disease is clinically required aspiration techniques may be employed to obtain cytologic material either from ascitic collections or from solid lesions.

In the long-term monitoring of patients with histologically proven ovarian malignancy ultrasound can now make a significant impact on patient management (Fig. 42).

COMMENT

Is ultrasound of practical value to the gynecologist in evaluating ovarian mass? In patients who are difficult to examine it may be the only noninvasive method of demonstrating ovarian pathology. It will confirm or question an initial clinical diagnosis and may radically alter patient management. In the patient with a clinically benign mass in whom laparotomy is contraindicated, or likely to be delayed, ultrasound should be used to confirm the diagnosis and to measure and monitor the lesion. In patients on specific treatment schedules ultrasound is an invaluable noninvasive method of serial assessment. It compares well with computed tomography in this application.

There are, however, diagnostic limitations imposed by restricted sensitivity and inadequate system resolution. There remains a lack of information on

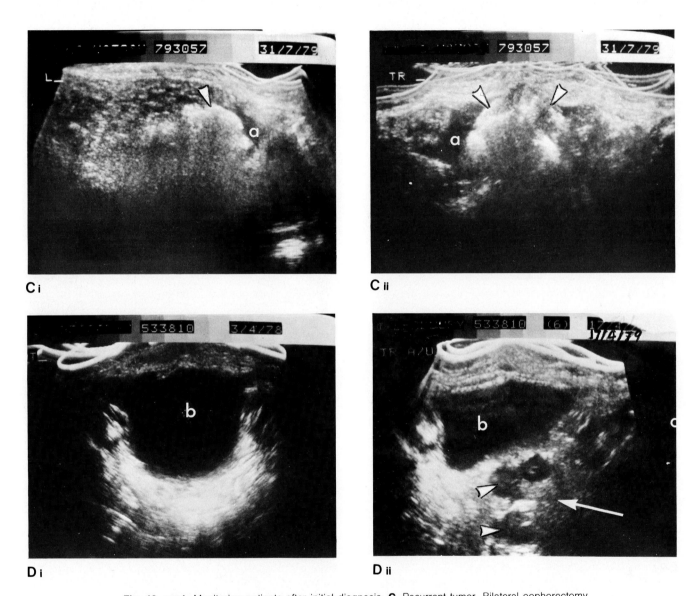

Fig. 42. cont. Monitoring patients after initial diagnosis. **C.** Recurrent tumor. Bilateral oophorectomy and hysterectomy for adenocarcinoma of ovary in 1971. Well until 1979 when presented with mass in right iliac fossa. Ultrasound demonstrated infiltrating mass in the right iliac fossa with associated ascites. i. Longitudinal. ii. Transverse. **D.** Solid tumor recurrence in the pelvis. Stage III bilateral papillary cystadenocarcinoma diagnosed in September 1977. Nodules were noted in the pouch of Douglas. Initial postoperative scan showed no pelvic abnormality and the pelvis remained clear until March 1979 when extensive solid recurrence was demonstrated in the pelvis (*cont.*). [a—Ascites, b—Bladder.]

512

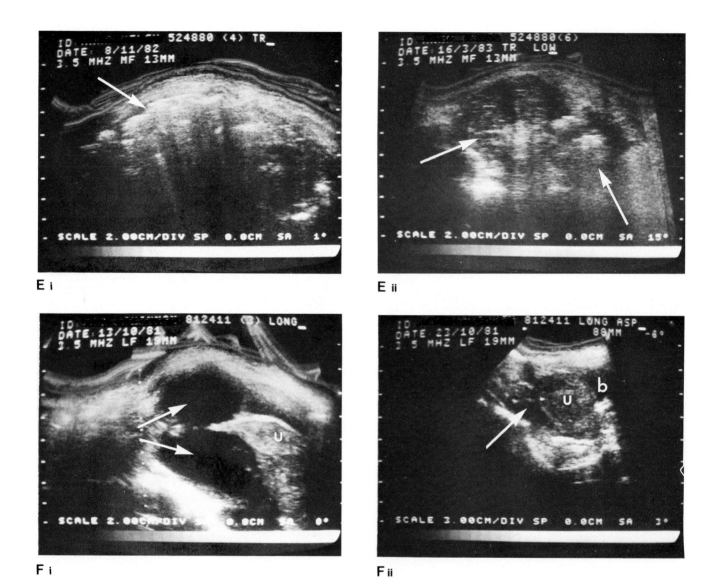

E i

E ii

F i

F ii

Fig. 42. cont. Monitoring patients after initial diagnosis. **E.** Frozen pelvis—Advanced carcinoma not controlled by chemotherapy. Bilateral salpingo-oophorectomy for ovarian adenocarcinoma in 1971. Recurrence March 1982 presenting with lower abdominal pain. At laparotomy the colon was found to be involved requiring sigmoid resection and a colostomy. The tumor failed to respond to chemotherapy and the patient developed a frozen pelvis and widespread dissemination. **F.** Aspiration of recurrent cystic tumor. Ovarian carcinoma resected in 1978. This patient was not scanned routinely and recurrence was diagnosed clinically in March 1981. The tumor failed to respond to radiotherapy and chemotherapy. To relieve the marked discomfort caused by the large cystic recurrence 900 ml³ of fluid was aspirated under ultrasonic control (*cont.*). [b—Bladder, u—Uterus.]

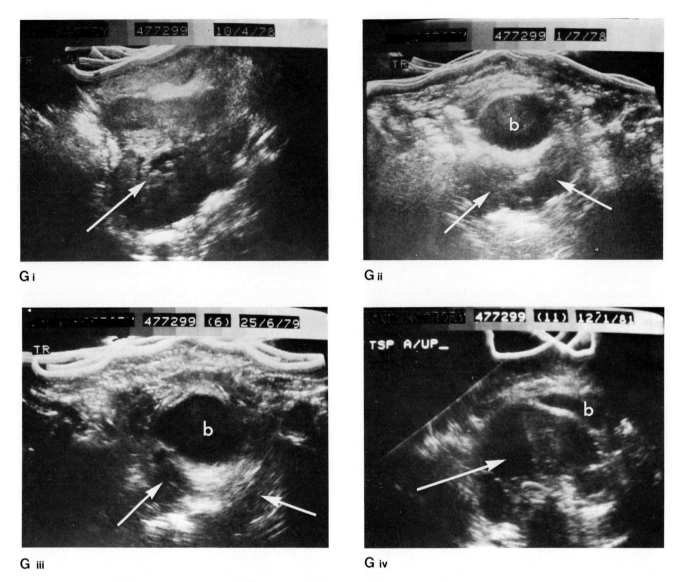

Fig. 42. cont. Monitoring patients after initial diagnosis. **G.** Regression of tumor. Papillary adenocarcinoma of the ovary diagnosed at laparotomy in March 1978. The postoperative scan in April 1978 showed a large mass of residual pelvic tumor. Interval ultrasonic examination demonstrated reduction in tumor volume by July 1978 and residual tumor in June 1979. At a second laparotomy in August 1980 the patient was considered to be "disease free" and to be in complete remission. The ultrasonic scans, however, remained suspicious—January 1980, March 1980, September 1980—and in January 1981 there was massive cystic pelvic recurrence. [b—Bladder.]

changes in the acoustic properties (tissue signature) of soft tissues in differing pathologic processes and there is no established method of quantifying these changes in vivo. Ultrasonic diagnosis is therefore based largely on assessing morphologic changes, ultrasonic tissue characterization is rudimentary. Improved instrumentation will give greater refinement in detail and the introduction of new methods of echoanalysis may result in a wider range of diagnostic applications.

REFERENCES

1. Donald I, MacVicar J, Brown TG: Investigation of abdominal masses by pulsed ultrasound. Lancet 1:1888, 1958
2. Cochrane WJ, Thomas MA: Ultrasonic diagnosis of gynaecological pelvic masses. Radiology 110:649, 1974
3. De Land M, Fried A, Van Nagell JR, et al: Ultrasonography in the diagnosis of tumours of the ovary. Surg Gynecol Obstet 148:346, 1979

4. Donald I: Use of ultrasonics in diagnosis of abdominal swellings. Br Med J 2:1154, 1963
5. Donald I: Diagnostic use of sonar in obstetrics and gynaecology. J Obstet Gynaecol Br Commonw 72:907, 1965
6. Kangarloo H, Sarti DA, Sample WF: Ultrasound of the paediatric pelvis. Semin Ultrasound 1:51, 1980
7. Kobayashi M, Hellman LM, Cromb E: Atlas of Ultrasonography in Obstetrics and Gynecology. New York, Appleton-Century-Crofts, 1972
8. Kratochwil A: Ultrasonic diagnosis in pelvic malignancy. Clin Obstet Gynecol 3:898, 1970
9. Lawson TL, Albarelli J: Diagnosis of gynecologic pelvic masses by gray scale ultrasonography—analysis of specificity and accuracy. Am J Roentgenol 128:1003, 1977
10. Mettler FA, Requard CK, Wicks JD: Preoperative sonography of malignant ovarian neoplasms. Am J Roentgenol 137:79, 1981
11. von Micsky LI: Gynecological ultrasonography, in King DL (ed), Diagnostic Ultrasound. St. Louis, Mosby, 1974
12. Mizuro J, Takenchi H, Nakano K: Diagnostic application of ultrasound in obstetrics and gynaecology, in Grossman CC, Holmes HH, Joyner C, et al (eds), Diagnostic Ultrasound. Proceedings of the First International Conference. New York, Plenum, 1966, p 452
13. Morley P, Barnett E: The use of ultrasound in the diagnosis of pelvic masses. Br J Radiol 43:602, 1970
14. Paling MR, Shawker TH: Abdominal ultrasound in advanced ovarian carcinoma. J Clin Ultrasound 9:435, 1981
15. Sarti DA, Sample WF: Diagnostic Ultrasound. Text and Cases. Boston, Hall, 1980
16. Thomas HE: Ultrasound techniques in pelvic cancer. Clin Obstet Gynecol 12:354, 1969
17. Thomas HE, Holmes JH, Gottesfield KR, et al: Ultrasound as a diagnostic aid in diseases of the pelvis. Am J Obstet Gynecol 98:472, 1967
18. Walsh JW, Rosenfield AT, Jaffe CC, et al: Prospective comparison of ultrasound and computed tomography in the evaluation of gynaecological pelvic masses. Am J Roentgenol 131:955, 1978
19. Walsh JW, Taylor KJW, Rosenfield AT: Gray scale ultrasonography in the diagnosis of endometriosis and adenomyosis. Am J Roentgenol 132:87, 1979
20. Walsh JW, Taylor KJW, Wasson JF McL, et al: Gray scale ultrasound in 204 proved gynaecologic masses: Accuracy and specific diagnostic criteria. Radiology 130:391, 1979
21. Kratochwil A, Urban G, Friedrichs F: Ultrasonic tomography of the ovaries. Ann Chir Gynaecol Fenn 61:211, 1972
22. Hackelöer BJ, Robinson HP: Ultraschalldarstellung des wachsenden Follikels und Corpus luteum im normalen physiologischen. Zyklus Geburtsh u Frauenheilk 38:163, 1978
23. Hall DA, Hann LE, Ferrucci JT, et al: Sonographic morphology of the normal menstrual cycle. Radiology 133:185, 1979
24. Merill JA: The morphology of the prepubertal ovary. South Med J 56:225, 1963
25. Goswamy RK, Campbell S, Whitehead MI: Establishment of normal ranges for ovarian volumes and identification of enlarged ovaries by real time sector sonar in post-menopausal women, in Lerski RA, Morley P (eds), Ultrasound 82. Proceedings of the Third Meeting of the World Federation for Ultrasound in Medicine and Biology. Oxford, Pergamon, 1983
26. Hackelöer BJ, Nitschke-Dabelstein S: Ovarian imaging by ultrasound: An attempt to define a reference plane. J Clin Ultrasound 8:497, 1980
27. Holm HH: Personal communication, 1982
28. Kratochwil A: Cross sectional ultrasonic tomography of the small pelvis and its clinical importance, in de Vlieger M, White DN, McReady VR (eds), Ultrasonics in Medicine. Amsterdam, Excerpta Medica, 1974, p 163
29. Morley P, Donald G, Sanders R: Ultrasonic Sectional Anatomy. Edinburgh, London, Churchill Livingstone, 1983
30. Sample WF, Lippe BM, Gyepes MT: Grey scale ultrasonography of the normal female pelvis. Radiology 125:477, 1977
31. Zemlyn S: Comparison of pelvic ultrasonography and pneumography for ovarian size. J Clin Ultrasound 2:331, 1974
32. Parisi L, Tramonti M, Casciano S, et al: The role of ultrasound in the study of polycystic ovarian disease. J Clin Ultrasound 10:167, 1982
33. Swanson M, Saverbrei E, Cooperberg PL: Medical implications of ultrasonically detected polycystic ovaries. J Clin Ultrasound 9:219, 1981
34. Van Nagell JR, Barber HRK: Modern Concepts of Gynaecologic Oncology. Bristol, Boston, London, John Wright PSG, 1982
35. Barnett E, Morley P: Abdominal Echography, in Trapnell DH (ed), Radiology in Clinical Diagnosis. London, Butterworths, 1974
36. Baum G (ed): Fundamentals of Medical Ultrasonography. New York, Putnam, 1975
37. Goldberg BB, Kotler MM, Ziskin MC, et al: Diagnostic Uses of Ultrasound. New York, Grune and Stratton, 1975
38. King DL (ed): Diagnostic Ultrasound. St. Louis, Mosby, 1974
39. Frank RT, Bolich P, Reichert J. Sonographic appearances of organized blood within a cyst. J Clin Ultrasound 3:233, 1975
40. Sandler MA, James JK: The spectrum of ultrasonic findings in endometriosis. Radiology 127:229, 1978
41. McGahon JP, Phillips HE, Di RH: Endometriomas in pregnancy. J Clin Ultrasound 10:180, 1982
42. Kalstone EC, Jaffe RB, Abel MR: Massive edema of the ovary stimulating fibroma. Obstet Gynecol 34:564, 1969
43. Kapadia R, Sternhill V, Schwartz E: Massive edema of the ovary. J Clin Ultrasound 10:469, 1982
44. Rowlands JB: Hyperreactio luteinalis: A case report. J Clin Ultrasound 6:327, 1978
45. Stein IF, Leventhal ML: Amenorrhoea associated with bilateral polycystic ovaries. Am J Obstet Gynecol 125:477, 1977

46. Ginsburg J, Havard CWH: Polycystic ovary syndrome. Br Med J 2:737, 1976
47. Yen SSC: The polycystic ovary syndrome. Clin Endocrinol 12:177, 1980
48. Schenker JG, Weinstein D: Ovarian hyperstimulation syndrome: A current survey. Fertil Steril 30:355, 1978
49. Rankin RN, Hutton LC: Ultrasound in the ovarian hyperstimulation syndrome. J Clin Ultrasound 9:473, 1981
50. McArdle CR, Sacks BA: Ovarian hyperstimulation syndrome. Am Roentgenol 135:835, 1980
51. Langley FA: The pathology of the ovary, in Fox H, Langley FA (eds), Postgraduate Obstetrical and Gynaecological Pathology. Oxford, Pergamon, 1973, p 198
52. Seale WB: Sonographic findings in a patient with pseudomyxoma peritonei. J Clin Ultrasound 10:441, 1982
53. Sandler MA, Silver TM, Karo JJ: Gray scale ultrasonic features of ovarian teratomas. Radiology 131:705, 1980
54. O'Malley BP, Richmond H: Struma ovarii. J Ultrasound Med 1:177, 1982
55. Anderson JC, Berry DL, Bickers GH, et al: Sonography of ovarian involvement in childhood acute lymphocytic leukemia. Am J Roentgenol 137:399, 1981
56. Asher WM, Freimanis AK: Echographic diagnosis of retroperitoneal lymph node enlargement. Am J Roentgenol

Radium Ther Nucl Med 105:438, 1969
57. Leopold GR: A review of retroperitoneal ultrasonography. J Clin Ultrasound 1:82, 1973
58. Taylor KJW, Carpenter DA, McCready VR: Gray scale echography in the diagnosis of intrahepatic disease. J Clin Ultrasound 1:284, 1973
59. Gilby ED, Taylor KJW: Ultrasound monitoring of hepatic metastases during chemotherapy. Br Med J 1:371, 1975
60. Brascho DJ: Clinical applications of diagnostic ultrasound in abdominal malignancy. South Med J 65:1331, 1972
61. Brascho DJ: Computerised radiation treatment planning with ultrasound, in de Vlieger M, White DN, McReady VR (eds), Abstracts of 2nd World Congress on Ultrasonics in Medicine. Amsterdam, Excerpta Medica, 1973, p 43
62. Brascho DJ, Shawker TH: Abdominal Ultrasound in the Cancer Patient. New York, Wiley, 1980
63. Brown RE, Bogardis CR, Sartin M: Ultrasound, computers, and radiation therapy planning, in de Vlieger M, White DN, McReady VR (eds), Abstracts of the 2nd World Congress on Ultrasonics in Medicine. Amsterdam, Excerpta Medica, 1973, p 43

37 Follicular Size Assessment by Ultrasound

B.J. Hackelöer

The use of ultrasound in the detection of adnexal masses and the demonstration of ovarian tumors is well known and is described in Chapter 36. Recent work has concentrated on the ultrasonic delineation of the physiologic development of the follicle and corpus luteum. Following an initial report in 1972,[1] we used sonography to observe ovarian changes in hormone-treated patients[2,3] in the search for a more efficient and reliable way of monitoring ovulation induction. High-resolution compound B-scan ultrasound equipment and the full bladder technique has made the visualization of ovaries and of clearly outlined cystic structures within the ovaries (follicles) possible. Good results can be obtained today with standard real-time scanners. Sector scanners are easier to use than linear array scanners, but for the demonstration of specific structural changes within the uterus and ovary some still consider a compound B-scan to be superior.

The demonstration of the presence of ovulation is the aim of ovarian cycle sonography. The ultrasonic changes seen are:

1. Demonstration of growing follicles with measurement of their number and size.
2. Demonstration of intrafollicular structures—cumulus oophorus, corpus luteum.
3. Demonstration of the uterine endometrial reaction to follicular growth.
4. Quantitative flow measurement in ovarian vessels.

DEMONSTRATION OF FOLLICULAR GROWTH

Using the full bladder technique and with the uterus as a landmark, serial longitudinal scans of the pelvis are made to either side of the midline. The follicle is recognized as a small cystic structure encompassed by tissue of relatively low amplitude echo (the ovary). The ovary is itself surrounded by the more dense echoes of the posterior and lateral pelvic walls and the inferior surface of the bladder. With electronic calipers the maximum diameter of the follicle may be measured in both longitudinal and transverse planes (Figs. 1–3). Others have used average dimensions. The ovary is an ovoid structure with a smooth outline and a hyporeflective characteristic texture. The normal size is approximately 2 × 3 × 2.5 cm, though it can measure up to 4.5 cm in any one axis.

Follicle growth may be followed from an initial 5 mm diameter. Normally only one follicle appears and grows but in cases stimulated by Clomid or Perganol more follicles are usually observed (average diameter 5 to 10 mm), forming a typical spoke-like structure (Fig. 4). The normal physiologic follicular growth is linear. The follicles have a squared off shape 4 to 5 days prior to ovulation and develop a round shape at ovulation (Figs. 5–7). The reported size of the mature (Graafian) follicle ranges between 20 and 27 mm in an average dimension (Table 1).[4] Some of the size difference found by different authors is explained by measurement techniques or by the use of different sound velocity (1500 to 1600 m/sec).

Since the follicle has an ovoid outline, maximum diameters should be taken (inside to inside of the follicle) transversally, longitudinally, and sagittally, and the mean used as an index of follicular size (Fig. 8). Graafian follicles seen following hormone treatment are in the same size range (18 to 25 mm). For many years it was thought that the size of the Graafian follicle was 13 to 15 mm; however, we and others have

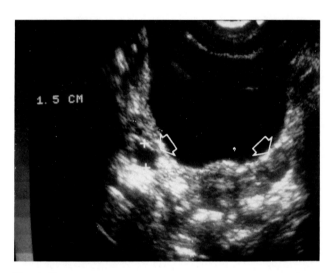

Fig. 1. Transverse scan; uterus and both ovaries (*arrows*) shown with 15-mm follicle in the right ovary.

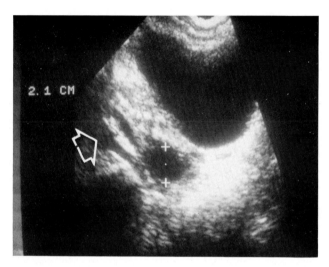

Fig. 2. Longitudinal scan; follicle 21 mm, ovarian vessels (*arrow*).

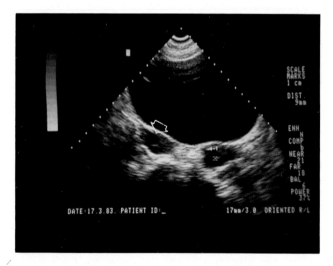

Fig. 3. Transverse scan; both ovaries with small follicles (*arrows*) less than 10 mm.

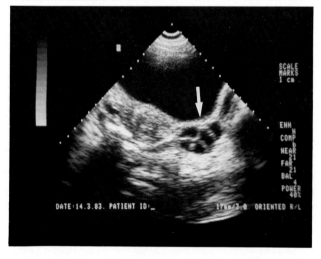

Fig. 4. Transverse scan; spoke-like structure of the right ovary (*arrow*) with several follicles.

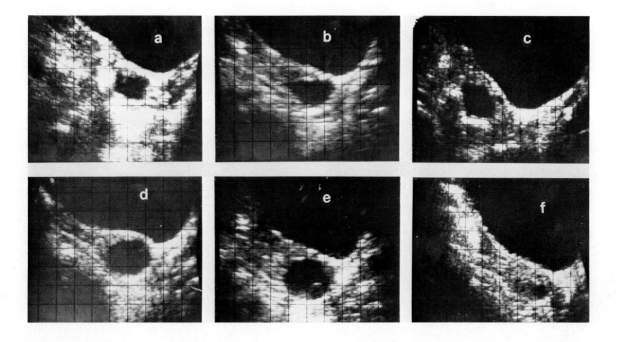

A

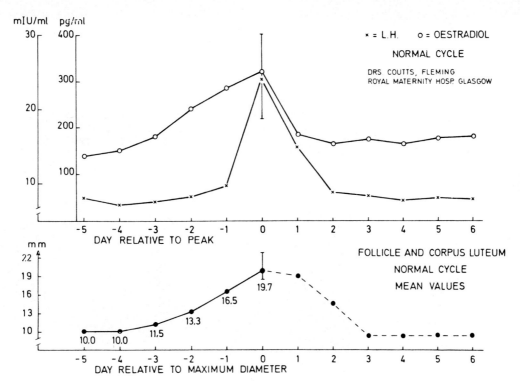

B

Fig. 5. A. Normal follicular growth. a. day 11, 11 mm. b. day 12, 13.5 mm. c. day 13, 16.5 mm. d. day 14, 20 mm. e. day 15, 21 + cumulus. f. day 20, solid parts, corpus luteum. **B.** Follicle growth and hormone profile. Demonstration of the follicular and corpus luteum growth measured ultrasonically in relation to hormonal values.

520

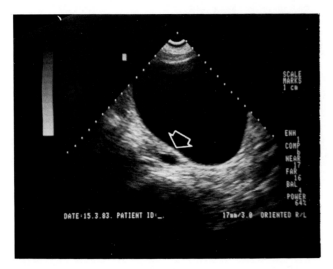

Fig. 6. "Edge-shaped" follicle, 10 mm, onset of cycle (*arrow*).

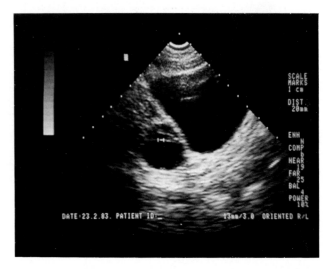

Fig. 7. Round follicle, 20 mm.

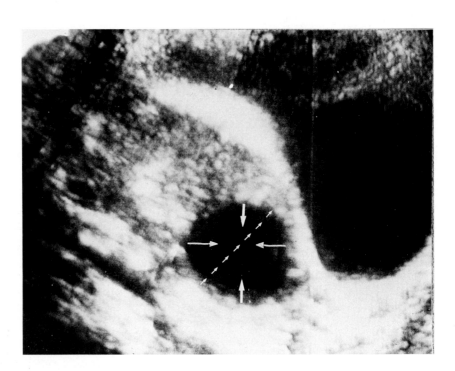

Fig. 8. Follicle measurement (transverse, longitudinal, sagittal).

TABLE 1
Size of the Graafian Follicle Prior to Ovulation in Spontaneous Ovulatory Cycles

Author	Size (mm)		Number of Cycles	Number of Patients	Technique of Measurement	Ultrasonic Equipment
Bryce et al (1980)	24.6 ± 2.3	SD	24	14	Maximum diameter	Comp. scanner
Hackelöer et al (1979)	20.0 ± 0.9	SEM	45	18	Mean derived from maximum transversal, longitudinal and sagittal diameter	Comp. scanner
Kerin et al (1981)	23.2 ± 0.3	SEM	6	56	Maximum diameter	Comp. scanner
Nilsson et al (1982)	21.4 ± 0.8	SD	16	?	Not mentioned	Comp. scanner (2.5 MHz)
	19.3 ± 1.1	SD	10	?	Not mentioned	
Nitschke-Dabelstein et al (1981)	20.9 ± 0.9	SEM	8	6	Mean derived from maximum transversal, longitudinal and sagittal diameter	Comp. scanner (2.5 + 3.5 MHz)
O'Herlihy at al (1980)	20.1 ± 1.6	SD	53	33	Mean derived from maximum transversal, longitudinal, and sagittal diameter	Real-time scanner (correspondent to nine cycles done with compound equipment)
	0.22	SEM				
Queenan et al (1979)	21.1 ± 3.5	SD	18	?	Mean derived from maximum transversal and longitudinal diameter	Sector scanner
Renaud et al (1980)	27 ± 0.3	SEM	10	10	Mean derived from maximum transversal and longitudinal diameter	Comp. scanner (2 MHz)
Robertson et al (1979)	25.0		12	11	Maximum diameter	Comp. scanner
Smith et al (1980)	25.5 ± 0.1	SEM	19	?	Not mentioned	Comp. scanner
Fleischer et al (1981)	20.0 (16–20)		45	15	Mean derived from maximum transversal and longitudinal diameter	Comp. scanner and Sector scanner

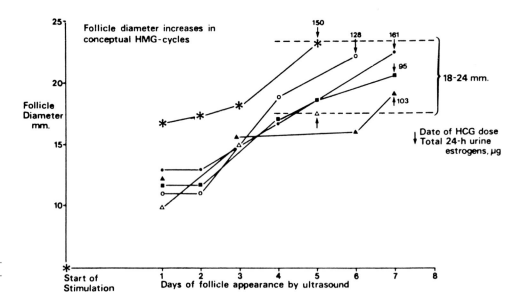

Fig. 9. Conceptual cycles. Follicular diameter increases in conceptual HMG/HCG cycles.

found a larger size on the basis of ultrasonic and laparoscopic findings.[5,6] A follicle size of at least 18 mm was present in those cycles that resulted in conception (Fig. 9).[7] The average time from the initial ultrasonic detection of the dominant follicle (in stimulated cases) to maturity was 6 to 9 days. A shorter time interval may result in only immature follicles!

With ovulation induction using human chorionic gonadotropin (hCG), there is usually a single dominant follicle. In such cases a singleton pregnancy results. Where two or three follicles of similar large diameter are present, multiple pregnancy may occur (Fig. 10). The premature appearance of multiple large follicles is a consequence of overstimulation. Stimulation is discontinued as soon as multiple follicles are seen. Our group and others have shown a high correlation between peripheral plasma hormone estradiol (E2) levels and ultrasonic size in following follicular development both in normal menstrual cycles and following hormonal stimulation.[2,8-10] The importance of ultrasound is even higher in stimulated multifollicular cycles because when estradiol levels are increased, it is otherwise impossible to differentiate between one big and many small follicles (Fig. 11).

DEMONSTRATION OF INTRAFOLLICULAR STRUCTURES

In a large number of cases structures with a reproducible position and shape that represent the cumulus oophorus are visible (Figs. 12–14). Bomsel-Helmreich, Bessis, and Lan Vu Huyen[11] examined sheep ovaries by ultrasound, concentrating on the cumulus struc-

tures, and compared the sonographic and histologic findings. The sonographic appearance of an echogenic area at one edge of the follicle—the cumulus—corresponded to the true cumulus oophorus. In our experience the appearance of the cumulus is followed by ovulation within the next 36 hours. Visualization of the cumulus oophorus allows one to state that the follicle contains an oocyte; this can be important for successful oocyte collection for an in vitro fertilization (IVF) program. Immediately prior to ovulation the cumulus mass becomes free within the follicle.

Immediately after ovulation with the development of the corpus luteum, a blurred margin can be seen around the follicle. Some internal echoes develop within the previously cystic lesion. These changes are

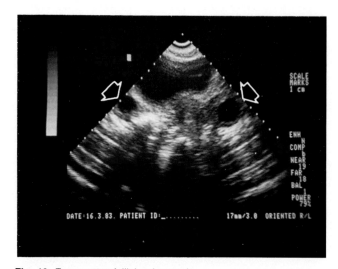

Fig. 10. Two mature follicles (*arrows*).

Demonstration of Mean Follicular Size, Plasma 17β-Estradiol, and Plasma Progesterone
on the Day prior to Ovulation in Stimulated Cycles

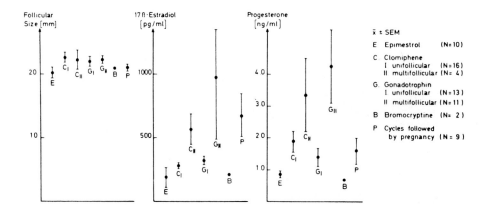

Fig. 11. Follicles and hormones in stimulated cycles.

also reproducible and correspond to the histologic image (Fig. 15).

The following structural changes in the follicle signal ovulation[12,13]:

1. Internal development of solid echoes with a slight decrease in diameter (Fig. 15).
2. Sudden collapse of the follicle with the development of either two cystic structures or one echogenic structure without a distinct outline (Figs. 16A,B).
3. A larger cyst with echogenic structures, in gonadotropin treatment often combined with large lutein cysts (Fig. 17).

The development of internal echoes within the follicle before it reaches the critical size (a minimum of 18 mm) or continuous cystic enlargement up to 30 or 40 mm prove ovulatory failure.

UTERINE ENDOMETRIAL REACTION TO FOLLICLE GROWTH

The normal uterine outline is smooth and its internal texture homogeneous. There is a central echogenic line derived from the superficial layers of the endometrium. During the course of the menstrual cycle the endometrial echo thickens and, based on the increasing fluid within the endometrium, hyporeflective areas develop around the echogenic line (Figs. 18–20).

At the moment of ovulation a sudden loss of fluid

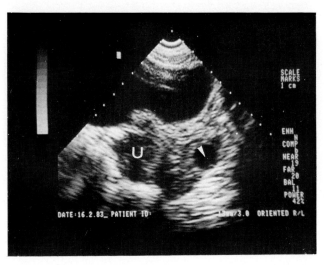

Fig. 12. Transverse scan. Uterus (U) and follicle (*left*) with cumulus oophorus (*arrowhead*).

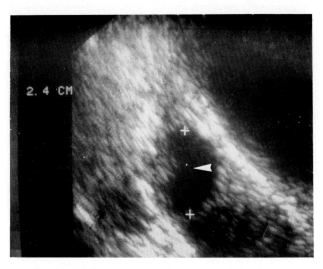

Fig. 13. Mature follicle (24 mm) and cumulus oophorus (*arrowhead*).

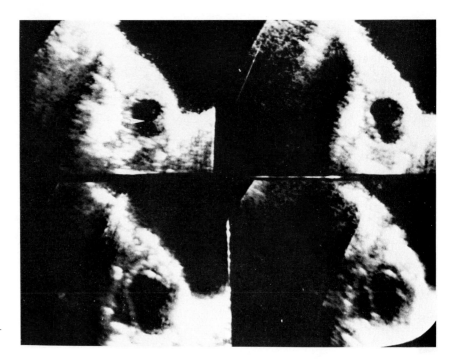

Fig. 14. Different longitudinal scans through follicle with cumulus oophorus (*arrowhead*).

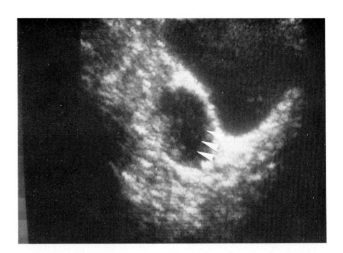

Fig. 15. Longitudinal scan. Early corpus luteum ("invasion" of solid parts).

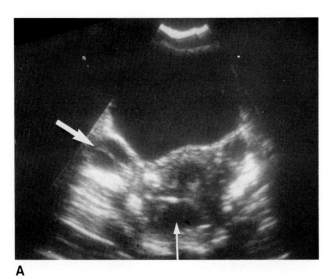

A

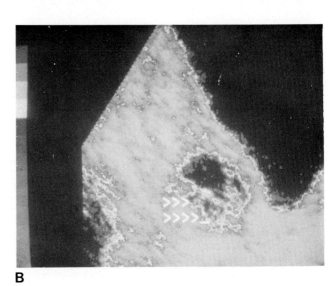

B

Fig. 16. A. Transverse scan. Collapsed follicle in the right ovary (*large arrow*) with fluid in the pouch of Douglas (*small arrow*). **B.** Postprocessed view of corpus luteum showing solid areas.

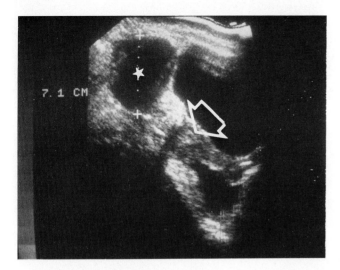

Fig. 17. Cystic corpus luteum (7.1 cm) (*star*) and uterine ring (*arrow*). Pregnancy? Fluid in cul de sac.

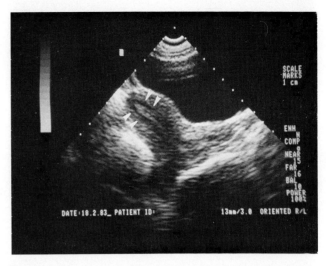

Fig. 18. Longitudinal scan. Thin endometrial line (*arrow*). Early follicle phase.

occurs and a "ring" structure appears within the fundal cavity (Figs. 21,22). This ring is similar to an early gestational sac and to the decidual cast sign in ectopic pregnancy. (The double sac sign can be used to identify an early intrauterine pregnancy as opposed to the endometrial reaction associated with ectopic pregnancy and with normal cyclic changes.[14]) This "ring" has never been seen in the absence of ovulation and is additional confirmation that ovulation has taken place within the previous 12 hours.

At the same time free fluid appears in the pouch of Douglas. The amount of fluid is variable and does not correlate with the volume of a mature follicle (4 to 6 ml). Perhaps a peritoneal reaction to ovulation causes more liquid than expected (Figs. 23 to 26).

Using these signs we believe that we can predict or confirm ovulation within ±12 hours. If serial examinations are performed, ovulation can be predicted within ±6 hours.

PROBLEMS, FAILURES, AND DIAGNOSTIC CLUES

It is sometimes difficult to differentiate between the more lateral part of the uterus, a possible fibroid, and the ovary. In particular, if the ovary is situated close to the uterus, it may be difficult to delineate the exact border between uterus and ovary. If the ovary is lateral and superior to the uterus the iliopsoas muscle and

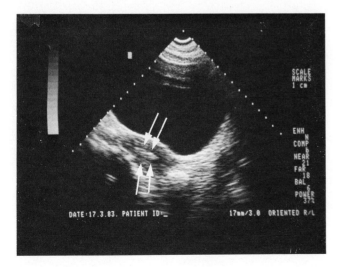

Fig. 19. Longitudinal scan. Thicker endometrial structure (4 to 5 mm) (*arrowheads*). Later follicle phase.

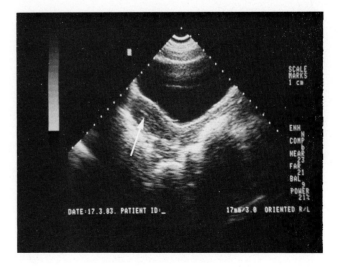

Fig. 20. Longitudinal scan. Thick endometrium surrounded by hyporeflective area (*arrowhead*). Late follicle phase.

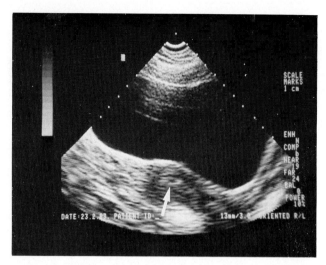

Fig. 21. Longitudinal scan. "Ring" structure (*arrow*). Preovulatory phase.

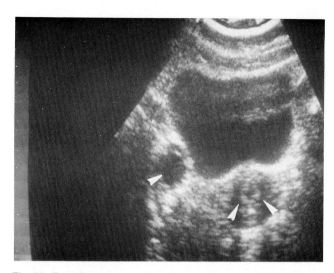

Fig. 22. Transverse scan. Follicle (*right*) and endometrial "ring" (*arrowheads*).

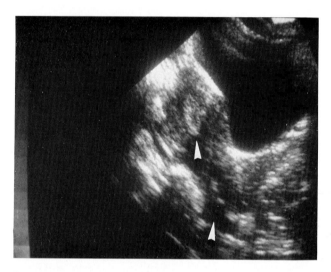

Fig. 23. Longitudinal scan. Ovulation. "Ring" and fluid in pouch of Douglas (*arrowhead*).

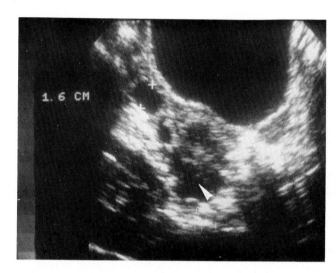

Fig. 24. Transverse scan. Postovulatory follicle with caliper measurements (16 mm) and increased fluid in the pouch of Douglas.

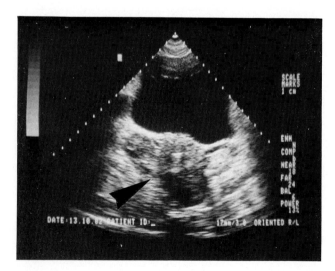

Fig. 25. Transverse scan. Ruptured follicle and fluid in the pouch of Douglas.

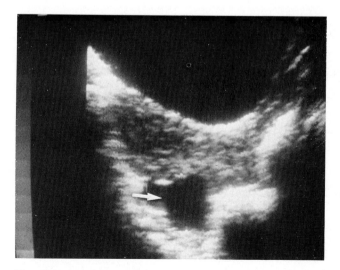

Fig. 26. Longitudinal scan. Large amount of liquid in the pouch of Douglas folowing ovulation (*arrow*).

526

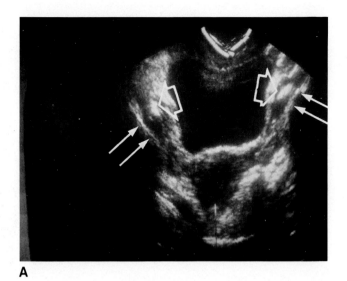

A

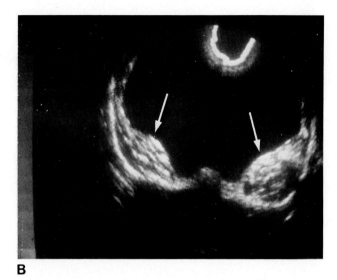

B

Fig. 27. A. Transverse scan. Uterus, ovaries and iliac crest (*arrows*). Note femoral nerve sheath (*open arrow*). **B.** Transverse scan. Iliopsoas muscles (*arrows*).

the iliac bone mimic ovary-like structures (Fig. 27). The ovary can be hidden behind a retroverted uterus, bowel, or lie in the pouch of Douglas. Liquid-filled bowel (especially following large fluid intake to fill the bladder) can mimic a follicle (Fig. 28), but a real-time examination will show peristaltic movement within bowel.

To be certain one is visualizing the unstimulated ovary, a thorough knowledge of the anatomic relationship of the ovary to neighboring structures is important. Two vessels with a close anatomic relationship to the ovary may indicate where the ovary is located by their pulsation. The ovarian arteries, which arise from the aorta, enter the true pelvis through the infundibulopelvic ligament by crossing the common iliac artery just before its bifurcation and reach the ovary

via the mesovarium. These vessels expand during the menstrual cycle and form an extensive vascular arcade that can reach a diameter of up to 11 mm. They can be seen as two parallel lines within the infundibulopelvic ligament (Fig. 29). The position of the ovarian vessels within the infundibulopelvic ligament is consistent in relation to the ovary, so these can be used as a reference plane for ovarian imaging.[15] A segment of the internal iliac artery can sometimes be visualized as well (Fig. 30A) as it passes beneath the ovary. However, the position of the ovary varies in relation to this vessel, so it cannot be used as a landmark.

We recently started to measure the average ovarian blood flow using a combination of a sector real-time scanner and Doppler equipment; it appears that there is an alteration in blood flow shortly before ovu-

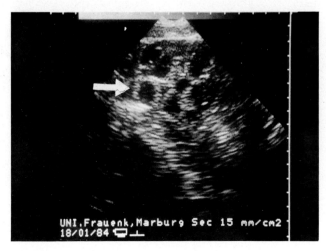

Fig. 28. Liquid-filled bowel mimicking follicles (*arrows*).

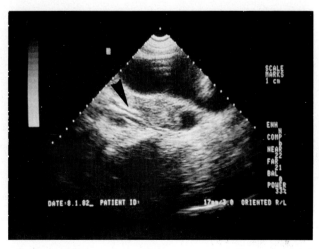

Fig. 29. Longitudinal scan. Ovary and ovarian vessels (*arrow*) in the infundibulopelvic ligament.

528

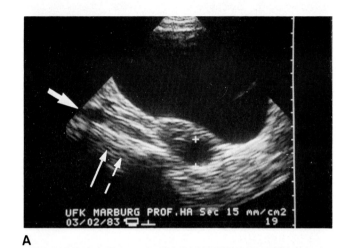

A

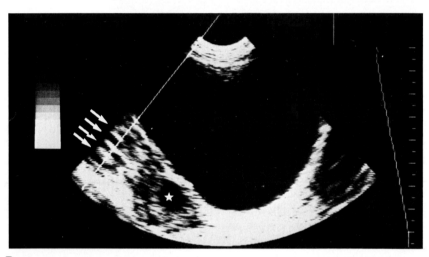

B

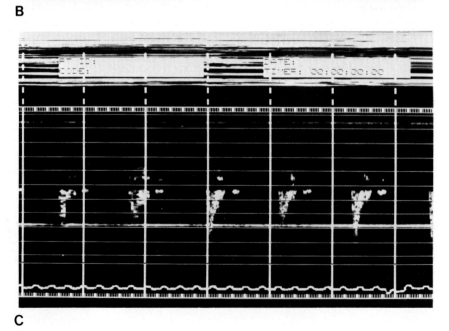

C

Fig. 30. A. Ovary, follicle of 199 mm and hypogastric artery (*arrows*). **B.** Ovarian vessels and,
C. Doppler signal for flow measurement.

lation. If this is correct, we shall have another criteria for predicting ovulation with greater precision and more certainty (Figs. 30B,C).

Ultrasound is an important aid in the treatment of the infertile woman. It more accurately predicts when the follicle is mature and when ovulation occurs than the basal body temperature and is faster than the hormone profile. With respect to in vitro fertilization, ultrasound has two other uses: first, oocyte collection can be undertaken by means of sonographically guided puncture[16,17] via the bladder. Second, replacement of the embryo can be controlled by sonographic visualization of the catheter.

REFERENCES

1. Kratochwil A, Urban G, Friedrich F: Ultrasonic tomography of the ovaries. Ann Chirur Gynaec Fenniae 61:211, 1972
2. Hackelöer BJ, Nitschke S, Daume E, et al: Ultrasonics of ovarian changes under gonadotrophin stimulation. Geburtsh u Frauenheilk 37:185, 1977
3. Hackelöer B-J, Fleming R, Robinson HP, et al: Correlation of ultrasonic and endocrinologic assessment of human follicular development. Am J Obstet Gynecol 135:122, 1979
4. Nitschke-Dabelstein S: Monitoring follicular development using ultrasonography, in Insler V, Lunenfeld B (eds), Infertility—Male and Female. Edinburgh, Churchill Livingstone, 1984
5. O'Herlihy C, De Crespigny L, Lopata A, et al: Preovulatory follicular size: A comparison of ultrasonic and laparoscopic measurement. Fertil Steril 34:24, 1980
6. Kerin JF, Edmonds DK, Warnes GM, et al: Morphological and functional relations of Graafian follicular growth to ovulation in women using ultrasonic, laparoscopic and biochemical measurements. Br J Obstet Gynecol 88:81, 1981
7. Hackelöer B-J: The ultrasonic demonstration of follicular development, in Kurjak A (ed), Recent Advances in Ultrasound Diagnosis. Amsterdam, Excerpta Medica Congress Series No 436, 1978, pp 122–128
8. Robertson R, Picker R, Wilson P, et al: Assessment of ovulation by ultrasound and plasma estradiol. Obstet Gynecol 54:686, 1979
9. Vargyas J, Marrs R, Kletzky O, et al: Correlation of ultrasonic measurement of ovarian follicle size and serum estradiol levels in ovulatory patients following clomiphene citrate for in vitro fertilization Am J Obstet Gynecol 144:569, 1982
10. Nitschke-Dabelstein S, Sturm G, Hackelöer B-J, et al: Ein Vergleich zwischen endocrinologischen und ultrasonographischen. Parametern Geburth u Frauenheilk 40:702, 1980
11. Bomsel-Helmreich O, Bessis R, Lan Vu Huyen R: Cumulus oöphorus of the preovulatory follicle by ultrasound and histology, in Christie AD (ed), Ultrasound and Infertility. Bromley, Chartwell-Bratt. p 105
12. Nitschke-Dabelstein S, Hackelöer B-J, Sturm G: Ovulation and corpus luteum formation observed by ultrasonography. Ultrasound Med Biol 7:33, 1981
13. Hackelöer B-J, Robinson HP: Ultrasound examination of the growing follicle and corpus luteum. Geburtsh u Frauenheilk 38:163, 1978
14. Bradley W, Filly RA, Fiske CE: The double sac sign of early intrauterine pregnancy: Use in exclusion of ectopic pregnancy. Radiology 143:223, 1982
15. Hackelöer B-J, Nitschke-Dabelstein S: Ovarian imaging by ultrasound: An attempt to define a reference plane. J Clin Ultrasound 9:275, 1980
16. Lenz S, Lauritsen JG: Ultrasonically guided percutaneous aspiration of human follicles under local anaesthesia: a new method of collecting oocytes for in-vitro fertilization. Fertil Steril 38:673, 1983
17. Wikland M, Nilsson L, Hamberger L: The use of ultrasound in a human in vitro fertilization program. Ultrasound Med Biol 8 (Suppl 1):208, 1982
18. Eik-Nes S, Marsal HK, Brubakk A, et al: Ultrasonic measurement of human fetal blood flow, in Kurjak A (ed), Recent Advances in Ultrasound Diagnosis 2. Amsterdam, Excerpta Medica International Congress Series 498, 1980, pp 233–240
19. Fleischer AC, Daniell J, Rodier J, et al: Sonographic monitoring of ovarian follicular development. J Clin Ultrasound 9:275, 1981
20. Queenan JT, O'Brien G, Bains L, et al: Ultrasound scanning of ovaries to detect ovulation in women. Fertil Steril 34:99, 1980
21. Ylöstalo P, Lindgren P, Nillius S: Ultrasonic measurement of ovarian follicles, ovarian and uterine size during induction of ovulation. Acta Endocrinol 98:592, 1981
22. Bryce RL, Shuter B, Sinosich MJ, et al: The value of ultrasound, gonadotropin, and estradiol measurements for precise ovulation prediction. Fertil Steril 37:42, 1982
23. Nilsson L, Wikland M, Hamberger BJ: Recruitment of an ovulatory follicle in the human following follicle-ectomy and luteectomy. Fertil Steril 37:30, 1982
24. Renaud R, Macler J, Dervain I, et al: Echographic study of follicular maturation and ovulation during the normal menstrual cycle. Fertil Steril 33:272, 1980
25. Smith D, Picker R, Sinosich M, et al: Assessment of ovulation by ultrasound and estradiol levels during spontaneous and induced cycles. Fertil Steril 33:387, 1980

38 Sonographic Evaluation of Uterine Malformations and Disorders

Arthur C. Fleischer
Stephen S. Entman
Saar A. Porrath
A. Everette James, Jr.

The ability of sonography to depict subtle changes in the myometrium and endometrium makes it the diagnostic modality of choice for the evaluation of many uterine disorders (Figs. 1A,B). With sonography, the uterus can be imaged in several scan planes. With real time, the sonographer can alter the scanning plane and gain settings for optimal depiction of the endometrium and myometrium (Fig. 1C).

Once a uterine lesion is suspected clinically, sonography can be used to establish the presence, size, extent, and internal consistency of the lesion, as well as to detect associated pathology such as liver metastases. Sonography has a major role in differentiating palpable uterine masses from those that arise from adnexal structures. The specific diagnosis can be confirmed by endometrial biopsy, through dilatation and curettage, by other imaging techniques such as hysterosalpingography, and, in some cases, even by direct hysteroscopic visualization.

This chapter discusses and illustrates the sonographic features of the most common uterine malformations and disorders. In order for the sonographer and sonologist to distinguish normal from pathologic findings, a short discussion of the sonographic features of the normal uterus follows pertinent comments concerning scanning technique.

SCANNING TECHNIQUE

Sonographic evaluation of the uterus should be performed when the patient has a fully distended bladder. A fully distended bladder displaces gas-filled bowel loops from the pelvis and places the uterus in a more horizontal plane. This orientation of the uterus relative to the transducer is advantageous since the uterus can be imaged utilizing the better characteristics of axial, rather than lateral, resolution. Occasionally, the urinary bladder can be overly distended, placing the uterus out of the focal range of a medium focused transducer. In these cases, partial voiding will place the uterus in a more optimal focal range. In some patients with very large uterine masses, full distension of the bladder may be impossible and adequate sonographic visualization of the uterus must be attempted without having the bladder fully distended.

When examining a pelvic mass, thought to be of uterine origin, it is important to establish the continuity of that mass with the uterus. Establishing that a mass is uterine involves (1) showing that the vagina leads into the mass and (2) that a linear echogenic interface in the uterus, the endometrium is present. Real-time sonography can be used to optimize depiction of these features.

A water enema can be utilized to further delineate possible masses arising from the posterior aspect of the uterus. In this technique, lukewarm water is slowly introduced into the rectum and followed utilizing real-time sonography. After about 50 to 100 ml of water are introduced, the rectosigmoid colon distends, thereby improving delineation of structures in the posterior pelvic compartment (Figs. 2A,B).[1]

The endometrium can be demonstrated in most patients. The superficial layer of the endometrium is especially prominent during menstruation (Figs. 1D,F). The thickness of the endometrium can usually be esti-

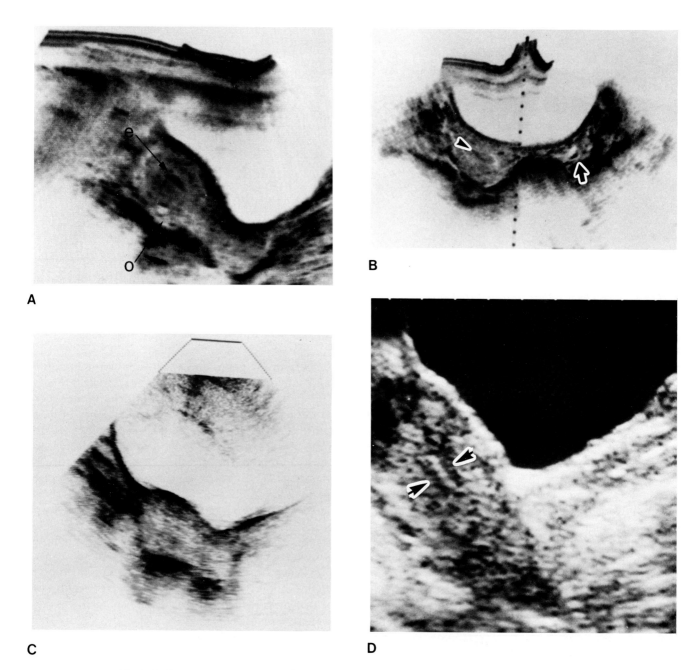

Fig. 1. A. Normal nulliparous uterus (longitudinal, midline). A normal uterus appears as a pear-shaped, mildly echogenic structure which is located immediately posterior to the bladder. The innermost layers of the endometrium (e) appear echogenic and are surrounded by a hypoechoic rim which probably corresponds to the spongiosa and basalis layers. The ovary (o) is also demonstrated posterior to the uterine body. A small sonolucent follicle can be seen within it. (*Reproduced with permission of publisher from Fleischer, James: Introduction to Diagnostic Sonography. New York, Wiley, 1980.*) **B.** Transverse static sonogram demonstrating the sonographic appearance of the uterus as imaged in transverse section through the uterine corpus. The endometrium appears as an echogenic interface (*arrowhead*) that is surrounded by less echogenic halo which probably corresponds to an area of endometrial edema. The uterus is slightly deviated to the right. The left ovary (*arrow*) is also delineated. **C.** Modified longitudinal real-time sonogram of normal uterus. Due to the ability to empirically alter the scan plane, the sonographer can angle the plane of the real-time sonogram to best depict the entire uterus. The thickness of the endometrium is apparent due to its relative hypoechogenicity when compared to the more echogenic myometrium. **D.** Early proliferative endometrium (*between arrow heads*) appearing as two hypoechoic layers on either side of the echogenic innermost surfaces (*cont.*).

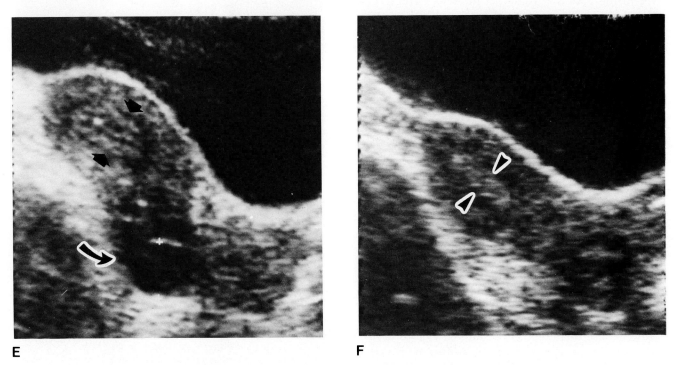

Fig. 1. cont. E. Mid-secretory endometrium appearing as echogenic, thick layer (*between arrowheads*). Several follicles are present within the ovary (*curved arrow*). **F.** Menstrual endometrium appearing as echogenic and irregular (*between arrowheads*).

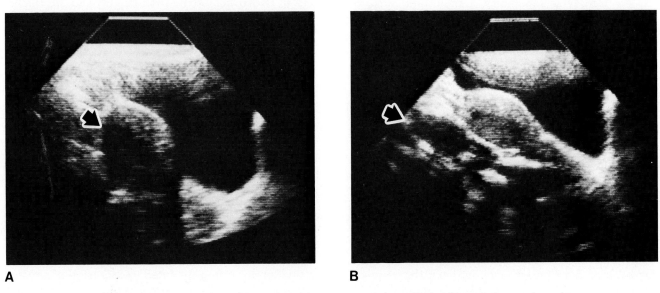

Fig. 2. Water enema. **A.** Longitudinal real-time sonogram demonstrating hypoechoic area (*arrow*) posterior to the uterus. Part of the shadowing distal to the uterus was probably due to reflection and refraction from the curved surface of the uterus. **B.** Longitudinal real-time sonogram taken from still frame during water enema. The rectosigmoid colon (*arrow*) is distended and contains some echogenic fecal material. With water distension of the rectosigmoid colon, the retrouterine area was delineated and the possibility of any mass in the retrouterine area was excluded.

mated by the distance from the echogenic superficial layer to the basalis–myometrial interface. The hypoechoic halo corresponds to edematous and hypertrophied glands within the compactum and spongiosa layers of the endometrium. The "natural contrast" provided by the endometrium can be used to definitively localize the uterus in relation to other masses that may surround or distort it.[2]

Sonographic Features of the Normal Uterus

Sonography can accurately depict the position, size, shape, and texture of the uterus. Each of these features should be carefully assessed and documented sonographically.

The position of the normal uterus is immediately posterior to the floor and dome of the urinary bladder. The fundus is usually anteriorly flexed when compared to the cervix (anteflexed) (Fig. 1A). Although a retroflexed uterus is sometimes a normal variant, this uterine configuration should raise suspicion of posterior compartment pathology (Fig. 3). Retroflexed uteri appear more lobular in contour than anteflexed uteri partly because there tends to be altered venous drainage with consequent myometrial suffusion. Because of the posterior position and curved surface of the fundus, it may be difficult to obtain detailed images of the fundal portion of a retroflexed uterus and the endometrial layer may not be seen.

On transverse sonograms, a significant range of variation in the right to left or anterior–posterior position of the uterus can be observed in normal individuals (Fig. 1B). These positional variants are in part dependent upon the degree of bladder and rectal distension present when the patient is examined.

Before discussing the size and shape of the uterus, the various anatomic segments of the uterus should be described. There are three main divisions of the uterus: the fundus, the corpus or body, and the cervix. The segment of the uterus that lies superior to the entrance of the uterine tubes is designated the fundus. Inferior to the fundus and superior to the internal cervix is the corpus. The lower portion of the corpus is sometimes termed the isthmus. Although the isthmus has been designated as a separate segment of the uterus this seems to be debatable since it is not distinct, on the basis of function or anatomy, from the corpus.[46] There is a transition from the smooth muscle wall of the fundus and corpus to the cervix, which consists of mostly fibrous tissue.

The size and shape of the uterus varies according to the patient's pubertal status, age, and parity.[3] Before puberty occurs, the uterus measures 1.0 to 3.3 cm in length and 0.5 to 1.0 cm in width (Fig. 4A). The cervix

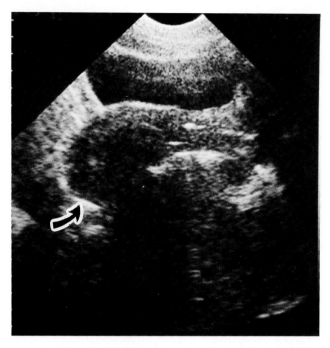

Fig. 3. Longitudinal real-time sonogram demonstrating retroflexed uterus. The uterine fundus (*arrow*) is directed posteriorly. It may be difficult to adequately depict the texture in the uterine fundus in a retroflexed uterus due to problems encountered in imaging tissue around a curved interface.

and isthmus comprise a greater proportion of the uterus (up to two-thirds of the total length) and are thicker than the fundus. In contrast, the nulligravidous, normal post- pubertal uterus measures 7 cm in length, 4 cm in width and height and has a relatively thicker fundus and shortened cervix (Fig. 4B). The multiparous woman typically has a uterus that measures an average of 1.2 cm greater in all directions as compared to the nulligravida individual (Fig. 4C).[4] A postmenopausal woman has a uterus that is smaller than the normal postpubertal woman. The average dimension of the postmenopausal uterus ranges from 3.5 to 6.5 cm long and 1.2 to 1.8 cm thick (Fig. 4D).[5]

The texture of the normal myometrium is consistent throughout all age groups and is of a homogenous, low to medium echogenicity. The innermost layers of the endometrium appear as a central linear echogenicity, most prominent during menses (Figs. 1A–E). Surrounding this echogenic interface is a band of sonolucency that, most likely, corresponds to the spongiosa and basal layers of the endometrium. The endometrium thickens from 2 to 3 mm in the proliferative phase to 3 to 6 mm in the secretory phase. The hypoechoic texture of the endometrium that is most frequently seen in the proliferative phase is related to the particular arrangement of the enlarging glands and stromal

535

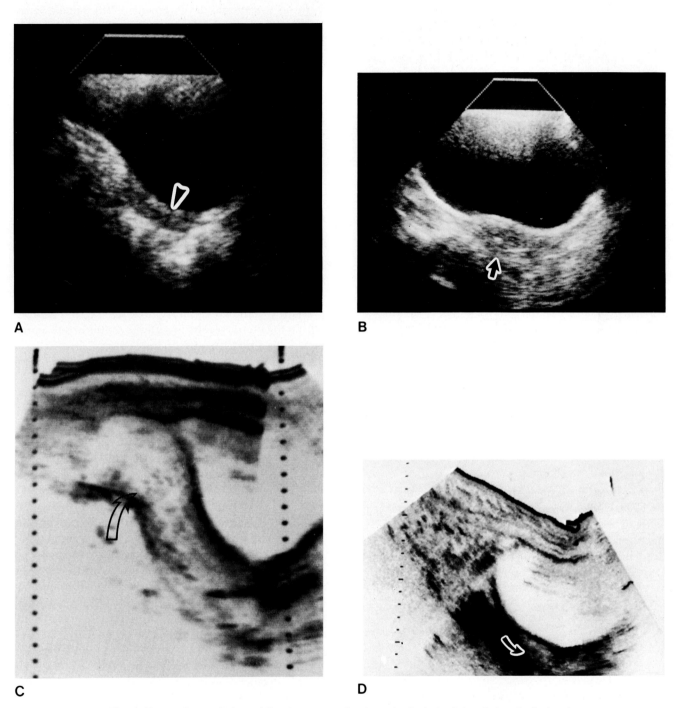

Fig. 4. Range of normal sizes of the uterus according to endocrinologic status. **A.** Longitudinal real-time sonogram of 1-year-old infant. The uterus is tubular and the uterine cervix (*arrowhead*) is slightly thicker than the fundus. **B.** Longitudinal real-time sonogram demonstrating normal postpubertal, nulliparous uterus with uterine fundus (*arrows*) thicker than uterine cervix. **C.** Multiparous uterus (longitudinal, midline). Multiparous (*curved arrow*) uteri are 2 to 3 cm longer than nulliparous uteri. Mild irregularity of the uterine outline may be observed following pregnancy. **D.** Longitudinal static sonogram of normal postmenopausal uterus (*curved arrow*). After menopause, the uterus undergoes atrophy (*cont.*).

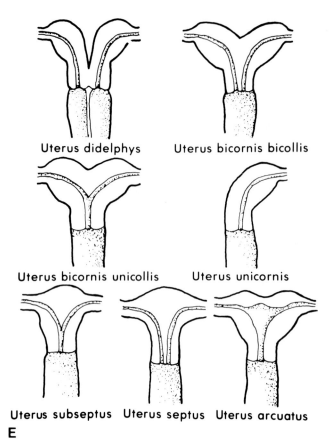

Uterus didelphys   Uterus bicornis bicollis

Uterus bicornis unicollis   Uterus unicornis

Uterus subseptus   Uterus septus   Uterus arcuatus

E

Fig. 4. cont. E. Diagram of various uterine malformations. (*Courtesy of Peter W. Callen, MD.*)

edema (Fig. 1D). A small amount of intraluminal fluid can be observed during the periovulatory and secretory phase of the cycle.[6,47] The endometrium appears thickened and echogenic during the secretory phase (Fig. 1E). The echogenic texture of the secretory endometrium is probably related to the hypertrophied and tortuous glands which contain a mucinous secretion.[48]

CONGENITAL MALFORMATIONS AND RELATED DISORDERS

On pelvic exam, a malformed uterus may be confused with an adnexal mass. Similarly, the sonographic appearance of malformations is sometimes mistaken for uterine fibroids. The most common congenital uterine malformations arise from anomalies of fusion (Fig. 4E). A T-shaped uterus is associated with a history of diethystilbesterol ingestion by the mother of the patient.[7] Hematometra can be secondary to congenital malformation,[8] but also can be acquired secondary to cervical stenosis.[9] Each of these entities is discussed in detail as it relates to sonographic findings.

Fusion Anomalies

Early in embryonic development of the female fetus, the Wolffian and Mullerian duct systems interact to form the internal genitalia. The Wolffian system regresses and the uterus, oviduct, ovary, and vagina are formed from paired Mullerian structures that eventually fuse in the midline.

The most common anomalies of the internal genitalia result from defects in fusion of the paired structures that form the uterus, cervix, and vagina. The degree of failure can range from partial to complete.[3] If there is total failure of fusion, a uterus didelphys will result. In patients with uterus didelphys, two vaginas, two cervices, and two uteri are present. Partial fusion of the Mullerian duct derivatives range from uterus bicornis bicollis (two uterine horns, two cervices), uterus bicornis unicollis (two uterine horns, one cervix), to uterus arcuatus (mildest fusion anomaly with saddle shaped lumen). In all of these fusion anomalies a common central wall between the two uteri is present. Incomplete resorption of the sagittal septum within the uterus results in a uterus septus or subseptus depending upon the size of the septum.

Uterine malformations are suspected from the findings on pelvic examination and are diagnosed definitively by hysterosalpingography. The lesions become important to the sonologist since they can be encountered on pelvic sonography as an incidental finding and confused with an adnexal mass.

Arrested development of the Mullerian ducts results in uterine aplasia; if this occurs unilaterally, a uterus unicornis unicollis is formed. The suffix "cornis" refers to the uterine horns; "collis" refers to the cervix.

Although it is usually not possible to distinguish with any confidence between the more subtle types of uterine anomalies on the basis of sonography, it is important to remember that other congenital defects may be associated with these uterine malformations. Specifically, renal anomalies, such as renal agenesis may be encountered on the same side as the uterine malformation.[10] Thus, if a uterine anomaly is suspected, one should scan the area of the kidneys.

Duplication of the uterus can be associated with an obstructed horn resulting in hematometra. A bicornuate uterus can mimic the sonographic appearance of a parauterine solid mass. However, the typical pear shape of the uterus can be recognized on multiple sagittal scans. Sonographic recognition of a uterine septum in a gravid patient is important because of the predisposition to premature labor, fetal malpresentation, and third trimester bleeding (Fig. 5D).

One of the most common uterine anomalies detected on sonography is the gravid bicornuate uterus. There are usually no symptoms to bring the patient to the attention of the physician and the anomaly is

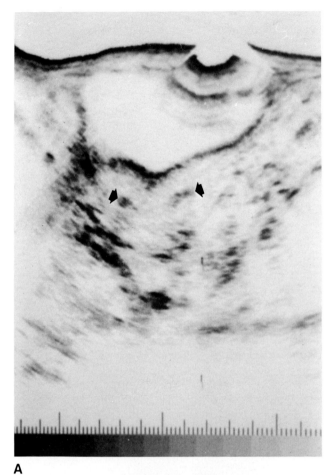

A

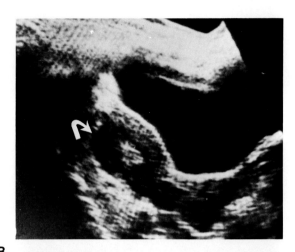

B

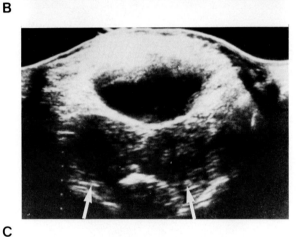

C

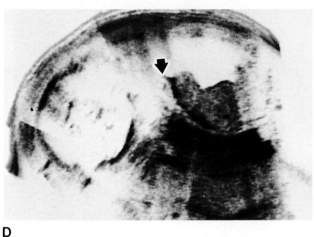

D

Fig. 5. Uterine malformations. **A.** Transverse static sonogram of patient with bicornuate uterus. The endometrium in both horns is echogenic (*arrows*). **B.** Bicornuate uterus (longitudinal, midline). In this longitudinal scan, the uterine outline appears normal (*arrow*). **C.** Transverse scan of patient in 5B, 6 cm above symphysis pubis. The uterine outline is binodular (*arrows*) representing separate horns of a bicornuate uterus. (*Courtesy of Thomas Lawson, MD.*) **D.** Transverse static sonogram showing a partial uterine septum arising from the posterior uterine wall (*arrow*). The fetal head is located within the right side of the fundus, the placenta on the left.

often first discovered when a nodular mass is palpated; the empty horn of the uterus can be mistaken for a parauterine mass on pelvic examination.

The nongravid bicornuate uterus usually appears sonographically as a binodular structure that is best delineated on transverse scans (Figs. 5A,B). It can appear quite similar to leiomyomata except that the myometrium has a homogeneous texture as opposed to

the "whorled" appearance of a leiomyoma. During menstruation two uterine lumina may be identifiable (Fig. 5A).

Hydrometrocolpos and Hematometrocolpos

These conditions can be associated with either congenital or acquired malformation of the uterus or vagina.[8,9] They result from accumulation of secretions

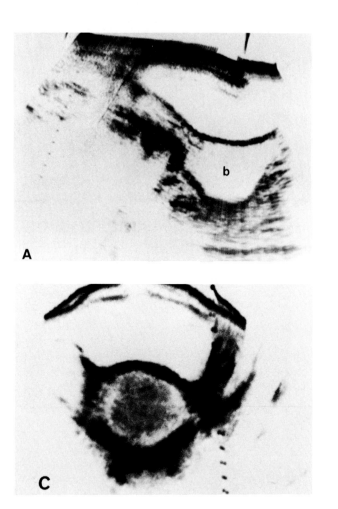

A

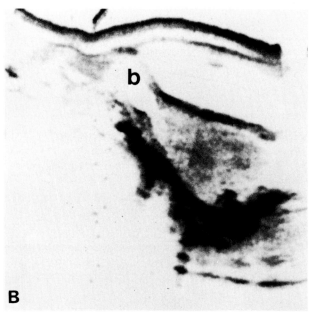

B

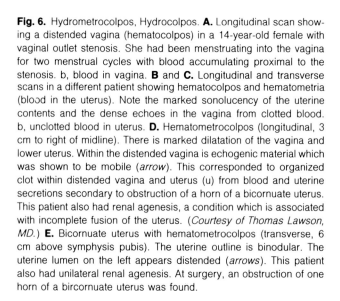

C

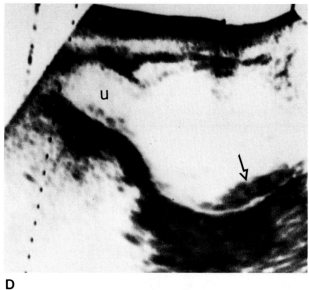

D

Fig. 6. Hydrometrocolpos, Hydrocolpos. **A.** Longitudinal scan showing a distended vagina (hematocolpos) in a 14-year-old female with vaginal outlet stenosis. She had been menstruating into the vagina for two menstrual cycles with blood accumulating proximal to the stenosis. b, blood in vagina. **B** and **C.** Longitudinal and transverse scans in a different patient showing hematocolpos and hematometria (blood in the uterus). Note the marked sonolucency of the uterine contents and the dense echoes in the vagina from clotted blood. b, unclotted blood in uterus. **D.** Hematometrocolpos (longitudinal, 3 cm to right of midline). There is marked dilatation of the vagina and lower uterus. Within the distended vagina is echogenic material which was shown to be mobile (*arrow*). This corresponded to organized clot within distended vagina and uterus (u) from blood and uterine secretions secondary to obstruction of a horn of a bicornuate uterus. This patient also had renal agenesis, a condition which is associated with incomplete fusion of the uterus. (*Courtesy of Thomas Lawson, MD.*) **E.** Bicornuate uterus with hematometrocolpos (transverse, 6 cm above symphysis pubis). The uterine outline is binodular. The uterine lumen on the left appears distended (*arrows*). This patient also had unilateral renal agenesis. At surgery, an obstruction of one horn of a bircornuate uterus was found.

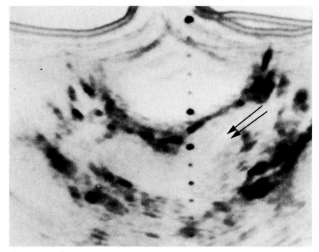

E

and/or blood within the uterus and/or vagina because of congenital or acquired obstruction of a uterine horn, cervix, or vaginal tract.

Obstruction of menstrual flow can be congenital and symptomatic, as in delayed menarche with imperforate hymen or vaginal atresia, or asymptomatic as in a blind horn. Previously healthy women may have neoplastic obstruction of the uterine outflow tract. In either case, retrograde menstruation can occur.[8]

Premenarchal girls may accumulate clear secretions in the vagina (Fig. 6A). Patients with this condition may be asymptomatic but can present with vague pelvic discomfort, pain during defecation or urination due to compression of the rectum or bladder by the pelvic mass. Similar to delayed menarche in the otherwise healthy girl, hematometrocolpos can be encountered in patients with an imperforate hymen or vaginal atresia.

Sonographically, the distended uterus and/or vagina appear as pear-shaped structures with either anechoic or echogenic internal contents. If clotted blood is contained within the uterus, echoes emanating from the clotted blood can be seen. These are usually mobile when the patient is scanned in various positions (Figs. 6B–E).

A small amount of fluid or blood can be present within the endometrial cavity during menstruation or in pelvic inflammatory disease.[9] However, the intraluminal collection encountered in hematohydrometra is quite extensive and should not be mistaken for the small intraluminal fluid collections that can occur around the time of menses.

T-Shaped Uterus

A specific uterine anomaly has been encountered in women whose mothers received diethylstilbestrol (DES) as a part of a therapeutic regimen. DES was widely prescribed to pregnant women between 1940 and 1960 as an antiabortifacient. A great many women who were exposed to DES in utero have multiple benign abnormalities of the genital tract.[11] Additionally, over 300 cases of clear-cell adenocarcinoma of the vagina have been reported to date.[4]

Sonography can be useful in detecting the so-called T-shaped uterus associated with DES exposure. The volume of the T-shaped uterus, calculated from length, width, and anterior–posterior dimension, has been reported to be significantly less than a control group of women at similar ages.[7] The T-shaped uterus derived its name from the hysterographic appearance of the uterine lumen. The abnormal shape and decreased size of the uterus can be detected sonographically by a greater than usual transverse dimension, as well as decreased thickness of the fundus[3] (Fig. 7A,B).

INFLAMMATORY DISORDERS

Pyometrium or suppurative endometritis may occur as a sequela to postpartum infection or after an attempted abortion with septic complications. Pyometrium may also result from cervical stenosis secondary to radiation treatment of the uterine cervix for cervical carcinoma.[9] Endometritis is occasionally seen with salpingitis.

The sonographic appearance of the postpartum uterus is discussed in Chapter 34. Normally, the linear intraluminal interface is centrally located and the endometrial layers are closely opposed.

Puerperal infection is usually caused by retrograde contamination of the uterine cavity by normal or pathogenic vaginal flora introduced during labor. Prolonged labor, premature rupture of membranes, retention of placental tissue, and cervical and vaginal lacerations are known risk factors. Clinically, this condition is suspected when a yellowish-green to black discharge is found in the lochia. The endometritis can progress to a myometritis, parametritis (pelvic lymphangitis), pelvic abscess, and septic pelvic thrombophlebitis.

It is clinically helpful to have a sonographic evaluation of the extent of the disease or involvement of the adnexa. The sonographic appearance of pelvic and adnexal inflammatory disease is discussed in Chapter 40. Endometrial inflammatory suppuration can be depicted as irregular sonolucencies in an enlarged uterine cavity (Fig. 8).

ACQUIRED ABNORMALITIES

Adenomyosis of the uterus is a condition in which clusters of endometrial tissue occur deep within the myometrium. During menstruation, significant pain can be caused by bleeding of the endometrial tissue within the muscle of the uterus. The uterus may be slightly enlarged. Occasionally, this condition can be diagnosed sonographically because of a thickened and "swiss cheese" appearance of the myometrium due to areas of hemorrhage and clot within the muscle (Fig. 9).

Endometrial hyperplasia typically follows prolonged endogenous or exogenous estrogenic stimulation. Adenomatous hyperplasia is thought to be a precursor of endometrial carcinoma.[12] Endometrial hyperplasia may be suspected sonographically because of an abnormal thickening (greater than 6 mm) of the endometrium. Pseudopolyps of endometrial tissue may appear to project into the uterine cavity. Because of the risk of endometrial hyperplasia and carcinoma, the sonographic finding of an abnormally thickened (over

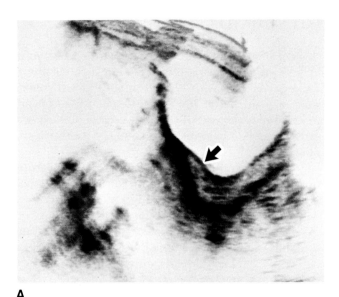

A

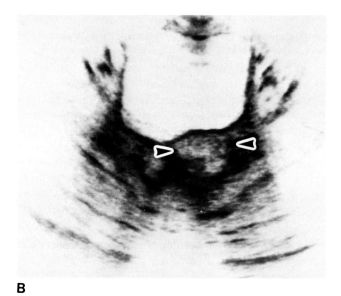

B

Fig. 7. T-shaped uterus. **A.** Longitudinal static sonogram of patient with T-shaped uterus whose mother took DES. The uterine fundus (*arrow*) is thinner than the cervix in this 26-year-old woman. **B.** Transverse sonogram of patient with T-shaped uterus demonstrating greater transverse dimension (*between arrowheads*) of the uterine corpus and fundus.

6 mm from superficial to basalis layers) and echogenic endometrium should prompt further clinical evaluation. Endometrial hyperplasia and carcinoma lead the differential diagnosis for this sonographic finding.

UTERINE LEIOMYOMATA

Clinical Aspects
Uterine leiomyomata are benign tumors that consist of smooth muscle and connective tissue. They are the

most common tumors encountered in gynecologic practice and are commonly referred to as fibroids. It is estimated that leiomyomata are present in 20 percent of women over 35 years of age. They are estrogen-dependent and usually regress after menopause. Leiomyomata are most prevalent in black women and other dark-skinned groups. The usual clinical picture is a palpable mass in a middle-aged woman, but leiomyomata may be associated with excessive menstrual bleedings and pelvic pain. They may cause infertility

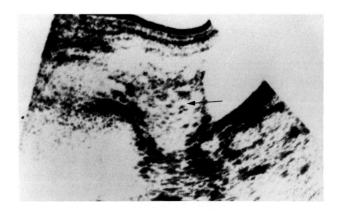

Fig. 8. Endometritis (longitudinal, 4 cm to left of midline). There are numerous sonolucent vesicular areas within the uterus representing small collections of inflammatory fluid within the myometrium (*arrow*). This case was the result of septic abortion. (*Courtesy of Thomas Lawson, MD.*)

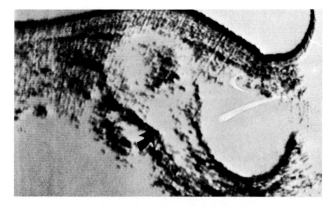

Fig. 9. Adenomyosis (longitudinal, 3 cm to right of midline). The uterine outline is enlarged and its texture is inhomogeneous. There is a sonolucent area along the posterior aspect of the uterus (*arrow*). This was found to be the result of infiltration of endometrial tissue within the myometrium resulting in adenomyosis. This condition is frequently associated with endometrial tissue outside of the uterus (endometriosis). (*Courtesy of Barry Goldberg, MD.*)

due to distortion of the isthmic portion of the tube. In addition, fibroids can contribute to uterine dystocia or pelvic obstruction in the laboring patient.

The fibroid is important to the sonologist for two reasons. First, as a neoplasm, fibroids do have a small malignant potential. More commonly, however, the clinician needs to differentiate a palpable mass of uterine origin from an adnexal mass. For these reasons, detailed sonographic examination of these tumors is warranted.

Leiomyomata usually develop in the myometrium of the upper contractile fundal and corporeal portions of the uterus. Only 3 percent of the leiomyomata are of cervical origin. Intramural leiomyomata cause the uterus to contract, and the resultant compression of these tumors is believed to displace them either toward the peritoneal surface to form subserous nodules or the endometrial cavity to produce submucous nodules. Intraligamentary nodules can arise by extrusion of the intramural nodule retroperitoneally into the areolar tissue between the leaves of the broad ligament. Additionally, rarely, leiomyomata can develop from fibromuscular structures in the round ligament or from those surrounding the vessels.

Leiomyomata of the uterus are usually multiple and of various sizes. A solitary nodule is found in only 2 percent of patients; the number of tumors in a uterus may reach hundreds. The size ranges from microscopic to massive, with 100 pounds being the largest single fibroid reported.[13] Microscopically, each nodule is delineated by a pseudocapsule through which vascular channels enter and arborize within the tumor. As the tumor increases in size, it may eventually outgrow the blood supply and central ischemia is followed by various stages of degeneration.

Degenerative processes may be benign or malignant, asymptomatic or symptomatic. Asymptomatic benign degenerative processes include atrophic, hyaline, cystic, myxomatous, lipomatous, and carneous degeneration.

The symptomatic group includes carneous degeneration, infarction, and infection. Under the effect of strong uterine contractions, rotation of nodules within the pseudocapsule may shear supplying vessels and result in necrobiosis of the tumor. This process is most frequently seen during pregnancy.

Both subserous and submucous nodules may become pedunculated and undergo torsion of the pedicle with subsequent infarction, degeneration, necrosis, and potential infection. For some pedunculated nodules whose circulation is occluded, attachment to the omentum or intestine allows the entry of new vessels and consequently a revitalized blood supply. Under these circumstances, the pedicle may atrophy and the nodule becomes completely detached from the uterus, giving rise to a so-called parasitic fibroid.

Submucous fibroids are prone to necrosis because their blood supply is frequently insufficient to support the tumor mass. More importantly, their exposed position subjacent to the uterine lumen predisposes them to ascending infection. Pelvic inflammatory diseases may involve adjacent fibroids by direct extension or through the lymphatics; curettage can injure submucous nodules and introduce bacteria. Occasionally, when the fibroid is infected, the central core may be filled with purulent material.

Malignant change in the tumor is a generative, not a degenerative process. Although the occurrence of leiomyosarcoma in preexisting leiomyomata is 0.2 percent or less, the prevalence of leiomyomata results in this form of sarcoma being the most common malignant stromal uterine tumor (25 percent). Malignancy in a fibroid is seldom diagnosed preoperatively because there are no characteristic symptoms to distinguish this entity from preexisting fibroid nodules. Sudden accelerated growth in a previously static tumor and postmenopausal enlargement should suggest the possibility of a superimposed malignant process.

The clinical manifestations of fibroids are variable and depend upon the size and number of the tumors, age of the patient, proximity of the tumor to the endometrial cavity, mobility of the fibroid (sessile or pedunculated), and the presence or absence of degenerative processes. Submucous tumors typically encroach on the endometrium and distort the endometrial cavity. Due to pressure necrosis, alteration in the vascular architecture of the endometrium may occur and excessive menstrual bleeding may be the presenting symptom. When submucous fibroids outgrow their blood supply, surface necrosis, slough, and bloody discharge may result. Pain is not a common symptom except in the presence of degenerative changes or torsion of the pedicle of a subserous nodule. Pelvic discomfort due to pressure on the surrounding organs may be present with large tumors, but often the only symptoms are abdominal enlargement and a palpable mass. Pedunculated submucous leiomyomas ("fibroid polyps") can be partially or completely extruded through the cervical canal and can cause infection, necrosis, and ascending endometritis. This event may also be associated with inversion of the uterus. Larger fibroids, particularly of the intraligamentous type, may compress the ureter with resultant hydroureter and hydronephrosis.

Sonographic Features

The typical sonographic appearance of leiomyomata consists of mildly to moderately echogenic intrauterine mass(es) that cause nodular distortion of the uterine outline (Fig. 10A). Small intramural or submucous leiomyomata may be recognized by their distortion of the normally linear central endometrial echoes (Figs. 10B,C). The solid nature of a fibroid often may cause an indentation on the bladder or rectum (Fig. 10D).

The echogenicity of a fibroid depends upon the relative ratio of fibrous tissue to smooth muscle. With a more fibrous component, there is increased echogenicity of the nodule. The sonographic texture of fibroids also depends on the type and presence of degeneration and upon the vascular supply. Interfaces between the normal myometrium and the pseudocapsule of the mass can sometimes be demonstrated (Fig. 10A). In some fibroids, the "whorled" internal architecture can be appreciated (Fig. 10E–G). The whorled appearance corresponds to bundles of smooth muscle and connective tissue that are arranged in a concentric pattern. In some cases, leiomyomas are only minimally echogenic and appear as cystic masses except that their posterior wall is not as prominent as expected (Fig. 10H). Irregular sonolucent areas may be seen within leiomyomata if cystic degeneration has occurred. Calcific degeneration within a leiomyoma is quite common and can be recognized as clusters of high-level echoes that are associated with distal acoustical shadowing (Fig. 10I).

The most common cause of calcification within the uterus is calcific degeneration within a fibroid. Twenty-five percent of one series of 75 cases of fibroids had calcifications.[13] The pattern of calcification varied from a few small foci to a large rim of globular calcification. If the calcification is extensive and is located along the anterior portion of the fibroid, it may prohibit complete sonographic delineation of the mass (Figs. 10J–L). Intrauterine calcifications can also be encountered in uterine sarcomas, but this condition is much less common than leiomyomata.

Other types of degeneration within leiomyomas that produce sonographically recognizable changes in uterine texture include cystic, myxomatous, and hyaline degeneration. Among these, hyaline degeneration is the most common and appears as anechoic areas within a fibroid. Areas of hyaline degeneration can be distinguished from areas of cystic degeneration in that areas of cystic degeneration will usually demonstrate distal wall enhancement (Figs. 10A,I).

Leiomyomas that are pedunculated can be confused with other adnexal masses if their pedicle is not visualized. The most common location of pedunculated leiomyomas is superior to the uterine fundus. In most cases, an echogenic interface corresponding to the tissue plane connecting the fibroid and the fundus can be delineated. Pedunculated subserosal fibroids can also extend into the broad ligament and thus appear as an extrauterine mass (Fig. 10M). However, the typical whorled configuration of the fibroid usually can be recognized (Fig. 10N). In order to ascertain whether or not a mass is connected to the uterus by a pedicle, applying slight pressure to the mass while scanning has been suggested.[14] The mass will move with the uterus if the two are connected. This procedure should be performed by an experienced gynecologist and monitored with real-time sonography.

Submucous leiomyomata may be difficult to differentiate from intramural leiomyomata. Both may produce distortion of the endometrial echoes. Submucosal fibroids are best documented by hysterosalpingography.

Fibroids may be particularly difficult to detect in the retroverted uterus. Because the uterine fundus curves posteriorly in the retroverted uterus, this area may appear to be relatively sonolucent. Appropriate gain settings and TCG curves should be used; a hypoechoic area within the fundus of a retroverted uterus may be technical in origin rather than a fibroid (Fig. 3).

Serial sonographic evaluation of leiomyomata can be of significant clinical value to the clinician. Follow-up scans of the fibroid uterus of a pregnant woman may help assess the growth and accelerated degeneration of this mass.[15,16] A recent study of fibroids during pregnancy revealed that the size of most fibroids remains stable during pregnancy[16] (see Chapter 33). Since fibroids should regress after menopause, serial sonograms can objectively document enlargement or regression of leiomyomata in the older woman.

Sonographic Mimics of Fibroids

Occasionally, solid masses that are adjacent to the uterus appear as masses within the uterine contour. This finding has been referred to as "the indefinite uterus sign."[17] In this setting, a retrouterine mass may be misdiagnosed as an enlarged uterus. The most common solid masses to simulate the sonographic appearance of a fibroid are the solid ovarian tumors (Fig. 11E). Metastases that settle and enlarge in the cul de sac, such as those associated with breast tumors, can also produce apparent enlargement of the uterine contour (Figs. 11A–D).

BENIGN LESIONS OF THE CERVIX

Condylomata accuminata or venereal warts can occasionally be depicted in pelvic sonography. They can appear as a solid mass, distorting the contour of the cervix (Fig. 12A,B,D). Epithelial inclusion cysts of the cervix (Nabothian cysts) appear as small cysts within the borders of the cervix (Fig. 12C).[18]

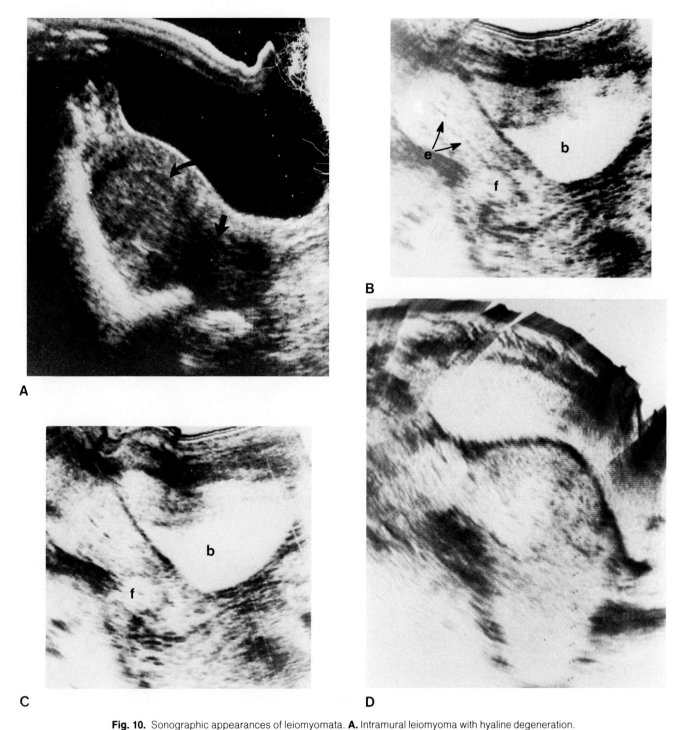

Fig. 10. Sonographic appearances of leiomyomata. **A.** Intramural leiomyoma with hyaline degeneration. There is an area of relatively diminished echogenicity along the posterior aspect of the uterine myometrium. This mass causes nodular enlargement of the uterine outline (*curved arrow*). There is a sonolucent area along its inferior aspect (*arrow*) which most likely represents hyaline degeneration within the mass. Hyaline and cystic types of degeneration appear as focal areas of relative sonolucency within leiomyomas. (*Courtesy of Thomas Lawson, MD.*) Longitudinal scan **B** in the midline and **C** 1 cm to the left, showing an anterior deviation of a portion of the endometrial canal (e) with a well-defined sonolucent area due to a fibroid (f), causing the deviation. The endometrial canal is seen better in **A** than in **B.** These and other cases show the need of multiple scans to fully recognize the extent of pathology. b, bladder. **D.** Longitudinal scan showing an enlargement extending from the inferior–posterior aspect of the uterus with decreased echoes and decreased transonicity, representing a fibroid (*cont.*).

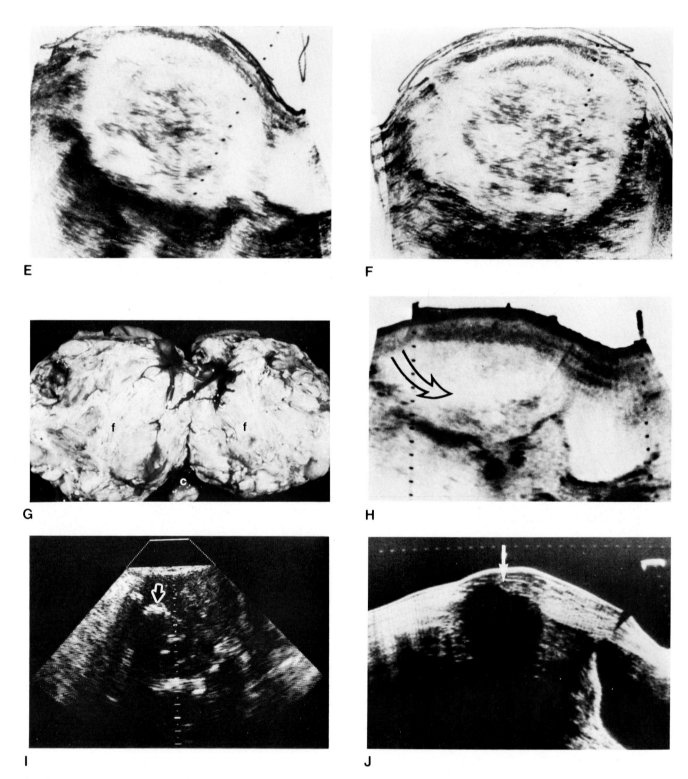

Fig. 10. cont. Longitudinal **(E)** and transverse **(F)** scans showing a "whorled" pattern of echoes within the large uterine fibroid. Echogenic and sonolucent areas are intermingled. **G.** Photograph of specimen bivalved. Note the cystic areas within the fibroid (f) which accounted for the sonolucent areas on the ultrasound. c, cervix. (*Courtesy of Phillip Ralls, MD.*) **H.** Parasitic leiomyoma with cystic internal degeneration (longitudinal, 4 cm to left of midline). This subserosal pedunculated leiomyoma had derived its blood supply from the mesentery. Infarction resulted in central cystic degeneration (*arrow*). **I.** Longitudinal real-time sonogram of fibroid containing multiple calcifications. Calcifications appear as echogenic foci (*arrow*) with distal shadowing. **J.** Calcified uterine leiomyoma (longitudinal, 4 cm to right of midline). This leiomyoma had extensive calcification along its anterior wall which produced posterior acoustical shadowing and limited delineation of the posterior aspect of the mass (*arrow*). These calcifications were demonstrated by abdominal radiographs (*Courtesy of Thomas Lawson, MD*). (*cont.*)

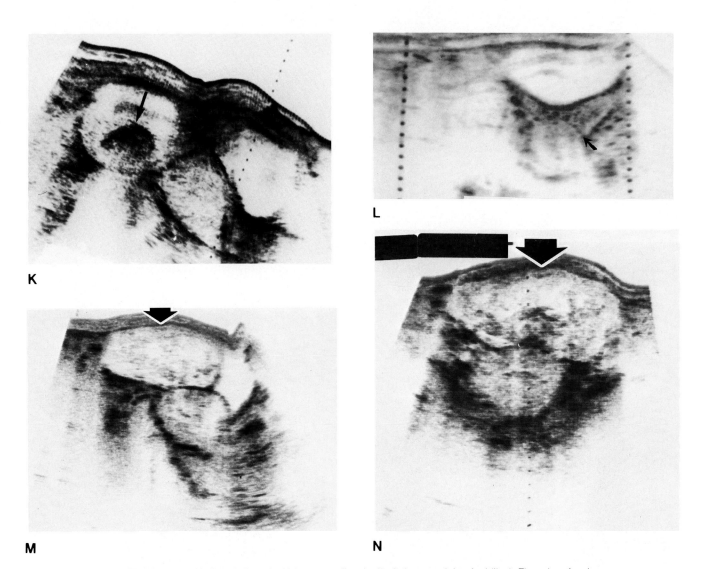

Fig. 10. cont. K. Calcified uterine leiomyoma (longitudinal, 6 cm to right of midline). There is a focal area of high-level echoes with posterior acoustical shadowing corresponding to an area of calcification within this leiomyoma (*arrow*). (*Courtesy of Roger Sanders, MD.*) **L.** Longitudinal static sonogram of subserosal pedunculated fibroid. There is an echogenic interface (*arrow*) between the uterine fundus and the subserosal fibroid (*cont.*). Intraligamentous fibroid (*arrow*) as depicted on this longitudinal **(M)** and transverse **(N)** static sonograms. The mass appears to be extrauterine but was identified as a fibroid due to its characteristic whorled appearance. The uterus is enlarged and had adenomyosis.

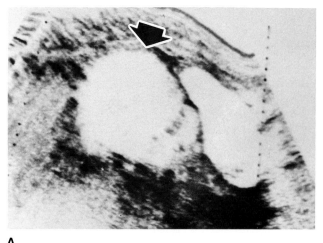

A

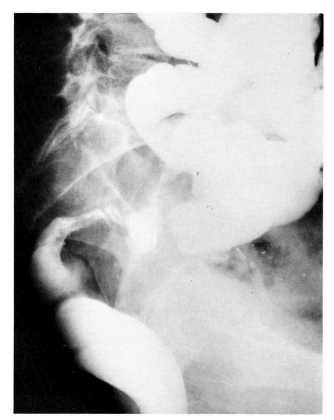

B i

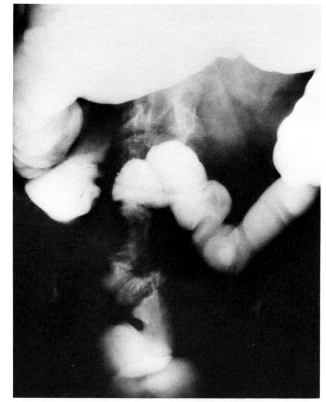

B ii

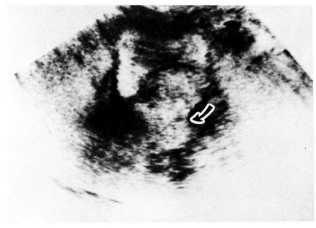

C

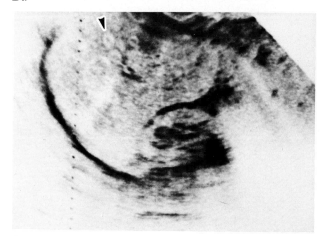

D

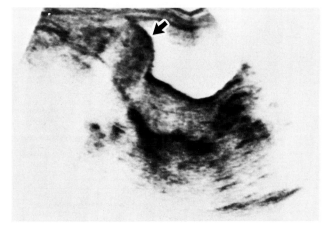

E

MALIGNANT TUMORS OF THE CERVIX AND UTERUS

With the increased use of ultrasound for the evaluation of uterine pathology, certain sonographic characteristics of the uterus and uterine tumors have been recognized.[19]

Changes in the ultrasonic configuration of the uterus that allow a tumor to be detected are:

1. Distortion or change of the uterine outline or contour
2. Distortion or deviation of the endometrial cavity or the cervical canal
3. Change in the sonographic texture of the uterus
4. Change in the transonicity, or attenuation properties of the uterus
5. The presence of calcium within the uterus
6. The presence of a mass adjacent to the uterus
7. Changes in other pelvic organs
8. Secondary tumor signs, such as dense echoes within the endometrial canal from the accumulation of blood

Several reviews of the use of ultrasound in gynecology exist[20-24] but few deal specifically with gynecologic malignancy.[25,26] Malignant tumors of the uterus that may be detected by ultrasound include:

1. Carcinoma of the cervix
2. Carcinoma of the endometrium
3. Tumors of connective tissue
   a. Leiomysarcoma
   b. Sarcoma
   c. Endometrial stromal sarcoma
4. Mixed tumors
   a. Carcinosarcoma
   b. Sarcoma botryoides
5. Rare tumors
   a. Lymphoma
   b. Malignant melanoma
6. Metastatic

Most malignant tumors of the uterus and cervix are small, and may not be detected by ultrasound. Most carcinomas of the cervix and half of the carcinomas of the endometrium are this small.[27] Nevertheless, sonologists should be alert to irregularities in the outline of the cervical canal and the uterine cavity for evidence of exophytic overgrowth of tissue or endophytic crateriform destruction of the tissue. This information can be useful to the clinician planning for a definitive diagnostic procedure.[28]

CARCINOMA OF THE CERVIX

Squamous cell carcinoma of the cervix is one of the common malignancies among American women. It is epidemiologically linked to lower socioeconomic status, early sexual exposure, multiple sexual partners, and positive herpesvirus type 2 titers. The incidence of the disease and the death rate have both decreased dramatically since the use of Pap smears for early detection of squamous cell abnormalities. Nevertheless, 16,000 women each year develop invasive cancer of the cervix. It is clear that early cancers are more readily treated successfully than advanced disease.

CLASSIFICATION OF SQUAMOUS CELL CARCINOMA OF THE CERVIX

Stage O	Carcinoma in situ, preinvasive carcinoma, intraepithelial carcinoma
Stage I	Carcinoma strictly confined to the cervix
Stage IA	Microinvasive
Stage IB	Carcinoma confined to the cervix
Stage IC	(Occult) carcinoma confined to the cervix, but clinically detectable
Stage II	Carcinoma extends beyond the cervix, but has not reached the pelvic wall or the lower third of the vagina
Stage IIA	Medial parametrial extension with vaginal involvement
Stage IIB	Lateral parametrial involvement

Fig. 11. Sonographic mimics of fibroids. **A.** Longitudinal static sonogram of Krukenberg tumor of the ovary (*arrow*) adjacent to the uterus. Due to its homogeneous texture and close apposition to the uterus, it was misinterpreted as a uterine fibroid. **B.** Barium enema of a patient with a cul de sac mass. The rectal mucosa appears intact. The rectum appears to be deformed by an extraluminal mass. **C.** Transverse sonogram patient depicted in **B** demonstrating a moderately echogenic mass (*arrow*) adjacent to the uterus mimicking a cervical fibroid. **D.** The patient also had intrahepatic metastasis (*arrowhead*). At surgery, the pelvic mass was found to represent metastases from breast carcinoma to the cul de sac region. **E.** Longitudinal static sonogram of solid teratoma superior to the uterus. This solid mass appeared to be contiguous with the uterus and simulated the appearance of a fibroid.

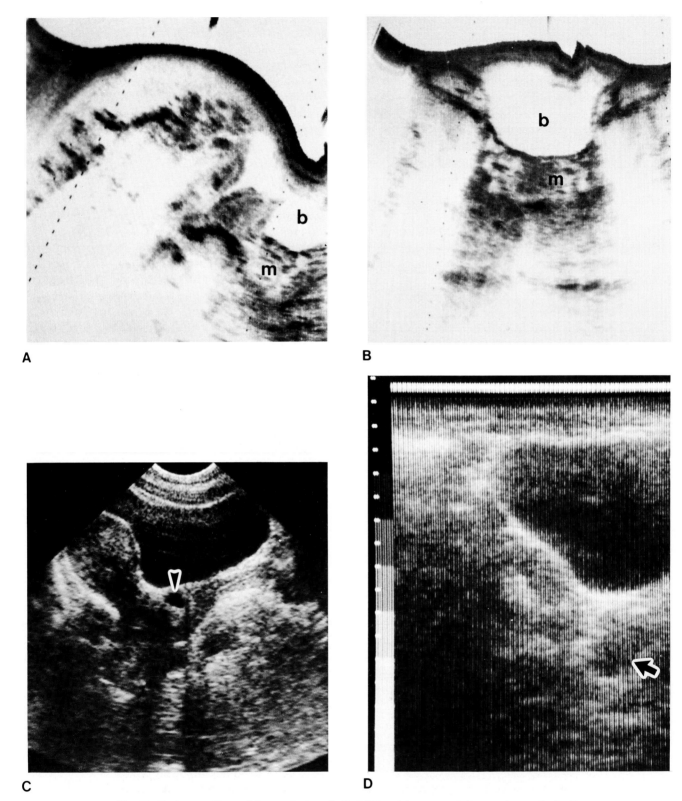

Fig. 12. Benign conditions of the cervix. Longitudinal **(A)** and transverse **(B)** scans in a patient with several condylomata of the cervix and vagina presenting as a vaginal mass (*m*) on ultrasound. Note concomitant intrauterine pregnancy. (*Courtesy of Caroline Yeager, MD.*) b, bladder. **C.** Longitudinal real-time sonogram depicting small cyst (*arrowhead*) in cervical region representing a Nabothian cyst. **D.** Longitudinal real-time sonogram demonstrating enlargement of the cervical area due to condylomata (*arrow*).

Stage III — Carcinoma has extended onto the pelvic wall or involves the lower third of the vagina

Stage IIIA — No extension onto the pelvic wall, but involvement of the lower third of the vagina

Stage IIIB — Carcinoma has extended onto the pelvic wall; hydronephrosis or nonfunctioning kidneys occurs

Stage IV — Carcinoma has extended beyond the true pelvis or has involved the mucosa of the bladder or rectum

Stage IVA — Biopsy-proven rectal or bladder involvement

Stage IVB — Distant metastases

The impact of stage of disease on 5-year survival is dramatic. Carcinoma in situ is essentially 100 percent curable, stage I is 80 percent curable, and Stage III is 40 percent curable. When the tumor is superficial, there is little role for ultrasound. Ultrasound is principally useful in the evaluation of advanced lesions. If there is a large exophytic or fungating tumor growth, there will be an ultrasonically detectable mass. For Stages II, III, and IV, ultrasound can demonstrate the extent of the disease.[29] It is helpful in the evaluation of distant metastases to organs such as the liver. Ureteral obstruction can be shown with noninvasive techniques. This common disease is now considered using the guidelines outlined at the beginning of the chapter.

Distortion or Change of the Cervical Outline or Contour

Carcinoma of the cervix even in the earlier stages may present as a large mass arising from the cervix. Sonographic identification of the cervix can sometimes be enhanced by the use of a fluid soaked tampon within the vagina (Fig. 13). As cervical carcinoma progresses from Stage I to other stages with involvement of the surrounding tissue, the size of the tumor mass may increase (Figs. 14A–D). The definition of the margin of the mass can be clarified by the use of the water enema.[30] Care must be taken to differentiate between normal variations in cervical size and true pathology. The cervix itself can be somewhat patulous and rather large without being abnormal. In addition, benign entities such as inflammatory changes or condylomata (venereal warts) of the cervix may cause cervical enlargement and irregularity. Postsurgical changes such as the cystic variation noted following cone biopsy may be confusing. The uterine fundus itself may sometimes become enlarged, which may suggest that the cancer has extended beyond the cervix and has involved the

endometrial cavity. Patients with other gynecologic lesions, such as fibroids or adenomyosis, can develop carcinoma of the cervix or of the endometrium so that the overall size of the uterus or distortion of the uterus does not necessarily mean tumor extension. Approximately one-third of our cases of carcinoma of the cervix had a normal sized uterus (Fig. 15).[31] Of the remaining third, about one-half had fibroids incidental to the cancer. Uterine enlargement due to tumor alone is not a common finding, although it is more likely to occur with advanced disease.

Distortion or Deviation of the Endometrial Canal

Little distortion or deviation of the endometrial cavity is seen since this type of tumor primarily involves the cervix. If distortion is present, it may well be due to other pathology.

Texture Changes

Changes in ultrasonic texture and transonicity are difficult to visualize because the cervix is not well delineated. Hypoechoic masses enlarging the cervix may be seen in diffuse neoplasms (Fig. 16).

Focal Echogenicities With or Without Shadowing Due to Calcium

Calcification in the area of the cervix is rare but may occur (Fig. 17). More frequently it is due to coincident leiomyoma. Calcified pheboliths may also appear as focal echogenicities near the adnexa.

Presence of a Mass Adjacent to the Uterus

This is not an uncommon finding. The tumor mass may extend from the cervix into the parametrium and appear as a contiguous mass. Occasionally, such a mass may appear somewhat removed from the uterus. The echo pattern of the mass may be totally different from either the texture of carcinoma of the cervix or that of the uterus. Lymph node metastases to the parametrium appearing as separate masses not contiguous with the uterus itself may also be seen.

Extension of tumor into the parametrium changes the clinical staging and is an important finding with sonography or computed tomography (Fig. 18). Not all adnexal parametrial masses represent tumor extension; concomitant leiomyomata or ovarian masses may simulate extension. Nodal metastases to more distant nodes along the iliac chain with apparent skip areas may be seen (Fig. 19). This finding is of significant practical importance in patient management, for pa-

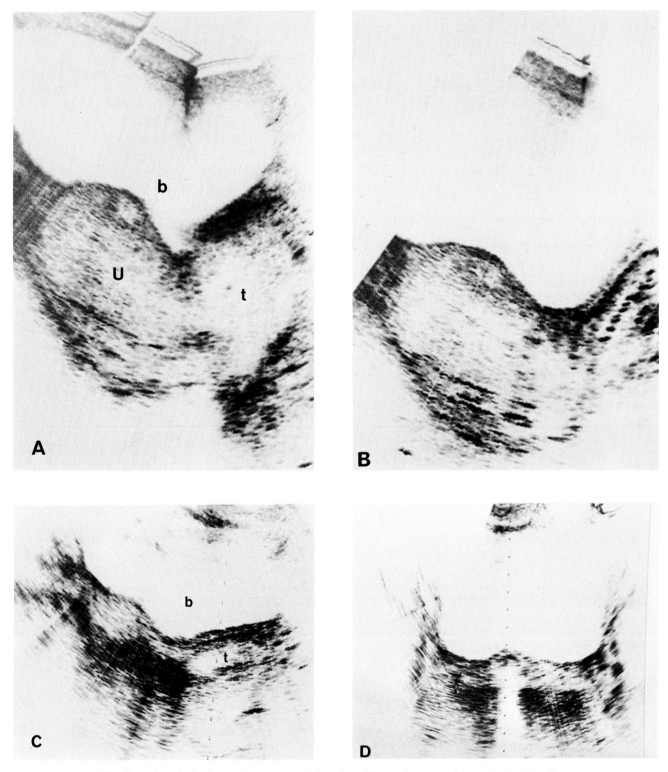

Fig. 13. A. Longitudinal scan showing poor delineation of the vagina caused by marked shadowing from a vaginal tampon (t). **B.** Same patient—longitudinal scan with the tampon removed. **C** and **D.** Longitudinal and transverse scans in another patient showing a sonolucent area posterior to the cervix. Shadowing is seen on the transverse scan. This represents a tampon soaked with blood. b, bladder; t, tampon.

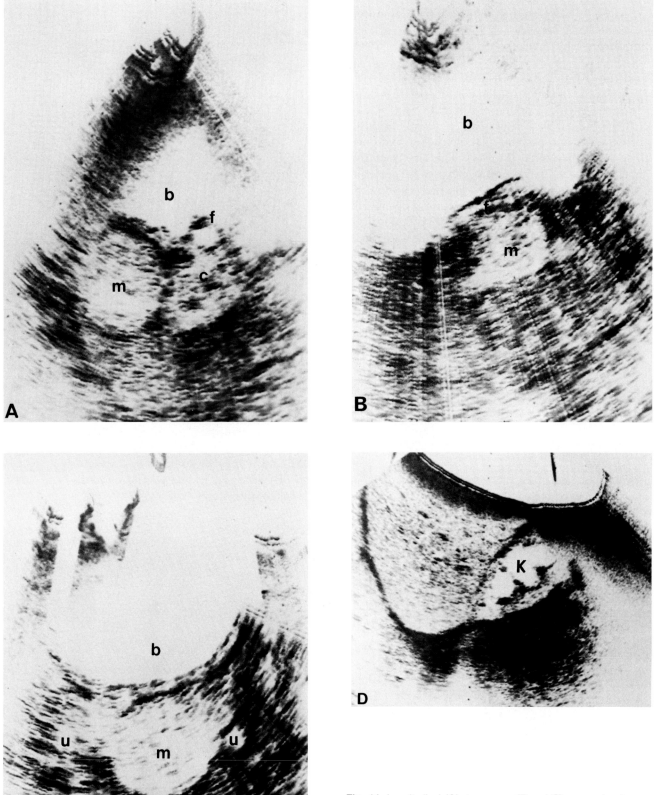

Fig. 14. Longitudinal **(A),** transverse **(B** and **C)** scans showing enlargement of the cervix (c) by carcinoma (m). There is a loss of the wall between the bladder and vagina with a large fistulous tract (f). Dilatation of the ureters is seen (u). b, bladder. **D.** Longitudinal section through the liver. The right kidney (k) is hydronephrotic.

tients with lymph node involvement will respond less satisfactorily to surgery than radiotherapy. Computed tomography has been shown to delineate associated lymphadenopathy much better than sonography.[32,33]

Effect on Other Pelvic Organs

With advanced tumors, invasion of other pelvic organs, such as the vagina, bladder, and rectum, can be detected on sonography. The ureter is frequently invaded or compressed, and ureteral dilation and/or hydronephrosis can be detected (Fig. 14). The effects of the neoplasm on other pelvic organs can also be depicted by conventional radiographic exams such as intravenous pyelography for the ureter or barium enema for the rectum. Computed tomography (CT) is better than ultrasound at detecting pelvic wall extension (Figs. 20A–C).[32,33]

Secondary Signs

Some bleeding may be associated with carcinoma of the cervix, and there may be dense echoes within the endometrial canal due to blood. This is a nonspecific finding. Tumor obstruction of the cervix can occur with carcinoma of the cervix, or cervical stenosis secondary to radiation therapy, may result in hematometra (Fig. 21).[9,34]

CARCINOMA OF THE UTERUS

Carcinoma of the uterus is a very different disease from carcinoma of the cervix, with a different progno-

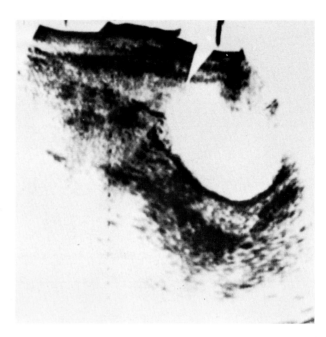

Fig. 15. Longitudinal scan showing an atrophic uterus with normal texture and transonicity. This 57-year-old woman had a Stage I carcinoma of the cervix.

sis, lymphatic pathways of spread, and treatment. Histologically, most carcinomas of the cervix are squamous cell carcinomas, whereas endometrial lesions are usually adenocarcinomas. An endometrial adenocarcinoma that extends into the cervix is designated corpus et colli, and it may be difficult to distinguish it from a primary adenocarcinoma of the endocervix, thereby confusing the site of origin.

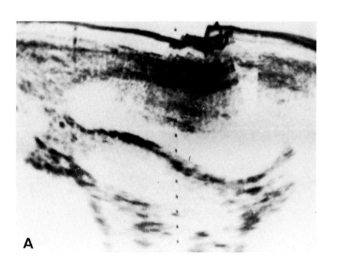

A

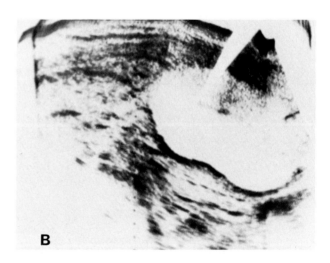

B

Fig. 16. A. Longitudinal scan showing enlarged uterus (10 cm in length) with decreased texture and transonicity. **B.** Same patient, longitudinal scan, 1 year later, showing a normal sized uterus (7 cm) with normal echogenicity. This followed a course of radiation therapy and radium implantation for Stage II A carcinoma of the cervix. Occasionally, the uterus will regain its normal size and echo pattern after radiation therapy.

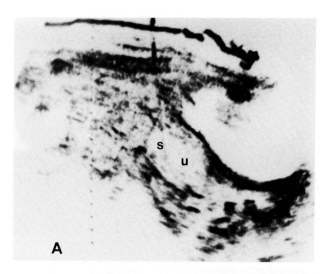
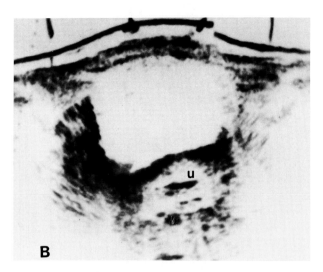

Fig. 17. Longitudinal **(A)** and transverse **(B)** scans in a woman with carcinoma of the cervix. There is uterine enlargement (u), probably due to the coexistence of cervical and fundal fibroids, which appear as dense calcifications in the cervix and a sonolucent area in the fundus (s). Note the shadowing of the cervical fibroids on the transverse scan.

Adenocarcinomas of the uterus is typically a disease of perimenopausal and postmenopausal women.[35] Epidemiologically, these patients tend to have had fewer pregnancies and a later first pregnancy than patients with cervical lesions. An association with estrogen therapy has been strongly suggested. Occasionally, endometrial carcinoma can occur in young women; 2 percent are under the age of 35 and 5 percent are under the age of 40.

Clinically, adenocarcinoma of the endometrium typically presents with a watery or bloody discharge. These tumors of the uterine corpus spread either by local invasion to surrounding organs, such as the bladder and rectum, or by lymphatic spread.

STAGING OF CARCINOMA OF THE UTERUS

Stage I	Carcinoma confined to the body of the uterus
Stage IA	Length of the uterine cavity is 8 cm or less
Stage IB	Length of the uterine cavity is greater than 8 cm
Stage II	Carcinoma has involved the body of the uterus and the cervix
Stage III	Carcinoma extends outside the uterus, but not outside the true pelvis
Stage IV	Carcinoma extends outside the true pelvis or has obviously involved the mucosa of the bladder or rectum

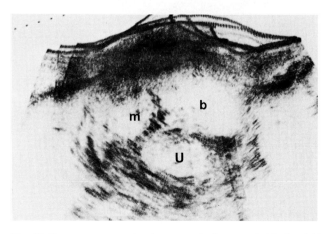

Fig. 18. Transverse scan showing a neoplastic mass (m) in the right adnexal area against the pelvic side wall representing nodal spread of cervical carcinoma. b, bladder; U, uterus.

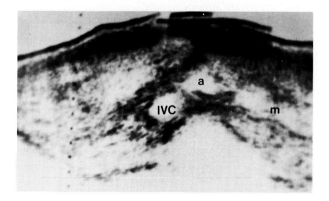

Fig. 19. Transverse scan in 78-year-old woman showing nodes at the bifurcation of the aorta (m). This means the patient has a Stage IV carcinoma of the cervix. a, aorta; IVC, interior vena cava.

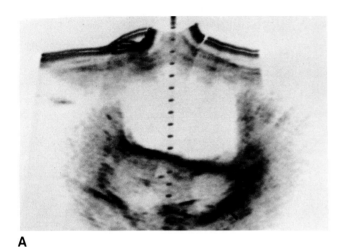

A

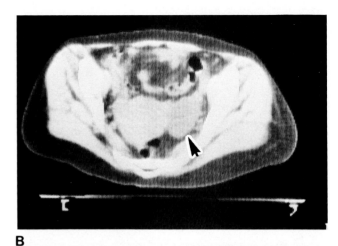

B

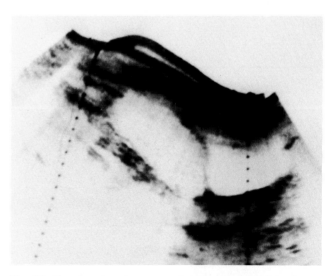

C

Fig. 20. A. Transverse static sonogram of patient with Stage IIB carcinoma of the cervix. The tumor (*arrow*) appears to extend into the left pelvic side wall. **B.** CT scan obtained at same level suggesting extension of tumor to left pelvic side wall (*arrow*). The surrounding fat planes are intact. **C.** The presence of associated lymphadenopathy in the right hypogastric lymph node group (*arrows*) was depicted on CT and not on sonography.

Sonography and computed tomography have a role in assessing the extent of disease. The more advanced stages of adenocarcinoma of the endometrium can be differentiated from the less extensive stages by sonography.[19,36-38] Specifically, patients with stages I and II are described as having a normal or bulbous uterus and a normal or hypoechoic parenchymal pattern. It is readily apparent that ultrasound can be useful in the distinction between Stage IA and IB by sizing the uterine lumen. Conventionally, this information is obtained by using a probe to sound the length of the endometrial canal, but ultrasound is an equally effective way of evaluating uterine size in a less invasive fashion. A patient with Stage III or IV cancer will usually have a globular uterus with a mixed echo pattern arising from the endometrium.[36] This distinction by sonography may be helpful in the pretreatment evaluation of patients with adenocarcinoma of the endometrium.

Fig. 21. Hematometrocolpos secondary to endometrial carcinoma (longitudinal, 2 cm to left of midline). The uterine lumen is filled with blood and secretions as the result of cervical obstruction by tumor.

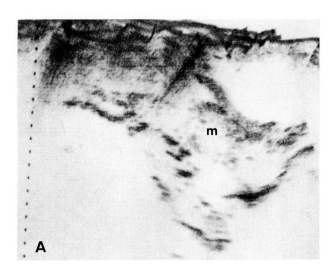
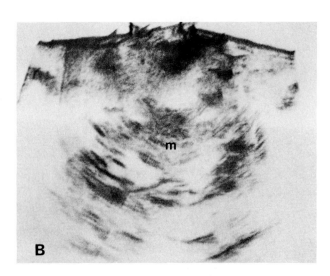

Fig. 22. Longitudinal **(A)** and transverse **(B)** scans showing a pelvic mass (m), posthysterectomy, representing a recurrent leiomyosarcoma. There are increased echoes and a disorganized pattern.

Of great clinical importance is that the uterus can be coincidentally enlarged by tumors other than carcinoma, such as fibroids, thereby influencing the clinical decision regarding therapy.

Although the extent of the invading carcinoma into the myometrium may be suggested by sonographic signs of invasion, computed tomography appears to be more precise in evaluating the extent of disease.[37,39] Invasion into the colon by an adenocarcinoma of the uterus is best shown on the barium enema. Bladder invasion may be detected by cystoscopy, contrast cystography, or computed body tomography. Moderately enlarged nodes (over 1.5 cm) can also be detected by sonography but are more reliably demonstrated by computed body tomography.[33,40] A different conclusion was reported in one study, but the investigators did not administer contrast media rectally when the CT examination was performed.[41]

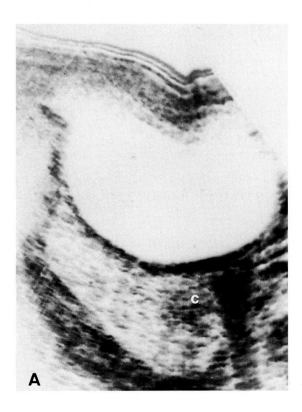
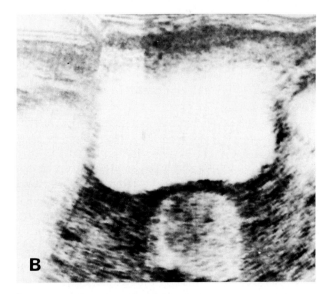

Fig. 23. Longitudinal **(A)** and transverse **(B)** scans in a 70-year-old female with carcinoma of the endometrium. The carcinoma extends into the cervix, making this a Stage II, corpus et collum. The uterus is enlarged for a 70-year-old. There are dense echoes in the lower uterine segment with a segmental enlargement of this portion of the uterus at the site of the tumor (c).

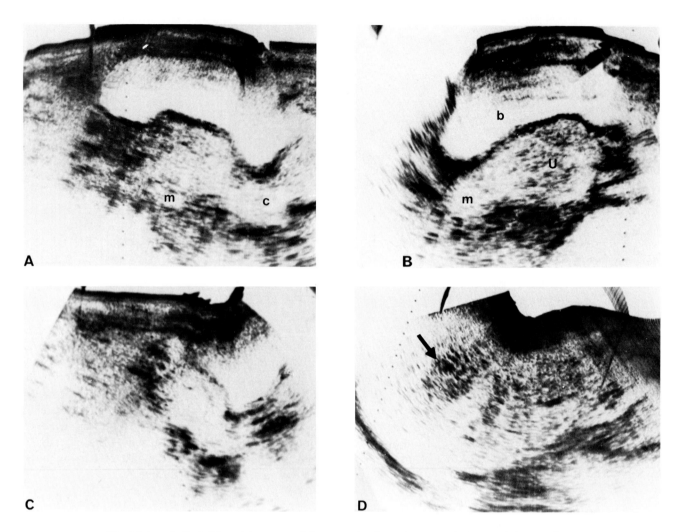

Fig. 24. Longitudinal **(A)** and transverse **(B)** scans showing a large cervical mass (m) extending into the vagina, enlargement of the uterus, and dense echo patterns throughout in a patient who has a Stage II carcinoma of the endometrium, corpus et collum. There is an eccentric convexity of the uterus (u) to the right in the transverse scan (m). c, cervix. **C.** Longitudinal scan in the same patient after radiation therapy and radium insertion. Note the marked decrease in the size of the masses and the change in the echo pattern. **D.** Longitudinal scan over the liver in the same patient six months later showing metastatic disease (*arrow*). There is no specific pattern to metastatic disease, although most metastases to the liver are echogenic.

The sonographic findings in uterine tumors will again be considered using the criteria enumerated at the beginning of the chapter.

Distortion or Change of the Uterine Outline or Contour

Adenocarcinoma of the endometrium may present with atrophy, normality, or enlargement of the uterus and with a normal or abnormal configuration (Fig. 22). There are benign processes that can enlarge the uterus coincidental to carcinoma of the endometrium. Local sonographic enlargement due to tumor may be detectable (Figs. 23, 24). A significant percentage of the patients in one series had carcinoma of the endometrium in association with uterine fibroids (Figs. 25,26).[31] It

is difficult to evaluate the extent of the tumor based on the sonographic findings of size or contour alone.

Distortion or Deviation of the Endometrial Layer

Distortion or deviation of the endometrial layer can occur with the development of a neoplasm. Again, this may be due to coincidental fibroids. Endometrial carcinoma generally involves the endometrial surface without significant deviation of this layer (Fig. 22). In advanced legions, the endometrium appears thickened (greater than 6 mm) and markedly irregular. Hypoechoic areas within the lumen may be seen with hematometria.

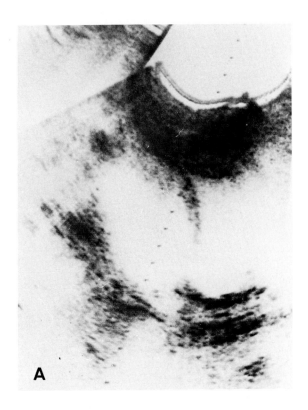

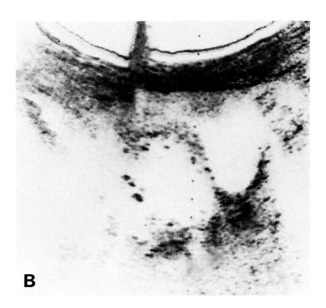

Fig. 25. Longitudinal **(A)** and transverse **(B)** scans in 89-year-old woman with Stage I B carcinoma of endometrium. There is marked sonolucency of the uterus. It was originally thought that this represented hematometria, but at surgery homogeneous tumor tissue was found.

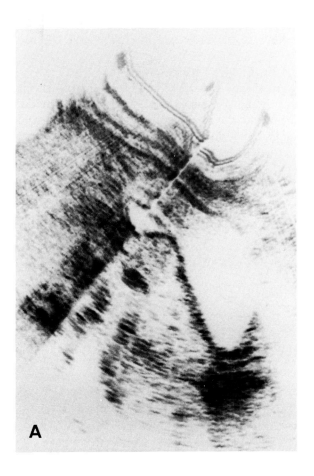

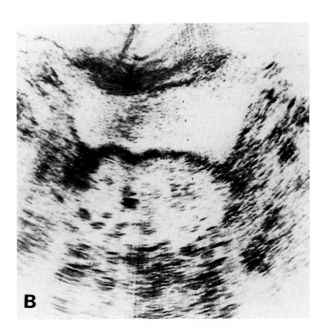

Fig. 26. Longitudinal **(A)** and transverse **(B)** scans in a Stage I B carcinoma of endometrium. The dense echoes with acoustic shadowing represent calcifications due to uterine fibroids. One cannot, therefore, tell if the endometrial carcinoma has enlarged the uterus.

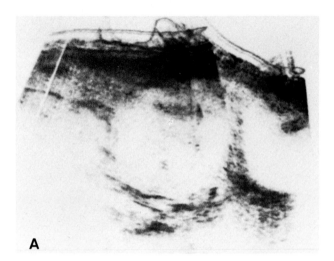
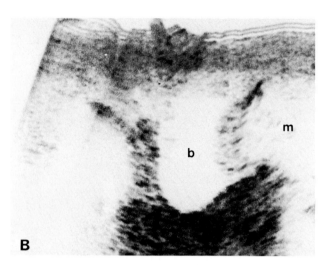

Fig. 27. Longitudinal **(A)** and transverse **(B)** scans in a Stage II carcinoma of the endometrium with extension to the left pelvic sidewall (m). There is evidence of bladder wall invasion. b, bladder.

Change in Ultrasonic Texture

Since early carcinomas are superficial lesions, it is impossible to detect texture changes. In a series of static scans of more advanced endometrial carcinomas, only 14 out of 50 could be evaluated for texture changes.[31] Most of the other cases were excluded because of (1) minimal involvement (early stages) in normal sized or atrophic uteri, or (2) the presence of other abnormalities, predominantly fibroids. Inadequate documentation of the anatomic location of the lesion is a common problem. Carcinoma of the endometrium can occur anywhere along the length of the endometrial canal, and the area of involvement does not necessarily correlate with the area of ultrasonic change. Areas of hemorrhage surrounding the tumor focus can mimic areas of actual tumor. Nonetheless, of the 14 cases evaluated, 6 showed increased echogenicity (Figs. 22, 23), 3 showed normal sonolucency, and 4 had decreased echogenicity (Figs. 22,25). In one case, there were areas of both increased and decreased echogenicity.

The technical advances of mechanical sector real-time scanners provide improved parenchymal detail, which enhances the ability to detect subtle changes in the early stages of endometrial carcinoma.

Change in Transonicity

As with texture changes, it was difficult to evaluate transonicity in our series.[31] Only 13 cases could be evaluated adequately. Two cases showed increased transonicity (Fig. 25), whereas the other 11 showed normal transonicity (Fig. 26). Decreased transonicity can be encountered in obstructed uteri filled with clotted blood resulting from cervical stenosis.[9]

Presence of a Mass Adjacent to the Uterus

Masses adjacent to the uterus in carcinoma of the uterus may arise from direct extension of the tumor, metastasis to other pelvic organs, lymphatic spread to pelvic nodes, or the presence of a coincidental benign or malignant lesion of the adnexa (Fig. 27). The sonogram can help delineate the anatomic relationship of the uterus to the mass and to characterize the mass.

Effect on Other Pelvic Organs

Invasion of the rectum is difficult to evaluate ultrasonically, although a water enema may be helpful. Invasion of the bladder is easier to assess since the irregular tumor margin is outlined by urine (Fig. 14). If the ureter is obstructed, hydronephrosis may be seen (Fig. 14).

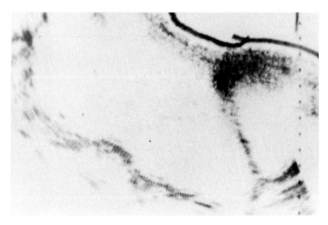

Fig. 28. Longitudinal scan in a patient with carcinosarcoma. There is massive uterine enlargement, with decreased echogenicity and increased transonicity due to tumor.

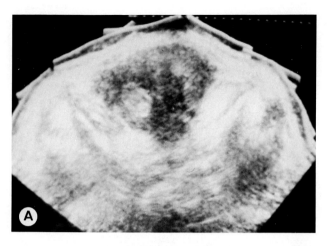 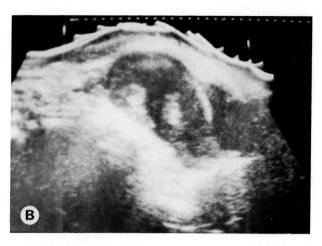

Fig. 29. Transverse **(A)** and longitudinal **(B)** scans showing an enlarged uterus containing multiple dense echo areas in a leiomyosarcoma. (*Courtesy of Barry Green, MD.*)

Occasionally, a large mass may involve the upper vagina (Fig. 14). As with carcinoma of the cervix, CT scanning more accurately detects and delineates pelvic wall extension, but ultrasound has some advantages in the evaluation of midline structures.

Secondary Effects
Carcinomas of the uterus bleed into the lumen of the uterus and may result in hematometra if the drainage path is obstructed by tumor or scarring of the canal.

CARCINOSARCOMAS

Carcinosarcomas are uncommon tumors of mixed origin, containing stromal and Mullerian elements. Patients tend to be in their 50s and 60s and are postmenopausal. The uterus is usually enlarged two to three times normal and is filled with polypoid masses. The two patients that we have encountered demonstrated massive enlargement of the uterus with decreased tumor echogenicity and increased transonicity (Fig. 28).[31]

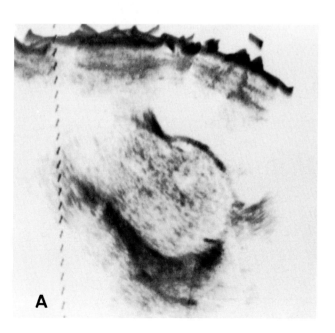 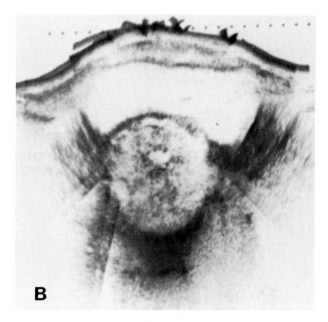

Fig. 30. Longitudinal **(A)** and transverse **(B)** scans showing an echogenic uterus with leiomyosarcoma.

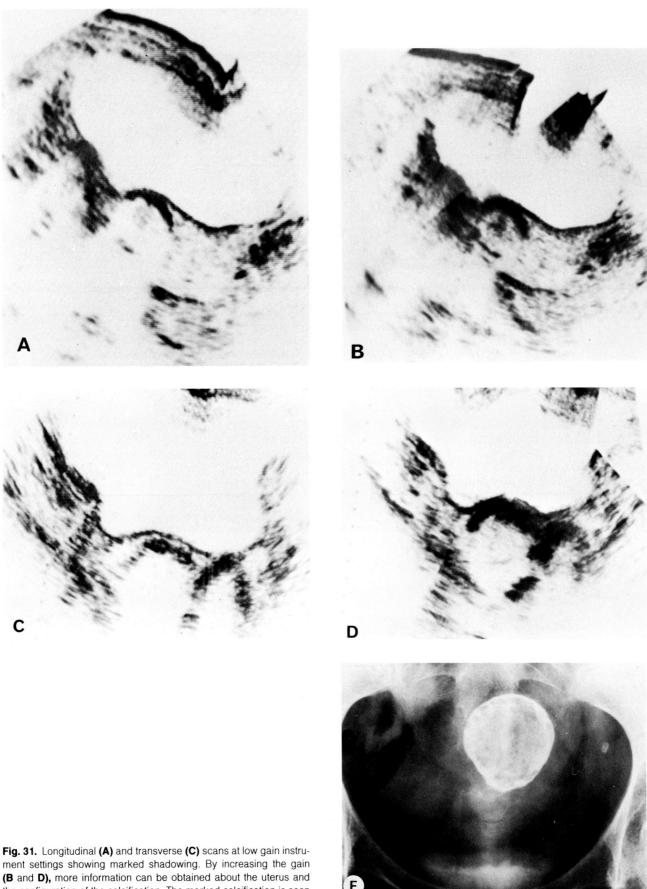

Fig. 31. Longitudinal **(A)** and transverse **(C)** scans at low gain instrument settings showing marked shadowing. By increasing the gain **(B** and **D),** more information can be obtained about the uterus and the configuration of the calcification. The marked calcification is seen in a radiograph of the pelvis **(E).**

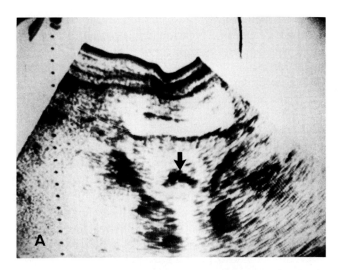
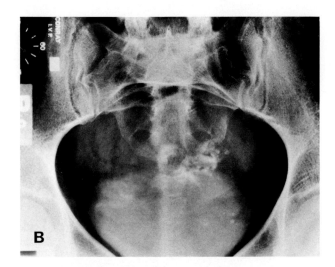

Fig. 32. A. Uterine sarcoma (longitudinal, 4 cm to right of midline). Nodular enlargement of the uterine outline is present. Within the uterus, there is a focus of high-level echoes with posterior acoustical shadow (*arrow*). This corresponded to a focus of calcification within this uterine sarcoma which had osteogenic components. (*Courtesy of Thomas Lawson, MD.*) **B.** Pelvic radiograph of uterine sarcoma demonstrating irregular calcification within uterine tumor. (*Courtesy of Thomas Lawson, MD and with permission from Am J Roentgenol, C Thomas, publisher.*)

SARCOMA BOTRYOIDES

Sarcoma botryoides is a rare tumor arising from the uterus in children. It is a mixed stromal tumor, predominantly rhabdomyosarcoma. Sarcoma botryoides is a soft, polypoid mass, frequently large, and often extruding from the cervix. Ultrasonographically, it appears as a complex mass deforming the uterine outline.[42]

LEIOMYOSARCOMAS

Leiomyosarcomas can arise from a preexisting leiomyoma or from muscle or connective tissue within the myometrium or blood vessels. The average age of patients is in the mid-50s. This is an infrequent development; less than 0.2 percent of all leiomyomas undergo sarcomatous change. However, due to the frequency of leiomyomas, leiomyosarcoma is a not uncommon uterine tumor.

Clinical findings in leiomyosarcoma can mimic those of a leiomyoma. A rapidly growing tumor at or after menopause, associated with pain and bleeding, should suggest leiomyosarcoma. Unless the tumor extends into the endometrial canal, a dilatation and curettage will not be diagnostic. Sonographically, the tumor may be too small to be seen or may be indistinguishable from a benign leiomyoma. In our experience, high-level echoes can be seen within the mass (Figs. 29–32) and may represent areas of calcification or ossification (Figs. 31,32), but these findings are nonspecific.

LYMPHOMA

Lymphomatous involvement of the uterus and cervix is a rare occurrence, with few reported cases.[43] In the patient shown in Figure 33, the diagnosis was made clinically. The ultrasonic pattern was that of a "normal sized," focally sonolucent uterus with a lobulated outline.

CARCINOMA OF THE OVIDUCT

Carcinoma of the oviduct is a rare gynecologic neoplasm. Most patients with this malignancy are undiagnosed both sonographically and clinically until the time of surgery. Sonographically, one patient presented with an ill-defined complex, fusiform mass concomitant with a large intramural leiomyoma. In another patient, a reniform, complex mass with a central echogenic core surrounded by a sonolucent halo was encountered. At surgery, the mass depicted by pelvic sonography corresponded to a loop of jejunum that was infiltrated by surrounding tumor (Fig. 34).

POSTHYSTERECTOMY EVALUATION

Patients who have undergone hysterectomy have altered anatomic relations in the pelvis and may be difficult to evaluate adequately by manual pelvic examination (Figs. 35,36).[44] Detection of pelvic mass in these

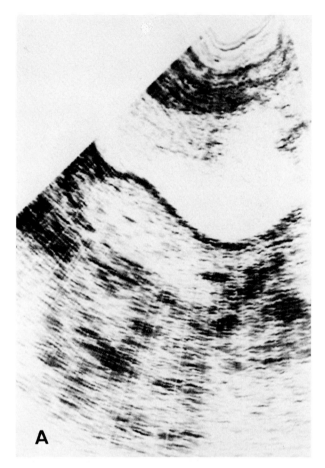

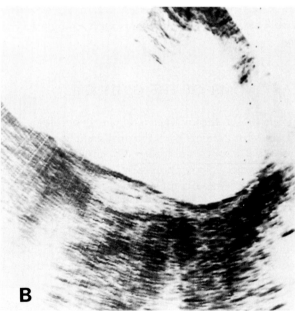

patients may require additional clinical and radiographic evaluation. Occasionally, a patient is encountered who has had a supracervical hysterectomy. This operation consists of removal of the uterus, leaving the cervix in place, creating the potential for clinical confusion and later development of cervical carcinoma.

Pelvic masses not related to the uterus can be encountered in the patient who has undergone hysterectomy and/or salpingo-oophorectomy. For instance, a small ovarian remnant may enlarge and produce a pelvic mass even though most of the ovary has been removed. The potential for resumption of ovulatory function remains, however, and the patient may resume production of ovarian sex steroids. The enlarged ovarian remnant is often adherent to the pelvic side wall and may also produce partial obstruction of the ureter due to compression.[45]

Hematomas and nondistended loops of bowel may appear as masses within the pelvis of a posthysterectomy patient, depending upon the organization of a hematoma. They appear as anechoic to hypoechoic masses (Fig. 37). In the postmenopausal patient, the ovary should be small and difficult to delineate (Fig. 36).

A portion of omentum may be rounded and appears as a soft tissue mass. This may be adherent to the vaginal cuff or cul de sac and mimic the appearance of an ovary. It is indeed difficult to distinguish these two entities by sonography (Figs. 36,38). Postoperative peritoneal adhesions may enclose fluid, causing a peritoneal retention cyst (Fig. 39).

The use of the water enema technique with simultaneous monitoring by real-time scanning is advocated for further evaluation of the posthysterectomy patient

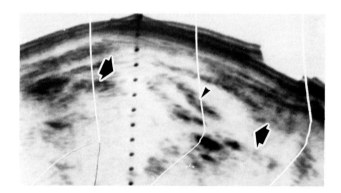

Fig. 33. A. Longitudinal scan in a young woman showing a sonolucent apparently normal sized uterus. In point of fact, the uterus is diffusely enlarged by lymphomatous deposition. **B.** Longitudinal scan following radiation therapy. This patient had endocrine dysfunction secondary to lymphoma and now a small atrophic uterus can be seen.

Fig. 34. Transverse static sonogram of fusiform mass resulting from massive thickening of the right oviduct due to carcinoma. The mass (*arrows*) mimicked the appearance of abnormally thickened bowel except it was oriented in a transverse, rather than longitudinal plane. The intraluminal surface (*arrowhead*) is thick and irregular. Processor artifacts are present on the print.

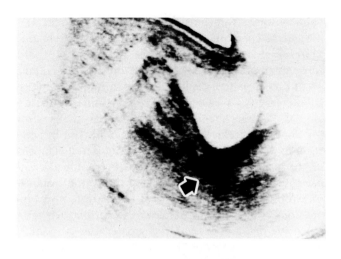

Fig. 35. Longitudinal static sonogram of posthysterectomy patient demonstrating close proximity of rectum to (*arrow*) bladder floor.

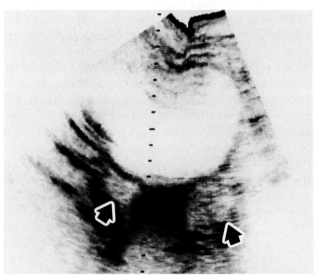

Fig. 36. Transverse static sonogram depicting normal ovaries (*arrows*) in a posthysterectomy patient. The ovaries are normal sized for this previously premenopausal patient.

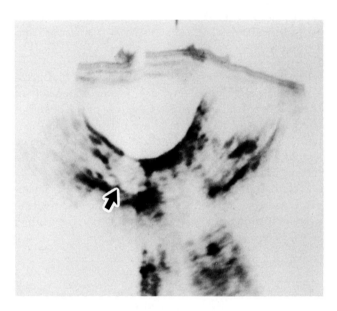

Fig. 37. Transverse static sonogram of patient 2 days after hysterectomy for fibroids. The hematoma (*arrow*) appears as a hypoechoic mass.

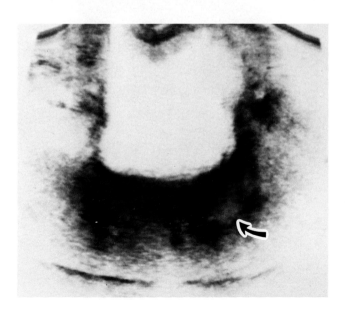

Fig. 38. Transverse static sonogram of posthysterectomy patient with rounded isoechoic mass (*arrow*). At surgery, a ball of omentum was found.

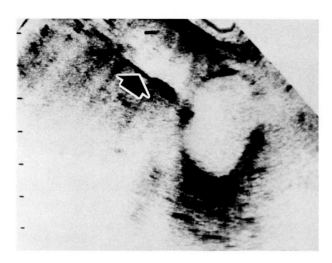

Fig. 39. Longitudinal static sonogram of posthysterectomy patient showing irregular cystic mass (*arrow*) superior to the bladder representing a peritoneal inclusion cyst.

when the initial sonographic study suggests that presence of a pelvic mass (Fig. 38). Water distension of the rectum affords a detailed evaluation of the posterior compartment of the pelvis of a posthysterectomy patient. Only small remnants of supravaginal tissue should be present between the urinary bladder and rectum of these patients.[44]

Radiation therapy, given to a patient with cancer, can cause areas of fibrosis, making pelvic examination even more difficult. With radiation therapy, the vaginal vault becomes foreshortened, stenotic, and rigid. It is difficult to examine the adnexa or the suprapubic area. Ultrasound and computed tomography may be, therefore, an important diagnostic adjunct in the follow-up of cancer patients.[44] Ideally, the initial examination should serve as a baseline for comparison with future studies. Because edematous changes in the cuff persist for about 6 weeks (Fig. 40), a delay in the baseline for 2 to 3 months after surgery is suggested. The size of the vagina and "cuff" will vary from patient to patient, depending upon the age of the patient, amount of atrophic changes, amount of irradiation, and type of surgery. In general, the older the patient, the more extensive the surgery, or the greater the amount of irradiation, the smaller the residual vagina. Cuff size is also dependent upon surgical technique. The degree of tissue incorporated and the type of suture used in closure will affect the cuff size. Usually, the cuff appears as a 1 to 1.5 cm structure along the upper pole of the vagina. Once the size and configuration of the vaginal cuff are established on baseline examination, the cuff should not enlarge on later studies (Fig. 41), and as the patient ages, the cuff size usually decreases. If an increase is noted on follow-up examination, the possibility of tumor recurrence should be considered (Figs. 42,43). Adherent bowel or an ovary adjacent to the upper vagina can mimic recurrent tumor around the cuff (Fig. 44). Whenever the appearances are unusual, a water enema should be performed.

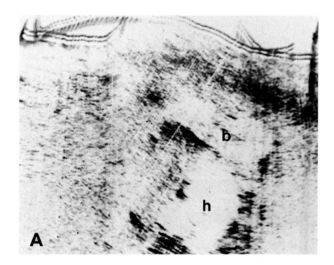

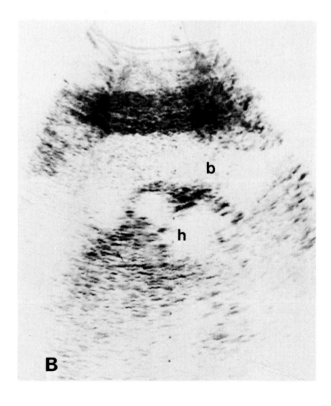

Fig. 40. Longitudinal (**A**) and transverse (**B**) scans of a posthysterectomy patient showing hematoma (h) at the vaginal cuff. The sonolucent areas represent blood accumulation. Good bladder distension is not always possible in postoperative patients, and sometimes scans will be suboptimal. b, bladder.

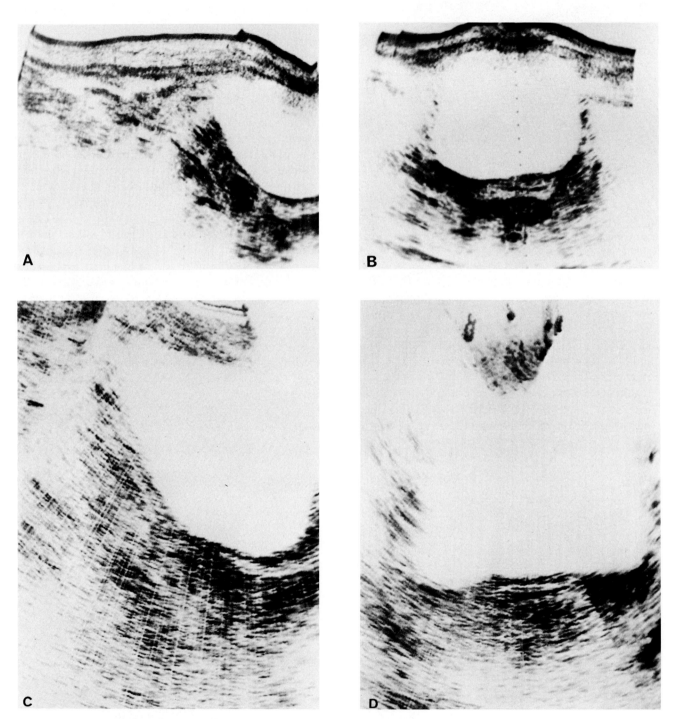

Fig. 41. Longitudinal **(A)** and transverse **(B)** scans showing a normal sized vaginal cuff. Longitudinal **(C)** and transverse **(D)** scans demonstrating a small vaginal cuff.

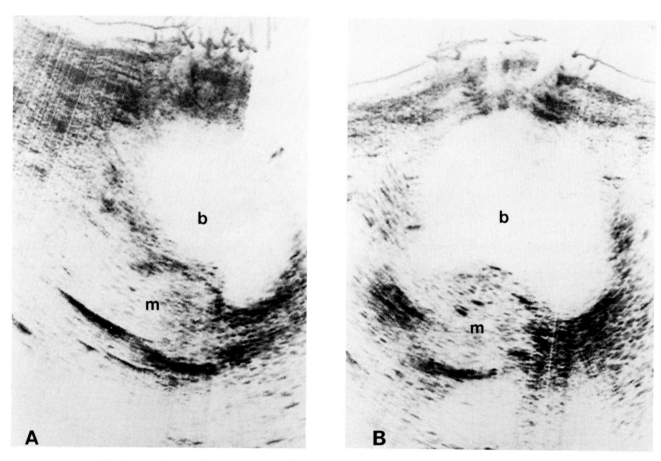

Fig. 42. Longitudinal **(A)** and transverse **(B)** scans showing a recurrence at the vaginal cuff (m) in a Stage II carcinoma of the endometrium. b, bladder.

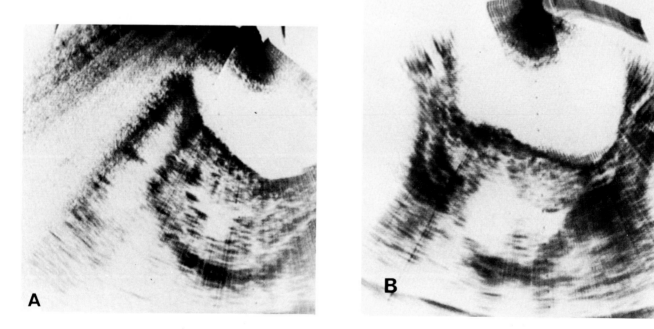

Fig. 43. Longitudinal **(A)** and transverse **(B)** scans which delineate recurrent tumor and fluid accumulation in the pelvis posthysterectomy in a patient with carcinoma of the cervix.

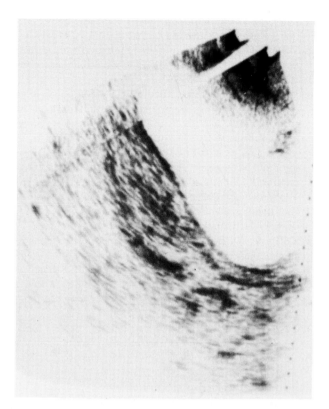

Fig. 44. Longitudinal scan posthysterectomy. Care must be taken not to misinterpret the echo pattern so as to make a uterus appear when one is not present. The phantom uterus seen here is a combination of bowel and pelvic soft tissues.

SUMMARY

Because of its ability to depict the location, size, and texture of the uterus, when the urinary bladder is distended, sonography has an important role in evaluating patients with suspected uterine malformations and disorders. This chapter has emphasized those uterine disorders in which sonographic examination can be helpful.

REFERENCES

1. Kurtz A, Rubin C, Kramer F, et al: Ultrasound evaluation of the posterior pelvic compartment. Radiology 132:677, 1974
2. Callen P, Demartini W, Filly R: The central uterine cavity echo: A useful anatomic sign in the ultrasonographic evaluation of the female pelvis. Radiology 131:187, 1979
3. Sample W, Lippe B, Gyepes M: Gray scale ultrasonography of the normal female pubis. Radiology 125:477, 1977
4. Gross B, Callen R: Ultrasound of the uterus, in Callen P (ed), Ultrasonography in Obstetrics and Gynecology. Philadelphia, Saunders, 1983, pp 227–247

5. Miller E, Thomas R, Cines P: The atrophic postmenopause uterus. J Clin Ultra 5:261, 1977
6. Laing F, Filly R, Marks W, et al: Ultrasonic demonstration of endometrial fluid collections unassociated with pregnancy. Radiology 137:471, 1980
7. Viscomi G, Gonzales R, Taylor K: Ultrasound detection of uterine anomalies after diethylstilbestrol (DES) exposure. Radiology 136:733, 1980
8. Wilson D, Stacy T, Smith E: Sonographic diagnosis of hydrocolpous and hydrometrocolpous. Radiology 128:451, 1978
9. Scott W, Rosenshein N, Seigelman S, et al: The obstructed uterus. Radiology 141:767, 1980
10. Fried A, Oliff M, Wilson E: Uterine anomalies associated with renal agenesis: Role of gray scale sonography. Am J Roentgenol 131:973, 1978
11. Kaufman R, Binder G, Gray P: Upper genital tract changes associated with exposure in utero to diethylstilbestrol. Am J Obstet Gynecol 128:51, 1971
12. Johnson M, Graham M, Cooperburg P: Abnormal endometrial echoes: Sonographic spectrum of endometrial pathology. J Clin Ultrasound Med 1:181, 1982
13. Von Micsky L: Sonographic study of uterine fibromyomas, in Sanders R, James AE, Jr (eds), Ultrasonography in Obstetrics and Gynecology. New York, Appleton-Century-Crofts, 1977
14. Bezjian A, Carretero M: Ultrasonic evaluation of pelvic masses in pregnancy. Clin Obstet Gynecol 20:325, 1977
15. Hassani S, Bard R: Ultrasonic changes of uterine fibroids in pregnancy and degeneration, in White D, Lyons E (eds), Ultrasound in Medicine. New York, Plenum, 1978, vol 4, p 259
16. Sanders R, Nelson M, Cavalieri R, et al: Myomas in pregnancy discovered by sonography (in preparation).
17. Bowie J: Ultrasound of gynecologic pelvic masses: The indefinite uterus sizes and other patterns associated with diagnostic error. J Clin Ultrasound 5:323, 1977
18. Fogel S, Slasky B: Sonography of Nabothian cysts. Am J Roentgenol 138:927, 1982
19. Walsh J, Brewer W, Schneider V: Ultrasound diagnosis in diseases of the uterine corpus and cervix. Semin Ultrasound 1:30, 1980
20. Carson SC: Ultrasound in obstetrics and gynecology. J Reprod Med 20:1, 1978
21. Cochrane WJ, Thomas MS: Ultrasound diagnosis of gynecologic pelvic masses. Radiology 110:649, 1974
22. Lawson TL, Albarelli JN: Diagnosis of gynecologic pelvic masses by gray scale ultrasonography: Analysis of specificity and accuracy. Am J Roentgenol 128:1003, 1977
23. Leopold GR, Asher WM: Ultrasound in obstetrics and gynecology. Radiol Clin N Am 12:127, 1974
24. Perlmutter GS, Goldberg BB: Ultrasound in obstetrics and gynecology. J Reprod Med 20:1, 1978
25. Levi S: Value of ultrasonic diagnosis of gynecologic tumors in 370 surgical cases. Acta Obstet Gynecol Scand 55:261, 1976
26. Samuels BI, Silver TM: Diagnostic ultrasound in the evaluation of patients with gynecologic cancer. Surg Clin N Am 58:3, 1978

27. Saig PJ, et al: Synopsis of Gynecologic Oncology. New York, Wiley, 1975

28. Rutledge F, et al: Gynecologic Oncology. New York, Wiley, 1976

29. Von Micsky L: Gynecologic ultrasonography, in King D (ed), Diagnostic Ultrasound. St. Louis, Mosby, 1975, p 207

30. Rubin C, Kurtz A, Goldberg B: Water enema: A new ultrasonic technique for defining pelvic anatomy. J Clin Ultrasound 6:28, 1978

31. Porrath SA, et al: Ultrasound in Endometrial Carcinoma. Presented at AIUM meeting, San Diego, October 1978

32. Coulam C, Julian C, Fleischer A: Clinical efficacy of CT and US in gynecologic tumors. Appl Radiol 11:79, 1982

33. Lee J, Stanley R, Sagel S, et al: Accuracy of computed tomography in detecting intra-abdominal and pelvic cystic node metastases from pelvic cancers. Am J Roentgenol 131:675, 1978

34. Breckenridge J, Kurtz A, Ritchie W, et al: Postmenopausal uterine fluid collection: Indication of carcinoma. Am J Roentgenol 139:529, 1982

35. Hertig A, Gore H: Tumors of the Female Sex Organs. Part 2, Tumors of the Vulva, Vagina and Uterus. Washington, D.C., Armed Forces Institute of Pathology, 1960

36. Requard L, Wilks J, Mettler F: Ultrasonography in the staging of endometrial adenocarcinoma. Radiology 140:781, 1981

37. Hamlin D, Burgnerm F, Becham J: CT of intramural endometrial carcinoma: Contrast enhancement is essential. Am J Roentgenol 137:551, 1982

38. Walsh J, Gopherud D: Computed tomography of primary, persistent, and recurrent endometrial malignancy. Am J Roentgenol 139:1149, 1982

39. Walsh J, Goplerud D: Computed tomography of primary, persistent, and recurrent endometrial malignancy. Am J Roentgerol 139:1149, 1982

40. Walsh J, Amendila M, Konerding K: Computed tomographic detection of pelvic and cystic node metastases from primary and pelvic malignant disease. Radiology 137:157, 1980

41. Walsh JW, et al: Gray-scale ultrasound in 204 proven gynecologic masses: Accuracy and specific diagnostic criteria. Radiology 130:465, 1979

42. Woodring J, Halberg D, Daff D: Sarcoma botryoides of the uterus presenting as an abdominal mass: A case report. J Clin Ultrasound 10:347, 1982

43. Rochester D, Bowei J, Kunzmann A, et al: Ultrasound in the staging of lymphoma. Radiology 124:483, 1977

44. Parulekar S: Ultrasound evaluation of the posthysterectomy pelvis. J Clin Ultrasound 10:265, 1982

45. Phillips H, McGahan J: Ovarian remnant syndrome: A case report. Radiology 142:477, 1982

46. Bassett D, Jacobson G: Gross anatomy of the female reproductive track, in Danforth D (ed), Textbook of Obstetrics and Gynecology. New York, Harper and Row, 1971, p 69

47. Hackeloer B: The role of ultrasound in female infertility management. Ultra Med Bio 10:35, 1984

48. Fleischer A, Pittaway D, Beard L, et al: Sonographic depiction of the endometrium in normal and stimulated cycles. J Ultra Med (in press), 1984

39 | Ultrasound in the Management of Gynecologic Malignancies

Damon D. Blake

Both ultrasound and computed tomography (CT) imaging modalities have been shown to be helpful in the diagnosis and management of tumors in most areas of the body[1-8] and in gynecologic tumors in particular.[6,9-17] Ultrasound imaging provides anatomic information in a format that can be very helpful in the treatment and management of patients with gynecologic malignancies.[6,15-17] In chemotheraphy treatment the most helpful procedure is the monitoring of tumor growth and response to drug therapy.[18] When treatment is with radiation therapy there are numerous ways in which ultrasound is useful (Table 1). A brief description of radiotherapy principles and procedures will serve as a background for demonstrating the needs that ultrasound can fulfill.

PRINCIPLES OF RADIATION THERAPY

The goal of radiation treatment of a malignancy has always been to deliver a cancerocidal dose of radiation to all of the tumor, while sparing the normal tissues. This goal can almost be reached when it is possible to implant radioactive material within the tumor; it is most difficult to attain when the tumor is deep seated and has to be treated with external beam radiation that must pass through normal tissues before reaching the tumor. The incidence of side effects of radiation and of complications of treatment rise with an increase in the volume of normal tissues receiving irradiation. Therefore, the *treatment volume* is kept as small as possible, while still containing the entire *tumor volume.* In instances in which the *radiation dosage* to the tumor can

be relatively low (very radiosensitive tumors, or palliative situations) the necessity for minimizing the treatment volume is not as great as it is with high-dose treatment. An important factor in determining the treatment volume is the *radiosensitivity of the normal tissues* in question and how critical it is to preserve their function. In the abdomen we are most often concerned about the kidneys, liver, and bowel. In the pelvis, the small bowel, bladder, and rectum may need to receive attention in treatment planning. The treatment volume can be shaped by the introduction of shielding or wedge filters into the radiation beam, and by using multiple beams appropriately placed.

RADIATION TREATMENT PLANNING

The application of computers in treatment planning has allowed rapid and accurate calculation and display of the distribution of radiation within the tissues. This is especially helpful when multiple treatment fields are used, but only if we also can accurately display the location and extent of the malignancy and location of sensitive normal tissue structures. Ultrasound and CT scan imaging can provide that information in a format that is easily incorporated into the treatment planning procedure.[15] Prior to the availability of these two imaging modalities, the localization of the tumor and of vital normal structures was indirect, from a variety of sources of information (physical examination, surgical findings, radiographic studies, and cross-sectional anatomy texts).

To enter patient contour and tumor localization

TABLE 1
Uses of Ultrasound in Management of Gynecologic Malignancies

A. Radiation treatment planning
   1. Obtaining patient contour
   2. Tumor localization
   3. Kidney localization
   4. Help in radioactive implants
B. Monitor response to treatment
   1. Radiotherapy
   2. Chemotherapy
C. Follow-up
   1. Local recurrence
   2. New disease sites

into a computer-generated treatment plan the ultrasound image is traced with a digitizer cursor that converts the graphic information into numerical coordinates for the computer (Fig. 1). The dose distribution of the proposed field arrangement is displayed on the cathode ray tube within the sonic contour (Fig. 2). Once a satisfactory plan is found, a life-sized hard copy is produced by the computer-controlled incremental plotter (Fig. 3). An example of a computer-generated three-field treatment plan is seen in Fig. 4.

INDICATIONS FOR CT SCANNING

CT scanning and ultrasound scanning overlap considerably in their ability to provide the kinds of information needed for radiation treatment planning. Both modalities should be available, since one may be successful when the other is not. In cases where either imaging method could provide the needed information it would seem to make sense to use ultrasound because of its greater accessibility, flexibility, and lesser cost. In general, the indications for use of CT imaging rather than ultrasound scans occur in these situations:

1. Marked obesity, which prevents adequate sonic imaging.
2. Extension of the tumor into pelvic bone, so that ultrasound does not demonstrate its full extent.
3. Failure of the ultrasound scan to depict as much of the disease as was seen on a previous CT scan or was suspected from physical examination and other studies.
4. Bowel gas or bone structures that prevent a satisfactory sonic scan.
5. A recent surgical wound that does not allow transducer contact with the skin.
6. The bladder cannot be adequately filled for one reason or another.

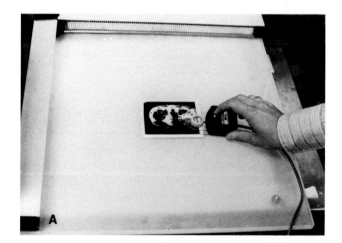
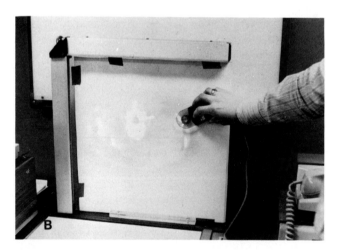

Fig. 1. Computerized treatment planning. **A.** Sonic digitizer in horizontal position. A Polaroid print of an ultrasound scan is laid on the digitizer, and the patient's contour and other pertinent structures are traced from the image with the cursor. This enters the graphic information into the treatment planning computer which then displays this information on the cathode ray screen. **B.** The sonic digitizer can also be placed in the upright position, so that the ultrasound or CT scan image can be projected onto it life-size. The correct amount of enlargement is determined by using the centimeter marker on the scan. Tracing with the cursor from this large image is somewhat more accurate than tracing directly from the original Polaroid. (*Reprinted with permission from Blake DD: Use of ultrasound in radiotherapy, in Reznick MI, Sanders RC (eds), Ultrasound in Urology, 2nd ed. Baltimore, Williams and Wilkins, 1984.*)

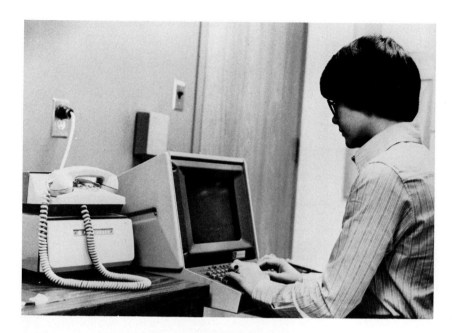

Fig. 2. Computerized treatment planning. The dosimetrist enters nongraphic data into the computer via the keyboard of the computer terminal pictured here. A computer-generated treatment plan is seen on the cathode ray display screen. (*Reprinted with permission from Blake DD: Use of ultrasound in radiotherapy, in Reznick MI, Sanders RC (eds), Ultrasound in Urology, 2nd ed. Baltimore, Williams & Wilkins, 1984.*)

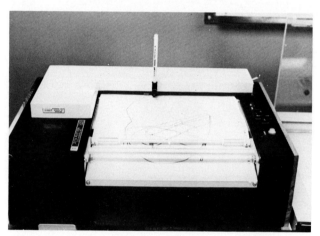

Fig. 3. Computerized treatment planning. The incremental plotter (digital plotter) prints out a life-size hard copy of the final approved treatment plan as it appears on the cathode ray display screen. (See Fig. 4.) (*Reprinted with permission from Blake DD: Use of ultrasound in radiotherapy, in Reznick MI, Sanders RC (eds), Ultrasound in Urology, 2nd ed. Baltimore, Williams & Wilkins, 1984.*)

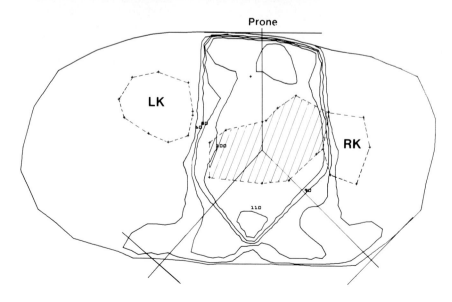

Fig. 4. Computer-generated three-field treatment plan. The patient's contour and location of tumor mass (*shaded*) and kidneys (LK, RK) were derived from ultrasound scan. Accurate anatomic information allows a plan that delivers adequate dose to the tumor while sparing the kidneys. (*Reprinted with permission from Blake DD: Use of ultrasound in radiotherapy, in Reznick MI, Sanders RC (eds), Ultrasound in Urology, 2nd ed. Baltimore, Williams & Wilkins, 1984.*)

7. When there is a special need for tissue inhomogeneity data in radiation dose distribution calculations. This is most likely to occur in chest treatment because of the aerated lung which absorbs less radiation than solid tissues.

INSTRUCTING THE ULTRASONOGRAPHER

The imaging information needed for radiotherapy purposes tends to be different from the usual diagnostic ultrasound information, and so it is necessary to instruct the ultrasonographer in the special requirements and techniques. Until that has been accomplished, a member of the radiotherapy team should be in attendance during the scanning. For treatment planning purposes:

1. Emphasis is on defining the margins of the disease rather than its internal echo pattern.
2. The true relationship of the tumor to the skin surface and to adjacent vital normal structures should be clearly evident on any given scan.
3. The location of the plane of the scan should be reproducible by proper labeling and by relating it to some external landmark such as the umbilicus. If the scan plane is other than a true transverse or sagittal one, it may be best to label according to the official recommendations drawn up by the Standards Committee of the AIUM.[19]
4. The patient should be scanned in treatment position when it is being done for radiation treatment planning purposes. This includes the position of the arms (up or down), since skin marks move significantly with change in arm position.
5. Special care should be taken to exactly center the transducer over any skin point that is being marked on the scan.
6. The accuracy of the scanning equipment should be maintained by regularly scheduled calibration tests.
7. Scanning for the *diagnosis* of tumors is often accomplished with sector scans or real-time scanning. For therapy purposes however, static B-scan images are needed.
8. The use of the top of the pubic bone as a reference level is not very accurate if it is determined by palpation, because the thickness of skin, subcutaneous tissue and muscle obscure the actual bony edge. It is better to use the umbilicus and indicate all other scans as plus or minus so many centimeters.

OBTAINING THE BODY CONTOUR

An accurate contour of the body at the level of the middle of the radiation treatment port is the starting

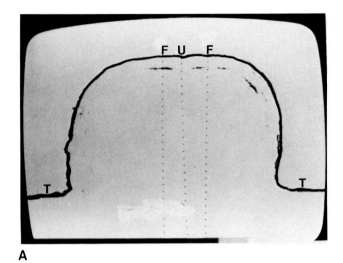

A

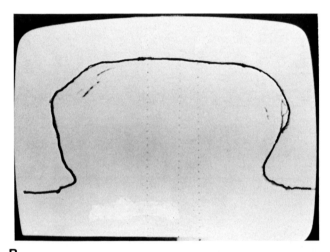

B

Fig. 5. Simple body contours obtained with gain turned down. **A.** Supine transverse scan with location of umbilicus (U), therapy field skin marks (F), and table top (T) indicated. **B.** Prone scan of same patient. Note the change in configuration compared with **A.** The contour used for a particular treatment field must be made with the patient in treatment position. (*Reprinted with permission from Blake DD: Use of ultrasound in radiotherapy, in Reznick MI, Sanders RC (eds), Ultrasound in Urology, 2nd ed. Baltimore, Williams & Wilkins, 1984.*)

point in most treatment planning procedures. The historical method of obtaining this contour consisted of wrapping a soft solder wire or a narrow strip of plaster of Paris partway around the patient and transferring this to a sheet of tracing paper. The contour can be more simply and accurately made with ultrasound and the image enlarged to life-size either with a digitizer (Fig. 1) or by projecting the image.[17] Certain precautions should be noted in making the contour: (1) If only an outline is needed, without display of deeper structures, the gain can be turned down (Fig. 5). (2) Care must be used to avoid depressing or deforming the tissues with the transducer. (3) No more padding

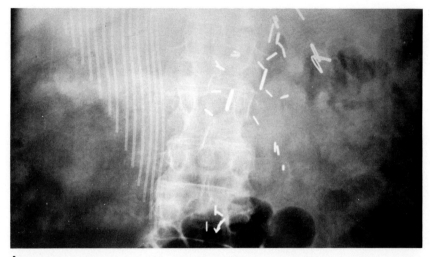

A

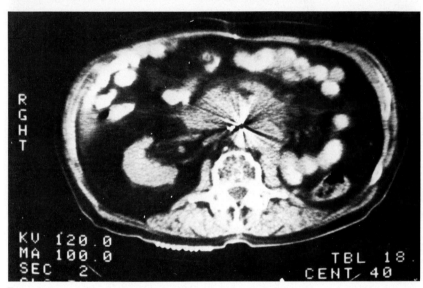

B

Fig. 6. Method of localizing the level at which a CT section was made. **A.** A radiograph is made with a row of radiopaque catheters taped to the patient's skin. There is a stepwise increment of catheter length of one centimeter. **B.** The catheters can be seen in cross section on the posterior skin surface of the CT section. These are counted, and the number of catheters is referred to the radiograph to determine the level of the cut. The method is cumbersome and subject to error. (*Reprinted with permission from Blake DD: Use of Ultrasound in Radiotherapy, in Reznick MI, Sanders RC (eds), Ultrasound in Urology, 2nd ed. Baltimore, Williams & Wilkins, 1984.*)

should be used on the scanning table top than is used on the treatment table, and the surface should be indicated on the contour scan on both right and left sides. (4) Both supine and prone scans are usually needed, since the configuration of the tissues changes with change in body position.

Whenever the contour crosses an external landmark, such as the umbilicus or the skin mark of a radiation treatment portal, that point should be indicated either by recording the centimeter marker or lifting the transducer from the skin. This should be done with great care to ensure that the transducer is directly over the point to be indicated. The ability to easily and directly mark external landmarks, or to project deep structures onto the external surface, is a particular advantage of ultrasound contour scanning.

TUMOR LOCALIZATION

The flexibility of ultrasound scanning allows a three-dimensional display of tumor masses and is the simplest and most direct way to project and mark this display onto the skin surface in order to set up radiation treatment ports. To do this with CT requires a cumbersome and indirect method (Fig. 6). Localization of the tumor for treatment planning may be helpful in a number of circumstances:

1. To check tumor coverage of therapy fields that have already been marked on the patient. A contour made at midfield level, containing the tumor image and location of field skin marks is sufficient (Fig. 7).
2. To aid in initial placement of therapy field by pro-

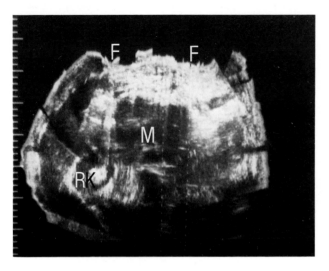

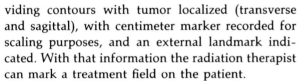

Fig. 7. Transverse scan to check coverage of radiation therapy field. It is made at the level of the widest diameter of the tumor (M), and the skin marks of the field margins are indicated with the centimeter marker (F). The relationships of the tumor, right kidney (RK), skin, and therapy field are all shown, and appropriate changes can be made. The left kidney is absent.

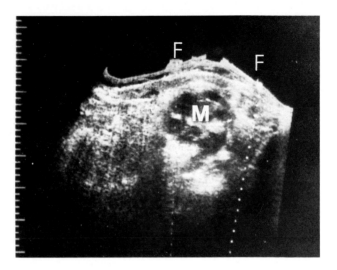

Fig. 8. Palpable superficial tumor mass. Transverse scan of mass (M) with therapy field margins (F) indicated, as they were initially set up by palpation. The field position needs to be changed for better tumor coverage. The thickness (depth) of the mass is useful for dosage calculation.

viding contours with tumor localized (transverse and sagittal), with centimeter marker recorded for scaling purposes, and an external landmark indicated. With that information the radiation therapist can mark a treatment field on the patient.

3. To check tumor coverage of therapy fields placed over superficial tumor masses by palpation (Fig. 8). The nonpalpable portions of the mass may extend beyond the palpable portion. The depth or thickness of the mass can also be measured for dose calculation.

4. Scanning superficial tumors that are to be treated with opposing tangential beams is uniquely helpful in determining beam positions and angles (Fig. 9).[8] It is preferable to mark tentative skin ports before doing the scan and then indicate their position on the scan. With this information the dosimetrist can prepare a treatment plan that covers the depths of the tumor, yet includes a minimum of normal tissue.

KIDNEY LOCALIZATION

Concern for the location of the kidneys in relation to the treatment volume arises when treating abdominal extensions of ovarian or endometrial tumors, or metastatic paraaortic node masses. This concern must be particularly prominent when one of the patient's kidneys is already compromised by ureteral obstruction or some other process. The radiation tolerance

of the kidney(s) varies with the amount of renal tissue irradiated and the dose received.[20] The highest dose is allowed if only a portion of one kidney receives radiation (with two normal kidneys). The least allowable dose occurs when all of both kidneys must receive radiation. These dose decisions must be tempered, of course, by other factors such as the question of whether tumor tissue would be shielded by the kidney block. The treatment ports for irradiation of moderately enlarged paraaortic nodes do not generally overlap the kidneys, whereas treatment of large areas of the abdomen for extensive ovarian carcinoma may require bilateral shields.

It is usually sufficient to provide kidney shields only for the posterior ports, providing the dose received via the anterior port does not exceed the kidney tolerance dose. The procedure involved in localizing the kidney with ultrasound and fashioning the kidney block has been described by Brascho.[21] The outline of the organ is projected onto the skin surface and transferred to a flat transparent sheet of plastic or cleared x-ray film, which has been marked with reference points corresponding to the patient's skin. From this, the therapy dosimetrist or physicist constructs the block of proper size and determines its precise location within the treatment beam according to the treatment geometry.

When ultrasound localization is done with care, the end results are more consistently reliable than other methods. Radioisotope renal scans or radiographic

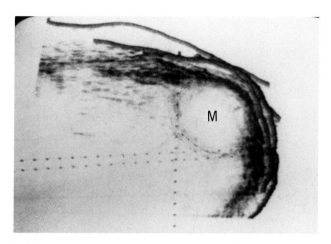

Fig. 9. Treatment planning for tangential beams. Transverse scan through tumor. Localization of the superficial tumor mass (M) is essential for planning the location and angles for opposing tangential beams.

studies to locate the kidney on the skin surface are less direct methods which are more subject to error (Fig. 10). It is important to have the patient in precise "treatment position," including the position of the arms, and to record the kidney outline points when the patient is in "passive expiration" phase of respiration.

At other times it may not be necessary to project the renal outline onto the skin surface, but only to provide a prone contour containing the kidney cross section images. If the radiation treatment fields are al-

ready marked on the skin, the intersections with the field marks should also be indicated on the contour by raising the transducer or recording the centimeter marker *precisely* at that point.

PELVIC SCANNING—SPECIAL ASPECTS

Ultrasound scanning of the pelvis can often provide the unique kinds of information needed in the radiation management of carcinomas of the cervix, endometrium, and ovary. An initial survey of the pelvis with a real-time device gives a quick orientation and can reduce the time necessary to make the appropriate static B-scans. The adequacy of filling of the bladder is noted, and the position and axis of the uterus determined so that a longitudinal scan can be made along that axis.

Anteverted Uterus
With the anteverted uterus in Figure 11A, a vertical transverse CT scan would not give a true picture of the dimensions of the organ. Chen[14] reported that with CT studies of uterine size, the longitudinal axis dimension was generally 30 to 60 percent smaller than the surgical specimen measurement. With ultrasound, the transverse scan plane can be tilted in order to approach a cross section of the uterus (Fig. 11C). Sometimes it is possible to push the uterus down into a more horizontal plane by distending the bladder (Fig. 11B), or even by doing it manually through the abdomen during the scan.

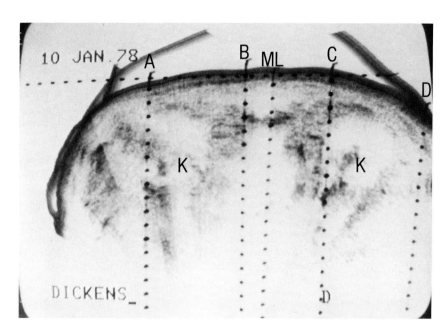

Fig. 10. Kidney localization. Prone transverse scan at level of kidneys (K) which had been initially localized by radioisotope renal scan. The supposed medial and lateral kidney margins were marked on the skin and those marks are indicated on the sonic scan at A, B, C, D. ML, midline. They do not agree with the actual kidney locations. Ultrasound localization is more direct and reliable. (*Reprinted with permission from Blake DD: Use of ultrasound in radiotherapy, in Reznick MI, Sanders RC (eds), Ultrasound in Urology, 2nd ed. Baltimore, Williams & Wilkins, 1984.*)

Cervix Carcinoma

When planning the intracavitary component of a radiotherapy program for cervix carcinoma the overall length of the cervix–fundus should be known. This dimension is on occasion not available by sounding the uterus, as, for example, when the disease destroys the os and canal, or when anteflexion or retroflexion of the uterus makes the sounding depth uncertain. A longitudinal scan allows a length measurement to be made. A vaginal obturator (see below) can be used to identify the distal end of the cervix if it is not clear-cut.

Our technique for painlessly dilating the cervical canal prior to insertion of a cervix applicator tandem involves (1) sounding the canal, (2) placement of a "laminaria" (Fig. 15) in the canal for a period of about 18 hours, (3) removing the swollen laminaria, and (4) introducing the tandem through the painlessly dilated canal.[22] The procedures are done in the radiotherapy department, obviating the need for anesthesia and operating room. If the uterine sounding has been difficult and there is some question as to whether the laminaria is properly situated in the cervical canal, an ultrasound scan will usually clarify the issue (Fig. 12). Likewise, when an unloaded tandem has been placed under difficult anatomic circumstances and there is question of perforation of the uterus, a scan will show the position of the tandem in relation to the uterine fundus.[17] A knowledge of the size and position of the fundus prior to these procedures will help a lot in preventing complications.

Endometrial Carcinoma

When endometrial carcinoma is apparently confined to the uterus, one method of treatment is to implant the cavity with radioactive sources to treat the organ prior to hysterectomy.[16] These are usually placed in the uterus at the time of dilatation and curettage, and if ultrasound measurements of the dimensions of the fundus are already available, an estimate of the number of sources needed can be made. Also, these dimensions can be used to calculate the hours necessary to deliver the prescribed dose to the serosal surface of the organ. Management of vaginal cuff recurrence after hysterectomy is discussed later.

Ovarian Carcinoma

This is a surgical disease, at least when in its earlier resectable stages. The second line of attack is chemotherapy. Radiation treatment can be used as an alternative to chemotherapy, or to manage disease that has failed chemotherapy. Ultrasound can usually demon-

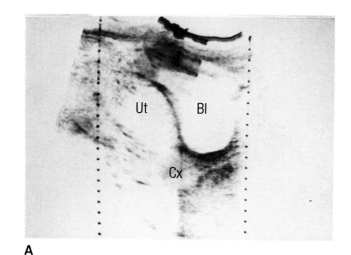

A

B

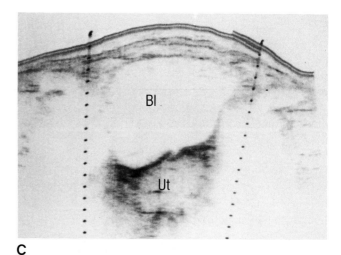

C

Fig. 11. Enlarged anteverted uterus. **A.** Longitudinal scan through anteverted uterus which is enlarged due to endometrial carcinoma. **B.** Increased bladder filling tends to correct the anteversion. **C.** When the transverse scan plane is angled 25 degrees cranially it shows a good cross section of the fundus, an example of the flexibility of ultrasound imaging. Bl, bladder. Ut, uterine fundus. Cx, cervix.

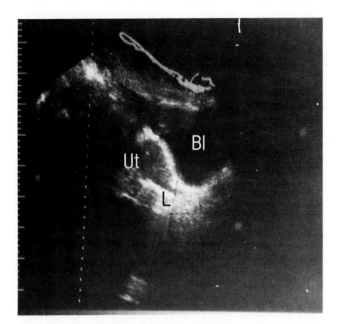

Fig. 12. Laminaria in cervix. Longitudinal scan through uterus to demonstrate location of a laminaria used to dilate the cervical canal prior to introduction of a cervix applicator tandem. It is properly situated in the cervix and lower uterine segment. Bl, bladder. Ut, uterus, L, laminaria.

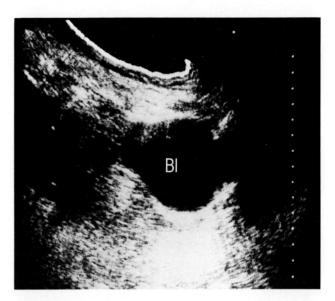

Fig. 13. Obscuring detail. Longitudinal scan in midline of posthysterectomy patient. The detail of tissues posterior to the bladder are obscured by the dense echo pattern caused by excessive transmission through full bladder, Bl. When that area is being studied, the gain needs to be turned down until there is good detail there.

strate the extent of the pelvic ovarian mass or masses very well for treatment planning with external beam therapy.[9,10,12] Even with extension of disease to the entire abdomen radiation therapy is one option for palliation. The "moving strip" technique treats a relatively small volume of tissue at any one time, gradually moving the volume up the abdomen. Ultrasound can demonstrate the position of the dome of the diaphragm, which would be the upper boundary of the treatment volume. "Half-body radiation," or in this case whole abdomen radiation, is another approach. Here, the entire abdomen–pelvis is irradiated at one sitting, to a high single increment dose, perhaps repeated once after an interval.

In this kind of widespread abdominal disease, the most helpful role of ultrasound might be monitoring the response of the disease to treatment (discussed below).

Posthysterectomy Patients

Ultrasound is sometimes more successful than CT in imaging small structures situated posterior to the bladder, such as a cervical stump, or small masses associated with the vaginal cuff in posthysterectomy patients (Fig. 14). However, it is easy to obscure detail in this area by dense recording of echoes caused by the increased transmission through the bladder (Fig. 13). As an alternative to surgical removal, a small cervical stump carcinoma or a vaginal cuff recurrence of a carcinoma can

be implanted with radioactive seeds or needles. Transverse and longitudinal depiction of the structure gives the dimensions necessary to determine the number of implant sources needed and their intended distribution. Precise localization of structures in that area may sometimes be helped by placing an "obturator" in the vagina with the inner end up against the cervix or the vaginal cuff (Fig. 14). The relationship of the structure with the end of the obturator precisely localizes it on longitudinal and transverse scans. A tampon has been used for this purpose in CT scans,[23] but for ultrasound imaging a "water bag" or a nylon vaginal dilator is preferable (Fig. 15). The nylon device stops transmission of the sound beam and produces recognizable dense echoes from its near surface plus a shadow effect (Fig. 16). The water bag is recognized as a discrete cystic tube and is the most satisfactory of the two (Fig. 14). A 6-inch segment of three-fourths-inch diameter rubber drain material (a flat hollow tube) is tied off at one end with suture material and then turned inside out. The open end is fitted over a water faucet and filled under a little pressure, and the tube twisted to prevent escape of water. A long-handled forcep is then clamped over the twisted portion and used to hold the tube for insertion. By wrapping the tube around the tip of the clamp, its diameter will increase as it is shortened. As an alternative, a large-size rubber finger cot can substitute for the drain material.

In the patient who has undergone hysterectomy

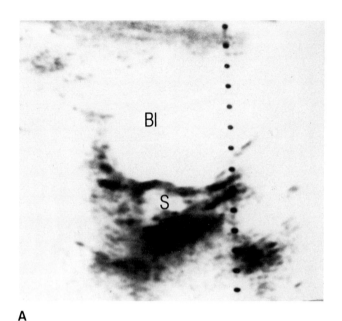

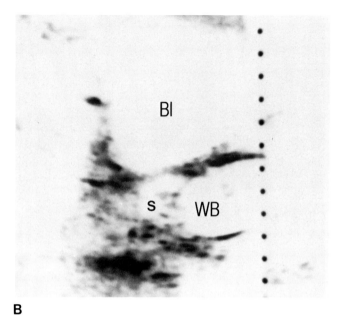

A   **B**

Fig. 14. Cervical stump carcinoma. **A.** A longitudinal midline pelvic scan demonstrates a 2 × 2-cm mass behind the bladder. **B.** The same scan after placement of a vaginal water bag, shows the relation of the mass to the vagina and provides information for planning treatment by radioactive implant through the vagina. Bl, bladder. S, stump ca. WB, water bag. (See Fig. 15.)

for endometrial or ovarian cancer, the tissues at the line of amputation of the vagina (vaginal cuff area) are at high risk for recurrence (Fig. 17). The recurrence may or may not be visible on speculum examination. For the first few months after hysterectomy there is invariably a small mass of indurated tissue at the cuff, which can be discerned on ultrasound scans. In some

patients a degree of mass effect remains indefinitely.[24] Imaging of this area after the initial healing of the vaginal wound will serve as a baseline for later comparison scans looking for recurrence. Any enlargement of the cuff tissues has to be viewed with suspicion.

MONITORING RESPONSE TO TREATMENT

Any tumor that can be imaged with ultrasound can be reexamined at appropriate times for assessment of its response to treatment by either radiation or chemotherapy. This assessment can be a major factor in making management decisions and is much more precise and quantitative than relying on written descriptions of physical examinations, especially if they are being done by more than one physician. Brascho,[17] with ultrasound equipment within the department, has regularly scanned his radiotherapy patients during and after their treatment course. Significant tumor shrinkage during treatment may allow a reduction in treatment volume, thus sparing some normal tissues the full dose of radiation. A "boost dose" of additional radiation delivered to a residual mass after completion of large field therapy is a common treatment technique (Fig. 17).

Shawker[25] has extensively described the uses and methods of ultrasound tumor monitoring, either for determining tumor growth rate or its response to a

Fig. 15. Vaginal obturators and cervix laminaria. **A.** Segment of Penrose rubber drain tubing. **B.** Tubing tied off and filled with water (water bag). **C.** Nylon vaginal dilator (obturator). **D.** Laminaria for dilating cervical canal. Usually, a smaller diameter laminaria is used (3 mm), which swells overnight to 7 or 8 mm, thus painlessly dilating the canal.

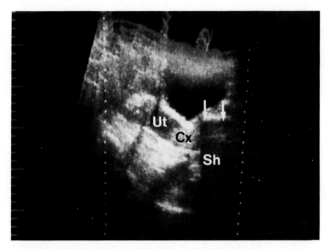

Fig. 16. Vaginal obturator as an aid in measuring uterine length for planning uterine implants. Longitudinal scan with nylon vaginal obturator against end of cervix. Arrows indicate anterior surface of obturator. The shadowing helps to localize the end of the obturator. Ut, fundus. Cx, cervix. Sh, shadowing.

particular treatment. A baseline image of the tumor size should be made at the start of a course of radiation therapy or chemotherapy in such a way that the same dimensions can be taken at subsequent monitoring scans. This is the time to decide just what measurements of the tumor mass are going to be used to follow its course. Gross changes in tumor size can be followed by measuring the largest diameter obtainable in a single reproducible plane. Multiple parallel scans are made through the tumor to find the largest dimension. This method is most valid for *spherical masses* (Fig. 18), in which case its relationship to the volume of the tumor is $V = 4.2\ (d/2),^3$ where d = diameter. If the mass is *ellipsoid*, volume calculation requires the three dimensions of length, width, and height — $V = 0.52$ (LxWxH). As an alternative, the "average tumor diameter" could be obtained by averaging the two perpendicular largest dimensions. With *irregularly shaped* masses a "tumor index value" can be obtained with a single sweep, always through the same portion of the tumor. A better index can be obtained by taking an arithmetic average of the three largest perpendicular dimensions.

True volume determination of an irregular mass requires making parallel images through the tumor at specific intervals, and then summing the areas of each image. The area can be obtained with a planimeter, but the effort is simplified with a computer program in which the areas are calculated and summed merely by drawing around the perimeter with a digitizer pen.[25] Volume determinations give a more precise picture of changes in tumor size, but in any case the measurements obtained serially should be plotted against time

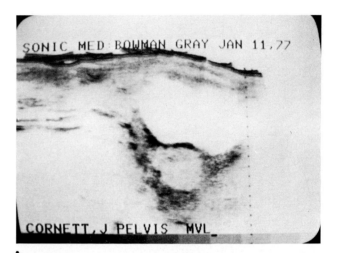

A

B

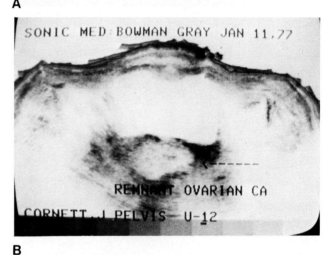

C

Fig. 17. Vaginal cuff recurrence of ovarian carcinoma. **A, B.** Longitudinal and transverse scans demonstrate size and location of a discrete 4 cm recurrent mass associated with the vaginal cuff. This could be treated with external beam therapy or needle implant or combination of the two. **C.** Transverse scan after external beam therapy shows small residual mass at the cuff which was subsequently implanted with needles. (*Reprinted with permission from Blake DD: Ultrasonography in the practice of radiotherapy. Appl Radiol 8:120, 1979.*)

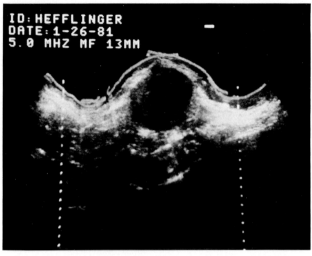

A

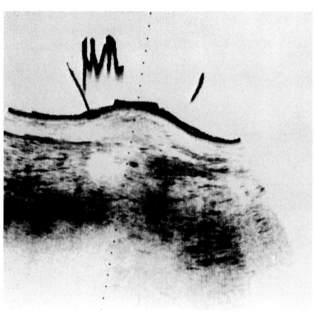

B

Fig. 18. Monitoring tumor response to chemotherapy. **A.** Pretreatment scan through a metastatic abdominal wall mass (ovarian cancer) which was treated with chemotherapy. The volume of a spherical mass can be calculated from just one diameter measurement. **B.** Reduced volume after one month of chemotherapy. Monitoring serial volumes of a mass is very helpful to the chemotherapist in making treatment decisions.

on graph paper. To this can be added any pertinent information about treatment.

When multiple tumors are present, such as may occur with abdominal extension of ovarian carcinoma, it is preferable to follow several masses rather than one. The rates of response of different tumor masses often vary within the same patient. Their locations

should be numbered and mapped out on an external body diagram, to be referred to at each monitoring visit. This is helpful to the physician who is managing the treatment as well as to the sonographer. Several recommendations can be made that will tend to reduce the incidence of errors in serial tumor monitoring:

1. The same sonographer should do all scans on a particular patient.
2. The same scanning machine and transducer should be used.
3. Maintain frequent calibration of scanning unit.

FOLLOW-UP AFTER TREATMENT

Scanning done at interval follow-up visits after completion of radiation or chemotherapy should include the entire pelvis and abdomen as well as the previously treated disease.[18] One should look for new tumor masses, enlarged pelvic or paraaortic nodes, or the presence of ascitic fluid (Fig. 17). If there is demonstrable residual or new disease, it should be documented quantitatively so that its response to subsequent treatment can be monitored, as described above.

REFERENCES

1. Ekstrand KE, Dixon RL, et al: The calculation of dose distribution for chest wall irradiation using B-mode ultrasonography. Radiology 111:185, 1974
2. Battista JJ, Van Dyk J, et al: Practical aspects of radiotherapy planning with computed tomography. Clin Invest Med 4:5, 1981
3. Spanos WJ Jr, Hogstram KR: An overview of radiation therapy planning systems. Appl Radiol 69, Mar–Apr 1982
4. Lee DJ, Leibel S, et al: The value of ultrasonic imaging and CT scanning in planning the radiotherapy for prostatic carcinoma. Cancer 45:724, 1980
5. Blake DD: Use of ultrasound in radiotherapy, in Resnick MI, Sanders RC (eds); Ultrasound in Urology. Baltimore, Williams and Wilkins, 1979, p 352
6. Carson PL, Wenzel WW, et al: Ultrasound imaging as an aid to cancer therapy—I & II. Int J Radiat Oncol Biol Phys 1:119, 335, 1975
7. Kratochwil A: Treatment planning, in Goldberg BB (ed), Ultrasound in Cancer. New York, Churchill Livingstone, 1981
8. Zagzebski JA, Wiley AL, et al: Ultrasonic B-scanning for radiation therapy planning and follow-up of superficial tumors. Int J Radiat Oncol Biol Phys 2:715, 1977
9. Coulam CM, Julian CG, et al: Clinical efficacy of CT and US in evaluating gynecologic tumors. Appl Radiol 79, Jan–Feb 1982

10. Walsh JW, Rosenfield AT, et al: Prospective comparison of ultrasound and computed tomography in the evaluation of gynecologic pelvic masses. Am J Roentgenol 131:955, 1978

11. Zaritzky D, Blake D, et al: Transrectal ultrasonography in the evaluation of cervical carcinoma. Obstet Gynecol 53:105, 1979

12. Walsh JW, Taylor KJW, et al: Gray-scale ultrasound in 204 proved gynecologic masses: Accuracy and specific diagnostic criteria. Radiology 130:391, 1979

13. Brizel HE, Livingston PA, et al: Radiotherapeutic applications of pelvic computed tomography. J Comp Assist Tomogr 3:453, 1979

14. Chen SS, Kumari S, et al: Contribution of abdominal computed tomography (CT) in the management of gynecologic cancer: Correlated study of CT image and gross surgical pathology. Gynec Oncol 10:162, 1980

15. Blake DD: Ultrasonography in the practice of radiotherapy. Appl Radiol 112, Jan–Feb 1979

16. Brascho DJ, Kim RY, et al: Use of ultrasonography in planning intracavitary radiotherapy of endometrial carcinoma. Radiology 129:163, 1978

17. Brascho DJ: Radiation treatment planning, in Brascho DJ, Shawker TH, Abdominal Ultrasound in the Cancer Patient. New York, Wiley, 1980

18. Paling MR, Shawker TH, et al: Ultrasonic evaluation of therapeutic response in tumors: Its value and implications. J Clin Ultrasound 9:281, 1981

19. Standards Committee, American Institute of Ultrasound in Medicine. Standard presentation and labeling of ultrasound images. J Clin Ultrasound 5:103, 1977

20. Blake DD: Radiobiologic aspects of the kidney. Radiol Clin N Am 3:75, 1965

21. Brascho DJ, Bryan JM, et al: Diagnostic ultrasound to determine renal size and position for renal blocking in radiation therapy. Int J Radiat Oncol Biol Phys 2:1217, 1977

22. Ferree CR, Raben M, et al: Use of laminaria in intracavitary applications for carcinoma of the cervix. Radiology 109:222, 1973

23. Cohen WN, Seidelmann FE, et al: Use of a tampon to enhance vaginal localization in computed tomography. Am J Roentgenol 128:1064, 1977

24. Parulekar SG: Ultrasound evaluation of the posthysterectomy pelvis. J Clin Ultrasound 10:265, 1982

25. Shawker TH: Monitoring response to therapy, in Brascho DJ, Shawker TH, Abdominal Ultrasound in the Cancer Patient. New York, Wiley, 1980

40 Pelvic Inflammatory Disease and Endometriosis: Conditions Affecting Both Uterus and Adnexa

Roger C. Sanders

INTRODUCTION

This chapter considers gynecologic diseases that do not conveniently fall into the category of an ovarian or uterine process and generally involve both the uterus and adnexa. The commonest conditions in which this situation occurs are pelvic inflammatory disease (PID) and endometriosis. Other conditions that may on occasion involve both adnexa and uterus, such as a ruptured corpus lutein cyst, are briefly discussed. Ectopic pregnancy is considered in Chapter 30.

PELVIC INFLAMMATORY DISEASE (PID)

There are few countries in the world in which pelvic inflammatory disease is not a major problem. This disease is increasing in frequency due to the venereal disease epidemic that is sweeping the globe. Although the usual cause of veneral PID is gonorrhea, other bacteria, notably *C. trachomitis* may be responsible. Less often a local pelvic source may be responsible for infection rather than a venereal contact. Possible local causes include ruptured appendiceal abscess with spread into the pelvis, diverticular abscess, Crohn's disease with accompanying abscess formation, surgery in the region of the pelvis and puerperal and postabortion complications. Intrauterine devices (IUDs) predispose to PID,[1-5] which occurs most often at the time of insertion or reinsertion or when there is perforation of the IUD into the surrounding tissues. PID among IUD users tends to be associated with actinomycosis.[1] With other types of PID of nonvenereal origin, bacterial de-

rived from the intestinal tract such as *E. coli* are usually responsible.

Clinical

Staging the severity of PID helps in management.[6] The typical clinical presentation of mild salpingitis is a woman who has a vaginal discharge, a temperature of greater than 37.8°C and a slightly elevated ESR. Patients with such a mild presentation are considered to have acute salpingitis without peritonitis. In more severe disease there is bilateral lower quadrant rebound tenderness and a very high ESR. This is considered to be acute salpingitis with peritonitis; culdocentesis is of value in this group. Triple rather than double drug therapy is usually given for this more severe variety of infection.

If, in addition to the signs already described, a pelvic mass can be felt, acute salpingitis with pyosalpinx is considered present. Drug therapy is given to this group for a relatively short period of time before surgery is adopted if antibiotic therapy is ineffective. When pelvic tenderness is disseminated and there are multiple masses, tuboovarian abscesses are considered present, in which case surgical removal of the infected organs has been recommended.[6]

Other Methods of Diagnosis

The usual way of establishing the diagnosis of PID is to perform a Gram stain on cervical vaginal material looking for gonorrhea or other bacteria. If no organism is seen, a culdocentesis may be required. Examination of the male partner may also allow culture of the offending organism. It may be necessary to proceed to laparoscopy to obtain infected material in the more subtle cases.[7]

Spread

Characteristically, venereal PID disseminates along the mucosa of the pelvic organs. After initial infection of the cervical area, spread is along the uterine endometrium (metritis) through the fallopian tubes (salpingitis) and into the region of both ovaries (oophoritis). Intraperitoneal spread then takes place with the formation of multiple abscesses. Venereal infections are almost always bilateral. If the abscess develops as a consequence of IUD migration out of the uterus,[5] following gut rupture, or pelvic operation, unilateral abscess development may take place and spread occurs in the region where the source of the infection is located, e.g., around a leaking anastomotic line or at the site of diverticular rupture.

Ultrasonic Technique

The ultrasonic techniques used in the investigation of PID are similar to those used elsewhere in the pelvis. As in the examination of any pelvic lesion, it is desirable to have a full bladder before the ultrasonic examination is performed. Unfortunately, due to the inflammatory disease and associated tenderness, optimal distension of the bladder may not be possible. In some cases, however, the abscess itself provides an adequate acoustical window.

Sonographic Findings

Acute PID. With venereal PID the first sonographic finding is endometrial involvement (endometritis). As a rule a more prominent decidual reaction is seen than usual; the consequent echogenic line may well be surrounded by a sonolucent zone not too dissimilar to the halo effect around the decidual reaction that occurs normally just before menstruation (Fig. 1). It has been suggested that uterine echogenicity may be generally decreased in the presence of acute uterine PID[4] but I have not seen this. The decidual reaction associated with endometritis may be so severe that fluid can be seen within the endometrial cavity (Fig. 2) or the endometrial echoes may be much more pronounced than usual (Fig. 3). Progression to pyocolpus does not occur in venereal PID but is occasionally seen in older women with cervical stenosis usually following irradiation of carcinoma of the cervix or in association with rare infective entities such as tuberculosis (Fig. 4). If gas is present in a pyocolpus, partial shadowing of a portion of the uterine wall will occur (Fig. 5).

Although spread into the tubes occurs next, in practice the earliest sonographic evidence that infection

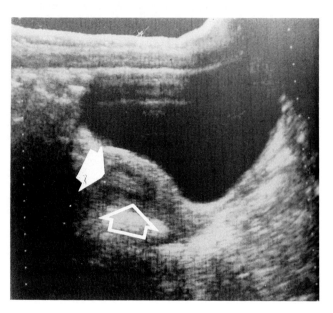

Fig. 1. Prominent decidual reaction within the uterus due to endometritis. Note the hypoechoic area (*open arrow*) around the decidual reaction (*solid arrow*).

has occurred, after the uterine involvement, is the development of a subtle line of fluid along the posterior aspect of the uterus (Fig. 6). This fluid often spreads to a more superior location than the small amount of cul de sac fluid seen at the time of ovulation. With more severe infection, a large fluid collection may develop in the cul de sac (Figs. 7, 8). In the earlier stages such a collection can be confused with midcycle fluid due to follicular rupture. Fluid in the cul de sac indistinguishable from PID can also be seen with ascites and hemorrhage. If much oral fluid is given to the patient before a sonographic examination, fluid may occur in the cul de sac area either associated with fluid-

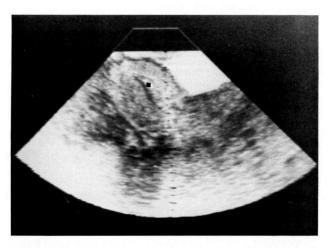

Fig. 2. Endometritis causing formation of fluid (*black square*) within the uterine cavity.

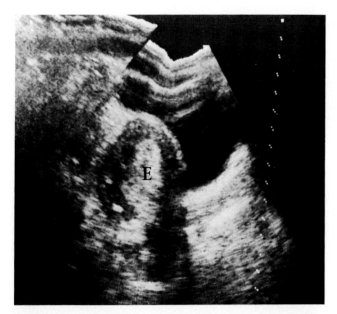

Fig. 3. Endometritis associated with a large echogenic decidual reaction (E).

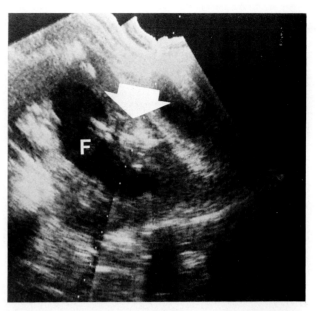

Fig. 4. Longitudinal section of a pyocolpus due to tuberculosis. Note the calcification within the myometrium (*arrow*) and the fluid (F) within the endometrial cavity.

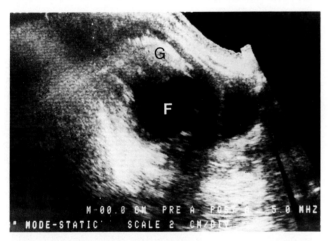

Fig. 5. Longitudinal section. Pyocolpus with gas formation due to cervical stenosis. There is fluid (F) within the uterus. Some gas (G) has caused acoustical shadowing.

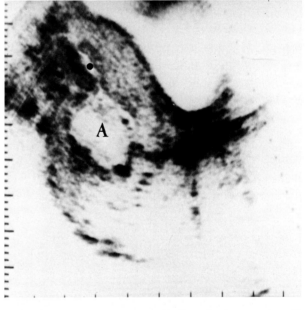

Fig. 6. Abscess in the cul de sac (A). There is also pus alongside the posterior aspect of the uterus (*black dot*)—a common early finding in pelvic inflammatory disease.

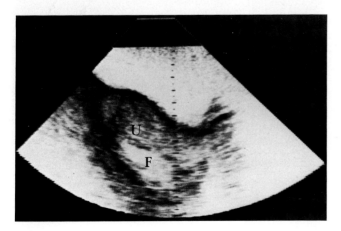

Fig. 7. Fluid in the cul de sac due to pelvic inflammatory disease. There is more fluid (F) in the cul de sac than is normally seen in association with the menstrual cycle and ovulation. U = uterus.

585

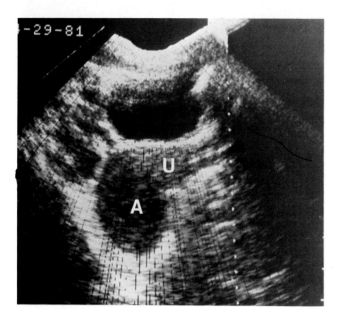

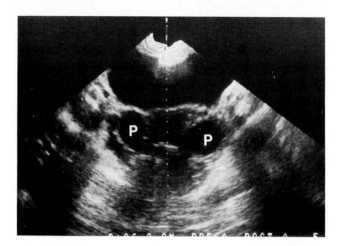

Fig. 9. Bilateral pyosalpinx. The two pyosalpinx are circular (P) and are similar in size.

Fig. 8. Subtle abscess in association with pelvic inflammatory disease in which the margin between the uterus (U) and the abscess (A) is not well seen. There is a slight difference in acoustical texture between the uterus and the abscess.

filled bowel loops or perhaps due to the development of intraperitoneal fluid.[8] Pus in the cul de sac may contain internal echoes and be hard to distinguish from the uterus (Fig. 8).

Pyosalpinx, pus filling the fallopian tube, occurs at a slightly later stage. Pus within a dilated tube is confined within a circular or more or less ovoid structure (Figs. 9, 10A, B). There may well be low-level echoes present within the fluid and a fluid–fluid level is a feature particularly suggestive of a pyosalpinx

(Figs. 11, 12) (a fluid–fluid level may also be seen with hematoma, dermoids and the occasional necrotic pelvic tumor). Usually the walls of a pyosalpinx are relatively smooth; there may be a variable echogenic pattern within although most are more or less echo-free. A configuration suggestive of an ectopic gestational sac may be seen and even apparently contain a fetal pole (Fig. 13). Pyosalpinx is commonly bilateral (Fig. 9).

With a worsening infection a tuboovarian abscess (TOA) develops. TOAs do not usually have the round shape of a pyosalpinx and may be multilocular. Several sonolucent areas may surround the ovary (Figs. 14, 15).[9] The ovary is relatively resistant to veneral infection. Low-level echoes within the collections are frequent (Fig. 16).

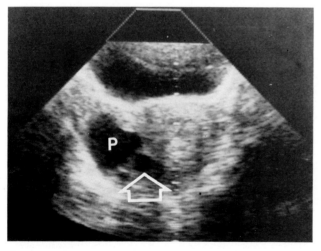

A

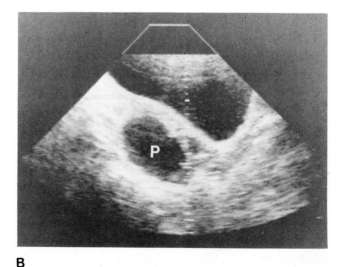

B

Fig. 10. Transverse and longitudinal views. Pyosalpinx with a less spherical shape (P) and a few internal echoes. A small abscess has formed behind the uterus (*arrow*).

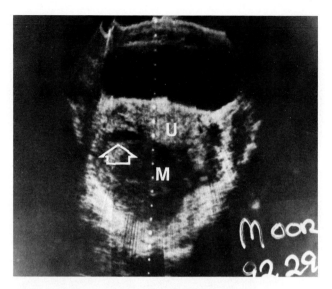

Fig. 11. Pyosalpinx containing a fluid–fluid level (*arrow*). The abscess is almost filled with somewhat echogenic material (M). The uterus is slightly deviated to the left (U).

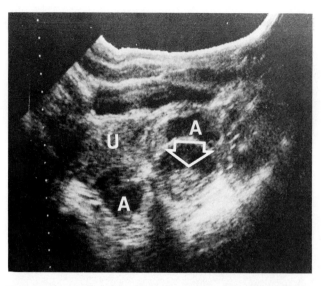

Fig. 12. Pyosalpinx with a fluid–fluid level (*arrow*). The uterus is deviated to the right (U). There are two other abscesses present (A).

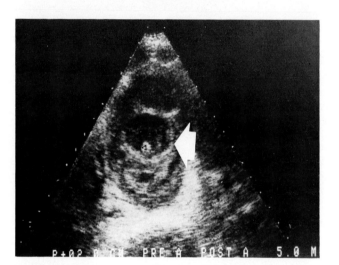

Fig. 13. Tuboovarian abscess resembling an ectopic pregnancy. There appears to be an adnexal ring (*arrow*) and even a small fetal pole (*black triangle*). This was purulent material within the abscess.

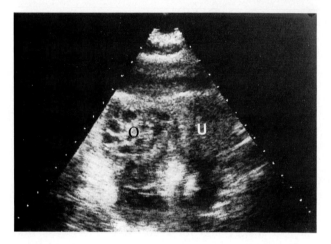

Fig. 14. Multiple small tuboovarian abscesses surround the ovary (O). The uterus (U) is deviated to the left and hard to distinguish from the surrounding infected area.

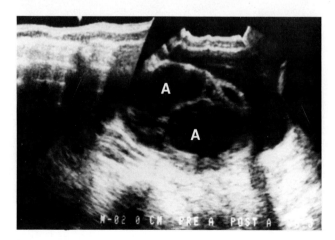

Fig. 15. Tuboovarian abscesses (A) with multiple loculations. Note the septa between the abscess components.

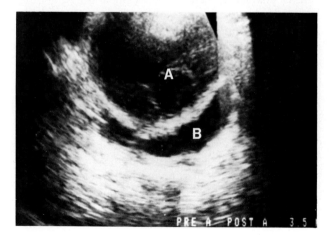

Fig. 16. Tuboovarian abscesses in an unusual location anterior to the bladder (B). The abscess (A) contains a number of low-level echoes.

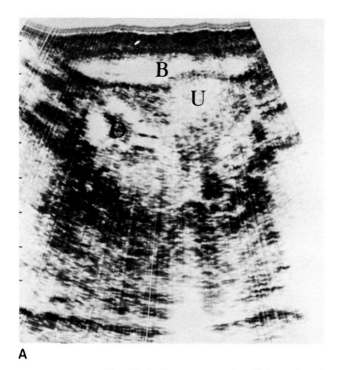

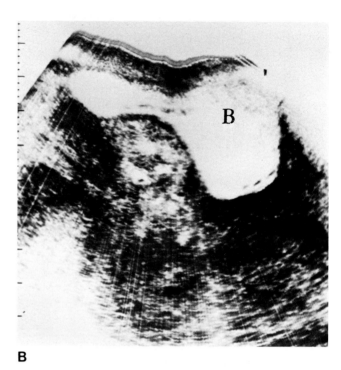

A   B

Fig. 17. A. Transverse section. Tuboovarian abscess with relative sparing of the ovary. The ovary (O) is surrounded by several small loculated cavities. There is widespread abscess formation so the uterus (U) cannot be easily made out. **B.** Sagittal section. Note the fixation of the bladder (B) on the sagittal section. The abscess bulges toward the bladder.

At a later stage multiple abscesses develop throughout the pelvis. The abscesses tend to form in a dependent site in the cul de sac (Figs. 17A, B). If generalized abscesses are present, the borders are irregular and shaggy and there are frequently areas that are less echogenic than the surrounding mesentery where inflammation without liquid material exists as opposed to the sonolucent areas where abscesses containing pus are present. Sonolucent areas sometimes containing septa are interspersed with slightly more echogenic regions that are, nevertheless, less echogenic than the mesentery. Gas may be present in some abscesses, which can either be seen as patchy dense echoes or, if there is a good deal of gas, as echoes associated with acoustical shadowing. When infection has spread out of the tubes into the neighboring tissues, the borders between the various adnexal organs become indistinct. The uterus develops an indefinite outline if a portion of the pelvic mass lies alongside the uterine border (Fig. 18). Confusion with fibroids can occur (Fig. 8).

Widespread PID can be confused with loops of fluid-filled bowel; distinction between these two entities depends on observation of peristaltic movement or the performance of a water enema (Figs. 19A, B).[10] In this procedure a tube is inserted into the rectum and a small amount of water is run into the gut while the area is examined with real time through the bladder. Paristalsis within bowel will be recognized by a fanlike movement as water moves through bowel.

The pubococcygeus muscle can be mistaken for an abscess if casual technique is used. Distinction can be made by noting that a second similar muscle mass

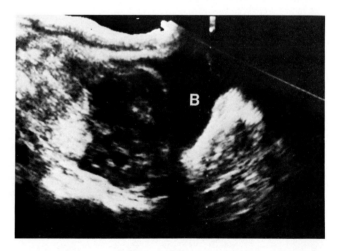

Fig. 18. Very severe pelvic inflammatory disease with loss of normal landmarks, multiple abscess formation and indentation of the bladder (B).

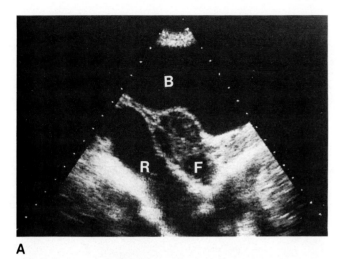

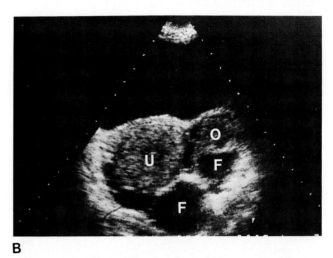

A

B

Fig. 19. A. Fluid-filled cystic structures (F) were seen posterior to the uterus (U) and the left ovary (O). It was uncertain whether these represented abscesses or fluid-filled bowel loops. **B.** A water enema was performed. There was evidence of a cul de sac fluid collection (F) in addition to gut. The rectum has a characteristic configuration (R).

is present on the contralateral side (Figs. 20A, B). Obliquing the patient away from the suspect area may help.

IUDs and Abscesses

Abscesses associated with IUDs tend to be unilateral. Abscesses occur with increased frequency even when the IUD is still present within the uterus (Figs. 21, 22).[11] It is unusual to be able to see the IUD responsible for an abscess if it has perforated out of the uterus (see Chapter 41). If the abscess is entirely pus filled and the IUD lies in the center, the IUD may occasionally be visible (Fig. 23). As already mentioned, IUD

abscesses are often due to actinomycosis. Abscesses associated with actinomycosis tend to have more septa than others (Fig. 24).

Chronic PID

With long-standing severe PID widespread fibrosis with adhesions occurs so that all of the contents of the pelvis merge in a central mass or an ovary becomes adhesed and lies in an unusual site. Both in acute and chronic PID obliteration of the margins between the various structures that lie in the pelvis (the adnexa and uterus) is commonplace (Fig. 25A, B).[12] A central ill-defined mass composed of all the adnexal organs

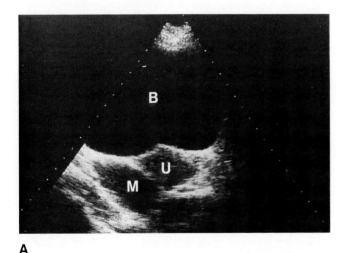

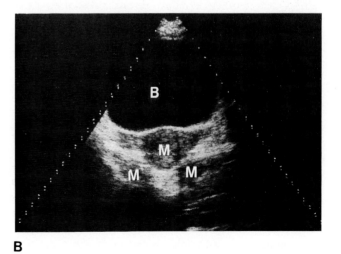

A

B

Fig. 20. A. A transverse section showing an apparent mass (M) just to the right of the uterus (U) that was initially considered to be an abscess. **B.** An examination at a slightly higher level shows the uterus and ovaries in front of the pubococcygeous muscles (M). The muscle mass was mistaken for an abscess. B = bladder.

590

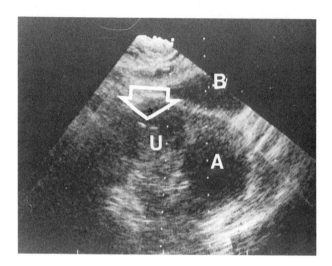

Fig. 21. Large pelvic abscess (A) due to a Dalcon shield. The Dalcon shield (*arrows*) can be seen within the uterus (U). B = bladder.

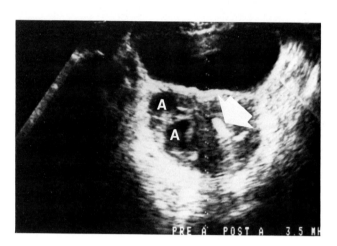

Fig. 22. Tuboovarian abscess due to Copper 7 IUD. Transverse section showing the Copper 7 (*arrow*) within the uterus with small abscess cavities in the right adnexa (A).

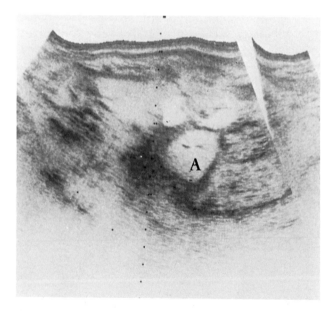

Fig. 23. Widespread pelvic inflammatory disease with multiple abscesses. The Dalcon shield can be seen within one of the abscesses (A) surrounded by fluid in the abscess; the IUD can be seen even though it lies outside the uterus.

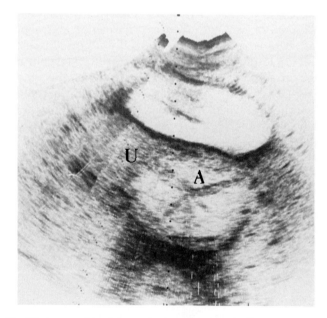

Fig. 24. Large pelvic abscess due to actinomycosis. Note the septations within the abscess cavity (A), a feature suggestive of actinomycosis. U = uterus.

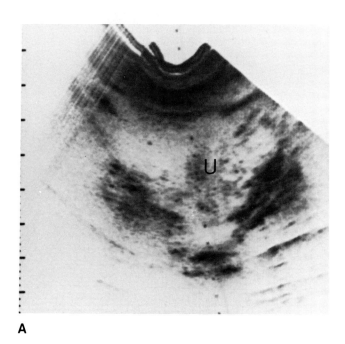

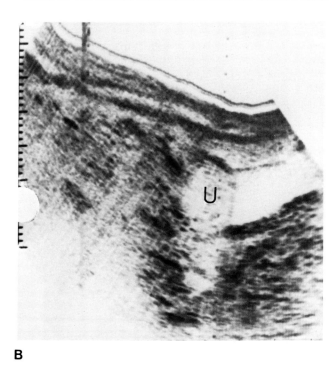

A   B

Fig. 25. A. Long-standing, very severe pelvic inflammatory disease with much fibrosis. The uterus (U) can barely be made out surrounded by multiple abscesses. A longitudinal section **(B)** shows the acute anteversion of the uterus (U) due to fixation and fibrosis.

and the uterus in which structures are indistinguishable may occur.

Hydrosalpinx

The long-term consequences of PID depend on severity. Hydrosalpinx may develop as a consequence of tubal adhesions, frequently on a bilateral basis.

Hydrosalpinx have a tendency to adopt a characteristic ultrasonic configuration. The ampullary segment of the tube expands more than the interstitial portion; a circle is formed with a tail pointing towards the uterus (Figs. 26, 27A, B). The tail may kink back on itself. The long tubular tail of the hydrosalpinx can be confused with a dilated ureter or vice versa. Internal echoes within a hydrosalpinx are unusual. Some hydrosalpinx appear as circular cystic structures and the proximal portion of the tube is never visualized. In other hydrosalpinx a tapered ovoid shape suggests a mass other than the standard ovarian cyst (Fig. 28). In chronic interstitial salpingitis, the tube becomes enlarged but has thick walls so the mass created appears solid. Peritoneal adhesions are commonplace in severe PID, with the consequent development of inflammatory cysts of the peritoneum (peritoneal retention cysts). These irregularly shaped cystic structures are usually anechoic.[13]

Ultrasound in Clinical Management

Ultrasound assists in the diagnosis and management

of PID in two ways. The patient with PID usually has an acutely tender pelvis that is hard to assess by clinical examination; satisfactory delineation of pelvic mass size and location can be made with an ultrasonic examination. In one study of 50 cases of PID a mass was found in 78 percent by sonography but only felt in 30 percent on a bimanual examination.[14] Since the extent of the disease, and in particular the presence of a mass, affects antibiotic selection (double versus triple therapy) and the possibility of surgery, sonogra-

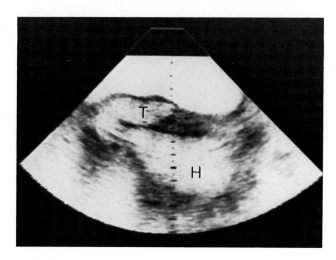

Fig. 26. Hydrosalpinx. The dilated fimbriated end (H) and much of the remainder of the tube (T) can be seen.

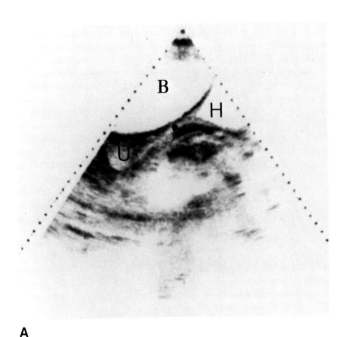

A

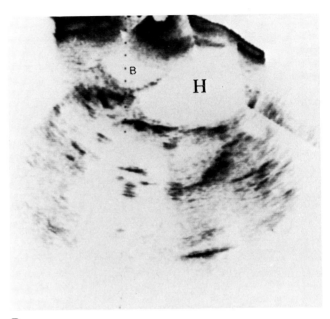

B

Fig. 27. A. Proximal end of hydrosalpinx. The uterus (U), fallopian tube and proximal end of the hydrosalpinx (H) can be made out. B = bladder. **B.** A section through the dilated fimbriated end shows the widened portion of the tube containing the hydrosalpinx (H). B = bladder.

phy becomes worthwhile when patient examination is suboptimal.

Once the abscess has been detected and measurements have been obtained, quantification of the response to antibiotic therapy can be provided. As a rule, response occurs within 2 to 5 days; if no clinical or sonographic response occurs, a change of antibiotic

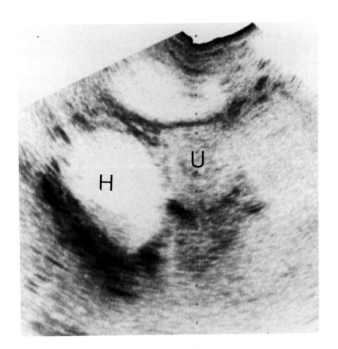

Fig. 28. Ovoid shaped hydrosalpinx (H). U = uterus.

therapy or surgery has to be considered.[7] If surgery is chosen, then sonography can help to decide whether the abscess can be easily drained. Multiple septations indicate a vaginal or rectal approach is unlikely to be satisfactory because the abscess is multilocular, whereas a single sonolucent area indicates that the abscess is appropriate for a puncture type drainage approach. The presence of internal echoes within an abscess does not necessarily mean that drainage will be unsuccessful. Pus can be echogenic.

Long-term consequences of abscess formation and PID include ectopic pregnancy and adhesions causing abdominal obstruction. Surprisingly, pregnancy is not totally incompatible with PID; presumably in such cases infection postdated the patient becoming pregnant (Fig. 29).

ENDOMETRIOSIS

A condition easily confused with PID from an ultrasonic viewpoint is endometriosis, although the clinical presentation is rather different. Endometriosis is a condition that affects, for the most part, women in their 30s who are infertile and of social class I. Its presentation may be occult, with little or no symptomatology except infertility or there may be dyspareunia, metromennorhagia, or dysmenorrhea. The condition is found in 8 to 30 percent of menstruating women at gynecologic surgery.

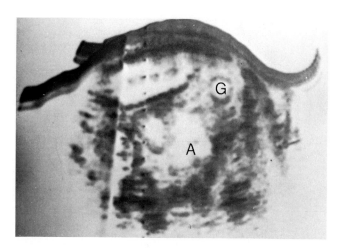

Fig. 29. A gestational sac (G) is present within the uterus which is deviated to the left. In addition there is a large pelvic abscess (A).

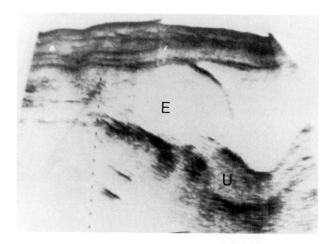

Fig. 30. Endometrioma. The large fluid-filled structure superior to the uterus (U) and bladder represents an endometrioma (E).

Ectopic endometrial tissue is laid down in a number of abnormal locations—typically around the ovaries and the broad ligament but also attached to other peritonealized organs such as bowel, ureter, and bladder. Endometrial tissue can occur within the myometrium when it is known as adenomyosis. The latter condition may cause a generalized enlargement of the uterus. Most of the time the abnormal endometrial tissue is deposited in relatively small amounts and is hard to detect with ultrasound; however, the secondary effects of the ectopic endometrial tissue may be detectable; every time the patient menstruates, the endometrial tissue bleeds with the formation of collections of blood known as "chocolate cysts."

Ultrasonic Features

The ultrasonic features are principally those of cystic structures containing blood.[15,16] Such "chocolate cysts" may in a minority of instances be totally echofree, with a relatively smooth border (Figs. 30, 31). The walls of endometrial cysts are, however, irregular as opposed to the smooth wall of the usual ovarian cyst. A common pattern is for the chocolate cyst to contain even low-level echoes (Fig. 32). Marginal echoes within an otherwise cystic structure may be seen.[17] Septa occur as an unusual feature.[17] Fluid–fluid levels are occasionally seen (Fig. 33). On other occasions the cysts contain clumps of dense high-level echoes representing clot (Figs. 34, 35). Several cysts may be seen simultaneously at different phases of the evolution of the blood clot (Fig. 36). In a minority of cases blood achieves a texture similar to that of a neoplastic mass or the uterus (Fig. 37). The discovery of what appears sonographically to be a solid ovarian neoplasm in a menstruating women is commonly due to endometriosis. As in pelvic inflammatory disease, masses due to endometriosis

may be hard to distinguish from the neighboring uterus. Pelvic inflammatory disease and endometriosis may coexist. Chocolate cysts can achieve a very large size and are occasionally seen in pregnancy.

The amount of abnormal endometrial tissue needs to be quite large before it can be seen with ultrasound. The small amounts that cause infertility and are appropriately treated with Danazol or other therapeutic agents rather than surgery are usually ultrasonically invisible.

It has been suggested that some of the lesions

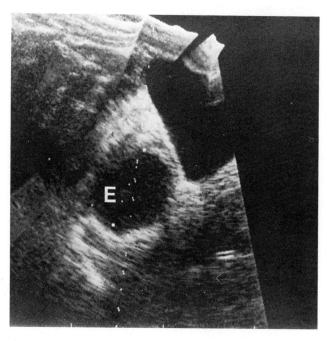

Fig. 31. This cystic endometrioma (E) could be mistaken for many other pelvic cystic masses such as a follicular cyst, serous cystadenoma, hydrosalpinx, etc.

594

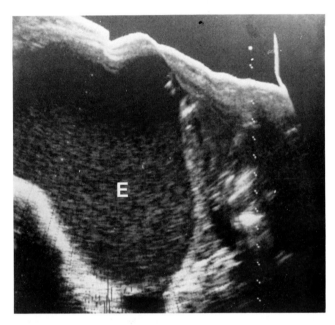

Fig. 32. Large endometrioma containing a number of low-level echoes (E). The rather even echogenic appearance is often seen in endometrioma. (*Courtesy of E. Lipsit M.D.*)

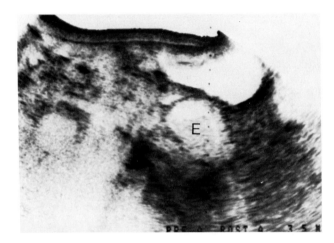

Fig. 33. Endometrioma (E) containing a number of low-level echoes in its more dependent portion with irregular fluid–fluid level.

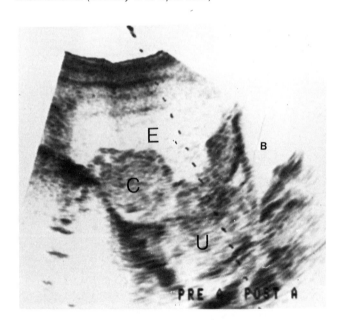

Fig. 34. Endometrioma (E) containing much echogenic clot (C) in addition to fluid-filled areas. U = uterus.

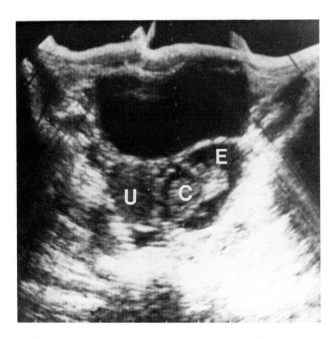

Fig. 35. Endometrioma (E) containing echogenic clot (C) with a relatively small fluid-filled area around the clot. U = uterus.

595

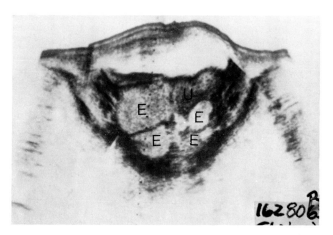

Fig. 36. Transverse views of multiple chocolate cysts (E) in varying stages of aging. Some are more echogenic than others. U = uterus.

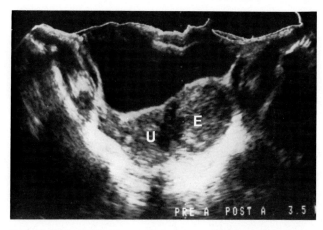

Fig. 37. Mass in the adnexa (E) thought prior to operation to be a solid ovarian neoplasm (E) but that proved to be an endometrioma. U = uterus.

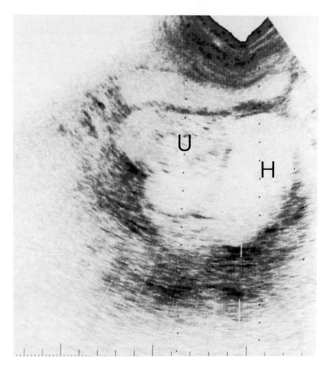

Fig. 38. Ruptured corpus lutein cyst with hematoma formation. The uterus (U) is deviated to the right and surrounded by a large fluid-filled area that represents blood (H). An identical appearance may be found with an ectopic pregnancy with a large bleed.

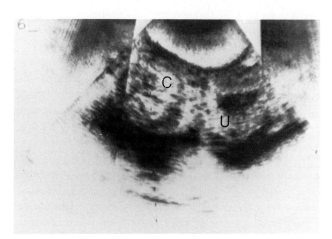

A

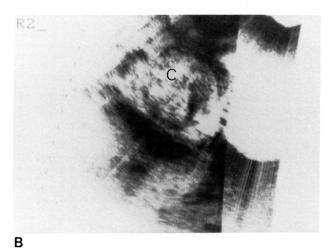

B

Fig. 39. A. Longitudinal section. **B.** Transverse section. Twisted hemorrhagic cyst. The cyst (C) contains numerous high-level echoes with echogenic material and resembles an endometrioma. There is a prominent decidual reaction within the uterus (U).

of adenomyosis, the form of endometriosis that involves the uterus, may be visible ultrasonically.[18] The finding said to indicate endometrioma deposits is the presence of small sonolucent areas within the uterus. This finding has not been duplicated by other authors.

OTHER CAUSES

There are a few other conditions in which involvement of the ovaries, adnexa, and uterus may occur with a confusing pattern that can be mistaken for PID. The commonest condition other than endometriosis that can mimic PID is ectopic pregnancy, which is dealt with in Chapter 30. Rupture of a corpus lutein cyst causes the formation of a pelvic hematoma; the consequent mass may be sonographically identical to ectopic pregnancy or PID (Fig. 38).[20] The contents of a twisted hemorrhagic cyst may resemble an endometrial chocolate cyst (Figs. 39 A, B). Severe bilateral ovarian cancer can spread to involve all the neighboring tissues so that distinction between the uterus, ovaries, and neoplastic tissue is difficult or impossible. Ovarian cancer may be multicystic in appearance resembling PID or endometriosis (see Chapter 36).

Although a specific diagnosis by ultrasound is often not possible in PID and endometriosis, accurate assessment of the extent and progress of the disease is feasible with ultrasound. An ultrasound examination is particularly useful when clinical examination is hindered by tenderness or obesity.

REFERENCES

1. Keebler C, Chatwani A, Schwartz R: Actinomycosis infection associated with intrauterine contraceptive devices. Am J Obstet Genecol 145:596, 1983
2. Edelman DA, Berger GS: Contraceptive practice and tuboovarian abscess. Am J Obstet Gynecol 138:541, 1980
3. Burkman RT, The Women's Health Study: Association between intrauterine device and pelvic inflammatory disease. Obstet Gynecol 57:269, 1981
4. Sample F: Pelvic inflammatory disease and endometriosis, in Sanders RC, James AE Jr (eds), The Principles and Practice of Ultrasonography in Obstetrics and Gynecology. New York, Appleton-Century-Crofts, 1980
5. Faulkner WL, Ory HW: Intrauterine devices and acute pelvic inflammatory disease. JAMA 235:1851, 1976
6. Monif GR: Clinical staging of acute bacterial salpingitis and its therapeutic ramification. Am J Obstet Gynecol 143:489, 1982
7. Spaulding LB, Gelman SR, Wood SD, et al: The role of ultrasonography in the management of endometritis/salpingitis/peritonitis. Obstet Gynecol 53:442, 1979
8. Sukov RJ, Whitcomb MJ: Rapid oral hydration: A cause of pelvic fluid collections at sonography. J Clin Ultrasound 9:115, 1981
9. Uhrich PC, Sanders RC: Ultrasonic characteristics of pelvic inflammatory masses. J Clin Ultrasound 4:199, 1976
10. Kurtz AB, Rubin CS, Kramer FL, et al: Ultrasound evaluation of the posterior pelvic compartment. Radiology 132:677, 1979
11. Westrom L, Bengtsson LP, Mardh PA: The risk of pelvic inflammatory disease in women using intrauterine contraceptive devices as compared to non-users. The Lancet 2:221, 1976
12. Bowie JD: Ultrasound of gynecologic pelvic masses: The indefinite uterus and other patterns associated with diagnostic error. J Clin Ultrasound 5:323, 1977
13. Lees RF, Feldman PS, Brenbridge NA, et al: Inflammatory cysts of the pelvic peritoneum. Am J Roentgenol 131:633, 1978
14. Spirtos HJ, Bernstine RL, Crawford WL, et al: Sonography in acute pelvic inflammatory disease. J Repro Med 27:312, 1982
15. Sandler MA, Kara JJ: The spectrum of ultrasonic findings in endometriosis. Radiology 127:229, 1978
16. Goldman SM, Minkin SI: Diagnosing endometriosis with ultrasound accuracy and specificity. J Reproduct Med 25:178, 1980
17. Coleman BG, Arger PH, Mulhern CB: Endometriosis: Clinical and ultrasonic correlation. Am J Roentgenol 132:747, 1979
18. Walsh JW, Taylor KJW, Rosenfield A: Gray scale ultrasonography in the diagnosis of endometriosis and adenomyosis. Am J Roentgenol 132:87, 1979
19. Hager WD, Eschenbach DA, Spence MR, et al: Criteria for diagnosis and grading of salpingitis. Obstet Gyncol 61:113, 1983
20. McCort JJ: Ruptured corpus luteum with hemoperitoneum. Radiology 116:65, 1975

41 | Ultrasound and the Intrauterine Device

William J. Cochrane

IUDs are more effective than any nonsurgical method, other than oral contraceptives, in preventing pregnancy. According to the most recent statistics, 8 to 10 percent of women practicing contraception use the IUD as the preferred method. It is estimated that 1.7 million women are currently using the IUD in the United States.[1,2] Five types of IUDs are presently available for use in this country: Lippes Loop, Saf-T-Coil, Cu7, CuT, and Progestasert (Fig. 1). The first two types are inert polyethylene devices, whereas the Cu7 and CuT have a fine copper wire wrapped around their proximal ends. The Progestasert, as the name suggests, has a core reservoir of progesterone which is released in constant minute amounts over a period of time. Bioactive types are reputed to have enhanced contraceptive qualities. Cumulative pregnancy rates range from 2 to 5 per 100 woman-years for all types currently in use. (Pooled data from manufacturer sources.)

MODE OF ACTION

The consensus of opinion suggests that the IUD prevents implantation of the fertilized egg by stimulating a nonspecific inflammatory reaction in the endometrium.[1,2] There is some additional evidence, however, that indicates that implantation may not be inhibited in some users. It is thought that implantation in these individuals is almost immediately followed by abortion.[2] In such cases human chorionic gonadotropin (hCG) testing may be transiently positive.[3]

Since ovulation and corpus luteum formation is not suppressed by IUD usage, the incidence of benign ovarian cysts is the same as in the general population (Fig. 2). This is in contradistinction to oral contraceptive users who have a markedly reduced incidence of physiologic ovarian cyst formation.

COMPLICATIONS

Although a popular means of contraception, the use of IUDs is not problem free. Among the expected complications are the following:

1. Lost IUD
2. Method failure
3. Associated pelvic inflammatory disease

All IUDs have a locator thread attached to their proximal ends. This thread extrudes from the cervical os and may be palpated or visualized on vaginal examination. If the thread is not located, then one of the following events has occurred:

1. Spontaneous unrecognized expulsion of the device
2. Detachment of the thread (very rare)
3. Migration of the thread into the cervical canal or uterine cavity (Often associated with an unsuspected pregnancy.)
4. Uterine perforation by the device

IUD RECOGNITION

In the majority of cases, if the IUD is present in the uterus, it can be visualized using sonography. Often a characteristic echo pattern is obtained from each type

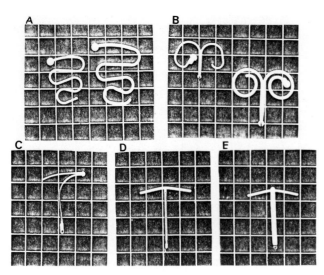

Fig. 1. A. Lippes Loop. **B.** Saf-T-Coil. **C.** Copper-7. **D.** Copper-T. **E.** Progestasert.

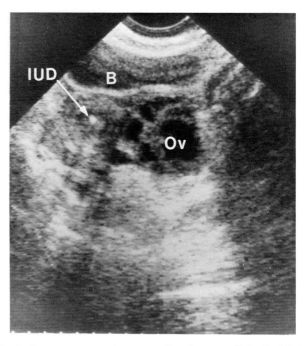

Fig. 2. Transverse scan shows a multicystic ovary (Ov) with IUD in situ. B, bladder.

of device (Fig. 3). If a typical echo pattern is not obtained, then strong echo activity with acoustical shadowing is highly suggestive of the presence of a device (Fig. 4). Without posterior shadowing, it can be difficult to distinguish endometrial echoes from echoes produced by an IUD, especially at the premenstrual stage, when the endometrium is most echogenic. This problem may be clarified by the use of postprocessing, which will eliminate the low level echoes produced by the endometrial lining (Fig. 5). If, as is unlikely, postprocessing is not available, then manipulation of the overall gain setting will aid in recognition. The high level echoes from the IUD will persist when echoes from other structures have disappeared.

There are several situations where IUD recognition can be problematic. When the uterus is retroverted or retroflexed, the ultrasound beam may not be in the ideal axis at right angles to the IUD and typical acoustical shadowing may not be demonstrated. Increased

bladder filling, however, will enable the examiner to alter the beam axis and increase the chances of recognition. Manual manipulation of the uterus during scanning to improve beam angle can be a valuable aid in such cases. Foci of uterine calcification or intrauterine gas bubbles can also produce strong echo activity with posterior shadowing. These processes can mimic the echo activity produced by an IUD. Calcifications are usually associated with myoma formation and a discrete tumor is often recognized (Fig. 6). Retained bone fragments from an incomplete abortion will produce highly reflective echoes similar to that of a device (Fig. 7). Where there is a coexisting pregnancy of more than 3 months, it is often impossible to distinguish the IUD

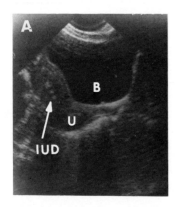
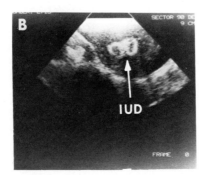
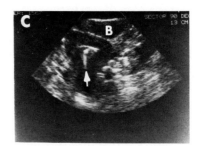

Fig. 3. Typical echo patterns of three types of devices. **A.** Lippes Loop. **B.** Saf-T-Coil. **C.** Copper-7. B, bladder. U, uterus.

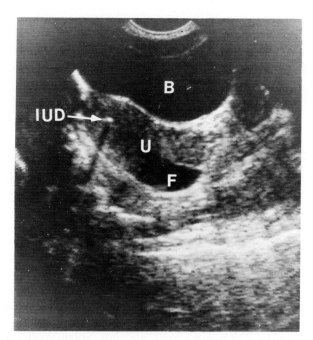

Fig. 4. Marked acoustical shadowing from an IUD which is not displaying any recognizable echo pattern. B, bladder. U, uterus. F, fluid in the cul de sac.

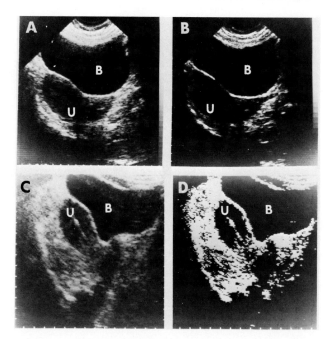

Fig. 5. Scan **A** shows an empty uterus with low level echoes from the endometrial cavity. In **B** postprocessing has attenuated completely the cavity. Compare **C** and **D** where the echoes produced by the IUD are not attenuated. B, bladder. U, uterus.

from the products of conception (see below). At times, the cervical canal, will produce a linear echo pattern simulating the presence of a Lippes type of IUD.

IUD PLACEMENT

In addition to locating the device, sonography can determine proper placement. The device should be situated in the fundal segment of the cavity, with the entire device distal to the internal cervical os. If the IUD is not placed in the fundus and lies in the mid-cavity or lower segment, expulsion or severe cramping and bleeding may ensue, necessitating removal (Fig. 8). Malplacement of the device will reduce its contraceptive effectiveness. Routine scanning of all patients having IUD insertions is not recommended, however, scanning of those patients at risk for malplacement, such as obese or postpartum patients, is suggested. Another group who may benefit from preinsertion scanning are women with retroverted or retroflexed uteri. These individuals have an increased risk of perforation.

PERFORATION

It is generally agreed that perforation most commonly occurs, or at least begins, at the time of insertion.[4] The diagnosis of complete perforation of the uterus

is made by displaying the uterus as sonographically empty with radiographic evidence of the presence of an IUD.[5] This may be confirmed by hysterography if the sonographic findings are uncertain (Fig. 9). Using hysterography as the only method of localization involves certain risks. It is an invasive technique involving the risk of infection and perforation. Recently the use of CAT scanning for localization of extrauterine IUDs has been reported.[6] This technique together with hysterography would present a biologic burden on an unsuspected pregnancy.

Partial perforation occurs when a portion of the

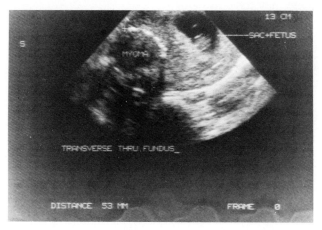

Fig. 6. Transverse scan of gravid uterus. There is a partially calcified myoma in the right fundal area. Note the acoustical shadowing.

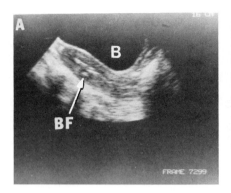
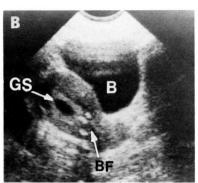

Fig. 7. A. A nonpregnant uterus containing bone fragment (BF) from an incomplete abortion. **B.** Gravid uterus with bone fragments (BF) in the lower segment. B, bladder. GS, gestational sac. Same patient as in **A.**

device remains within the myometrium. This can be difficult to diagnose sonographically. An incomplete echo pattern with an IUD placement eccentric to the endometrial cavity is suggestive of partial perforation.[5] If incomplete perforation is suspected, diagnostic laparoscopy is recommended for confirmation.

EMBEDMENT

When the IUD is eccentrically placed in the uterus, embedment of the device may have occurred. This means a portion of the device has intruded into the myometrium but has not perforated the serosal surface of the uterus (Fig. 10). It should be kept in mind that uterine myomas can displace the cavity, also resulting in an eccentrically positioned IUD (Fig. 11). Also congenital abnormalities such as a bicornate uterus can give rise to an eccentric sonographic localization. Embedment may also be suspected when the "central uterine cavity echo," consistent with the endometrium, is not seen surrounding the device.[7] Despite recent improvement in ultrasound resolution, uterine embedment by a device is still a difficult diagnosis to make. Other techniques such as hysteroscopy and hysterography may have to be used.

METHOD FAILURE

As mentioned previously, pregnancy rates of 2.8 to 5.3 per 100 woman-years have been reported with an IUD in place. Bioactive devices have a significantly lower rate (1.6 to 1.8 per woman-years).[2] The potential hazards of an IUD pregnancy are spontaneous abortion and sepsis. The spontaneous abortion rate in pregnancies where the IUD is not removed is about 50 percent. This is more than twice the abortion rate in those women whose IUDs have been removed or have spontaneously been expelled (23 percent).[8] The spontaneous abortion rate in the general population is about 18 percent.[9]

In 1974, the following recommendation was made by the American College of Obstetricians and Gynecologists: "Because of the increased risk of septic abortion, the IUD should be removed if the string is visible, or interruption of the pregnancy should be considered or offered as an option." Often as a pregnancy progresses the locator thread is drawn into the uterus, making removal impossible. It is therefore imperative to make an early diagnosis of a coexisting pregnancy. Ultrasound confirmation of an intrauterine pregnancy can be made from 5 menstrual weeks on. Most often the IUD is extragestational and in the lower or upper

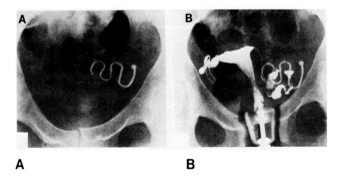

Fig. 8. Longitudinal **(A)** and transverse **(B)** scans showing a malpositioned IUD in the lower uterine segment. The left adnexal mass is a large endometrioma. B, bladder. U, uterus. E, endometrioma.

Fig. 9. A. Flat plate showing the presence of an IUD. **B.** Hysterosalpingogram confirming the extrauterine location of the IUD.

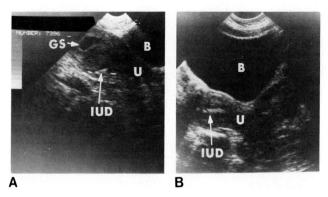

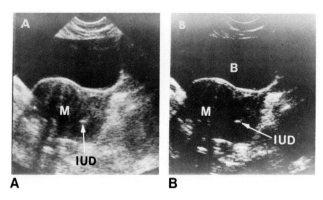

Fig. 10. A. Gravid uterus with the IUD just beneath the posterior serosal surface of the uterus. **B.** Embedded IUD. Distal third of the device is in the myometrium. GS, gestational sac. U, uterus. B, bladder.

Fig. 11. A. Eccentrically placed IUD in a myomatous uterus. **B.** Display of the device is enhanced by post processing. M, myoma. B, bladder.

segment of the uterus (Fig. 12). Occasionally the device appears closely related to the developing pregnancy and at times even intraamniotic (Fig. 13). One would presume that the more distant the IUD is from the developing pregnancy the more favorable the outcome. The available current information shows that there appears to be no increased risk in IUD pregnancies of congenital abnormalities.[2]

ECTOPIC PREGNANCY

There is a general belief that the use of an IUD increases the risk of an ectopic pregnancy. This is not the case. Only the relative frequency of ectopic pregnancies is higher in IUD users. In other words since the uterine implantations are markedly reduced by IUD use, those pregnancies that do occur are more likely to be extrauterine. In fact during the first 2 years of use, the IUD user has less chance of an ectopic pregnancy than women not using any contraception. The risk of ectopic pregnancy, however, increases with the length of use. This can be explained by the fact that,

with time, histologic changes associated with IUD use affect the fallopian tube. Women who present with an accidental pregnancy after more than three years use of an IUD have about a 1 in 10 chance of having an ectopic pregnancy. Despite this frequency the level of risk of an ectopic pregnancy in these long-term users is about the same as the general population not using contraceptives.[10,11]

A point that should be kept in mind is that an IUD user is at greatest risk of ectopic pregnancy immediately after the removal of the device. Up to 1 year after removal the foreign body reaction remains at a sufficient level to alter tubal function but not to prevent implantation.[11]

A proportion of IUD users will have a history of irregular bleeding. This makes accurate assessment of their menstrual history difficult and the possibility of a coexisting pregnancy should always be kept in mind. Any ultrasound examination done for localization of an IUD should include careful study of both adnexal areas to rule out the presence of a coexisting extrauterine pregnancy. Figure 14 shows an early ectopic pregnancy with an IUD in utero.

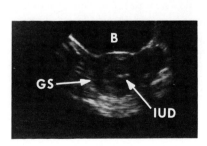
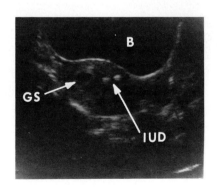
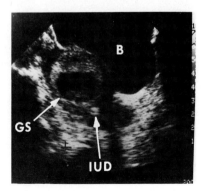

Fig. 12. A sequence of scans of a progressing pregnancy with the IUD remaining extragestational and in the lower segment. GS, gestational sac. B, bladder.

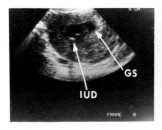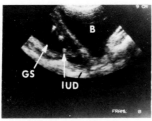

Fig. 13. Both scans show IUDs which are apparently in an intra-amniotic location.

PELVIC INFLAMMATORY DISEASE

Users of IUDs appear to have a two to three times greater risk of pelvic inflammatory disease over nonusers.[12,13] This risk is found to be the same for all types of IUDs. Advanced disease may take the form of a unilateral tuboovarian abscess.[14] Most often an associated infection is of an acute nature, either an endometritis or a salpingitis, conditions in which ultrasound offers little diagnostic help. However, if an abscess is present, sonography can accurately locate it and monitor response to treatment.

Recent evidence suggests that long-term use of any device may be associated with actinomycosis infection of the uterus.[15] It is now recommended that all types of IUDs should be periodically replaced. Previously this recommendation was only made for bioactive devices.

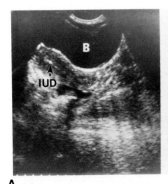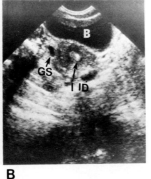

A   B

Fig. 14. Longitudinal **(A)** and transverse **(B)** scans displaying a right ectopic pregnancy with the IUD in situ. GS, gestational sac. B, bladder.

CONCLUSION

The IUD is a major method of contraception. Related complications such as malposition, expulsion, perforation, pregnancy, and infection have been discussed. Within certain limits ultrasonography can aid in the diagnosis and management of these complications.

REFERENCES

1. Forrest TD, Tietze C, Sullivan E: Abortion in the United States, 1976–1977. Fam Plan Perspect 10:271, 1978
2. Hubers SC, Piotrow PT, Orlans FB: Intrauterine devices, in Population Reports, Series B, No 2. Washington, D.C., George Washington University Medical Center, 1975, B21
3. Hogen GD, Chern HC, Dufay ML: Transitory hCG-like activity in the urine of some IUD users. J Clin Endocrinol Metab 46:469, 1978
4. Ledger WJ, Wilson JR: Intrauterine contraceptive devices: The recognition and management of uterine perforation. Obstet Gynecol 806:811, 1966
5. Cochrane WJ, Thomas MA: The use of ultrasound B-scanning in localization of intrauterine devices. Radiology 104:632, 1972.
6. Richardson M, Kinard RE, Watters DH: Localization of intrauterine devices: Evaluation of computerized tomography. Radiology 142:690, 1982
7. Callen PW, De Martini WJ, Filly RA: The central uterine cavity echo: A useful anatomic sign in ultrasonography evaluation of the female pelvis. Radiology 131:187, 1979
8. Vessey MP, Johnson B, Doll R: Outcome of pregnancy in women using intrauterine devices. Lancet i:495, 1974
9. Shine RM, Thompson JF: The in situ IUD and pregnancy outcome. Am J Obstet Gynecol 57:137, 1981
10. Ory HW: Ectopic pregnancy and intrauterine devices, new perspectives. Obstet Gynecol 57:137, 1981
11. Vessey MP, Yates D, Flanel R: Risk of ectopic pregnancy and duration of use of intrauterine devices. Lancet ii:501, 1979
12. Golditch IM, Huston JE: Serious pelvic infections associated with the intrauterine device. Int J Fertil 18:156, 1973
13. Luukkainew T, Neilson NC, Nygren KG, et al: Nulliparous women, IUD and pelvic infection. Am Clinical Res 11:121, 1979
14. Taylor ES, McMillan JH, Greer BE, et al: The intrauterine device and tubo-ovarian abscess. Am J Obstet Gynecol 123:338, 1975
15. Wagner M, Kiselow MC, Goodman JJ, et al: The relationship of IUD, actinomycosis infection and bowel abscess. Wisc Med J 78:23, 1979

42 | The Use of Ultrasound in Breast Evaluation

Catherine Cole-Beuglet

Two methods are currently utilized in ultrasound evaluation of breast abnormalities. The first is insonation of a palpable breast mass, and the second is B-scan imaging of the entire mammary gland, utilizing dedicated breast equipment. Initial attempts by many investigators utilizing A- and B-mode techniques to categorize benign and malignant breast mass lesions were disappointing. Patients who presented with palpable breast masses were examined with ultrasound equipment available at that time in an attempt to differentiate benign from malignant mass lesions. It was found there was considerable overlap in the criteria of breast mass lesions and it was not possible to make a specific histopathologic diagnosis. Ultrasound imaging of palpable breast masses could reliably distinguish fluid-filled masses from solid mass lesions. This information continues to be a valuable adjunct to physical examination of the breast and x-ray mammography.

The recent development of specialized equipment capable of evaluating the large volume of soft tissue comprising the breast has made ultrasound mammography possible. This term indicates the complete evaluation of the mammary gland using ultrasound imaging. The history of whole breast ultrasound imaging, the scan techniques, and the indications for ultrasound mammography are discussed.

DEDICATED BREAST ULTRASOUND EQUIPMENT

Various investigators throughout the world have developed different methods of immobilizing the breast.

Wells, in Great Britain, suggested the use of transducers mounted at the base of a water tank.[1] The patient, in a prone position, would immerse the breast within an open water bath. In Japan, Wagai and Kobayashi developed enclosed water-path systems.[2,3] One contained a 5-MHz transducer mechanically driven at preset increments to obtain sequential transverse B-scans of approximately one quadrant of the breast. With this system, the patient, in a supine position, had the enclosed water path placed over a quadrant of the breast. The size and weight of the instrumentation provided adequate immobilization of the breast against the anterior chest wall. In Australia, Kossoff and associates developed an automated static water-path scanner for general obstetric and abdominal use, and a second smaller unit for breast imaging.[4,5] In the United States, two types of dedicated breast scanners using water-path techniques were developed. One type has single or multiple transducers mounted at the base of the water bath and the patient, in a prone position, immerses the breast. The transducers are mechanically moved to obtain simple or compound B-scan images of the gland. These images are recorded for either static or real-time viewing.[6,7] A second type has transducers mounted within an enclosed water path that is placed over the breast of a patient in a supine position.[8] In Europe, a third type of dedicated breast scanner uses one or several linear array transducers mounted in an enclosed water bath. The patient sits with one breast opposed to the scanner head. Several types of dedicated breast scanners are now commercially available and these allow B-scan imaging of the entire mammary gland with rapid playback and viewing capabilities.

TECHNIQUE FOR ULTRASOUND EXAMINATION OF THE BREAST

Patients referred for ultrasound evaluation of the breast are examined clinically by a physician or a medical ultrasound technologist who has been trained in breast physical examination. Sites of mass lesions, other palpable abnormalities, thickening, biopsy scars, and retraction are diagrammed on paper for subsequent correlation with the ultrasound and x-ray mammograms. At the time of the physical examination, a history is obtained of past breast diseases in the patient and/or her family.

AUTOMATED WHOLE BREAST EXAMINATION

The patient is then instructed to lie prone and immerse one breast at a time in an open water-path scanner. All patients are scanned with breast compression; a thin polyethylene membrane is used to flatten the breast tissue against the anterior chest wall. The water acts as a coupling agent. The pulsed sound waves from the transducers at the base of the water tank travel through the water and into the breast. Sagittal B-scans can be obtained at 1- to 5-mm increments and recorded on a multiformat imager. With a multitransducer, multipurpose, water-path scanner, compound scans are obtained using three or four of the eight transducers. In areas of mass lesions or other abnormalities, single-sector scans may be obtained using a single transducer. Real-time sector imaging at 10 frames per second can be obtained over areas of palpable masses utilizing one of the eight transducers.

Using a large-aperture single transducer dedicated automated breast scanner with real time capability, sagittal B-scans in real time can be imaged and recorded without interruption from the medial to the lateral breast margins. This continuous imaging and recording of the total breast is termed the "swim through" technique.[9] The large soft-tissue volume of the breast can be imaged in less than 1 minute. For a permanent record, freeze-frame B-scan images can be recorded on a multiformat imager at preset increments, usually 1 to 5 mm. The spatial resolution of available systems is approximately 2 mm in the axial direction.

LIMITED EXAMINATION OF A PALPABLE ABNORMALITY

For an examination of a palpable abnormality by contact gray scale[10] or real-time water-path B-scanning

techniques,[11] the patient is placed in a supine oblique position with a pillow or other support under the shoulder of the breast to be examined. With the patient in this position, the breast lies naturally flattened over the anterior chest wall. The site of the palpable mass is marked on the overlying skin. If the mass is located in the upper outer quadrant or axillary tail of the breast, the arm is extended under the patient's head to stretch the breast over the thoracic wall. A coupling agent, mineral oil or sonic gel, is applied directly to the skin over the mass. The mass may be immobilized with one hand while making sector contact scans over the mass using the other hand. Alternatively, real-time linear array or water-path scanners can be placed directly over the mass. The weight of the scanner head results in some compression of the breast tissue against the chest wall and prevents the mass from moving.

For optimal resolution, medium- and high-frequency transducers (5, 7.5, and 10 HMz) are utilized. The optimum transducer is determined by the size and position of the palpable breast mass and the depth of penetration required. When the ultrasonic image is examined, the area of the mass is compared with the adjacent glandular tissue to determine whether the mass is fluid-filled or solid. The ultrasound criteria of the various mass lesions for patients examined in the supine and prone positions have been outlined.[8,10-17]

BREAST ANATOMY

The breast is composed of four major types of tissue: fat, parenchyma (ducts and alveoli), loose connective tissue, and dense connective tissue. The relative amounts of these tissues change according to age and body habitus, resulting in differing sonic attenuation effects. Of the normal anatomic structures, the connective tissue septa of the breast have the highest acoustic impedance. The amplitude of the echo produced by an ultrasound reflection at tissue interfaces is a function of the relative difference in acoustic impedance of the tissues forming the interface. The greatest difference occurs at fat–fibrous connective tissue interfaces, which appear as strong echogenic lines. The fat–parenchyma interfaces, with a smaller difference in acoustic impedance, present as intermediate echo-reflective areas.

The angle of incidence of the ultrasonic beam on the reflecting interface is an important factor in the relative echogenicity of the various interfaces within the breast. When perpendicular to the beam, the interfaces appear as bright echogenic lines. When parallel to the beam, the interfaces are imaged poorly or not at all. The fibrous connective tissue septa of the breast are arranged in a radial fashion from the subcutaneous fat to the retromammary fascia. Much of the ultrasonic beam is absorbed and reflected by dense connective tissue, resulting in reduced sound transmission to the deeper areas of the breast. In the free-hanging position, the inferior surface of the breast is more steeply curved than the superior surface. The surface and peripheral breast structures may be well imaged; however, the central structures may be obscured because of reflection, absorption, and attenuation.[18]

In a normal B-scan over the nipple, there is a cone-shaped shadow, the apex of which is directly below the nipple. This shadow differs from the nipple shadowing represented by a narrow, echo-free zone less than 1.0 cm wide directly below the nipple. Nipple shadowing results from sound absorption by the dense connective tissue stroma of the retroareolar ducts, in combination with reflection and/or refraction from the obliquely oriented sides of the protruding nipple.

In a recent investigation at Thomas Jefferson University Hospital, 2 cadaver breasts and 20 mastectomy specimens were sectioned in the sagittal plane. The histologic sections of normal and pathologic structures were correlated with the in vivo preoperative sagittal B-scan images to yield the following anatomic findings.[19]

The subcutaneous fat immediately beneath the skin is clustered in lobules surrounded by connective tissue walls and septa that are usually less than 1 mm thick. Smaller fat lobules occupy the retromammary zone overlying the chest wall muscles. The connective tissue of the subcutaneous septa are continuous superficially with the connective tissue of the dermis (Cooper ligaments). The parenchyma is situated between the superficial and deep connective tissue fascial planes. The retromammary zone separates the deep mammary fascia from the fascia overlying the pectoralis major muscle.

The parenchyma is made up of lobules, each of which contains a lactiferous duct. These ducts are usually collapsed in the nonlactating female, but may attain a diameter from 2 to 8 mm at the level of the lactiferous sinuses immediately below the nipple. The deeper lactiferous ducts and their lobular branches gradually curve radially into a plane paralleling the skin surface. They also enter the connective tissue planes surrounding the parenchyma as well as the connective tissue septa between the fat lobules and the parenchyma. The lobular ducts and the terminal alveolar ducts are surrounded by loose intralobular connective tissue. On a B-scan image of a functional breast, the tissues of the parenchyma are manifested as intermediate-strength echoes in a fine homogeneous pattern (Fig. 1). In postmenopausal breasts, lobules of fat even-

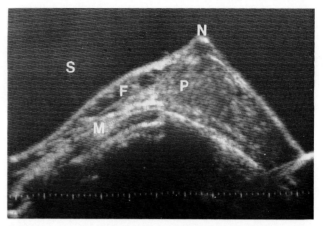

A

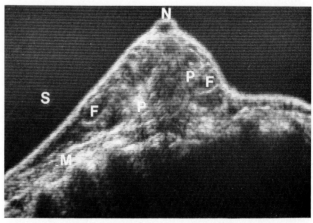

B

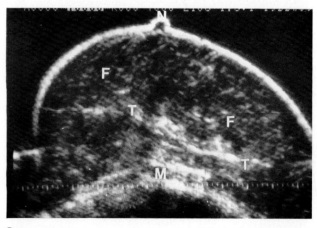

C

Fig. 1. Typical breast patterns. Sagittal B-scans. **A.** The breast of a 24-year-old woman contains parenchyma (P) of intermediate echogenicity in uniform distribution and a small amount of subcutaneous fat (F). S, superior; N, nipple; M, pectoralis major muscle. **B.** The breast of a 36-year-old woman contains a deeper layer of subcutaneous fat (F). **C.** The breast of a 56-year-old postmenopausal woman contains predominantly adipose tissue (F) and echogenic fibrous tissue strands (T).

tually replace the functioning parenchyma, resulting in images containing round to oval areas of low acoustic impedance, with curvilinear lines of dense connective tissue interspersed with Cooper ligaments (Fig. 2).

ULTRASOUND BREAST PARENCHYMAL PATTERNS

Wolfe has correlated the varying x-ray mammographic breast parenchymal patterns with age.[20] Ongoing evaluation of ultrasound mammograms has led to recognition of several dominant ultrasound breast patterns based on the arrangement and brightness of the echoes.[21]

In a breast B-scan, the skin line and the fibrous tissue of the retromammary fascia manifest the brightest echoes. Subcutaneous fat is weakly echogenic and interspersed with strongly echogenic Cooper ligaments. Functional breast parenchyma is intermediate in echogenicity. In the younger patient, it has a fine, uniform, "tightly packed" echogenic pattern. Coalescence of these echoes may result in a sheetlike configuration of the glandular tissue extending in a radial fashion from the subareolar area throughout the gland. The subcutaneous and retromammary fat may be 5 mm or less in depth. In the older patient, fatty replacement of the parenchyma extends into the central core of the breast, and the echo amplitude of the glandular tissue decreases. Oval to round areas of weak echogenicity representing fat lobules are interspersed between sheetlike areas of higher-amplitude parenchymal echoes.[22]

Fluid-filled lactiferous ducts may be imaged as echo-free tubular structures radiating for variable distances from the nipple into the breast parenchyma. The dimensions of these ducts can be measured, and the extent of their penetration into the breast parenchyma recorded. In the majority of women they are less than 2 mm in width (Fig. 3). When the ducts are overdistended with fluid (as in late pregnancy or lactation), their diameter increases. Whereas in x-ray mammograms the visualized ducts comprise the lumen, epithelial lining, and periductal collagen tissue,[20] in ultrasound mammograms, the lumen alone is responsible for the image.

In B-scans, the middle-aged breast may show sheetlike areas of bright echogenic tissues immediately beneath the subcutaneous fat. This tissue has scalloped anterior margins paralleling the skin surface and arching toward the skin where traversed by Cooper ligaments. The fibrous tissue cap has a cone-shaped or triangular configuration, with the apex beneath the

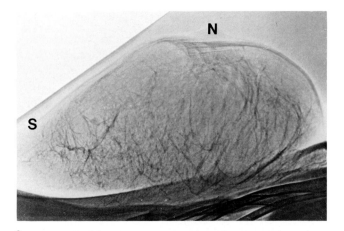

A

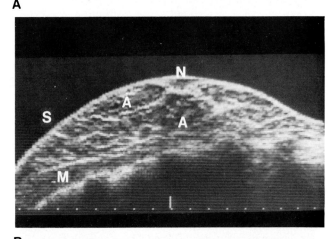

B

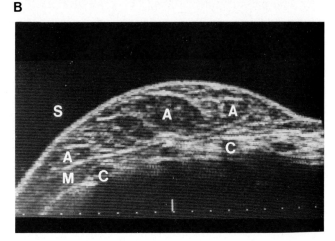

C

Fig. 2. Postmenopausal breast, 66-year-old-woman. **A.** Medial lateral right xeromammogram. S, superior; N, nipple. Sagittal B-scans of the right breast: **B.** At the nipple (N). S, superior; A, adipose tissue; M, pectoralis major muscle. **C.** One centimeter medial to the nipple. A, adipose tissue; C, costal cartilage.

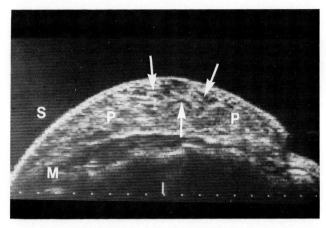

Fig. 3. Prominent fluid filled ducts in a 30-year-old woman who presented with breast nodularity without evidence of dominant mass. Sagittal B-scan adjacent to the right nipple demonstrates echo free tortuous tubular structures (*arrows*) within the breast parenchyma (P). S, superior; M, muscle.

nipple, and may manifest great echo attenuation. The central core of glandular tissue may be echo free because of considerable overlying fibrous stroma and therefore may not be imaged. In these cases, compressing the breast against the chest wall with a thin sheet of plastic often realigns the dense fibrous tissue so that it becomes incidental to the insonating beam. Rescanning with compression then allows imaging of the central cone of breast tissue previously shadowed by fibrous tissue (Fig. 4).[23]

ULTRASOUND EVALUATION OF BREAST MASS LESIONS

Familiarity with normal breast anatomy and parenchymal patterns enhances the ability to detect abnormal areas. Mass lesions can be identified as fluid-filled or solid.

FLUID-FILLED MASSES

Fluid-filled cysts have well-defined smooth margins, echo-free interior, well-defined posterior walls, and enhanced sound transmission distally (Fig. 5). Regardless of sensitivity setting, the central area should remain echo-free. Cysts are generally round or oval, but if multiple, they may manifest a lobulated appearance. In many cases, palpable abnormalities are not appreciated clinically and an ultrasound examination shows multiple variable-sized fluid collections throughout the breast parenchyma (Fig. 6). When a patient with a known history of fibrocystic disease develops a palpable mass, ultrasound mammography will delineate the characteristics of the mass, and designate the area as fluid-filled or solid in nature. Occasionally, septations are noted within a fluid-filled area. Two adjacent cysts may give the appearance of a larger cyst with an internal septation. Chronic fibrocystic disease may result in thickening of the cyst walls. Needle aspiration may lead to a distorted shape of the cyst or hemorrhage within it, giving internal echoes. The finding of thick

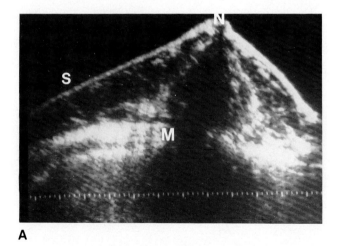

A

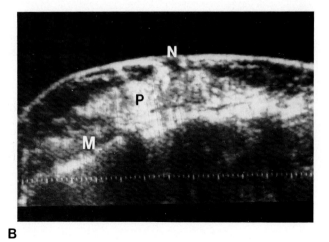

B

Fig. 4. Effect of compression. A 35-year-old woman with dysplastic glandular tissue on x-ray mammography. **A.** Sagittal B-scan of the left breast through the nipple area (N) with the breast hanging free within the water bath. Cone-shaped acoustic shadow extends from the subareolar area beneath the nipple (N) through the pectoralis major muscle (M). S, superior. **B.** Sagittal B-scan at the same position with the breast tissue compressed towards the chest wall. The echogenic parenchyma (P) is imaged between the anterior skin surface and the pectoralis major muscle (M).

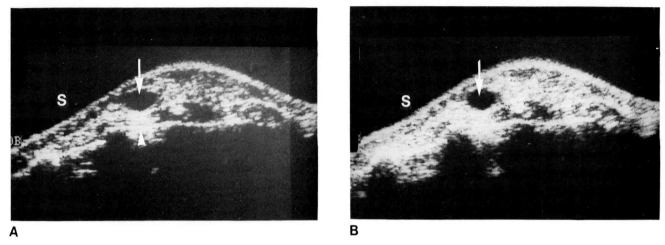

Fig. 5. Cyst in the upper outer quadrant of the right breast of a 37-year-old woman who presented with pain and tenderness in her breasts in the premenstrual period. **A.** Sagittal B-scan shows an oval shaped 1.5-cm mass (*arrow*) in the superior (S) parenchyma which is echo free, has smooth well-defined margins and exhibits acoustic enhancement (*arrowhead*). S, superior. **B.** Rescan at a higher sensitivity shows the mass remains echo-free.

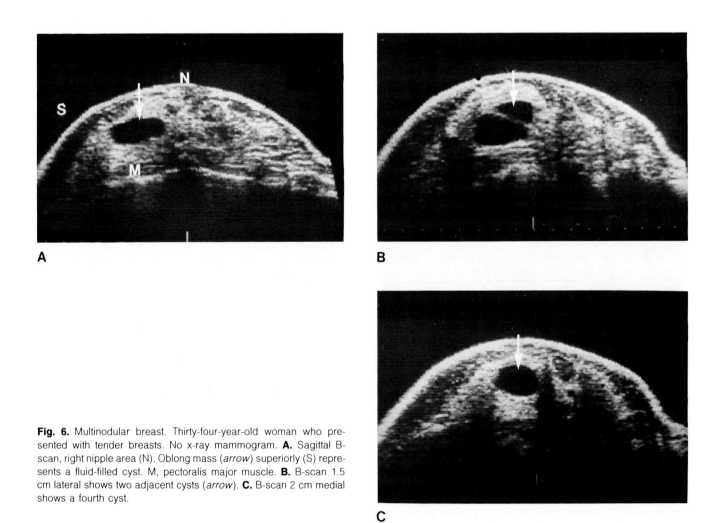

Fig. 6. Multinodular breast. Thirty-four-year-old woman who presented with tender breasts. No x-ray mammogram. **A.** Sagittal B-scan, right nipple area (N). Oblong mass (*arrow*) superiorly (S) represents a fluid-filled cyst. M, pectoralis major muscle. **B.** B-scan 1.5 cm lateral shows two adjacent cysts (*arrow*). **C.** B-scan 2 cm medial shows a fourth cyst.

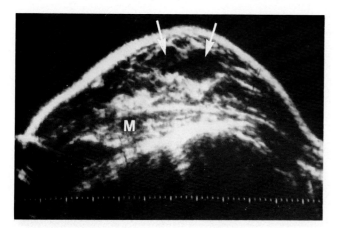

Fig. 7. Hematoma. Blunt trauma to the right breast 10 days previously. Ecchymosis on the skin surface. Transverse B-scan shows a lobulated mass (*arrows*) which contains scattered weak internal echoes. Aspiration confirmed a resolving hematoma. M, pectoralis major muscle.

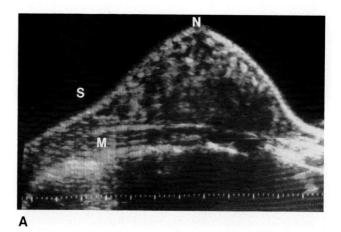

A

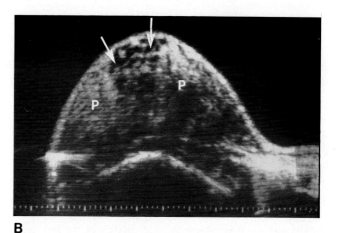

B

Fig. 8. Twenty-eight-year-old woman, breast feeding for 3 months presented with a multinodular breast. **A.** Sagittal B-scan at the nipple level shows radiating echo-free tubular structures converging under the nipple (N), milk-filled ducts. S, superior; M, pectoralis major muscle. **B.** Transverse B-scan above the nipple shows the echogenic hypertrophied parenchyma (P) and the fluid-filled ducts (*arrows*).

septations, internal papillary projections from the cyst wall, and/or echogenic debris within the cyst warrants cytologic and histopathologic investigation, as carcinoma may rarely arise in the wall of a cyst. In these cases, needle aspiration usually yields hemorrhagic fluid containing atypical and/or malignant cells. Jellins et al. have reported a 98 percent accuracy in their detection of fluid-filled masses in the breast.[24]

Ducts, abscesses, and hematomas may also be fluid-filled. Abscesses are usually periareolar and, when localized, have irregular margins and are relatively echo-free. Surgical drainage or antibiotic therapy lead to reduction in diameter. Increased thickness and brightness of surrounding Cooper ligaments may persist for several months after treatment. Retraction of the overlying skin may mark the site of a previous abscess.

A hematoma can usually be related to a history of trauma and evidence of overlying skin discoloration. A hematoma may occur following needle aspiration biopsy of a palpable mass (Fig. 7). On a B-scan performed within days of the trauma, the area appears as a weakly echogenic region of architectural distortion. As the hematoma becomes organized, 1 to 3 weeks later, the involved area manifests greater amplitude echoes and thickened Cooper ligaments. A large hematoma may require many months to resolve. In such cases, sequential B-scans show a gradual decrease in size of the distorted area as well as a decrease in intensity of echo reflections, ultimately returning to a normal pattern.

In the late pregnancy and postpartum periods, when the ducts are filled with protein-rich colostrum, their internal diameter enlarges and during lactation may attain a diameter of 6 to 8 mm. On B-scans, the echo free branching tubular structures are surrounded by uniformly echogenic hyperplastic breast parenchyma (Fig. 8).[19]

Galactoceles, localized accumulations of milk behind an obstructed duct, may be seen during lactation. On B-scans, the galactocele is a mass with poorly defined margins containing low-level uniform echoes. The high-protein fluid contents of a galactocele are weakly echogenic, in contrast with the echo-free contents of a cyst.

SOLID MASSES

The ability of ultrasound to reveal the nature of areas of breast thickening, hardening, or lumpiness can

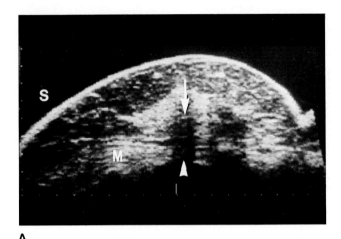

A

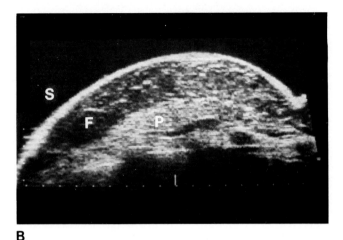

B

Fig. 9. A. Infiltrating duct carcinoma manifests as an irregular margined architectural disruption (*arrow*) in the superior (S) breast of a 58-year-old woman. Great acoustic attenuation manifest as shadowing (*arrowhead*) extends through the pectoralis major muscle layer (M). **B.** Sagittal B-scan of the opposite breast in the same area. F, subcutaneous fat; P, parenchyma.

greatly assist the clinician. Although it is useful to distinguish benign from malignant solid masses ultrasonically, the distinction may be difficult. Clinicians therefore are advised to biopsy any solid mass.

When a palpable mass images as a solid lesion, the ultrasound B-scan criteria are applied to determine if the solid is a malignant-appearing or a benign-appearing solid.[13,15] From a retrospective review of 117 confirmed breast carcinomas of all histologic types, the majority (77 percent) of malignant solids demonstrated an irregular contour and contained weak internal echoes. Some degree of significant acoustic attenuation was evident in over two-thirds of the tumors (Fig. 9).[17] Infiltrating duct carcinoma comprises the majority of infiltrating breast carcinomas in the United States, and these tumors elicit a desmoplastic reaction as they grow in stellate fashion into the breast parenchyma. For this reason, they are called scirrhous carcinomas. On a B-scan, they image as irregular-margined variable-shaped masses containing weak, nonuniform internal echoes. These tumors exhibit great acoustic attenuation, imaged on a B-scan as a central shadow distal to the mass.

A small percentage of breast carcinomas are termed cellular, as opposed to the previously described acellular carcinomas. Medullary carcinoma is an example of a cellular lesion. These are bulky tumors and growth from the periphery occurs in a smooth fashion compared to the tentacle stellate peripheral growth from an infiltrating duct carcinoma. When these malignancies are imaged on ultrasound, they have a smooth or slightly lobulated margin and contain weak internal echoes. The distribution of the echoes within the mass

may be inhomogeneous. These mass lesions do not exhibit significant acoustic attenuation; thus, echoes are usually recorded distal to the mass (Fig. 10).[17]

Besides these criteria for benign versus malignant solid masses, additional criteria have been encountered in the evaluation of 5000 ultrasound mammograms performed at Thomas Jefferson University Hospital. In premenopausal or postmenopausal women, an area of persistently strong acoustic attenuation may represent an infiltrating carcinoma (Fig. 11).[3,13,15,17] Areas of architectural distortion or areas that appear different from the normal parenchyma may represent malig-

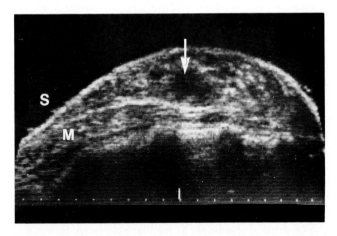

Fig. 10. Medullary carcinoma. Forty-four-year-old woman presented with a palpable right superior breast mass. Sagittal B-scan shows a solid mass (*arrow*) that contains weak internal echoes. The mass does not exhibit acoustic attenuation and appears to demonstrate some acoustic enhancement. Biopsy confirmed a 2-cm medullary carcinoma. S, superior; M, pectoralis major muscle.

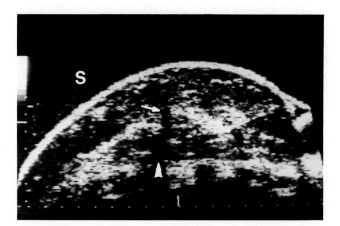

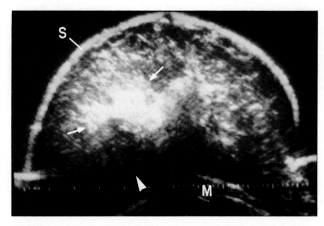

Fig. 11. Occult carcinoma, infiltrating duct. A 74-year-old woman with no palpable masses. Sagittal B-scan 6 mm lateral to the left nipple. Area of acoustic attenuation (*arrow*) originates from the subcutaneous fat, parenchymal junction and extends through the chest wall (*arrowhead*). X-ray mammography confirmed a stellate density characteristic of carcinoma. Biopsy revealed an 8 mm infiltrating duct carcinoma. S, superior.

Fig. 12. Ultrasound findings in advanced infiltrating carcinoma. Sixty-eight-year-old woman presented with a red inflamed breast. No mass palpable. Transverse B-scan shows thickened skin (S) and thickened echogenic Cooper ligaments (*arrows*) extending from the skin towards the chest wall (M). The tumor causes acoustic attenuation distally (*arrowhead*).

nancy. Bilateral subareolar asymmetry may also indicate malignancy. Thickened or retracted Cooper ligaments and/or skin thickening on ultrasound images are signs of advanced infiltrating carcinoma (Fig. 12) in the absence of a history of prior surgery.

In contrast, when a palpable mass images as a smooth-margined solid, usually with a round or oval shape, and demonstrates intermediate or no significant acoustic attenuation, it is likely that this represents a benign tumor (Fig. 13). The majority of benign-appearing solid mass lesions represent fibroadenomas. Generally, a younger patient presents to her clinician with

a recently discovered mobile palpable mass in the breast. Occasionally, x-ray mammography will image such a mass separate from the dense glandular tissue, normally present with the young breast. Ultrasound mammography will image these as smooth margined, weakly echogenic masses within the strongly echogenic breast parenchyma.[16] During an evaluation of 240 biopsy-confirmed solid breast masses examined with a dedicated breast scanner, 6 cases that exhibited the characteristic benign-appearing criteria proved on biopsy to be infiltrating duct carcinomas.[17] For this reason, the ultrasound B-scan criteria have been ex-

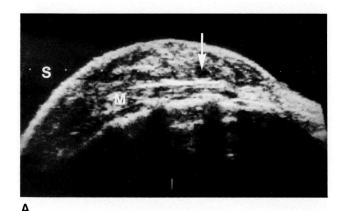

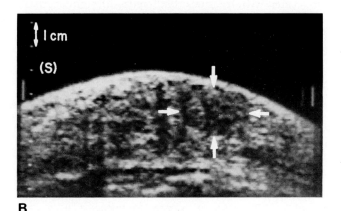

A

B

Fig. 13. A. Fibroadenoma within dysplastic breast of a 26-year-old woman. Sagittal B-scan of the left breast with compression of the breast towards the chest wall. The 1-cm round mass (*arrow*) has well-defined margins and contains weak internal echoes in a uniform distribution. Biopsy confirmed a 1-cm fibroadenoma. S, superior; M, pectoralis major muscle. **B.** Palpable mass in the left lower inner quadrant of a 36-year-old woman's breast. Sagittal B-scan with compression shows a lobulated solid mass (*arrows*) with smooth margins which contains internal echoes in a uniform distribution. (S) superior. Biopsy confirmed a 3-cm fibroadenoma.

TABLE 1
Indications for Ultrasound Mammography

1. Patients with a palpable breast mass
2. X-ray mammography shows dense breasts
3. Symptomatic adolescent patients
4. Symptomatic pregnant and breast feeding patients
5. Inflammatory conditions of the breast—mastitis, abscess
6. Breast trauma—hematoma, fat necrosis
7. Recurrent masses in a patient with fibrocystic disease
8. Differentiation of a true abnormality from normal breast tissue
9. Patients with positive axillary node biopsies
10. Augmented breast
11. Male breast
12. Patients with cancerophobia

panded to include all imaged solid mass lesions within the breast as potentially malignant. Thus, histopathology of a dominant solid mass lesion must be confirmed by a fine-needle or open-excisional biopsy.

PITFALLS IN DIAGNOSIS

Possible additional sources of foci of abnormally increased acoustic attenuation include normal diffuse dense fibrous connective tissue, biopsy scar, or clustered calcifications.[25] The coarse benign calcifications seen within mature fibroadenomas in x-ray mammograms are imaged on ultrasound B-scans as discrete, bright echoes on their anterior surface, with acoustic shadowing posteriorly. Due to the limited resolution of current ultrasound mammography, only calcifications 2 mm or greater in diameter can be identified. Microcalcifications within ducts and vascular calcifications in the micron-size range are not usually imaged. Such calcifications may rarely be evident when they are located within tissues that have a different acoustic impedance than the surrounding normal breast tissue (e.g., carcinomas). Then the microcalcifications appear

as small, brightly echogenic foci with acoustic shadowing distally. These calcifications may be partly responsible for the great acoustic attenuation observed in some breast cancers.

INDICATIONS FOR ULTRASOUND MAMMOGRAPHY

The indications for ultrasound mammography are listed in Table 1. These indications were formulated during an evaluation of 5000 ultrasound mammograms performed at Thomas Jefferson University Hospital using water-path techniques.

When a mass lesion is imaged on an ultrasound B-scan, the area of the mass lesion is compared with the surrounding glandular tissue. Mass lesions are designated as fluid-filled or solid. The breast mass diagnostic ultrasound B-scan criteria established in the literature are used to differentiate fluid-filled and solid mass lesions (Table 2).

When a patient presents with a radiographic diagnosis of a dense breast, masses may not be delineated. Ultrasound mammography may be able to demonstrate lesions within the uniformly echogenic glandular tissue. Frequently, these patients are less than 40 years of age. The American College of Radiology does not recommend periodic mammogram of the breast to detect carcinoma in patients less than 40 years of age. As a result, ultrasound shows promise of becoming a method to image dense breasts. Frazier et al. reported confirmation of four carcinomas imaged on ultrasound mammography and not detected on x-ray mammography.[26] One hundred thirty-five patients with questionable palpable breast nodularity were diagnosed as dysplastic (DY) breasts radiographically. No tumors or microcalcifications were imaged. Ultrasound exami-

TABLE 2
Breast Mass Diagnostic Ultrasound B-scan Criteria

	Fluid Filled	Solid	
		Benign Appearing	Malignant Appearing
Contour	Smooth	Smooth	Irregular
Shape	Round or Oval	Round or Oval	Round, Lobulated, Tubular
Internal Echoes	None	Weak, Uniform	Weak, Non-Uniform
Anterior Border	Strong	Strong to Intermediate	Intermediate
Posterior Border	Strong	Strong to Intermediate	Weak to Absent
Distal Echoes	Enhanced, Lateral Wall Shadows	Intermediate	Central Shadow, Interrupted Shadow
Attenuation Effect	Minimal	Intermediate	Great

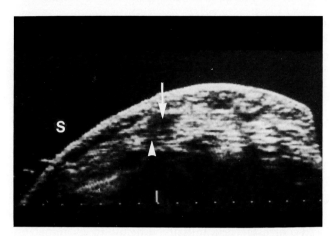

Fig. 14. Infiltrating duct carcinoma. Forty-two-year-old woman presented with a palpable nodule in the left upper inner breast quadrant. Mammogram showed dysplastic parenchyma. Sagittal B-scan in the area of the nodule shows an irregular margined solid mass (*arrow*). It contains weak internal echoes and exhibits acoustic attenuation manifest as shadowing (*arrowhead*). S, superior.

nation of the 135 patients detected four abnormalities that on aspiration or excision biopsy were malignant tumors (Fig. 14).[26]

During pregnancy and lactation, the proliferation of the terminal ducts within the mammary gland causes increased density on x-ray. These patients are not ideal candidates for x-ray evaluation of the breast during this period. Pregnant patients who develop palpable breast masses or questionable abnormalities are good candidates for ultrasound examination of the breast. The hyperplastic glandular tissue changes are imaged on sonomammography as uniform fine echoes throughout the gland. There is also a decrease in the amount of adipose tissue imaged. In late pregnancy and during the lactating period, the breast duct lumens increase in diameter and are fluid-filled. These ducts image as tubular, branching echo-free structures radiating from the nipple into the breast parenchyma. Fluid-filled masses may represent cysts, abscesses, or galactoceles. Solid mass lesions, benign fibroadenomas and infiltrating carcinomas have been imaged sonically in the breasts of pregnant and lactating women.

Frequently, clinicians palpate areas of breast parenchymal thickening or nodularity, and a clear distinction between a palpable mass and an area of normal breast parenchyma cannot be made on the basis of a physical examination. Ultrasound images of this area can be compared to the surrounding breast parenchyma, and to a similar area in the contralateral breast for evaluation of a true abnormality.

Mastitis is a term applied to diffuse inflammation of the breast. This is seen most frequently in a patient in the postpartum period, during lactation, or in the perimenopausal period. The inflammation of the breast may be diffuse or localized. When localized, the abscess typically occurs in the subareolar area. X-ray mammography is difficult to perform and interpret. To apply compression to an inflamed breast causes considerable patient discomfort. Inflammation images as an irregular-margined radiodensity similar to infiltrating carcinomas. Ultrasound mammography images the breast parenchyma and localized fluid collections. Abscesses image as irregular-margined, fluid-filled regions containing weak internal echoes. During lactation, or in an older woman, diffuse inflammation of the breast can occur as a result of rapid growth of an infiltrating duct carcinoma. The resultant inflammatory response within the breast parenchyma is termed an inflammatory carcinoma. Skin thickening occurs, either localized or diffuse, as a result of both inflammation or tumor infiltration. On an ultrasound B-scan, the volume of the breast parenchyma is generally increased compared to the opposite breast. The supporting structures of the breast, Cooper ligaments, and the breast parenchyma may appear altered and spread apart. Thickening of the fibrous connective tissue strands can often be imaged as brightly echogenic curvilinear lines extending to the skin surface.

The normal skin of the breast has a thickness of less than 2 mm in diameter. When thickened, the skin images as an increased echo-dense line measuring greater than 2 mm in diameter and has been recorded up to 12 mm. Occasionally, the thickened skin will demonstrate a narrow echolucent line within the center, giving the appearance of a relatively echo-dense outer and inner surface and a narrow echolucent center.[27] X-ray mammography, of course, is also capable of imaging thickened skin. Occasionally, the site of the inflammatory tumor within the inflamed breast cannot be appreciated on the x-ray mammogram. However, indirect signs on an ultrasound study, such as thickening of Cooper ligaments, straightening of the ligaments in a direction towards the tumor site, and an area of acoustic attenuation, can indicate the site of the tumor.

Trauma to the breast can occur as a result of a direct blow, an automobile accident or surgical intervention. Hemorrhage within the breast may present clinically as a bruise on the skin surface. When imaged ultrasonically within a few days of occurrence, the area immediately below the skin surface may show an irregular-margined weakly echogenic mass. Serial imaging at 3 and 6 months demonstrates a gradual fill-in of the margins and center with bright echoes until the mass effect is no longer evident. Thickening of the fibrous connective tissue ligaments in the area may be the only residue of the hematoma. Fat necrosis, also occurring as a result of trauma, can be recorded as an area of increased echogenicity with variable degrees of distal acoustic attenuation. It is usually difficult to differentiate the appearance of fat necrosis from infiltrating malignancy. A history of breast trauma or a recent surgical procedure is needed before such a specific diagnosis can be suggested.[24]

Augmentation of the breast is performed for cosmetic reasons or postsubcutaneous mastectomy for minimal or in situ breast carcinoma. Silicone gel prostheses are inserted in the retromammary space for enlargement of a small breast. The breast parenchyma is located over the surface of the conical prosthesis. Clinical evaluation of the glandular tissue over the prosthesis is frequently difficult due to fibrous changes, which occasionally occur in the tissue immediately adjacent to the envelope of the silicone gel. Nodularity along the incision sites may represent scar tissue formation, granulomas, or mass lesions. Using x-ray mammography, the glandular tissue overlying the prosthesis is incompletely imaged due to the high radiodensity of the silicone. Ultrasound examination of an augmented breast readily images both the overlying glandular tissue and the prosthesis. Because the speed of sound in silicone is slower than the speed of sound in the breast parenchyma, the posterior surface of the silicone prosthesis will project posteriorly into the chest wall. This geometric distortion is an artifact and it presents no diagnostic problems. Of course, if the prosthesis is saline-filled, there will be no such posterior margin displacement. A small percentage of patients develop a hard fibrous capsule around the silicone bag prosthesis. When this occurs, the prosthesis may assume a distorted shape. This images ultrasonically as a thickened bright line at the margin of the flattened or distorted silicone bag. The prosthesis may develop wrinkles on the surface or cracks within it which can be imaged on ultrasound examination.[28]

Enlargement of the soft tissues in the region of the nipple in the male may represent deposition of adipose tissue on the anterior chest wall or proliferation of the breast ducts in the subareolar area. This latter condition is termed gynecomastia. Localized duct proliferation in the subareolar area can clinically present as a palpable mass. Carcinoma of the breast in the male also presents as a palpable mass in the subareolar area, and it is, thus, difficult to differentiate from true gynecomastia. X-ray imaging of the soft tissues of the anterior chest wall in the male can be technically difficult. Ultrasound imaging of the enlarged male breast using water-path techniques permits evaluation of the tissues of the anterior chest wall. Both localized and diffuse duct proliferation can be imaged in the subareolar area.[29] Imaged masses are evaluated according to the criteria for mass lesions in the female breast.

ADVANTAGES AND LIMITATIONS OF ULTRASOUND MAMMOGRAPHY

The primary attraction of ultrasound mammography is its ability to image the breast repeatedly with no known deleterious effects.[30] In addition, some of the information obtained is unavailable from any other imaging technique. Palpable breast masses can be conclusively determined to be fluid-filled or solid. Whole-breast ultrasound mammography permits evaluation of the parenchymal pattern. Data are being collected that may enable us to correlate the different ultrasonic parenchymal patterns with risk for breast cancer. Large fatty breasts were initially difficult to examine, but with breast compression this ceased to be a problem. Since malignant tumors are weakly echogenic, an emphasis on appreciating architectural distortion and other subtle abnormalities of the parenchyma is proving useful in distinguishing between fat lobules and small carcinomas.

The major limitation of ultrasound mammograms is poor spatial resolution. Modern x-ray mammograms provide superb resolution of microcalcifications that may be the only sign of early carcinoma. At the present, state of the art ultrasound mammography, with a best resolution of 2 mm, cannot reliably detect microcalcifications. Thus, ultrasound mammography should not be performed as the initial imaging breast examination for the detection of cancer in asymptomatic women. This may change in the future with advancements in technology. In addition, repeated ultrasound examinations are possible at any age without known health hazards. This factor is of importance to young women when x-ray mammography demonstrates dysplastic breasts. For this age group x-ray mammography is less accurate and radiation exposure is a concern. Hopefully, the combination of ultrasound mammography and x-ray mammography will lead to increased accuracy in the diagnosis of breast disease.

REFERENCES

1. Wells PNT, Evans KT: An immersion scanner for two-dimensional ultrasonic examination of the human breast. Ultrasonics 6:220, 1968
2. Wagai T, Takahashi S, Ohashi H, et al: A trial for quantitative diagnosis of breast tumor by ultrasono-tomography. Jpn Med Ultrasonics 5:39, 1967
3. Kobayashi T: Gray-scale echography for breast cancer. Radiology 122:207, 1977
4. Kossoff G, Carpenter DA, Robinson DE, et al: Octoson—A new rapid general purpose echoscope, in White D, Barnes R (eds): Ultrasound in Medicine. New York, Plenum, 1976
5. Jellins J, Kossoff G, Buddee FW, Reeve TS: Ultrasonic

visualization of the breast. Med J Austral 1:305, 1971

6. Cole-Beuglet C, Kurtz A, Rubin C, et al: Ultrasound mammography: A comparison with radiographic mammography. Radiology 139:693, 1981

7. Maturo VG, Zusmer NR, Gilson AJ, et al: Ultrasound of the whole breast utilizing a dedicated automated breast scanner. Radiology 137:457, 1980

8. Harper P, Kelly-Fry E: Ultrasound visualization of the breast in symptomatic patients. Radiology 137:465, 1980

9. Cole-Beuglet C, Goldberg BB, Kurtz AB, et al: Clinical experience with a prototype real-time dedicated breast scanner. Am J Roentgenol 139:905, 1982

10. Texidor HS, Kazam E: Combined mammographic-sonographic evaluation of breast masses. Am J Roentgenol 128:409, 1977

11. Cole-Beuglet C, Beique RA: Continuous ultrasound B-scanning of palpable breast masses. Radiology 117:123, 1975.

12. Kobayashi T: Clinical Ultrasound of the Breast. New York, Plenum, 1978

13. Kobayashi T: Diagnostic ultrasound in breast cancer: Analysis of retrotumorous echo patterns correlated with sonic attenuation by cancerous connective tissue. J Clin Ultrasound 7:471, 1979

14. Jellins J, Kossoff G, Reeve T, et al: Ultrasonic gray-scale visualization of breast tissue. Ultrasound Med Biol 1:393, 1975

15. Harper PA, Kelly-Fry E, Noe JS, et al: Ultrasound in the evaluation of solid breast masses. Radiology 146:731, 1983

16. Cole-Beuglet C, Soriano RZ, Kurtz AB, et al: Fibroadenoma of the breast: Sonomammography correlated with pathology of 122 patients. Am J Roentgenol 140:369, 1983

17. Cole-Beuglet C, Soriano RZ, Kurtz AB, et al: Ultrasound analysis of 104 primary breast carcinomas classified according to histopathologic type. Radiology 147:191, 1983

18. Kossoff G, Jellins J: The physics of breast echography. Semin Ultrasound 3:5, 1982

19. Schneck CD, Lehman DA: Sonographic anatomy of the breast. Semin Ultrasound 3:13, 1982

20. Wolfe JN: Breast patterns as an index of risk for developing breast cancer. Am J Roentgenol 26:1130, 1976

21. Rubin CS, Kurtz AB, Goldberg BB, et al: Ultrasonic mammographic parenchymal patterns. Radiology 130:515, 1979

22. Picker RH, Fulton AJ: Maturational and physiological changes in the female breast. Semin Ultrasound 3:34, 1982

23. Ezo MG: Tissue compression for the optimization of images in water-path breast scanning. Med Ultrasound 5:113, 1981

24. Jellins J, Kossoff G, Reeve TS: Detection and classification of liquid-filled masses in the breast by gray-scale echography. Radiology 125:205, 1977

25. Cole-Beuglet C, Soriano RZ, Kurtz AB, et al: Ultrasound mammography evaluation of postoperative breast changes. Radiological Society of North America, November 1982, Chicago, Illinois

26. Frazier TG, Cole-Beuglet C, Kurtz AB, et al: Further evaluation by ultrasound of mammographically determined breast dysplasia. J Surg Oncology 19:69, 1982

27. Kopans DB, Meyer JE, Proppe KH: Double line of skin thickening on sonograms of the breast. Radiology 141:485, 1981

28. Cole-Beuglet C, Schwartz GF, Kurtz AB, et al: Ultrasound mammography for the augmented breast. Radiology 146:737, 1983

29. Cole-Beuglet C, Schwartz GF, Kurtz AB, et al: Ultrasound mammography for male breast enlargement. J Ultrasound Med 1:301, 1982

30. Lele PP: Review: Safety and potential hazards in the current applications of ultrasound in obstetrics and gynecology. Ultrasound Med Biol 5:307, 1979

43 | Certain Legal Aspects of Obstetric and Gynecologic Ultrasound

A. Everette James, Jr.
Albert L. Bundy
Burton A. Johnson
Arthur C. Fleischer
Frank C. Boehm
Roger C. Sanders

In recent years, the application of biomedical techniques in diagnostic sonography has had a significant impact on the practice of obstetrics and gynecology.[1,2] Improvements in instrumentation have resulted in more extensive employment of this diagnostic modality.[3] With this have come heightened patient and physician expectations, increased awareness of the virtues of this technology, and, appropriately, concerns regarding its application. Legal, ethical, and economic issues have arisen that must be appropriately addressed by both the groups responsible for the development, introduction, and continued utilization of diagnostic ultrasound. These multifaceted responsibilities are ones that must be shared by physicians requesting and sonographers performing the examinations. Particularly complex is the determination of the various roles that are assumed by the physician as individual purveyor and patient-advocate for the technology, those entrusted with public policy regarding allocation and distribution of the instrumentation, and the patient as consumer of these biomedical engineering advances.

Ultrasound related problems give rise to legal difficulties in five principal ways: (a) absence of performance of an ultrasound examination when the standard of care would have suggested that one was appropriate; (b) faulty performance of the sonographic equipment, with resultant failure to diagnose a lesion that should have been evident or an inadequate study with failure of the sonographer to identify a lesion; (c) failure to inform the physician or patient adequately of the sonographic findings; (d) overinterpretation of the sonogram so that a lesion is invented with subsequent negatively perceived results by the patient; and

(e) complications arising from an improperly performed invasive procedure (e.g., amniocentesis).

This chapter addresses the principal issues from a large body of potential topics concerning obstetric and gynecologic ultrasound. We have selected those topics that have the greatest possibility of affecting the practitioner.

FAILURE TO PERFORM ULTRASOUND

Situations in which the potential of legal action have occurred when ultrasound was not performed include:

1. Defining the legal limits for an abortion procedure.[4] In one state (Louisiana) it has been legislated that ultrasound should be performed prior to any abortion procedure. Performance of an ultrasound when the patient is approximately 20 weeks pregnant is a desirable maneuver prior to an abortion so that an unexpectedly viable infant is not aborted.
2. When there is a significant risk of intrauterine growth retardation (IUGR) based on the patient's history. Studies have suggested that up to 40 percent of the "high risk" obstetric population may develop intrauterine growth retardation (see Chapter 11). Precisely which indications mandate the performance of an obstetrical ultrasound study in a subsequent pregnancy is unclear. Indications such as two prior small infants, a maternal history of severe medical disease (e.g., chronic renal failure), heavy smoking history, and preeclamptic toxemia make the performance of an ultrasound examination desirable.

3. In the presence of a previous ectopic pregnancy when the patient has symptoms suggestive of a subsequent ectopic pregnancy. These risks are well known with a subsequent pregnancy in patients who have had a previous ectopic pregnancy (see Chapter 30).

4. Prior to amniocentesis. This is a controversial area, but when an amniocentesis fails or results in an abortion and no prior ultrasound study has been performed, litigation has ensued.

5. In the management of multiple pregnancy. Multiple pregnancies are known to be at risk for a number of problems such as IUGR, a clinical problem that should be followed by a series of ultrasonic examinations.

FAILURE TO DIAGNOSE OR MISDIAGNOSIS

Particular risk areas where mistakes in ultrasound interpretation are likely relate to ectopic pregnancy and multiple pregnancy and may result in litigation. Ectopic pregnancy represents a difficult diagnostic entity for the ultrasound expert, and many ectopic pregnancies show little or no sonographic evidence of their presence (see Chapter 30). Whether failure to diagnose an ectopic pregnancy is truly ultrasonic negligence is questionable. In certain instances, because ectopic pregnancy was not mentioned in the differential diagnosis, physicians have been cited as being negligent.

The literature suggests that a number of multiple pregnancies are not recognized (see Chapter 24). One may perform a limited ultrasound survey study and fail to be comprehensive in a routine pregnancy study, as there is a tendency to concentrate one's observations and attention on the fetus itself. Failure to recognize twins is probably more likely to occur when a real-time examination alone is performed, rather than combined static and real-time studies. If there is a family history of multiple pregnancy, particular care must be taken to perform a thorough sonographic examination, but in the absence of a family history of multiple pregnancy, failure to detect a multiple pregnancy does not appear to be an acceptable failure.

Fetal anomalies such as hydrocephalus, encephalocele, or spina bifida have been the subject of potential litigation when these have not been properly detected by ultrasound examination (see Chapters 18 and 19). This is a situation where the concept of level 1 and level 2 ultrasound is of assistance because the relatively inexperienced physicians employing ultrasound in their office or clinic with moderately priced and unsophisticated equipment may not be expected to diagnose subtle anomalies such as spina bifida. Under these circumstances, one may do well to qualify one's report with a statement that an examination does not exclude fetal malformations less than a certain size, such as 5 mm. Level 1 and 2 examinations refer to the completeness of the examination. The criteria and regulations referring to these types of studies have not been adopted by the AIUM and are still under consideration.

IATROGENIC OR SO-CALLED INVENTED LESIONS

Incorrect interpretations of a real observation are not common in obstetric ultrasound studies. Particular problems relate to the overdiagnosis of fetal death in obese individuals, misdiagnosis of a normal pregnancy as a molar pregnancy when the placenta is particularly large, and the "invention" of an IUD in the presence of pregnancy. When a fetal anomaly is thought to be present, it is prudent to refer the patient for a second opinion since the legal and psychological consequences may be grave if a normal fetus is subsequently terminated.

STANDARD OF CARE

One of the time-honored traditions in consideration of medical malpractice and negligence is the concept of "standard of care."[5] In our rather complex social and medical environment, it is difficult to determine the criteria for standard of care. Most subspecialists would be expected to maintain the standard of care of their colleagues with similar training in other geographic areas. This also has implications for antitrust considerations discussed later in this chapter.[6]

A joint committee with representatives from the Association of Ultrasound in Medicine, the American College of Radiology, and the American College of Obstetrics and Gynecology has recommended that minimum training for someone to perform real-time sonographic procedures is a 1-month period of concentrated training and experience. This is to be required before a physician attempts to perform a definitive study using real-time ultrasound. This 1-month training period should be followed by 2 months of practice (personal communication, Barry Goldberg).

In reviewing the legal and medical literature, there is almost no assistance with regard to development of a concept of "standard of care" as it applies to sonographic procedures.[7] At this time, it seems that ultrasound should be performed only in selected obstetric cases and not as a routine for obstetric practice. An appropriate indicator exists when there is any uncertainty in the mind of the referring physician relating to a clinical problem that may affect the management of the pregnancy or have a deleterious effect on the pregnancy. For example, if there is a discrepancy between the conception dates given in the patient's history and the size of the fetus by physical examination, then ultrasound should be performed. Also, if there are genetic problems in the family history placing a patient at high risk, a sonographic study should be obtained. Presently, it does not appear that an ultrasound study of a routine pregnancy is an absolute requirement for good obstetric care.

The question of "who should perform ultrasound?" is a very difficult one and is made more complex by whether one is discussing "level 1" or "level 2" examinations. There are no present guidelines and no particular position statements with regard to the qualifications of a sonologist. Legally, sonographic technology may be utilized by anyone who is willing to assume the responsibilities and the attendant risks.

FAILURE TO COMMUNICATE ADEQUATELY WITH CLINICIAN OR PATIENT

It is axiomatic that a failure of communication with patient or physician is present to a greater or lesser degree in most medical malpractice and other forms of litigation involving the healing arts. There are numerous instances in which the communication problem was the sole cause of litigation.[8] When placenta previa or ectopic pregnancy is diagnosed and there may be a delay in the written report reaching the clinician, telephone or direct verbal communication is essential. In two instances, dangerous and almost fatal hemorrhages have ensued when lesions were detected by ultrasound but the clinician did not receive a report of the findings until days later, at which time the hemorrhage had occurred. In many other instances, it is clear that verbal or written contact with the clinician or patient would have improved the subsequent management of the cases. Communication is becoming even more essential as the complexity of medicine increases and agency and subagency arrangements are utilized.[9]

THE ROLE OF THE TECHNOLOGIST SONOGRAPHER

Many ultrasound examinations are performed by a technologist sonographer when the physician is not present and a report is issued by a physician at a later time. The legal responsibilities of the sonographer are unusual because a necessary part of the performance of the sonogram may involve rendering an interpretation at the time the study is performed, especially if real-time instrumentation is used. This differs from the role of the technologists in other imaging disciplines. The technologist sonographer, however, is acting as the "agent" of the physician. Therefore, anything of significant consequence that the sonographer does in the course of her/his normal duties (scope of employment) is the responsibility of the physician.[9] If she/he makes an incorrect diagnosis and issues an erroneous preliminary report, this remains the ultimate responsibility of the physician. Conversely, if the sonographer becomes intoxicated at work and attacks a patient, this is not the normal practice of a sonographer's duties and results from this type of behavior becomes the responsibility of the sonographer. The physician is, thus, not accountable for activities of an agent outside of the scope of employment. This concept is discussed in the following section.

APPLICATIONS OF AGENCY TO ULTRASOUND

The considerations of agency law regarding the performance of procedures by technologists on behalf of the diagnostic sonographer are important ones. According to agency law, any individual who is performing an activity that will benefit another party becomes an agent of that party, the principal. This may even occur without the active consent of the principal or physician in charge. In fact, technologists and other personnel involved in diagnostic sonography may act as agents of the Director of the Ultrasound Section, even without the Director's knowledge under both standard and agency law. So long as the circumstance of employment exists that would make the activity reasonable and no efforts have been made by the principal to bar the activities of the agent, the principal is then held liable.[9] This is also known as the "captain of the ship" or "*respondeat superior*" doctrine.

There is also the doctrine of implied agency. If one sets up a set of circumstances that creates a reasonable image and belief in the public's view that an agency relationship exists, then the principal is bound by the actions of the apparent agent. Agency law is becoming more important as individuals with all levels of training and health care have become involved in its delivery.

WRONGFUL CONCEPTION OR WRONGFUL PREGNANCY

Diagnostic sonography also may have a role in cases of wrongful conception or wrongful pregnancy. In these particular issues, it would appear that causes of action might involve the diagnostic sonographer in the substantiation of a viable pregnancy (wrongful conception), the inclusion or exclusion of a congenital defect (initiation of later case involving wrongful life), and in the misdiagnosis of the circumstance of pregnancy following a sterilization procedure.

Women have a right to voluntary sterilization as protected by the U.S. Constitution (Fourteenth Amendment interpretation). There are legally and medically accepted methods of birth control that have no attendant civil or criminal liability for their performance. For example, no state may restrict voluntary sterilization without establishing a compelling reason to do so.[10] Women have a fundamental right to privacy in matters of reproduction; however, hospitals may refuse to permit a particular procedure that will alter the reproductive process, such as sterilization or abortion. A private hospital may also require spousal consent from the wife for an abortion but not from the husband, as noted in *Fisher v. Sibley Hospital.*[11,12] Although these procedures could be performed as a matter of hospital policy and have proper informed consent, litigation could result from other causes.

Tubal ligation is the most commonly employed surgical procedure for sterilization of the female and, when competently done, will result in a 1 to 2 percent chance of natural reunification of the tube and subsequent pregnancy. There is, however, a higher risk of tubal pregnancy following a ligation. Thus, while a well accepted and efficacious technique, tubal ligation is imperfect. This fact has legal implications with regard to the topics of wrongful conception, wrongful birth, and informed consent as related to the performance and interpretation of ultrasound procedures.

A wrongful birth case in which parents bring suit against a physician should be distinguished from a wrongful life claim in which the infant brings suit against the physician whose negligence caused its birth. In the case of wrongful life, the plaintiff (infant with attorney initiating the lawsuit) will most often bring the action by the child seeking damages for being born. The most common circumstance, of course, is that of a child with a congenital defect which may or may not be detectable by ultrasound. To date, there have been a number of cases instituted which involve the concept of wrongful life, but in the courts these claims have met with little success because of the difficulties

in comparing the value of life with that of nonexistence or not having life at all, which is the alternative.[13-18]

This dilemma of the courts comparing compromised life with none at all does not result in consistent rulings. Two recent cases have accepted wrongful life as a viable cause of action (Turbin v. Sortini, Habeson v. Parke-Davis).[19,20] The rise in the number of lawsuits of this kind can be partially attributed to the 1973 U.S. Supreme Court decision sanctioning the right to early term abortion (Roe v. Wade).[4] Since a decade later abortion is viewed as such an acceptable alternative to an unwanted infant for any cause, then seeking redress through litigation is also acceptable and a natural consequence.[22]

Regarding the topics of wrongful birth and wrongful life, one would anticipate more precedent decisions in the future when the topic reaches the appelate court level. In action for wrongful birth, most courts appear to deny a cause of action of an unwanted healthy child if the infant is deemed healthy. In *Miller v. Duhart,*[23] the court ruled that it was impossible to ascertain the damage for such a cause of action and felt that it would be against public policy to do so. They reasoned that all others born into the world under adverse conditions would be encouraged to initiate litigation should the suit of Miller be successful. In the case of *Hickman v. Myers,*[24] it was noted that an involuntary benefit of parenthood should far outweigh the monetary burdens of rearing a child. In *Morris v. Fruderfeld,*[25] the benefits of motherhood were felt to offset any damages sustained by the mother due to an imperfect birth or an unwanted one.

Generally, a plaintiff can recover for medical expenses and the related cause of pregnancy and childbirth, but not for the cost of rearing the child. This would force the physician to bear the enormous cost of providing for a child until it reached majority, thus constituting a windfall to the parents and an unreasonable financial burden to the physician. General logic in these rulings is that the results would be out of proportion to the degree of liability involved.[26,27]

Benefit analysis, of course, is quite a widespread topic of consideration in medicine today, in that it can be applied to the allocation of legal damages. This type of value analysis generally comes under the rubric of a "weighing test," which is well discussed in the case of *Troppi v. Scarf.*[28] Using this test for the fairness of supporting an impaired life, the plaintiff is never assured of recovering anything beyond the expenses of pregnancy and delivery. There are exceptions if the delivery is complicated by the circumstances of an unmarried mother, a mother or parents with additional small children, or a child with a genetic defect that decreases the benefits of parenthood. Ultrasound will be involved in the failure to diagnose the expression of a genetic defect.

Wrongful life actions in which a child with a congenital abnormality is born requiring additional expenditures of rearing have received a great deal of attention, but very little in the way of legal precedents have arisen.[29] In *Speck v. Feingold,*[30] a negligently performed vasectomy resulted in a child born with neurofibromatosis. The court ruled that it felt inadequate to compare between a life of an impaired state versus nonexistence, but upheld the cause of action for wrongful birth. Where diagnostic ultrasound becomes a part of this action is when there is a question as to whether a study should have been performed or if an abnormality could have been detected.

In *Turpin v. Sortini,*[19] a child was born deaf and the state ruled that a child may not recover from being born impaired as opposed to not being born at all but did allow the child to recover special damages for extraordinary expenses to treat the ailment. Again, the court ruled that the law is incapable of stating that an imperfect life is worse than having no life at all. Awards for sustaining an impaired life can be substantial and requests have been in the millions of dollars.

INFORMED CONSENT

The issue of informed consent has received widespread attention recently in the medical field.[8] (See also Reuters' statement Legal Committee, American College Radiology, 1983.) We have moved in this particular topic from one of total physician dominance to that of consumer participation with increased advocate activity through litigation.[31] In any ultrasound-related procedure with a significant risk (e.g., intrauterine transfusion), the woman should be advised regarding all material risks of the procedure.[1,3,33] In general, the logic of cases of informed consent have applied the reasonable person standard in determining whether a specific risk is material and should be disclosed to the patient. This concept attempts to apply the logic that the actions and reactions should be those expected by a reasonable person in the circumstance at issue.

It was held in *Nathanson v. Kline*[33] that the physician's judgment with regard to the material aspect will only be upheld if considered in *medical terms* of the physiologic and anatomic consequences and in *lay terms* regarding the reasonable person standard. Thus, if a decision could be reduced to lay terms and be understood by the average person, then the physician is obligated to present the facts in such a manner to the patient.

A significant issue is that of "what constitutes informed consent?" Should all ultrasound procedures be preceded by informed consent utilizing detailed consent forms that the patient may read and sign, or should informed consent be limited to only those patients who are undergoing invasive procedures with a significant risk. Real-time ultrasound has increased the ability to engage in procedures of this type.[34]

Certain jurisdictions have extended the doctrine of informed consent to include the right to be informed of the available medical alternatives.[31] This discussion concerns the differences in frames of reference of physicians, patients, attorneys, and the courts when presented with an identical set of facts and an analysis of the concept of what constitutes being "informed" regarding consent. This difference in attitude has led to geographic inconsistencies which have been noted as "majority rule" and "minority rule" states. In the majority rule states, the community standard rule applies and physicians must inform their patients of risks and benefits of a particular procedure as like practitioners would do in similar circumstances in that community. In minority rule jurisdictions, it is required that physicians anticipate the attitudes of patients and effectively inform patients so that, given the patient's frame of reference, the patient can render an informed consent. To obtain an informed consent for an invasive ultrasound procedure, the physician should indicate those risks that are significant. If this is done, then concerns of litigation should be minimal.

With the minority ruling, it becomes evident that a new type of action for malpractice and negligence has evolved. In addition to the battery claim (violation of one's body) and to the more common claim of negligence, there arises a third type of actionable activity— failure to inform or fully and reasonably inform. This differs from ordinary negligence in that no consideration or question of skill, competence, or deviation from standard of medical care is involved. Thus, the new type of action differs in matter of causation. The sonologist must now reveal all that the patient needs to know to render an informed decision.

In considering a technology that is evolving as rapidly as ultrasound, the data base of information is consistently expanding. Therefore, to provide the information for an informed consent is problematical. We are entering a much more innovative and exploratory era. For this reason, our knowledge of consequences of some of the more invasive procedures is incomplete.[35]

Although it does not appear from the survey of Sanders and Hohler that many actions arise from failure to obtain informed consent with the more invasive ultrasound procedures, this will predictably change.[36] Based upon experience with the surgical and radiologic applications of technology, we would make the following recommendation: In those procedures requiring significant risk, such as drainage of fluid collections, intrauterine surgery, and amniocentesis, informed consent should be obtained from the patient after an explanation of the procedure and its risks by a physician member of the team performing the procedure. The explanation should include the major risks, alternative procedures, if any, and should be delivered in clear, precise language.

Among the more common reasons for failure of physicians to inform their patients adequately are the following: (1) Fear of patient refusal for clinically necessary procedures. (2) Fear of precipitation of untoward psychologic or physical reaction. (3) Difficulty with establishing a relative frame of reference for the patient and the physician. (4) The extraordinary requirement of physician time and the logistics of providing information. However, communication appears to be the most reliable preventive measure regarding malpractice and negligence suits. In this age of consumerism, one must strive to improve communication and relationships with patients.

Ultrasound has been presented to the public as a safe, simple technology with a minimum of biologic implications. Thus, the sonographer and sonologist can with conviction reassure apprehensive patients but should also point out that the methodology is not infallible and not entirely without biologic implications (see Chapter 2).

A question arises as to whether or not detailed consent forms may circumvent many of these problems. The Commission on Liability and Malpractice of the American College of Radiology has issued a position statement on the use of detailed consent forms. Beginning with a discussion of *Karp v. Cooley,*[37] there is an extensive review of the case law regarding detailed consent forms. These forms can provide significant protection to diagnostic sonologists or obstetricians defending against a claim of inadequately informed consent. The information in the consent form must conform to the standard of care in the community, the statutory or common law requirements for informed consent in that jurisdiction, and a full description of the procedure in lay terms. Also, if one is to detail the severe complications, it is recommended that the incidence of those complications be conveyed to the patient.

One caveat should be interjected, however. That is, if an individual other than the obstetrician or radiologist performing the procedure obtains the consent from the patient, the obstetrician and/or radiologist will bear the liability for any inadequacies in the consent under ordinary rules of agency law.[9]

Detailed consent forms have some value of memorializing the information given to the patient. They have their greatest value in complex procedures such as amniocentesis, intrauterine treatment of congenital disorders with ultrasound guidance, and other techniques involving instrumentation and manipulation. These detailed consent forms are clearly superior to standard hospital forms. In simple ultrasound procedures, consent forms do not appear to have significant value, if one can extrapolate from the radiologic literature.

EQUIPMENT MALFUNCTIONS AND PATIENT INJURY

Although the physicians performing the ultrasound studies are ultimately responsible for those procedures, there is an opportunity for action against the manufacturer of the product if the untoward event resulted purely from the inadequacies or inappropriate design of the device employed.

In *Dubin v. the Michael Reese Hospital,*[38] the Illinois Supreme Court ruled that radiation therapy administered to a patient by a hospital was not a product subject to strict liability in tort. The professional performing the therapeutic examination was not looked upon as manufacturing a particular product. Hospitals and physicians do not normally sell products and have not been held to a standard of warranty.

In *Silverhart v. The Mount Zion Hospital,*[39] the court ruled that physicians and hospitals furnish services and must rely upon the judgment of the manufacturer who should have superior control and responsibility regarding product quality and performance. One might add that this does not appear to be a license to utilize equipment with which a physician usually is not familiar. Conversely, injury from instrumentation inappropriately employed will result in physician exposure to litigation.

CERTIFICATES OF NEED AND HOSPITAL PRIVILEGES

Regarding the issue of costly and sophisticated medical technology, resource allocation and distribution have in recent years been a major medical, social, and economic issue.[7] Granting of hospital privileges to physicians following the landmark decision of *Darling v. Charleston Community Hospital*[40] have decidedly changed the status of this activity and it has become increasingly difficult to be certified to practice in any particular hospital.[41] In this case, it was decided that the ultimate responsibility for the physician's actions may well reside in the Hospital Board. The so-called "expanded agency" rule has profound implications not only for governing bodies, but also for those responsible for medical care. Given the circumstance of limited distribution of sophisticated and costly technology, the effect of denial of hospital privileges will predictably result in causes of action brought by physicians for denial of the marketplace or denial of access to certain technology such as ultrasound in behalf of their patients.[6,7]

Although most ultrasound instrumentation is sufficiently inexpensive that it does not involve certificate of need application, combination units of pulsed Doppler real-time and static ultrasound, and breast dedicated units may.[7] Antitrust issues will be important in future considerations of who should be responsible for the acquisition and utilization of sonographic devices within hospital groups, a community of hospitals, or an individual institution.[42,43,44]

There are obviously many other topics with regard to the legal implications of the application of diagnostic sonography to the specialty of obstetrics. We are entering into an area of accountability, public awareness, and generally aggressive consumerism. It is encumbent that users of this technology address the issues in a concerned manner, according them the same respect that we would our patients. They will become increasingly the fabric of medicine.

ACKNOWLEDGMENTS

We are appreciative of the encouragement of Deans of Law and Medicine, Dent Bostick and John Chapman. Discussions with James Blumstein (School of Law) and Frank Sloan (Institute for Public Policy Studies) and Richard Zaner (Chair in Medical Ethics) were most helpful. We also gratefully acknowledge the comments of attorneys Karen Rothenberg, Landon Feazell, Donald Hall, Paul Gephart, Ed Hollowell, James Neal, and physicians Joseph Holmes, Ken Gottesfeld, Tommy Thompson, Lonnie Burnett, Alan C. Winfield, and Alan Kaufman. The editorial office of the Department of Radiology and Radiological Sciences at Vanderbilt University Medical Center (Mary Henry, Director) was responsible for the preparation and editing of the manuscript.

REFERENCES

1. Fleischer AC, James AE: Introduction to Diagnostic Sonography. New York, Wiley, 1980
2. James AE, Coulam CM, et al: Newer diagnostic medical imaging techniques: Their implications as evidence. J Legal Med 2:151, 1981
3. Fleischer AC, James AE: Real-Time Sonography. Norwalk, CT, Appleton-Century-Crofts, 1984
4. Roe v. Wade, 410 U.S. 113 (1973)
5. James AE (ed): Legal Medicine with Special Reference to Diagnostic Imaging. Baltimore, Urban & Schwarzenberg, 1980
6. Calvani T, James AE: Antitrust law and the practice of medicine, in James AE (ed): Legal Medicine with Special Reference to Diagnostic Imaging. Baltimore, Urban & Schwarzenberg, 1980
7. James AE: Law and medicine. The Vanderbilt Lawyer 13:20, 1983
8. James AE et al: Informed consent. Radiology 123:809, 1977
9. James AE, Sherrard TJ: Agency, in James AE (ed): Legal Medicine with Special Reference to Diagnostic Imaging. Baltimore, Urban & Schwarzenberg, 1980.
10. Griswold v. Conn., 381 U.S. 479 (1965)
11. Fisher v. Sibley Memorial Hospital, 403 A 2d 1130 (D.C. Cir. 1979)
12. Bundy AL, James AE et al: Wrongful life and ultrasound. J Cont Ob Gyn, (in press), 1984
13. Becker v. Schwartz, 60 App. Div. 2d 587 400 NYS 2d 119 (1977)
14. Berman v. Allan, 80 N.J. 421 404 A 2d 8 (1979)
15. Park v. Chessin, 387 N.Y.S. 2d 204 (Sup. Ct. 1976)
16. Stormeier v. Assoc. in Ob and Gyn, No. 5830 (Minn. Sup. Ct. 1982)
17. Gleitman v. Cosgrove, 49 N.J. 22; 227 A 2d 689 (1967)
18. Brocato v. Leggio, 393 So 2d 183 (La. App. 1980)
19. Turpin v. Sortini, 643 P. 2d 954 (Cal. Sup. Ct. 1982)
20. Harbeson v. Parke-Davis, Inc., 51 L.W. 2421 (Wash. Sup. Ct. 1983)
21. Curlender v. Bio-Science Lab., 165 Cal. Rptr. 477 (Cal. App. 1980)
22. Roe v. Wiley: Abortions because of unavailability of prenatal diagnosis. Lancet 2:936, 1981
23. Miller v. Duhart, 637 S.W. 2d 183 (1982)
24. Hickman v. Myers, 632 S.W. 2d 86 (1982)
25. Morris v. Fruderfeld, 185 Cal. Report (1978)
26. White v. U.S., 510 F Supp. 146 (Kan. 1981)
27. Coleman v. Garrison, 327 A 2d 757 (Del. Sup. 1974)
28. Troppi v. Scarf, 643, P 2d, 954 (Cal. 1982)
29. City of Akron v. Akron Center for Reproductive Health, Inc., 103 Sup. Ct. 2481 (1983)
30. Speck v. Feingold, 408 A 2d 486 (1979)
31. Johnson B, James AE: The radiologist and informed consent: A review, comments and proposals. Curr Prob Diag Radiol 8:3, 1979
32. Canterbury v. Spence, 464 F. 2d 772 (D.C. Cir.), Cert. denied, 409 U.S. 1064 (1972)

33. Nathanson v. Kline, 186 Kan. 393, 350 P. 2d 1093 (1960)

34. Hubbard R: Legal and Policy Implications of Recent Advances in Prenatal Diagnosis and Fetal Therapy. Women's Rights Law Reporter 7(3): 1982

35. James AE et al: The Legal Right of Abortion: Implications for Ultrasound. (in press), 1984

36. Sanders R, Hohler CW: Guest editorial: Legal suits involving ultrasound. J Ultra Med 2:R26, 1983

37. Karp v. Cooley, 419 U.S. 845 (1977)

38. Dubin v. Michael Reese Hospital, 83 Ill. 2d 277 (1980)

39. Silverhart v. Mt. Zion Hospital, 20 Cal. App. 3d, 1022 (1980)

40. Darling v. Charleston Community Hospital, 33 Ill. 2d 326, 211 N.E. 2d 253 (1965)

41. James AE, Sloan F, Blumstein J, et al: CON in an antitrust context. J Health Policy and Law 8:314, 1983

42. Partain CL, James AE, Rollo FD, et al: NMR Imaging. Philadelphia, Saunders, 1983

43. James AE et al: Legal implications associated with new medical imaging technology. Int Workshop PACS 318:464, 1982

44. James AE et al: Exclusive Contracts: The Implications of Hyde (in press), 1984

Appendix

APPENDIX 1

Correlation of Predicted Menstrual Age Based Upon Biparietal Diameters

Menstrual Age (weeks)	BPD Mean Values (mm)			
	Kurtz et al.[1] 1974	Hadlock et al.[2] 1982	Shepard & Filly[3] 1982	Jeanty & Romero[4] 1984
14	26	27	28	28
15	29	30	31	32
16	33	33	34	36
17	36	37	37	39
18	40	40	40	43
19	43	43	43	46
20	46	46	46	49
21	50	50	49	52
22	53	53	52	55
23	56	56	55	58
24	59	58	57	61
25	61	61	60	64
26	64	64	63	67
27	67	67	65	70
28	70	70	68	72
29	72	72	71	74
30	75	75	73	77
31	77	77	76	79
32	79	79	78	82
33	82	82	80	84
34	84	84	83	86
35	86	86	85	88
36	88	88	88	90
37	90	90	90	94
38	92	91	92	
39	94	93	95	
40	95	95	97	

[1] Kurtz AB, Wapner RJ, Kurtz RJ, et al: Analysis of biparietal diameter as an accurate indicator of gestational age. J Clin Ultrasound 8:319, 1980

[2] Hadlock RP, Deter RL, Harrist RB, et al: Fetal biparietal diameter: A critical reevaluation of the relation to menstrual age by means of real-time ultrasound. J Ultrasound Med 1:97, 1982

[3] Shepard M, Filly RA: A standardized plane for biparietal diameter measurement. J Ultrasound Med 1:145, 1982

[4] Jeanty P, Romaro R: Obstetrical Ultrasound. New York, McGraw Hill, 1984

APPENDIX 2

Predicted Normal Values for Measurements of the Fetus in Utero

Menstrual Age (weeks)	Head Circumference (HC)			Abdominal Circumference (AC)			Femur Length			HC/AC Ratio			Estimated Weight Percentiles		
	−2SD (cm)	Mean (cm)	+2SD (cm)	−2SD (cm)	Mean (cm)	+2SD (cm)	−2SD (cm)	Mean (cm)	+2SD (cm)	−2SD	Mean	+2SD	10th (kg)	50th (kg)	90th (kg)
12	5.1	7.0	8.9	3.1	5.6	8.1	0.2	0.8	1.4	1.12	1.22	1.31			
13	6.5	8.9	10.3	4.4	6.9	9.4	0.5	1.1	1.7	1.11	1.21	1.30			
14	7.9	9.8	11.7	5.6	8.1	10.6	0.9	1.5	2.1	1.11	1.20	1.30			
15	9.2	11.1	13.0	6.8	9.3	11.8	1.2	1.8	2.4	1.10	1.19	1.29			
16	10.5	12.4	14.3	8.0	10.5	13.0	1.5	2.1	2.7	1.09	1.18	1.28			
17	11.8	13.7	15.6	9.2	11.7	14.2	1.8	2.4	3.0	1.08	1.18	1.27			
18	13.1	15.0	16.9	10.4	12.9	15.4	2.1	2.7	3.3	1.07	1.17	1.26			
19	14.4	16.3	18.2	11.6	14.1	16.6	2.3	3.0	3.6	1.06	1.16	1.25			
20	15.6	17.5	19.4	12.7	15.2	17.7	2.7	3.3	3.9	1.06	1.15	1.24			
21	16.8	18.7	20.6	13.9	16.4	18.9	3.0	3.6	4.2	1.05	1.14	1.24	0.28	0.41	0.86
22	18.0	19.9	21.8	15.0	17.5	20.0	3.3	3.9	4.5	1.04	1.13	1.23	0.32	0.48	0.92
23	19.1	21.0	22.9	16.1	18.6	21.1	3.6	4.2	4.8	1.03	1.12	1.22	0.37	0.55	0.99
24	20.2	22.1	24.0	17.2	19.7	22.0	3.8	4.4	5.0	1.02	1.12	1.21	0.42	0.64	1.08
25	21.3	23.2	25.1	18.3	20.8	23.3	4.1	4.7	5.3	1.01	1.11	1.20	0.49	0.74	1.18
26	22.3	24.2	26.1	19.4	21.9	24.4	4.3	4.9	5.5	1.00	1.10	1.19	0.57	0.86	1.32
27	23.3	25.2	27.1	20.4	22.9	25.4	4.6	5.2	5.8	1.00	1.09	1.18	0.66	0.99	1.47
28	24.3	26.2	28.1	21.5	24.0	26.5	4.8	5.4	6.0	0.99	1.08	1.18	0.77	1.15	1.66
29	25.2	27.1	29.0	22.5	25.0	27.5	5.0	5.6	6.2	0.98	1.07	1.17	0.89	1.31	1.89
30	26.1	28.0	29.9	23.5	26.0	28.5	5.2	5.8	6.4	0.97	1.07	1.16	1.03	1.46	2.10
31	27.0	28.9	30.8	24.5	27.0	29.5	5.5	6.1	6.7	0.96	1.06	1.15	1.18	1.63	2.29
32	27.8	29.7	31.6	25.5	28.0	30.5	5.7	6.3	6.9	0.95	1.05	1.14	1.31	1.81	2.50
33	28.5	30.4	32.3	26.5	29.0	31.5	5.9	6.5	7.1	0.95	1.04	1.13	1.48	2.01	2.69
34	29.3	31.2	33.1	27.5	30.0	32.5	6.0	6.6	7.2	0.94	1.03	1.13	1.67	2.22	2.88
35	29.9	31.8	33.7	28.4	30.9	33.4	6.2	6.8	7.4	0.93	1.02	1.12	1.87	2.43	3.09
36	30.6	32.5	34.4	29.3	31.8	34.3	6.4	7.0	7.6	0.92	1.01	1.11	2.19	2.65	3.29
37	31.1	33.0	34.9	30.2	32.7	35.2	6.6	7.2	7.8	0.91	1.01	1.10	2.31	2.87	3.47
38	31.9	33.6	35.5	31.1	33.6	36.1	6.7	7.3	7.9	0.90	1.00	1.09	2.51	3.03	3.61
39	32.2	34.1	36.0	32.0	34.5	37.0	6.9	7.5	8.1	0.89	0.99	1.08	2.68	3.17	3.75
40	32.6	34.5	36.4	32.9	35.4	37.9	7.0	7.6	8.2	0.89	0.98	1.08	2.75	3.28	3.87

Reprinted with permission from Hadlock FP, Deter RL, Harrist RB: Sonographic detection of fetal intrauterine growth retardation. Applied Radiology 12:28, 1983.

APPENDIX 3

Fetal Kidney and Abdominal Parameters by Gestational Age Group in Normal Fetuses

Variable	Gestational Age (wk)					
	<16 (n = 9)	17–20 (n = 18)	21–25 (n = 7)	26–30 (n = 11)	31–35 (n = 19)	>36 (n = 25)
Fetal Kidney:						
Anteroposterior (cm)						
Mean	0.84	1.16	1.49	1.93	2.20	2.32
S.D.	0.24	0.24	0.37	0.19	0.32	0.32
Transverse (cm)						
Mean	0.86	1.13	1.64	2.00	2.34	2.63
S.D.	0.14	0.25	0.40	0.28	0.42	0.50
Circumference (cm)						
Mean	2.79	3.80	5.40	6.58	7.86	8.42
S.D.	0.64	0.72	0.68	0.67	0.86	1.39
Fetal Abdomen:						
Anteroposterior (cm)						
Mean	2.92	3.73	5.12	6.74	8.50	8.88
S.D.	0.62	0.72	0.80	0.58	0.82	0.94
Transverse (cm)						
Mean	2.93	3.68	5.12	7.09	8.76	9.68
S.D.	0.59	0.56	0.49	0.61	0.89	1.44
Circumference (cm)						
Mean	9.66	12.37	17.36	22.03	28.11	30.45
S.D.	1.88	2.28	1.77	1.77	2.31	3.45
KC/AC Ratio						
Mean	0.28	0.30	0.30	0.29	0.28	0.27
S.D.	0.02	0.03	0.02	0.02	0.03	0.04

Calculations of ratio used variables measured to eight decimal places.

Reprinted with permission from Grannum P, Bracken M, Silverman R, et al: Assessment of fetal kidney size in normal gestation by comparison of ratio of kidney circumference to abdominal circumference. Am J Obstet Gynecol 136:253, 1980.

APPENDIX 4

Predicted Biparietal Diameter and Weeks' Gestation from the Inner and Outer Orbital Diameters

Biparietal Diameter (cm)	Weeks' Gestation	Inner Orbital Diameter (cm)	Outer Orbital Diameter (cm)	Biparietal Diameter (cm)	Weeks' Gestation	Inner Orbital Diameter (cm)	Outer Orbital Diameter (cm)
1.9	11.6	0.5	1.3	5.7	23.8	1.5	4.1
2.0	11.6	0.5	1.4	5.8	24.3	1.6	4.1
2.1	12.1	0.6	1.5	5.9	24.3	1.6	4.2
2.2	12.6	0.6	1.6	6.0	24.7	1.6	4.3
2.3	12.6	0.6	1.7	6.1	25.2	1.6	4.3
2.4	13.1	0.7	1.7	6.2	25.2	1.6	4.4
2.5	13.6	0.7	1.8	6.3	25.7	1.7	4.4
2.6	13.6	0.7	1.9	6.4	26.2	1.7	4.5
2.7	14.1	0.8	2.0	6.5	26.2	1.7	4.5
2.8	14.6	0.8	2.1	6.6	26.7	1.7	4.6
2.9	14.6	0.8	2.1	6.7	27.2	1.7	4.6
3.0	15.0	0.9	2.2	6.8	27.6	1.7	4.7
3.1	15.5	0.9	2.3	6.9	28.1	1.7	4.7
3.2	15.5	0.9	2.4	7.0	28.6	1.8	4.8
3.3	16.0	1.0	2.5	7.1	29.1	1.8	4.8
3.4	16.5	1.0	2.5	7.3	29.6	1.8	4.9
3.5	16.5	1.0	2.6	7.4	30.0	1.8	5.0
3.6	17.0	1.0	2.7	7.5	30.6	1.8	5.0
3.7	17.5	1.1	2.7	7.6	31.0	1.8	5.1
3.8	17.9	1.1	2.8	7.7	31.5	1.8	5.1
4.0	18.4	1.2	3.0	7.8	32.0	1.8	5.2
4.2	18.9	1.2	3.1	7.9	32.5	1.9	5.2
4.3	19.4	1.2	3.2	8.0	33.0	1.9	5.3
4.4	19.4	1.3	3.2	8.2	33.5	1.9	5.4
4.5	19.9	1.3	3.3	8.3	34.0	1.9	5.4
4.6	20.4	1.3	3.4	8.4	34.4	1.9	5.4
4.7	20.4	1.3	3.4	8.5	35.0	1.9	5.5
4.8	20.9	1.4	3.5	8.6	35.4	1.9	5.5
4.9	21.3	1.4	3.6	8.8	35.9	1.9	5.6
5.0	21.3	1.4	3.6	8.9	36.4	1.9	5.6
5.1	21.8	1.4	3.7	9.0	36.9	1.9	5.7
5.2	22.3	1.4	3.8	9.1	37.3	1.9	5.7
5.3	22.3	1.5	3.8	9.2	37.8	1.9	5.8
5.4	22.8	1.5	3.9	9.3	38.3	1.9	5.8
5.5	23.3	1.5	4.0	9.4	38.8	1.9	5.8
5.6	23.3	1.5	4.0	9.6	39.3	1.9	5.9
				9.7	39.8	1.9	5.9

Reprinted with permission from Mayden KL, Tortora M, Berkowitz RL, et al: Orbital diameters: A new parameter for prenatal diagnosis and dating. Amer J Obstet Gynecol 144:292, 1982.

APPENDIX 5

Comparison of Predicted Femur Lengths at Points in Gestation

Menstrual Age (weeks)	Femur Length (mm)			
	Filly et al.[1] 1981	Jeanty et al.[3] 1981†	Hadlock et al.[2] 1982*	Hadlock et al.[2] 1982†
12		09	14	08
13		12	16	11
14	16	15	19	15
15	19	19	21	18
16	22	22	23	21
17	25	25	26	24
18	28	28	28	27
19	32	31	30	30
20	35	33	33	33
21	38	36	35	36
22	41	39	38	39
23	44	41	40	42
24	47	44	42	44
25	50	46	45	47
26	53	49	47	49
27	55	51	49	52
28	57	53	52	54
29	61	56	54	56
30	63	58	57	58
31		60	59	61
32		62	61	63
33		64	64	65
34		65	66	66
35		67	69	68
36		69	71	70
37		71	73	72
38		72	76	73
39		74	78	75
40		75	80	76

* Linear function
† Linear quadratic function

[1] Filly RA, Golbus MS, Carey JC, et al. Short-limbed dwarfism: Ultrasonographic diagnosis by mensuration of fetal femoral length. Radiology 138:653, 1981
[2] Fetal femur length as a predictor of menstrual age: Sonographically measured. Am J Roentgenol 138:875, 1982
[3] Jeanty P, Kirkpatrick C, Dramaix-Wilmet M, et al: Ultrasonic evaluation of fetal limb growth. Radiology 140:165, 1981

Reprinted with permission from Jeanty P, Romero R: Obstetrical Ultrasound. New York, McGraw Hill, 1984, p 327.

APPENDIX 6

Length of Fetal Long Bones in mm

Week No.	Humerus Percentile			Ulna Percentile			Femur Percentile			Tibia Percentile		
	5	50	95	5	50	95	5	50	95	5	50	95
12	4	9	13	3	7	11	4	8	13	3	7	12
13	7	11	15	5	10	14	6	11	16	5	10	14
14	10	14	18	8	13	17	9	14	18	8	12	16
15	13	17	21	11	15	20	12	17	21	10	15	19
16	16	20	24	14	18	22	15	20	24	13	17	21
17	18	22	27	16	21	25	18	23	27	15	20	24
18	21	25	29	19	23	28	21	25	30	18	22	27
19	24	28	32	22	26	30	24	28	33	21	25	29
20	26	30	34	24	28	33	26	31	36	23	27	32
21	29	33	37	26	31	35	29	34	38	26	30	34
22	31	35	39	29	33	37	32	36	41	28	32	37
23	33	38	42	31	35	39	35	39	44	31	35	39
24	36	40	44	33	37	42	37	42	46	33	37	42
25	38	42	46	35	39	44	40	44	49	35	40	44
26	40	44	48	37	41	46	42	47	51	37	42	46
27	42	46	50	39	43	47	45	49	54	40	44	48
28	44	48	52	41	45	49	47	52	56	42	46	50
29	46	50	54	43	47	51	50	54	59	44	48	52
30	47	51	56	44	48	53	52	56	61	46	50	54
31	49	53	57	46	50	54	54	59	63	47	52	56
32	51	55	59	47	52	56	56	61	65	49	54	58
33	52	56	60	49	53	57	58	63	67	51	55	60
34	54	58	62	50	55	59	60	65	69	53	57	61
35	55	59	63	52	56	60	62	67	71	54	58	63
36	56	61	65	53	57	61	64	68	73	56	60	64
37	58	62	66	54	58	63	65	70	74	57	61	66
38	59	63	67	55	59	64	67	71	76	59	63	67
39	61	65	69	56	60	65	68	73	77	60	64	69
40	62	66	70	57	61	66	70	74	79	61	66	70

Reprinted with permission from Jeanty P, Romero R: Obstetrical Ultrasound. New York, McGraw Hill, 1984, p 233.

APPENDIX 7

Estimated Fetal Weights

Biparietal Diameters	Abdominal Circumferences											
	15.5	16.0	16.5	17.0	17.5	18.0	18.5	19.0	19.5	20.0	20.5	21.0
3.1	224	234	244	255	267	279	291	304	318	332	346	362
3.2	231	241	251	263	274	286	299	312	326	340	355	371
3.3	237	248	259	270	282	294	307	321	335	349	365	381
3.4	244	255	266	278	290	302	316	329	344	359	374	391
3.5	251	262	274	285	298	311	324	338	353	368	384	401
3.6	259	270	281	294	306	319	333	347	362	378	394	411
3.7	266	278	290	302	315	328	342	357	372	388	404	422
3.8	274	286	298	310	324	337	352	366	382	398	415	432
3.9	282	294	306	319	333	347	361	376	392	409	426	444
4.0	290	303	315	328	342	356	371	386	403	419	437	455
4.1	299	311	324	338	352	366	381	397	413	430	448	467
4.2	308	320	333	347	361	376	392	408	424	442	460	479
4.3	317	330	343	357	371	387	402	419	436	453	472	491
4.4	326	339	353	367	382	397	413	430	447	465	484	504
4.5	335	349	363	377	393	408	425	442	459	478	497	517
4.6	345	359	373	388	404	420	436	454	472	490	510	530
4.7	355	369	384	399	415	431	448	466	484	503	523	544
4.8	366	380	395	410	426	443	460	478	497	517	537	558
4.9	376	391	406	422	438	455	473	491	510	530	551	572
5.0	387	402	418	434	451	468	486	505	524	544	565	587
5.1	399	414	430	446	463	481	499	518	538	559	580	602
5.2	410	426	442	459	476	494	513	532	552	573	595	618
5.3	422	438	455	472	489	508	527	547	567	589	611	634
5.4	435	451	468	485	503	522	541	561	582	604	627	650
5.5	447	464	481	499	517	536	556	577	598	620	643	667
5.6	461	477	495	513	532	551	571	592	614	636	660	684
5.7	474	491	509	527	547	566	587	608	630	653	677	701
5.8	488	505	524	542	562	582	603	625	647	670	695	719
5.9	502	520	539	558	578	598	619	642	664	688	713	738
6.0	517	535	554	573	594	615	636	659	682	706	731	757
6.1	532	550	570	590	610	632	654	677	700	725	750	777
6.2	547	566	586	606	627	649	672	695	719	744	770	797
6.3	563	583	603	624	645	667	690	714	738	764	790	817
6.4	580	600	620	641	663	686	709	733	758	784	811	838
6.5	597	617	638	659	682	705	728	753	778	805	832	860

Estimated Fetal Weights

Abdominal Circumferences

21.5	22.0	22.5	23.0	23.5	24.0	24.5	25.0	25.5	26.0	26.5	27.0	27.5
378	395	412	431	450	470	491	513	536	559	584	610	638
388	405	423	441	461	481	502	525	548	572	597	624	651
397	415	433	452	472	493	514	537	560	585	611	638	666
408	425	444	463	483	504	526	549	573	598	624	652	680
418	436	455	475	495	517	539	562	587	612	638	666	695
429	447	466	486	507	529	552	575	600	626	653	681	710
440	458	478	498	519	542	565	589	614	640	667	696	725
451	470	490	510	532	554	578	602	628	654	682	711	741
462	482	502	523	545	568	592	616	642	669	697	727	757
474	494	514	536	558	581	606	631	657	684	713	743	773
486	506	527	549	572	595	620	645	672	700	729	759	790
498	519	540	562	585	609	634	660	688	716	745	776	807
511	532	554	576	600	624	649	676	703	732	762	793	825
524	545	567	590	614	639	665	692	719	749	779	810	843
538	559	581	605	629	654	680	708	736	765	796	828	861
551	573	596	620	644	670	696	724	753	783	814	846	880
565	588	611	635	660	686	713	741	770	801	832	865	899
580	602	626	650	676	702	730	758	788	819	851	884	919
594	617	641	666	692	719	747	776	806	837	870	903	938
610	633	657	683	709	736	765	794	824	856	889	923	959
625	649	674	699	726	754	783	812	843	876	909	944	980
641	665	690	717	744	772	801	831	863	895	929	964	1,001
657	682	708	734	762	790	820	851	883	916	950	986	1,023
674	699	725	752	780	809	839	870	903	936	971	1,007	1,045
691	717	743	771	799	828	859	891	924	958	993	1,030	1,068
709	735	762	789	818	848	879	911	945	979	1,015	1,052	1,091
727	753	780	809	838	869	900	933	966	1,001	1,038	1,075	1,114
745	772	800	829	858	889	921	954	989	1,024	1,061	1,099	1,139
764	792	820	849	879	911	943	977	1,011	1,047	1,085	1,123	1,163
784	811	840	870	900	932	965	999	1,035	1,071	1,109	1,148	1,189
804	832	861	891	922	955	988	1,023	1,058	1,095	1,134	1,173	1,214
824	853	882	913	945	977	1,011	1,046	1,083	1,120	1,159	1,199	1,241
845	874	904	935	967	1,001	1,035	1,071	1,107	1,145	1,185	1,226	1,268
867	896	927	958	991	1,025	1,059	1,096	1,133	1,171	1,211	1,253	1,295
889	919	950	982	1,015	1,049	1,084	1,121	1,159	1,198	1,238	1,280	1,323

Estimated Fetal Weights (*cont.*)

Biparietal Diameters	Abdominal Circumferences											
	15.5	16.0	16.5	17.0	17.5	18.0	18.5	19.0	19.5	20.0	20.5	21.0
6.6	614	635	656	678	701	724	748	773	799	826	853	882
6.7	632	653	675	697	720	744	769	794	820	848	876	905
6.8	651	672	694	717	740	765	790	816	842	870	898	928
6.9	670	691	714	737	761	786	811	838	865	893	922	952
7.0	689	711	734	758	782	807	833	860	888	916	946	976
7.1	709	732	755	779	804	830	856	883	912	941	971	1,002
7.2	730	763	777	801	827	853	880	907	936	965	996	1,027
7.3	751	775	799	824	850	876	904	932	961	991	1,022	1,054
7.4	773	797	822	847	874	901	928	957	987	1,017	1,049	1,081
7.5	796	820	845	871	898	925	954	983	1,013	1,044	1,076	1,109
7.6	819	844	870	896	923	951	980	1,009	1,040	1,072	1,104	1,137
7.7	843	868	894	921	949	977	1,007	1,037	1,068	1,100	1,133	1,167
7.8	868	894	920	947	975	1,004	1,034	1,065	1,096	1,129	1,162	1,197
7.9	893	919	946	974	1,003	1,032	1,062	1,094	1,126	1,159	1,193	1,228
8.0	919	946	973	1,002	1,031	1,061	1,091	1,123	1,156	1,189	1,224	1,259
8.1	946	973	1,001	1,030	1,060	1,090	1,121	1,153	1,187	1,221	1,256	1,292
8.2	974	1,001	1,030	1,059	1,089	1,120	1,152	1,185	1,218	1,253	1,288	1,325
8.3	1,002	1,030	1,059	1,089	1,120	1,151	1,183	1,217	1,251	1,286	1,322	1,359
8.4	1,032	1,060	1,090	1,120	1,151	1,183	1,216	1,249	1,284	1,320	1,356	1,394
8.5	1,062	1,091	1,121	1,151	1,183	1,216	1,249	1,283	1,318	1,355	1,392	1,430
8.6	1,093	1,122	1,153	1,184	1,216	1,249	1,283	1,318	1,354	1,390	1,428	1,467
8.7	1,125	1,155	1,186	1,218	1,250	1,284	1,318	1,353	1,390	1,427	1,465	1,505
8.8	1,157	1,188	1,220	1,252	1,285	1,319	1,354	1,390	1,427	1,465	1,504	1,543
8.9	1,191	1,222	1,254	1,287	1,321	1,356	1,391	1,428	1,465	1,503	1,543	1,583
9.0	1,226	1,258	1,290	1,324	1,358	1,393	1,429	1,456	1,504	1,543	1,583	1,624
9.1	1,262	1,294	1,327	1,361	1,396	1,432	1,468	1,506	1,544	1,584	1,624	1,666
9.2	1,299	1,332	1,365	1,400	1,435	1,471	1,508	1,546	1,586	1,626	1,667	1,709
9.3	1,337	1,370	1,404	1,439	1,475	1,512	1,550	1,588	1,628	1,668	1,710	1,753
9.4	1,376	1,410	1,444	1,480	1,516	1,554	1,592	1,631	1,671	1,712	1,755	1,798
9.5	1,416	1,450	1,486	1,522	1,559	1,597	1,635	1,675	1,716	1,758	1,800	1,844
9.6	1,457	1,492	1,528	1,565	1,602	1,641	1,680	1,720	1,762	1,804	1,847	1,892
9.7	1,500	1,535	1,572	1,609	1,547	1,686	1,726	1,767	1,809	1,852	1,895	1,940
9.8	1,544	1,580	1,617	1,654	1,693	1,733	1,773	1,815	1,857	1,900	1,945	1,990
9.9	1,589	1,625	1,663	1,701	1,740	1,781	1,822	1,864	1,907	1,951	1,996	2,042
10.0	1,635	1,672	1,710	1,749	1,789	1,830	1,871	1,914	1,958	2,002	2,048	2,094

Estimated Fetal Weights (*cont.*)

Abdominal Circumferences

21.5	22.0	22.5	23.0	23.5	24.0	24.5	25.0	25.5	26.0	26.5	27.0	27.5
911	942	973	1,006	1,039	1,074	1,110	1,147	1,185	1,225	1,266	1,308	1,352
935	965	997	1,030	1,065	1,100	1,136	1,174	1,213	1,253	1,294	1,337	1,381
958	990	1,022	1,056	1,090	1,126	1,163	1,201	1,241	1,281	1,323	1,367	1,411
983	1,015	1,048	1,082	1,117	1,153	1,190	1,229	1,269	1,310	1,353	1,397	1,442
1,008	1,040	1,074	1,108	1,144	1,181	1,219	1,258	1,298	1,340	1,383	1,427	1,473
1,033	1,066	1,100	1,135	1,171	1,209	1,247	1,287	1,328	1,370	1,414	1,459	1,505
1,060	1,093	1,128	1,163	1,200	1,238	1,277	1,317	1,358	1,401	1,445	1,491	1,538
1,087	1,121	1,156	1,192	1,229	1,267	1,307	1,348	1,390	1,433	1,478	1,524	1,571
1,114	1,149	1,184	1,221	1,259	1,297	1,338	1,379	1,421	1,465	1,511	1,557	1,605
1,143	1,178	1,214	1,251	1,289	1,328	1,369	1,411	1,454	1,499	1,544	1,592	1,640
1,172	1,207	1,244	1,281	1,320	1,360	1,401	1,444	1,487	1,533	1,579	1,627	1,676
1,202	1,238	1,275	1,313	1,352	1,393	1,434	1,477	1,522	1,567	1,614	1,663	1,712
1,232	1,269	1,306	1,345	1,385	1,426	1,468	1,512	1,557	1,603	1,650	1,699	1,749
1,264	1,301	1,339	1,378	1,418	1,460	1,503	1,547	1,592	1,639	1,687	1,737	1,787
1,296	1,333	1,372	1,412	1,453	1,495	1,538	1,583	1,629	1,676	1,725	1,775	1,826
1,329	1,367	1,406	1,446	1,488	1,531	1,575	1,620	1,666	1,714	1,763	1,814	1,866
1,363	1,401	1,441	1,482	1,524	1,567	1,612	1,657	1,704	1,753	1,803	1,854	1,906
1,397	1,436	1,477	1,518	1,561	1,605	1,650	1,696	1,744	1,793	1,843	1,895	1,948
1,433	1,473	1,513	1,555	1,599	1,643	1,689	1,735	1,784	1,833	1,884	1,936	1,990
1,469	1,510	1,551	1,594	1,637	1,682	1,728	1,776	1,825	1,875	1,926	1,979	2,033
1,507	1,548	1,589	1,633	1,677	1,722	1,769	1,817	1,866	1,917	1,969	2,022	2,077
1,545	1,586	1,629	1,673	1,717	1,764	1,811	1,859	1,909	1,960	2,013	2,067	2,122
1,584	1,626	1,669	1,714	1,759	1,806	1,854	1,903	1,953	2,005	2,058	2,113	2,169
1,625	1,667	1,711	1,756	1,802	1,849	1,897	1,947	1,998	2,050	2,104	2,159	2,216
1,666	1,709	1,753	1,799	1,845	1,893	1,942	1,992	2,044	2,097	2,151	2,207	2,264
1,708	1,752	1,797	1,843	1,890	1,938	1,988	2,039	2,091	2,144	2,199	2,255	2,313
1,752	1,796	1,841	1,888	1,936	1,984	2,035	2,086	2,139	2,193	2,248	2,305	2,363
1,796	1,841	1,887	1,934	1,982	2,032	2,083	2,135	2,188	2,242	2,298	2,356	2,414
1,842	1,887	1,934	1,982	2,030	2,080	2,132	2,184	2,238	2,293	2,350	2,407	2,467
1,889	1,935	1,982	2,030	2,080	2,130	2,182	2,235	2,289	2,345	2,402	2,460	2,520
1,937	1,984	2,031	2,080	2,130	2,181	2,233	2,287	2,342	2,398	2,456	2,515	2,575
1,986	2,033	2,082	2,131	2,181	2,233	2,286	2,340	2,396	2,452	2,510	2,570	2,631
2,037	2,085	2,133	2,183	2,234	2,286	2,340	2,395	2,451	2,508	2,567	2,627	2,688
2,089	2,137	2,186	2,237	2,288	2,341	2,395	2,450	2,507	2,565	2,624	2,684	2,746
2,142	2,191	2,241	2,292	2,344	2,397	2,452	2,507	2,564	2,623	2,682	2,743	2,806

Estimated Fetal Weights (*cont.*)

Biparietal Diameters	Abdominal Circumferences											
	28.0	28.5	29.0	29.5	30.0	30.5	31.0	31.5	32.0	32.5	33.0	33.5
3.1	666	696	726	759	793	828	865	903	943	985	1,029	1,075
3.2	680	710	742	774	809	844	882	921	961	1,004	1,048	1,094
3.3	695	725	757	790	825	861	899	938	979	1,022	1,067	1,114
3.4	710	740	773	806	841	878	916	956	998	1,041	1,087	1,134
3.5	725	756	789	823	858	896	934	975	1,017	1,061	1,107	1,154
3.6	740	772	805	840	876	913	953	993	1,036	1,080	1,127	1,175
3.7	756	788	822	857	893	931	971	1,012	1,056	1,101	1,147	1,196
3.8	772	805	839	874	911	950	990	1,032	1,076	1,121	1,168	1,218
3.9	789	822	856	892	930	969	1,009	1,052	1,096	1,142	1,190	1,240
4.0	806	839	874	911	949	988	1,029	1,072	1,117	1,163	1,212	1,262
4.1	828	857	892	929	968	1,008	1,049	1,093	1,138	1,185	1,234	1,285
4.2	841	875	911	948	987	1,028	1,070	1,114	1,159	1,207	1,256	1,308
4.3	859	893	930	968	1,007	1,048	1,091	1,135	1,181	1,229	1,279	1,331
4.4	877	912	949	987	1,027	1,069	1,112	1,157	1,204	1,252	1,303	1,355
4.5	896	932	969	1,008	1,048	1,090	1,134	1,179	1,226	1,275	1,326	1,380
4.6	915	951	989	1,028	1,069	1,112	1,156	1,202	1,249	1,299	1,351	1,404
4.7	934	971	1,010	1,049	1,091	1,134	1,178	1,225	1,273	1,323	1,375	1,430
4.8	954	992	1,031	1,071	1,113	1,156	1,201	1,248	1,297	1,348	1,401	1,455
4.9	975	1,013	1,052	1,093	1,135	1,179	1,225	1,272	1,322	1,373	1,426	1,482
5.0	996	1,034	1,074	1,115	1,158	1,203	1,249	1,297	1,347	1,399	1,452	1,508
5.1	1,017	1,056	1,096	1,138	1,181	1,226	1,273	1,322	1,372	1,425	1,479	1,535
5.2	1,039	1,078	1,119	1,161	1,205	1,251	1,298	1,347	1,398	1,451	1,506	1,563
5.3	1,061	1,101	1,142	1,185	1,229	1,276	1,323	1,373	1,425	1,478	1,533	1,591
5.4	1,084	1,124	1,166	1,209	1,254	1,301	1,349	1,399	1,452	1,506	1,562	1,620
5.5	1,107	1,148	1,190	1,234	1,279	1,327	1,376	1,426	1,479	1,534	1,590	1,649
5.6	1,131	1,172	1,215	1,259	1,305	1,353	1,402	1,454	1,507	1,562	1,619	1,678
5.7	1,155	1,197	1,240	1,285	1,332	1,380	1,430	1,482	1,535	1,591	1,649	1,709
5.8	1,180	1,222	1,266	1,311	1,358	1,407	1,458	1,510	1,564	1,621	1,679	1,739
5.9	1,205	1,248	1,292	1,338	1,386	1,435	1,486	1,539	1,594	1,651	1,710	1,770
6.0	1,231	1,274	1,319	1,366	1,414	1,464	1,515	1,569	1,624	1,682	1,741	1,802
6.1	1,257	1,301	1,346	1,393	1,442	1,493	1,545	1,599	1,655	1,713	1,773	1,835
6.2	1,284	1,328	1,374	1,422	1,471	1,522	1,575	1,630	1,686	1,745	1,805	1,868
6.3	1,311	1,356	1,403	1,451	1,501	1,552	1,606	1,661	1,718	1,777	1,838	1,901
6.4	1,339	1,385	1,432	1,481	1,531	1,583	1,637	1,693	1,751	1,810	1,872	1,935
6.5	1,368	1,414	1,462	1,511	1,562	1,615	1,669	1,725	1,784	1,844	1,906	1,970

Estimated Fetal Weights (*cont.*)

Abdominal Circumferences

34.0	34.5	35.0	35.5	36.0	36.5	37.0	37.5	38.0	38.5	39.0	39.5	40.0
1,123	1,173	1,225	1,279	1,336	1,396	1,458	1,523	1,591	1,661	1,735	1,812	1,893
1,143	1,193	1,246	1,301	1,358	1,418	1,481	1,546	1,615	1,686	1,761	1,838	1,920
1,163	1,214	1,267	1,323	1,381	1,441	1,504	1,570	1,639	1,711	1,786	1,865	1,946
1,183	1,235	1,289	1,345	1,403	1,464	1,528	1,595	1,664	1,737	1,812	1,891	1,973
1,204	1,256	1,311	1,367	1,426	1,488	1,552	1,619	1,689	1,762	1,839	1,918	2,001
1,226	1,278	1,333	1,390	1,450	1,512	1,577	1,645	1,715	1,789	1,865	1,945	2,029
1,247	1,300	1,356	1,413	1,474	1,536	1,602	1,670	1,741	1,815	1,893	1,973	2,057
1,269	1,323	1,379	1,437	1,498	1,561	1,627	1,696	1,768	1,842	1,920	2,001	2,086
1,292	1,346	1,402	1,461	1,523	1,586	1,653	1,722	1,794	1,870	1,948	2,030	2,115
1,315	1,369	1,426	1,486	1,548	1,612	1,679	1,749	1,822	1,898	1,977	2,059	2,145
1,338	1,393	1,451	1,511	1,573	1,638	1,706	1,776	1,849	1,926	2,005	2,088	2,174
1,361	1,417	1,475	1,536	1,599	1,664	1,733	1,804	1,878	1,954	2,035	2,118	2,205
1,385	1,442	1,500	1,562	1,625	1,691	1,760	1,832	1,906	1,984	2,064	2,148	2,236
1,410	1,467	1,526	1,588	1,652	1,718	1,788	1,860	1,935	2,013	2,094	2,179	2,267
1,435	1,492	1,552	1,614	1,679	1,746	1,816	1,889	1,964	2,043	2,125	2,210	2,298
1,460	1,518	1,579	1,641	1,706	1,774	1,845	1,918	1,994	2,073	2,156	2,241	2,330
1,486	1,545	1,605	1,669	1,734	1,803	1,874	1,948	2,024	2,104	2,187	2,273	2,363
1,512	1,571	1,633	1,697	1,763	1,832	1,904	1,978	2,055	2,136	2,219	2,306	2,396
1,539	1,599	1,661	1,725	1,792	1,861	1,934	2,009	2,086	2,167	2,251	2,339	2,429
1,566	1,626	1,689	1,754	1,821	1,891	1,964	2,040	2,118	2,200	2,284	2,372	2,463
1,594	1,655	1,718	1,783	1,851	1,922	1,995	2,071	2,150	2,232	2,317	2,406	2,498
1,622	1,683	1,747	1,813	1,882	1,953	2,027	2,103	2,183	2,266	2,351	2,440	2,532
1,651	1,713	1,777	1,843	1,913	1,984	2,059	2,136	2,216	2,299	2,386	2,475	2,568
1,680	1,742	1,807	1,874	1,944	2,016	2,091	2,169	2,250	2,333	2,420	2,510	2,604
1,710	1,773	1,838	1,906	1,976	2,049	2,124	2,203	2,284	2,368	2,456	2,546	2,640
1,740	1,803	1,869	1,938	2,008	2,082	2,158	2,237	2,319	2,403	2,491	2,582	2,677
1,770	1,835	1,901	1,970	2,041	2,115	2,192	2,272	2,354	2,439	2,528	2,619	2,714
1,802	1,866	1,934	2,003	2,075	2,150	2,227	2,307	2,390	2,475	2,564	2,657	2,752
1,834	1,899	1,966	2,037	2,109	2,184	2,262	2,342	2,426	2,512	2,602	2,694	2,790
1,866	1,932	2,000	2,071	2,144	2,219	2,298	2,379	2,463	2,550	2,640	2,733	2,829
1,899	1,965	2,034	2,105	2,179	2,255	2,334	2,416	2,500	2,588	2,678	2,772	2,869
1,932	1,999	2,069	2,140	2,215	2,291	2,371	2,453	2,538	2,626	2,717	2,811	2,909
1,967	2,034	2,104	2,176	2,251	2,328	2,408	2,491	2,577	2,665	2,757	2,851	2,949
2,001	2,069	2,140	2,213	2,288	2,366	2,446	2,530	2,616	2,705	2,797	2,892	2,991
2,037	2,105	2,176	2,250	2,326	2,404	2,485	2,569	2,656	2,745	2,838	2,933	3,032

Estimated Fetal Weights (*cont.*)

Biparietal Diameters	Abdominal Circumferences											
	28.0	28.5	29.0	29.5	30.0	30.5	31.0	31.5	32.0	32.5	33.0	33.5
6.6	1,397	1,444	1,492	1,542	1,594	1,647	1,702	1,759	1,817	1,878	1,941	2,006
6.7	1,427	1,474	1,523	1,574	1,626	1,679	1,735	1,792	1,852	1,913	1,976	2,042
6.8	1,458	1,505	1,555	1,606	1,658	1,713	1,769	1,827	1,887	1,949	2,012	2,078
6.9	1,489	1,537	1,587	1,639	1,692	1,747	1,803	1,862	1,922	1,985	2,049	2,116
7.0	1,521	1,570	1,620	1,672	1,726	1,781	1,839	1,898	1,959	2,022	2,087	2,154
7.1	1,553	1,603	1,654	1,706	1,761	1,817	1,875	1,934	1,996	2,059	2,125	2,193
7.2	1,586	1,636	1,688	1,741	1,796	1,853	1,911	1,971	2,044	2,098	2,164	2,232
7.3	1,620	1,671	1,723	1,777	1,832	1,890	1,948	2,009	2,072	2,137	2,203	2,272
7.4	1,655	1,706	1,759	1,813	1,869	1,927	1,987	2,048	2,111	2,176	2,244	2,313
7.5	1,690	1,742	1,795	1,850	1,907	1,965	2,025	2,087	2,151	2,217	2,265	2,354
7.6	1,727	1,779	1,833	1,888	1,945	2,004	2,065	2,127	2,192	2,258	2,326	2,397
7.7	1,764	1,816	1,871	1,927	1,985	2,044	2,105	2,168	2,233	2,300	2,369	2,440
7.8	1,801	1,855	1,910	1,966	2,025	2,085	2,146	2,210	2,275	2,343	2,412	2,484
7.9	1,840	1,894	1,949	2,006	2,065	2,126	2,188	2,252	2,318	2,386	2,456	2,528
8.0	1,879	1,934	1,990	2,048	2,107	2,168	2,231	2,296	2,362	2,431	2,501	2,574
8.1	1,919	1,975	2,031	2,089	2,149	2,211	2,275	2,340	2,407	2,476	2,547	2,620
8.2	1,960	2,016	2,073	2,132	2,193	2,255	2,319	2,385	2,462	2,522	2,594	2,667
8.3	2,002	2,059	2,116	2,176	2,237	2,300	2,364	2,431	2,499	2,569	2,641	2,715
8.4	2,045	2,102	2,160	2,220	2,282	2,345	2,410	2,477	2,546	2,617	2,689	2,764
8.5	2,089	2,146	2,205	2,266	2,328	2,392	2,457	2,525	2,594	2,665	2,739	2,814
8.6	2,134	2,192	2,251	2,312	2,375	2,439	2,505	2,573	2,643	2,715	2,789	2,864
8.7	2,179	2,238	2,298	2,359	2,423	2,488	2,554	2,623	2,693	2,765	2,840	2,916
8.8	2,226	2,285	2,346	2,408	2,472	2,537	2,604	2,673	2,744	2,817	2,892	2,968
8.9	2,274	2,333	2,394	2,457	2,521	2,587	2,655	2,725	2,796	2,869	2,944	3,021
9.0	2,322	2,382	2,444	2,507	2,572	2,639	2,707	2,777	2,849	2,923	2,998	3,076
9.1	2,372	2,433	2,495	2,559	2,624	2,691	2,760	2,830	2,903	2,977	3,053	3,131
9.2	2,423	2,484	2,547	2,611	2,677	2,744	2,814	2,885	2,958	3,032	3,109	3,187
9.3	2,475	2,536	2,599	2,664	2,731	2,799	2,869	2,940	3,014	3,089	3,166	3,245
9.4	2,527	2,590	2,653	2,719	2,786	2,854	2,925	2,997	3,070	3,146	3,224	3,303
9.5	2,582	2,644	2,709	2,774	2,842	2,911	2,982	3,054	3,129	3,205	3,283	3,362
9.6	2,637	2,700	2,765	2,831	2,899	2,969	3,040	3,113	3,188	3,264	3,343	3,423
9.7	2,693	2,757	2,822	2,889	2,958	3,028	3,099	3,173	3,248	3,325	3,404	3,484
9.8	2,751	2,815	2,881	2,948	3,017	3,088	3,160	3,234	3,309	3,387	3,466	3,547
9.9	2,810	2,874	2,941	3,009	3,078	3,149	3,222	3,296	3,372	3,450	3,529	3,611
10.0	2,870	2,935	3,002	3,070	3,140	3,211	3,285	3,359	3,436	3,514	3,594	3,676

Estimated Fetal Weights (*cont.*)

Abdominal Circumferences

34.0	34.5	35.0	35.5	36.0	36.5	37.0	37.5	38.0	38.5	39.0	39.5	40.0
2,073	2,142	2,213	2,287	2,364	2,443	2,524	2,609	2,696	2,786	2,879	2,975	3,075
2,109	2,179	2,251	2,326	2,403	2,482	2,564	2,649	2,737	2,827	2,921	3,018	3,117
2,147	2,217	2,290	2,365	2,442	2,522	2,605	2,690	2,778	2,869	2,964	3,061	3,161
2,184	2,255	2,329	2,404	2,482	2,563	2,646	2,732	2,821	2,912	3,007	3,104	3,205
2,223	2,295	2,368	2,444	2,523	2,604	2,688	2,774	2,863	2,955	3,050	3,149	3,250
2,262	2,334	2,409	2,485	2,564	2,646	2,730	2,817	2,907	2,999	3,095	3,193	3,295
2,302	2,375	2,450	2,527	2,607	2,689	2,773	2,861	2,951	3,044	3,140	3,239	3,341
2,343	2,416	2,491	2,569	2,649	2,732	2,817	2,905	2,996	3,089	3,186	3,285	3,388
2,384	2,458	2,534	2,612	2,693	2,776	2,862	2,950	3,041	3,135	3,232	3,332	3,435
2,426	2,501	2,577	2,656	2,737	2,821	2,907	2,996	3,088	3,182	3,279	3,380	3,483
2,469	2,544	2,621	2,700	2,782	2,866	2,953	3,042	3,134	3,229	3,327	3,428	3,531
2,513	2,588	2,666	2,746	2,828	2,912	3,000	3,090	3,182	3,277	3,376	3,477	3,581
2,557	2,633	2,711	2,792	2,874	2,959	3,047	3,137	3,230	3,326	3,425	3,526	3,631
2,603	2,679	2,757	2,838	2,921	3,007	3,095	3,186	3,279	3,376	3,475	3,576	3,681
2,649	2,725	2,804	2,886	2,969	3,056	3,144	3,235	3,329	3,426	3,525	3,627	3,733
2,695	2,773	2,852	2,934	3,018	3,105	3,194	3,286	3,380	3,477	3,577	3,679	3,785
2,743	2,821	2,901	2,983	3,068	3,155	3,244	3,336	3,431	3,529	3,629	3,732	3,838
2,791	2,870	2,950	3,033	3,118	3,206	3,296	3,388	3,483	3,581	3,682	3,785	3,891
2,841	2,920	3,001	3,084	3,169	3,257	3,348	3,441	3,536	3,634	3,735	3,839	3,945
2,891	2,970	3,052	3,135	3,221	3,310	3,401	3,494	3,590	3,688	3,790	3,894	4,000
2,942	3,022	3,104	3,188	3,274	3,363	3,454	3,548	3,644	3,743	3,845	3,949	4,056
2,994	3,074	3,157	3,241	3,328	3,417	3,509	3,603	3,700	3,799	3,901	4,005	4,113
3,047	3,128	3,210	3,295	3,383	3,472	3,565	3,659	3,756	3,855	3,958	4,063	4,170
3,101	3,182	3,265	3,351	3,438	3,528	3,621	3,716	3,813	3,913	4,015	4,120	4,228
3,155	3,237	3,321	3,407	3,495	3,585	3,678	3,773	3,871	3,971	4,074	4,179	4,287
3,211	3,293	3,377	3,464	3,552	3,643	3,736	3,832	3,930	4,030	4,133	4,239	4,347
3,268	3,350	3,435	3,522	3,611	3,702	3,795	3,891	3,989	4,090	4,193	4,299	4,408
3,326	3,409	3,494	3,581	3,670	3,761	3,855	3,951	4,050	4,151	4,254	4,361	4,469
3,384	3,468	3,553	3,641	3,738	3,822	3,916	4,013	4,111	4,213	4,316	4,423	4,532
3,444	3,528	3,614	3,701	3,791	3,884	3,978	4,075	4,174	4,275	4,379	4,486	4,595
3,505	3,589	3,675	3,763	3,854	3,946	4,041	4,138	4,237	4,339	4,443	4,550	4,659
3,567	3,651	3,738	3,826	3,917	4,010	4,105	4,202	4,302	4,404	4,508	4,615	4,724
3,630	3,715	3,802	3,890	3,981	4,074	4,170	4,267	4,367	4,469	4,573	4,680	4,790
3,694	3,779	3,866	3,956	4,047	4,140	4,236	4,333	4,433	4,536	4,640	4,747	4,857
3,759	3,845	3,932	4,022	4,113	4,207	4,303	4,400	4,501	4,603	4,708	4,815	4,924

Log 10 (birth weight) = −1.7492 + 0.166(BPD) + 0.046(AC) − 2.646 (AC × BPD)/1,000. SD = ±106.0 gm/kg of birth weight.
Reprinted with permission from Shepard MJ, Richards VA, Berkowitz RL, et al: An evaluation of two equations for predicting fetal weight by ultrasound. Am J Obstet Gynecol 142:48, 1982.

Fetal Crown - Rump Length Against Gestational Age
Mean ± 2SD

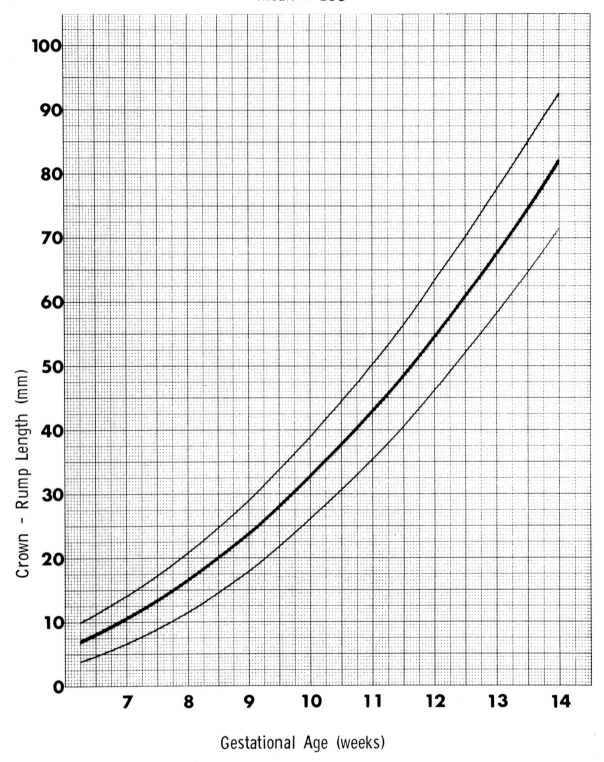

From Metreweli: Practical Clinical Ultrasound. Chicago, Heinemann, 1978.

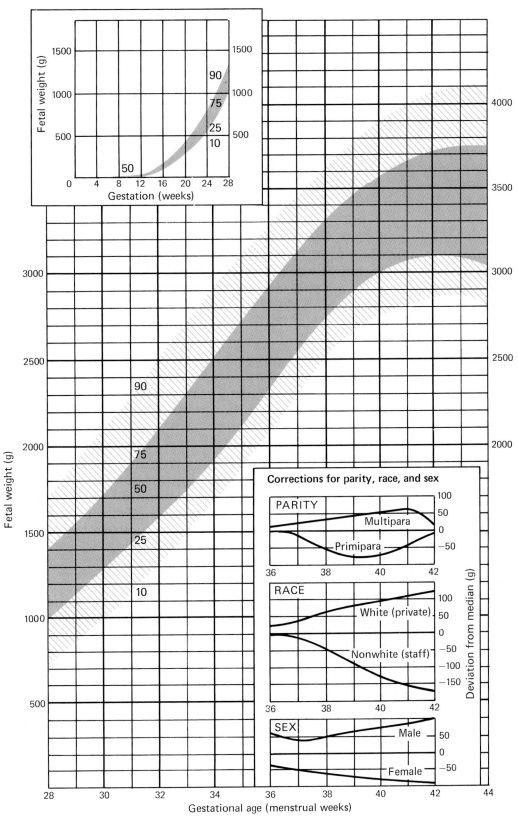

Increase in fetal weight with gestational age. (*Reprinted with permission from Brenner WE, Edelman DA, Hendricks CH: A standard of fetal growth for the United States of America. Am J Obstet Gynecol 126:555, 1976.*)

APPENDIX 10

Estimated Fetal Weight: Values Derived from the Birnholz Equation

BPD	Abdominal Perimeter																						
	40	45	50	55	60	65	70	75	80	85	90	95	100	105	110	115	120	125	130	135	140	145	150
30	58	62	67	73	79	85	92	100	108	117	126	135	146	156	167	179	191						
31	58	63	68	74	80	87	94	102	110	119	129	139	149	160	172	184	196	210	223				
32			69	75	81	88	96	104	112	122	131	142	153	164	176	188	201	215	229				
33			70	76	83	90	97	106	115	124	134	145	156	168	180	193	206	221	235				
34			71	77	84	91	99	108	117	127	137	148	159	172	184	198	212	226	241	257	273		
35					85	93	101	110	119	129	140	151	163	175	189	202	217	231	247	263	280		
36					86	94	103	112	121	132	143	154	166	179	193	207	222	237	253	269	287		
37					88	96	104	114	124	134	145	157	170	183	197	211	227	242	259	276	293	312	331
38							106	116	126	137	148	160	173	187	201	216	232	248	265	282	300	319	339
39							108	118	128	139	151	164	177	191	205	221	237	253	270	288	307	326	346

BPD	70	75	80	85	90	95	100	105	110	115	120	125	130	135	140	145	150	155	160	165	170	175	180
40	109	119	130	142	154	167	180	195	210	225	242	259	276	295	314	334	354						
41			132	144	157	170	184	198	214	230	247	264	282	301	321	341	362	384	406				
42			135	147	160	173	187	202	218	234	252	269	288	307	328	348	370	392	415				
43			137	149	162	176	191	206	222	239	257	275	294	314	334	356	378	401	424				
44			139	152	165	179	194	210	226	244	262	280	300	320	341	363	386	409	433	458	483		
45					168	182	198	214	231	248	267	286	306	326	348	370	393	417	442	467	494		
46					171	186	201	218	235	253	272	291	312	333	355	378	401	426	451	477	504		
47					174	189	205	221	239	257	277	297	317	339	362	385	409	434	460	486	514	542	571
48							208	225	243	262	282	302	323	345	368	392	417	442	469	496	524	553	582
49							212	229	247	267	287	308	329	352	375	400	425	451	478	505	534	563	593

BPD	100	105	110	115	120	125	130	135	140	145	150	155	160	165	170	175	180	185	190	195	200	205	210	215	220
50	215	233	252	271	292	313	335	358	382	407	433	459	486	515	544	574	605	636	669						
51			256	276	297	318	341	364	389	414	440	467	495	524	554	584	616	648	682						
52			260	280	302	324	347	371	396	421	448	476	504	534	564	595	627	660	694						
53			264	285	307	329	353	377	403	429	456	484	513	543	574	606	638	672	707	742	779				
54					312	335	359	384	409	436	464	492	522	553	584	616	650	684	719	755	792				
55					317	340	365	390	416	443	472	501	531	562	594	627	661	696	732	769	806				
56					322	346	370	396	423	451	479	509	540	571	604	638	672	708	744	782	820	860	900		
57							376	403	430	458	487	518	549	581	614	648	684	720	757	795	834	874	916		
58							382	409	437	465	495	526	558	590	624	659	695	732	769	808	848	889	931		
59									443	473	503	534	567	600	634	670	706	744	782	822	862	904	946	990	1034

Rows 60–69

	140	145	150	155	160	165	170	175	180	185	190	195	200	205	210	215	220	225	230	235	240	245	250
60	450	480	511	543	575	609	644	680	717	755	795	835	876	918	962	1006	1051						
61	457	487	519	551	584	619	654	691	729	767	807	848	890	933	977	1022	1068						
62			526	559	593	628	664	702	740	779	820	861	904	947	992	1038	1085	1133	1182				
63			534	568	602	638	674	712	751	791	832	874	918	962	1008	1054	1102	1151	1200				
64			542	576	611	647	685	723	762	803	845	888	932	977	1023	1070	1119	1168	1219				
65					620	657	695	734	774	815	857	901	946	991	1038	1086	1135	1186	1237	1290	1343		
66					629	666	705	744	785	827	870	914	959	1006	1054	1102	1152	1203	1256	1309	1363		
67					638	676	715	755	796	839	882	927	973	1021	1069	1118	1169	1221	1274	1328	1383	1440	1498
68							725	766	808	851	895	941	987	1035	1084	1134	1186	1239	1292	1347	1404	1461	1519
69							735	776	819	863	908	954	1001	1050	1100	1151	1203	1256	1311	1367	1424	1482	1541

Rows 70–79

	170	175	180	185	190	195	200	205	210	215	220	225	230	235	240	245	250	255	260	265	270	275	280	285	290
70	745	787	830	874	920	967	1015	1064	1115	1167	1220	1274	1329	1386	1444	1503	1563	1624	1687						
71			841	886	933	980	1029	1079	1130	1183	1236	1291	1348	1405	1464	1524	1585	1647	1711						
72			853	898	945	993	1043	1094	1146	1199	1253	1309	1366	1424	1484	1544	1606	1670	1734						
73					958	1007	1057	1108	1161	1215	1270	1327	1384	1443	1504	1565	1628	1692	1758	1824	1892				
74					970	1020	1071	1123	1176	1231	1287	1344	1403	1463	1524	1586	1650	1715	1781	1849	1918				
75					983	1033	1085	1137	1192	1247	1304	1362	1421	1482	1544	1607	1672	1737	1805	1873	1943	2014	2086		
76							1099	1152	1207	1263	1321	1379	1440	1501	1564	1628	1693	1760	1828	1898	1968	2040	2114		
77							1112	1167	1222	1279	1337	1397	1458	1520	1584	1649	1715	1783	1852	1922	1994	2067	2141		
78							1126	1181	1238	1295	1354	1415	1476	1539	1604	1670	1737	1805	1875	1946	2019	2093	2168	2245	2323
79									1253	1311	1371	1432	1495	1559	1624	1691	1759	1828	1899	1971	2044	2119	2195	2273	2352

Rows 80–89

	210	215	220	225	230	235	240	245	250	255	260	265	270	275	280	285	290	295	300	305	310	315	320	325	330
80	1268	1327	1388	1450	1513	1578	1644	1711	1780	1851	1922	1995	2070	2145	2223	2301	2381								
81			1405	1467	1532	1597	1664	1732	1802	1873	1946	2020	2095	2172	2250	2330	2411	2493	2577						
82			1422	1485	1550	1616	1684	1753	1824	1896	1969	2044	2120	2198	2277	2358	2440	2523	2608						
83			1438	1503	1568	1635	1704	1774	1845	1918	1993	2068	2146	2224	2304	2386	2469	2553	2639	2727	2815				
84					1587	1655	1724	1795	1867	1941	2016	2093	2171	2251	2332	2414	2498	2584	2671	2759	2849				
85					1605	1674	1744	1816	1889	1964	2040	2117	2196	2277	2359	2443	2528	2614	2702	2791	2882				
86							1764	1837	1911	1986	2063	2142	2222	2303	2386	2471	2557	2644	2733	2824	2916	3009	3104		
87							1784	1858	1932	2009	2087	2166	2247	2330	2414	2499	2586	2675	2765	2856	2949	3044	3140		
88							1804	1878	1954	2031	2110	2191	2272	2356	2441	2527	2615	2705	2796	2888	2983	3078	3175	3274	3374
89									1976	2054	2134	2215	2298	2382	2468	2556	2645	2735	2827	2921	3016	3113	3211	3311	3412

Rows 90–100

	255	260	265	270	275	280	285	290	295	300	305	310	315	320	325	330	335	340	345	350	355	360	365	370	375
90	2044	2097	2151	2207	2264	2323	2383	2445	2508	2573	2639	2707	2778	2849	2923	2999									
91		2145	2199	2256	2313	2372	2433	2495	2559	2624	2692	2760	2831	2903	2977	3054	3132	3212							
92		2193	2249	2305	2364	2423	2484	2547	2611	2677	2745	2814	2885	2958	3033	3109	3188	3268							
93		2243	2299	2356	2415	2475	2537	2600	2665	2731	2799	2869	2941	3014	3089	3166	3245	3326	3409	3494					
94				2408	2467	2528	2590	2654	2719	2786	2855	2925	2997	3071	3147	3224	3304	3385	3468	3554					
95				2461	2521	2582	2645	2709	2775	2842	2912	2982	3055	3129	3205	3283	3363	3445	3528	3614					
96						2637	2701	2765	2832	2900	2969	3041	3114	3188	3265	3343	3423	3505	3590	3676	3764	3854			
97						2694	2757	2823	2890	2958	3028	3100	3173	3248	3325	3404	3485	3567	3652	3738	3827	3918			
98								2881	2949	3018	3088	3160	3234	3310	3387	3466	3547	3630	3715	3802	3891	3982	4075	4170	
99								2941	3009	3078	3149	3222	3296	3372	3450	3530	3611	3695	3780	3867	3956	4047	4141	4236	
100								3002	3071	3141	3212	3285	3360	3436	3514	3594	3676	3760	3845	3933	4022	4114	4207	4303	4401

Estimated Fetal Weight: Values Derived from the Formula of Shepard et al.

Rows = BPD (biparietal diameter); Columns = Abdominal perimeter

BPD 30–39 × Abdominal perimeter 40–150

BPD	40	45	50	55	60	65	70	75	80	85	90	95	100	105	110	115	120	125	130	135	140	145	150
30	80	83	87	91	95	99	104	108	113	118	123	129	135	141	147	154	161						
31	83	86	90	94	98	103	107	112	117	122	128	133	139	145	152	159	166	173	181				
32			93	97	102	106	111	116	121	126	132	138	144	150	157	164	171	178	186				
33			97	101	105	110	115	120	125	130	136	142	148	155	162	169	176	184	192				
34			100	104	109	114	119	124	129	135	141	147	153	160	167	174	182	190	198	206	215		
35					113	118	123	128	134	139	145	152	158	165	172	180	187	195	204	213	222		
36					117	122	127	132	138	144	150	157	163	170	178	185	193	202	210	219	229		
37					121	126	131	137	143	149	155	162	169	176	183	191	199	208	217	226	235	245	256
38							136	142	148	154	160	167	174	182	189	197	206	214	223	233	243	253	263
39							141	146	153	159	166	173	180	187	195	203	212	221	230	240	250	260	271

BPD 40–49 × Abdominal perimeter 70–180

BPD	70	75	80	85	90	95	100	105	110	115	120	125	130	135	140	145	150	155	160	165	170	175	180
40	145	152	158	164	171	178	186	193	202	210	219	228	237	247	257	268	279						
41			163	170	177	184	192	200	208	217	226	235	245	255	265	276	288	299	312				
42			169	176	183	190	198	206	215	223	233	242	252	262	273	284	296	308	321				
43			174	182	189	197	205	213	222	231	240	250	260	270	281	293	305	317	330				
44			180	188	195	203	211	220	229	238	247	257	268	279	290	302	314	326	340	353	368		
45					202	210	218	227	236	245	255	265	276	287	299	311	323	336	349	363	378		
46					208	217	225	234	244	253	263	274	285	296	308	320	333	346	359	374	389		
47					215	224	233	242	251	261	271	282	293	305	317	329	342	356	370	384	400	415	432
48							240	250	259	269	280	291	302	314	326	339	352	366	381	395	411	427	444
49							248	258	268	278	289	300	312	324	336	349	363	377	392	407	422	439	456

BPD 50–59 × Abdominal perimeter 100–220

BPD	100	105	110	115	120	125	130	135	140	145	150	155	160	165	170	175	180	185	190	195	200	205	210	215	220
50	256	266	276	287	298	309	321	334	346	360	374	388	403	418	434	451	468	486	505						
51	266	276	285	296	307	319	331	344	357	370	385	399	414	430	447	464	481	500	519						
52			294	305	317	329	341	354	368	381	396	411	426	443	459	477	495	513	533						
53			304	315	327	339	352	365	379	393	408	423	439	455	472	490	508	527	547	568	589				
54					337	350	363	376	390	405	420	435	451	468	486	504	522	542	562	583	605				
55					348	360	374	388	402	417	432	448	464	482	499	518	537	557	577	598	620				
56					359	372	385	399	414	429	445	461	478	495	513	532	552	572	593	614	637	660	684		
57							397	412	426	442	458	474	492	509	528	547	567	587	609	631	654	677	702		
58							409	424	439	455	471	488	506	524	543	562	583	604	625	648	671	695	720		
59									453	469	485	503	520	539	558	578	599	620	642	665	689	713	739	765	792

Block 1 (rows 60–69)

	140	145	150	155	160	165	170	175	180	185	190	195	200	205	210	215	220	225	230	235	240	245	250
60	466	483	500	517	536	554	574	594	615	637	659	683	707	732	758	784	812						
61	480	497	514	532	551	570	590	611	632	654	677	701	725	751	777	804	832						
62			530	548	567	587	607	628	650	672	696	720	745	770	797	825	853	883	913				
63			545	564	583	603	624	645	668	691	714	739	764	790	818	846	875	905	936				
64			561	580	600	621	642	664	686	709	734	759	784	811	839	867	897	927	959				
65					617	638	660	682	705	729	753	779	805	832	860	889	919	950	982	1015	1050		
66					635	657	678	701	725	749	774	800	826	854	882	912	942	974	1006	1040	1075		
67					654	675	698	721	745	769	795	821	848	876	905	935	966	998	1031	1065	1100	1137	1174
68							717	741	765	790	816	843	870	899	928	959	990	1023	1056	1091	1127	1164	1202
69							738	762	786	812	838	865	893	922	952	983	1015	1048	1082	1117	1154	1191	1230

Block 2 (rows 70–79)

	170	175	180	185	190	195	200	205	210	215	220	225	230	235	240	245	250	255	260	265	270	275	280	285	290
70	758	783	808	834	861	888	917	946	977	1008	1041	1074	1109	1144	1181	1219	1258	1299	1340						
71			830	857	884	912	941	971	1002	1034	1067	1101	1136	1172	1209	1248	1287	1328	1371						
72			853	880	908	936	966	996	1028	1060	1094	1128	1164	1200	1238	1277	1317	1359	1402						
73					932	961	991	1022	1054	1087	1121	1156	1192	1229	1268	1307	1348	1390	1433	1478	1524				
74					958	987	1018	1049	1081	1115	1149	1185	1221	1259	1298	1338	1379	1422	1466	1511	1558				
75					983	1013	1044	1076	1109	1143	1178	1214	1251	1290	1329	1370	1411	1455	1499	1545	1592	1641	1691		
76							1072	1104	1138	1172	1208	1244	1282	1321	1361	1402	1444	1488	1533	1579	1627	1676	1727		
77							1100	1133	1167	1202	1238	1275	1313	1353	1393	1435	1478	1522	1568	1615	1663	1713	1764		
78							1129	1163	1197	1233	1269	1307	1346	1385	1426	1469	1512	1557	1603	1651	1700	1750	1802	1855	1910
79									1228	1264	1301	1339	1379	1419	1461	1503	1547	1593	1639	1688	1737	1788	1840	1894	1950

Block 3 (rows 80–89)

	210	215	220	225	230	235	240	245	250	255	260	265	270	275	280	285	290	295	300	305	310	315	320	325	330
80	1260	1296	1334	1373	1412	1453	1495	1539	1583	1629	1677	1725	1775	1827	1880	1934	1990								
81			1367	1407	1447	1488	1531	1575	1620	1667	1715	1764	1814	1866	1920	1975	2032	2090	2150						
82			1402	1441	1482	1524	1568	1612	1658	1705	1753	1803	1854	1907	1961	2017	2074	2133	2193						
83			1437	1477	1519	1561	1605	1650	1697	1744	1793	1843	1895	1948	2003	2059	2117	2176	2237	2300	2365				
84					1556	1599	1643	1689	1736	1784	1834	1885	1937	1991	2046	2103	2161	2221	2282	2346	2411				
85					1594	1638	1683	1729	1776	1825	1875	1927	1979	2034	2090	2147	2206	2266	2328	2392	2458				
86							1723	1770	1818	1867	1918	1970	2023	2078	2134	2192	2252	2313	2375	2440	2506	2574	2644		
87							1764	1811	1860	1910	1961	2014	2068	2123	2180	2238	2298	2360	2423	2488	2555	2623	2694		
88							1806	1854	1903	1954	2005	2059	2113	2169	2227	2286	2346	2408	2472	2538	2605	2674	2745	2817	2892
89									1947	1998	2051	2104	2160	2216	2274	2334	2395	2457	2522	2588	2656	2725	2797	2870	2945

Block 4 (rows 90–100)

	250	255	260	265	270	275	280	285	290	295	300	305	310	315	320	325	330	335	340	345	350	355	360	365	370	375
90	1993	2044	2097	2151	2207	2264	2323	2383	2445	2508	2573	2639	2707	2778	2849	2923	2999									
91			2145	2199	2256	2313	2372	2433	2495	2559	2624	2692	2760	2831	2903	2977	3054	3132	3212							
92			2193	2249	2305	2364	2423	2484	2547	2611	2677	2745	2814	2885	2958	3033	3109	3188	3268							
93			2243	2299	2356	2415	2475	2537	2600	2665	2731	2799	2869	2941	3014	3089	3166	3245	3326	3409	3494					
94					2408	2467	2528	2590	2654	2719	2786	2855	2925	2997	3071	3147	3224	3304	3385	3468	3554					
95					2461	2521	2582	2645	2709	2775	2842	2912	2982	3055	3129	3205	3283	3363	3445	3528	3614					
96							2637	2701	2765	2832	2900	2969	3041	3114	3188	3265	3343	3423	3505	3590	3676	3764	3854			
97							2694	2757	2823	2890	2958	3028	3100	3173	3248	3325	3404	3485	3567	3652	3738	3827	3918			
98									2881	2949	3018	3088	3160	3234	3310	3387	3466	3547	3630	3715	3802	3891	3982	4075	4170	
99									2941	3009	3078	3149	3222	3296	3372	3450	3530	3611	3695	3780	3867	3956	4047	4141	4236	
100									3002	3071	3141	3212	3285	3360	3436	3514	3594	3676	3760	3845	3933	4022	4114	4207	4303	4401

APPENDIX 11

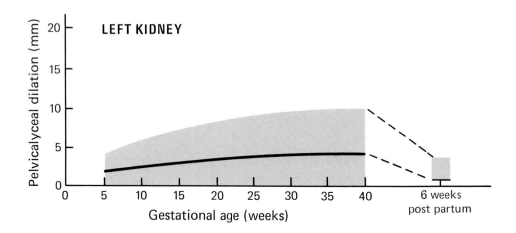

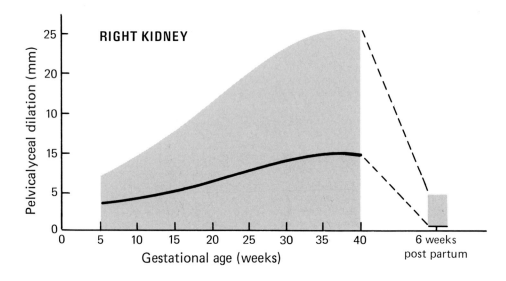

Patterns of sequential dilatation for right and left kidneys. The general trend is toward progressive dilatation more extensive on the right but with broad ranges for both. Dotted lines merely extend mean and maximum values to the postpartum period. (*Reproduced with permission from Fried A, Woodring JH, Thompson DJ: Hydronephrosis of pregnancy. J Ultrasound Med 2:225, 1983.*)

Index